*Progress in*
*Cancer Research and Therapy*
*Volume 17*

# NUTRITION AND CANCER:
# ETIOLOGY AND TREATMENT

# Progress in Cancer Research and Therapy

Progress in
Cancer Research and Therapy
Volume 17

# Nutrition and Cancer:
# Etiology and Treatment

## Editors

**Guy R. Newell, M.D.**
*Department of Cancer Prevention*
*The University of Texas System Cancer*
*Center*
*M. D. Anderson Hospital and Tumor*
*Institute*
*Houston, Texas*

**Neil M. Ellison, M.D.**
*Department of Hematology-Oncology*
*Geisinger Medical Center*
*Danville, Pennsylvania*

Raven Press ■ New York

**Raven Press, 1140 Avenue of the Americas, New York, New York 10036**

Made in the United States of America

International Standard Book Number 0–89004-631-x
Library of Congress Catalog Card Number 79-66-730

# Preface

Evidence from *in vitro* animal, and human studies shows that diet and nutrition play a role in the etiology and treatment of cancer. "Diet" means all substances ingested during the course of eating; "nutrition" refers to those essential dietary elements that the body is unable to synthesize *de novo*.

Although man is constantly exposed to varying amounts of cancer-causing agents, only a few are probably carcinogenic at the very low levels found in the diet. Most require activation and become carcinogenic through cocarcinogenesis or by tumor promotors. Carcinogens may be found as inherent components of food—naturally, through methods of food preparation, or as contaminants of foods. Carcinogens may also be produced endogenously from ingested foodstuffs. Thus, the relationship between nutrition and cancer ranges from the induction of cancer—to cancer prevention—to cancer treatment. Nutritional assessment plays an important part in determining the etiology and treatment of cancer.

This volume combines the current knowledge of etiology, assessment, and treatment of cancer and nutrition. It will serve as a valuable reference for understanding the relationship between nutrition and cancer.

Epidemiologists and nutritionists interested in the cancer problem, as well as oncologists or other practitioners concerned with the relationship between cancer and nutrition, will find this volume useful.

# Acknowledgments

The editors wish to thank all of the authors in this volume for their cooperation and hard work on a short deadline. We also want to thank Colleen M. Hubona and Diane C. Culhane of The University of Texas System Cancer Center's Department of Scientific Publications for their untiring assistance in editing manuscripts. We especially want to thank W. Bryant Boutwell for coordinating the many daily details involved in this publication.

# Contents

**Nutritional Treatments of the Cancer Patient**

# Contributors

**George L. Blackburn, M.D., Ph.D.**
Nutrition and Metabolism Laboratory
Cancer Research Institute
New England Deaconess Hospital and
  Harvard Medical School
Boston, Massachusetts 02215

**W. Bryant Boutwell, M.P.H.**
Department of Cancer Prevention
The University of Texas System Cancer
  Center, M. D. Anderson Hospital and
  Tumor Institute
Houston, Texas 77030

**Selwyn A. Broitman, Ph.D.**
Nutrition-Pathology Unit
Department of Microbiology
Mallory Institute of Pathology
Boston University School of Medicine
Boston, Massachusetts 02118

**Stephen K. Carter, M.D.**
Northern California Cancer Program
P. O. Box 10144
Palo Alto, California 94303

**Leonard A. Cohen, Ph.D.**
Division of Nutrition
American Health Foundation
Naylor Dana Institute for Disease Preven-
  tion
Valhalla, New York 10595

**Edward M. Copeland, III, M.D.**
Department of General Surgery
The University of Texas Medical School
  at Houston and The University of Texas
  System Cancer Center, M.D. Anderson
  Hospital and Tumor Institute
Houston, Texas 77030

**Pelayo Correa, M.D.**
Department of Pathology
Louisiana State University Medical Center
New Orleans, Louisiana 70112

**Wayne E. Criss, Ph.D.**
Department of Oncology-Biochemistry
Howard University Medical Center
Cancer Center
Washington, D.C. 20059

**John M. Daly, M.D.**
Department of General Surgery
The University of Texas Medical School
  at Houston and The University of Texas
  System Cancer Center
Houston, Texas 77030

**William DeWys, M.D.**
Nutrition, Cancer Therapy Evaluation
  Program
Division of Cancer Treatment
National Cancer Institute
Bethesda, Maryland 20205

**Sarah S. Donaldson, M.D.**
Department of Radiology
Stanford University Medical School
Stanford, California 94305

**Harry Drasin, M.D.**
University of California
San Francisco, California 94143

**Stanley J. Dudrick, M.D.**
Department of General Surgery
The University of Texas Medical at Hous-
  ton
Houston, Texas 77030

**Neil M. Ellison, M.D.**
Department of Hematology-Oncology
Geisinger Medical Center
Danville, Pennsylvania 17821

**Katherine M. Flegal, M.D.**
Division of Nutritional Science
Cornell University
Ithaca, New York 14853

**Leonard S. Gottlieb, M.D.**
Nutrition-Pathology Unit
Department of Pathology
Mallory Institute of Pathology
Boston University School of Medicine
Boston, Massachusetts 02118

**Saxon Graham, Ph.D.**
Department of Sociology and Social and
  Preventive Medicine
State University of New York at Buffalo
Buffalo, New York 14261

**Jere D. Hass, Ph.D.**
Division of Nutritional Sciences
Cornell University
Ithaca, New York 14853

**Steven B. Heymsfield, M.D.**
Department of Medicine
Clinical Research Facility
Emory University School of Medicine
Atlanta, Georgia 30332

**Peter Hill, Ph.D.**
Division of Nutrition
American Health Foundation
Naylor Dana Institute for Disease Preven-
  tion
Valhalla, New York 10595

**Laurie Hoffman-Geotz, Ph.D.**
Nutrition and Metabolism Laboratory
Cancer Research Institute
New England Deaconess Hospital and
  Harvard Medical School
Boston, Massachusetts 02215

**Ole Møller Jensen, M.D., Dr. Med.
Sci.**
Danish Cancer Registry
Strandboulevarden 49
DK 2100 Copenhagen Ø
Denmark

**Takashi Kawachi, M.D., Dr. Med.
Sci.**
National Cancer Center Research Institute
5–1–1, Tsukiji, Chou-ku
Tokyo 104, Japan

**Daniel L. Kisner, M.D.**
Nutrition, Cancer Therapy Evaluation
  Program
Division of Cancer Treatment
National Cancer Institute
Bethesda, Maryland 20205

**David M. Klurfeld, Ph.D.**
Wistar Institute
Philadelphia, Pennsylvania 19104

**Susanna H. Krey, R.D., M.Ed.**
Clinical Nutrition Unit
Boston University School of Medicine
University Hospital
Boston, Massachusetts 02118

**David Kritchevsky, Ph.D.**
Wistar Institute
Philadelphia, Pennsylvania 19104

**Harold Londer, M.D.**
Minneapolis, Medical Specialists
Minneapolis, Minnesota 55440

**G. David McCoy, Ph.D.**
Division of Nutrition
American Health Foundation
Naylor Dana Institute for Disease Preven-
  tion
Valhalla, New York 10595

**Curtis Mettlin, Ph.D.**
Department of Epidemiology
Roswell Park Memorial Institute
Buffalo, New York 14263

**Suresh Mohla, Ph.D.**
Department of Oncology-Biochemistry
Howard University Medical Center
Cancer Center
Washington, D.C. 20059

**James L. Mullen, M.D.**
Department of Surgery
University of Pennsylvania School of Medi-
  cine
Philadelphia, Pennsylvania 19104

**Minako Nagao, Ph.D.**
Biochemistry Division
National Cancer Center Research Institute
5–1–1, Tsukiji, Chou-ku
Tokyo 104, Japan

**Paul M. Newberne, D.V.M., Ph.D.**
*Department of Nutrition and Food Science*
*Massachusetts Institute of Technology*
*Cambridge, Massachusetts 02139*

**Guy R. Newell, M.D.**
*Department of Cancer Prevention*
*The University of Texas System Cancer*
*  Center, M. D. Anderson Hospital and*
*  Tumor Institute*
*Houston, Texas 77030*

**Robert A. Noel, B.S.**
*Department of Medicine*
*Clinical Research Facility*
*Emory University School of Medicine*
*Atlanta, Georgia 30332*

**Rulon W. Rawson, M.D.**
*Bonneville Center for Research on Cancer*
*  Cause and Prevention*
*University of Utah Research Institute*
*Salt Lake City, Utah 84108*

**Bandaru S. Reddy, Ph.D.**
*Division of Nutrition*
*American Health Foundation*
*Naylor Dana Institute for Disease Preven-*
*  tion*
*Valhalla, New York 10595*

**Adrianne E. Rogers, M.D.**
*Department of Nutrition and Food Science*
*Massachusetts Institute of Technology*
*Cambridge, Massachusetts 02139*

**Ernest H. Rosenbaum, M.D.**
*Mount Zion Hospital and Medical Center*
*San Francisco, California 94115*

**Isadora R. Rosenbaum**
*1515 Scott Street*
*San Francisco, California 94115*

**Thomas J. Slaga, Ph.D.**
*Cancer and Toxicology Program*
*Oak Ridge National Laboratory*
*Oak Ridge, Tennessee 37830*

**Neil E. Spingarn, Ph.D.**
*Division of Nutrition*
*American Health Foundation*
*Naylor Dana Institute for Disease Preven-*
*  tion*
*Valhalla, New York 10595*

**William P. Steffee, M.D., Ph.D.**
*Clinical Nutrition Unit*
*Boxton University School of Medicine*
*University Hospital*
*Boston, Massachusetts 02118*

**Carol Stitt, R.D.**
*Washoe Medical Center*
*Reno, Nevada 89502*

**Mason G. Stout, M.D., Ph.D.**
*Department of Internal Medicine*
*LDS Hospital*
*Salt Lake City, Utah 84143*

**Takashi Sugimura, M.D., Dr. Med.**
**  Sci.**
*National Cancer Center Research Institute*
*5–1–1, Tsukiji, Chou-ku*
*Tokyo 104, Japan*

**Michael H. Torosian, M.D.**
*Department of Surgery*
*University of Pennsylvania School of Medi-*
*  cine*
*Philadelphia, Pennsylvania 19104*

**Jan van Eys, M.D., Ph.D.**
*Department of Pediatrics*
*The University of Texas System Cancer*
*  Center, M. D. Anderson Hospital and*
*  Tumor Institute*
*Houston, Texas 77030*

**Joseph J. Vitale, Sc.D., M.D.**
*Nutrition-Pathology Unit*
*Department of Pathology*
*Mallory Institute of Pathology*
*Boston University School of Medicine*
*Boston, Massachusetts 02118*

**John H. Weisburger, Ph.D.**
*Division of Nutrition*
*American Health Foundation*
*Naylor Dana Institute for Disease Preven-*
  *tion*
*Valhalla, New York 10595*

**Ernst L. Wynder, M.D.**
*American Health Foundation*
*New York, New York 10017*

**Takie Yahagi, Ph.D.**
*Biochemistry Division*
*National Cancer Center Research Institute*
*5–1–1, Tsukiji, Chou-ku*
*Tokyo 104, Japan*

# Introduction

During recent years there has been a growing awareness by the oncologic community about the important association between nutrition and cancer—as a means of prevention and treatment. In the past, preventive efforts were virtually neglected or overlooked. The major focus in supportive care was directed toward systems of blood product replacement and treatment of infectious complications. We now recognize that this was not enough.

It is currently estimated that malnutrition in hospitalized patients may range from 20% to 50% and if divided into disease categories, cancer patients often make up the significant portion of these malnourished patients. Increasing evidence demonstrates that good nutrition, or lack of it, affects cancer patients just as it affects other patients with acute or chronic illnesses. Yet, while it is realized that good nutrition may enhance a beneficial cancer treatment, it cannot make a poor therapy effective.

In the area of prevention, epidemiologic correlations demonstrate definite patterns of neoplastic occurrence associated with nutrition as addressed in the first two chapters. For example, it hardly seems surprising that studies show diets high in total fat and low in certain fibers are associated with an increased incidence of large bowel cancer. For many of the more common cancers in this country (oral, esophagus, colon, breast, prostate, and stomach cancer), each individual does exert a certain amount of control over his own cancer risk through diet and lifestyle. As more is learned about the mechanisms of mutagens and carcinogens, and as inroads are made in the newly developing field of chemoprevention, it may be routinely possible to inhibit, block, or reverse the cellular processes involved in carcinogenesis by dietary modifications. Studies examining possible cancer associations for fat, fiber, vitamins, minerals, trace elements, alcohol, food additives, and contaminants as well as the timely topic of artificial sweeteners are all included in the first half of this volume.

Because diet as an environmental variable must be measured to accurately quantify its impact on the development of human cancer, an entire section covers the approaches to nutritional assessment. Despite the multitude of biochemical, immunologic, anthropometric, and body compositional parameters used for nutritional assessment, a single test has not yet emerged as the sole accurate indicator of nutritional status. Likewise, there is no generally accepted method of measuring the dietary intake of individuals. Considering the critical importance of accurate nutritional assessment, all of these topics are dealt with in detail.

In the treatment and care of cancer patients, malnutrition plays a dual role.

First, malnutrition can create a detrimental effect on multiple aspects of the treatment process. Malnutrition may adversely affect a patient before he or she receives medical care, interfere with the delivery of optimal oncologic therapy, prolong the morbidity of therapeutic complications, and have a detrimental effect on the patient's quality of life.

Second, optimal nutritional care can, in many instances, reverse these negative influences. Nutrition is now considered a positive therapeutic tool to complement advances in more traditional therapies such as chemotherapy, radiotherapy, surgery, and immunotherapy for cancer patients. Nutritional problems associated with cancer chemotherapy and radiation therapy are addressed in separate chapters as is the topic of nutrition for the pediatric cancer patient. Because many of the factors of diet and dietary contaminants in the etiology of adult cancer pertain in a very special way only to the pediatric age group, it is essential that the topic receives a chapter of its own dealing primarily with the effects of nutrition on the course of childhood cancer.

Finally, a discussion addressing the important contribution of enteral chemically defined diets and intravenous hyperalimentation, completes the section on nutrition as a positive therapeutic tool. Since its introduction in the early 1960s, this intravenous technique for nutritional replenishment has drawn international attention. Only during the last 5 years has the significance of nutritional rehabilitation and maintenance of the cancer patient before, during, and after treatment been scientifically addressed. Nutritional replenishment is now possible to some degree in almost all cancer patients, and the roles that adequate building blocks such as carbohydrates, amino acids, vitamins, minerals, and fats play in the management of acute and chronic illnesses are being increasingly recognized and appreciated.

It is only appropriate that all of the topics mentioned here be handled under one cover. The biological relationships between nutrition and cancer are multifaceted and intricate. Included among these relationships are identifications of dietary risk factors, improving patient care, and possibly enhancing treatment effectiveness. Perhaps this new appreciation of the impact of nutrition on cancer will lead to not only improved patient care and treatment but, more importantly, also to preventive efforts that affect the disease at the causal or development stage and lead to tremendous savings in both economic terms and in human lives.

W. Bryant Boutwell
Guy R. Newell
Neil M. Ellison

*Nutrition and Cancer: Etiology and Treatment,*
edited by G. R. Newell and N. M. Ellison.
Raven Press, New York © 1981.

# Nutrition and Cancer: Epidemiologic Correlations

## Pelayo Correa

*Department of Pathology, Louisiana State University Medical Center,
New Orleans, Louisiana 70112*

In the search for factors related to cancer etiology investigators have frequently taken advantage of data on the availability of foods among different populations. International data based on the "disappearance" of food items from the marketplace are collected and published by the Food and Agriculture Organization (FAO) (11). Within a given country, these data are usually collected by the Department of Agriculture or by special surveys (36). Occasionally, enough internal variation exists to justify their use in studies dealing with cancer etiology. National figures on food intake can be correlated with cancer frequency based on mortality data collected by the World Health Organization (31), or with incidence figures published by the International Association of Cancer Registries and the International Agency for Research on Cancer (38). Both sets of data are available for a limited number of countries.

This chapter will include a brief review of the published work on international correlations, an update on some of the results, and a discussion of their possible usefulness in the search for etiologic factors and preventive measures.

## BRIEF REVIEW OF CORRELATION STUDIES

The notion that nutrition and cancer might be interrelated is an old one. In modern times, one of its most articulate advocates has been Tannenbaum (34). His many contributions were mainly in the experimental field, but he also performed some correlation studies, mostly based on the statistics of life insurance companies, in which he found a positive association between overweight and several types of cancer. He simulated this human situation in numerous animal experiments and firmly established the fact that excessive nutrition enhances cancer development and progression (35).

Intercountry data on dietary intake were utilized on a large scale for correlation studies with coronary heart disease before similar studies were performed for neoplastic disease. An initial positive correlation between coronary heart disease and total fat intake was later found to be even stronger when saturated fats alone were considered (21). Many studies primarily concerned with cancer have also included coronary heart disease in their analyses because of its well-known correlation with certain neoplasms (39).

Cancer correlation studies were greatly facilitated by the pioneer work of Segi, who collected data and adjusted cancer death rates to the now widely used "world" population model (31). Lea, in 1967, correlated cancer death rates, as adjusted for age by Segi, with the availability of foods, as provided by the FAO publications (23). He was impressed by the fact that neoplasms seemed to fall into two groups: Group 1 was positively correlated with the ingestion of fat, sugar, animal protein, eggs, and milk; prominent neoplasms in this group were cancers of the breast, ovary, large bowel, and prostate. Group 2 consisted principally of cancers of the stomach and liver, and showed a negative association with such food items.

Wynder and co-workers (39,40), in reporting on studies of analytical epidemiology of colon cancer, concluded that dietary factors, and especially the high intake of fat, appeared to be associated with the etiology of colon cancer. A positive correlation between death rates from colon cancer and myocardial infarction was reported, again pointing toward possibly related dietary etiologies for both diseases.

Death rates for gastrointestinal cancer were correlated by Gregor and co-workers with food intake, in an effort to explain the negative correlation between death rates from gastric cancer and colon cancer (14). They reported that animal protein intake correlated positively with the death rate from colon cancer and negatively with gastric cancer. They corroborated previous findings by Dunn and Buell, who reached similar conclusions about the role of diet in gastrointestinal cancer while studying time trends in Japanese immigrants to California (7). A positive correlation between breast cancer death rates and the intake of fat and calories was reported by Carroll and co-workers (4), who were of the opinion that fat intake was the most relevant parameter.

The relationship of dietary intake to breast cancer during the premenopausal and postmenopausal periods has been reported by Hems (16). He concluded that the intake of sugar and fat accounted for three-quarters of the intercountry variation in postmenopausal breast cancer, whereas in premenopausal breast cancer genetic factors appeared to have a stronger influence.

Updated studies of incidence and mortality by Draser and Irving found no correlation of dietary items with gastric cancer, but found a positive correlation between breast and colon cancer rates and total intake of fat, animal protein, eggs, and sugar (6). Correlations with other indicators of affluence, such as income and number of automobiles and television sets, were also positive. No correlation with fiber intake was found.

The correlation between colorectal cancer and diet was analyzed by Howell (18,19), using international dietary data, data of a case-control study conducted by Haenszel et al. (15), and data on food consumption within the United States. Her correlation studies were based on incidence and mortality rates, and again showed a positive association of colorectal cancer frequency with fat and animal protein intake. In her opinion, correlation studies did not provide an adequate base from which to consider one dietary component more suspicious than the other. In case-control studies, milk and eggs were not differentiated, and stood out as the composite food item most consistently associated with colon cancer. A strong negative correlation between rice consumption and frequency of colon cancer was also reported.

The availability of new data on cancer incidence, refined statistical techniques, and indicators of data reliability were utilized by Armstrong and Doll for a critical reexamination of the question of diet–cancer correlations (1). They found gastric cancer to be negatively correlated with fat consumption; this negative association explained previously reported associations with protein consumption. Meat and animal protein consumption were the variables most highly correlated with colon cancer. Controlling for these variables substantially reduced the correlations with other variables, including total fat, whereas no other variable reduced the correlation coefficient with meat to less than 0.70. In the case of cancers of the breast, corpus uteri, and ovary, total fat intake provided the highest and most consistent correlation coefficients. Cereal and "pulses" (edible seeds) showed negative associations with these three endocrine-related cancers. Total fat consumption was also found to be positively correlated with cancers of the prostate, testicle, kidney, and nervous system, but some of these correlations were weak or inconstant.

Time trends of colon cancer and food consumption in Connecticut from 1935 to 1965 confirmed the positive correlation with beef consumption and also called attention to the fact that increases in fat and protein in the diet are accompanied by other changes, notably a reduction in consumption of cereal and potatoes in the United States (24). This study revealed a very strong negative correlation between colon cancer and intake of cereals and potatoes. Correlations of this type have contributed to the present interest in studying the possible role of fiber in preventing colon cancer (22), originally proposed by Burkitt and based on observations of high dietary fiber and low colon cancer frequency in Africa (3). Enstrom (9) failed to find positive correlation between fat consumption and colon cancer rates while examining data for the United States, where excessive fat intake can be traced several decades back. This has resulted in a rather homogeneous situation as far as fat intake and colon cancer rate are concerned.

The correlation between diet and death rates for breast cancer in 41 countries, as well as the influence of childbearing, was studied by Hems (17). He found a positive correlation with total fat, animal protein, and animal calories, but since these three items were closely correlated with one another, it was not possible to assign an etiologic role to one of them independently of the other two. Differences in childbearing per se contributed little to the international variation. Hems also reported a positive correlation between breast cancer rates and height of women in 29 countries. This confirmed results of previous case-control studies in Holland (5), Greece (37), Slovenia (30), and Brazil (28). Since nutrition influences height, this could be an indirect indication of nutritional status, but genetic factors most probably also have a strong influence on body height.

Gaskill and collaborators (12) analyzed the data for the main regions of the United States based on a 1965–1966 household food consumption survey. Again, they found the positive association of breast cancer rates with milk consumption. In addition, they found a previously undetected negative correlation between breast cancer rates and egg consumption. High egg consumption could be an indicator of poor socioeconomic status at the present time in the United States, or else could have some unknown biological significance. The lack of consistency with other international data should caution the investigator against assigning a causal role to such a negative correlation. Although consumption of eggs has declined in the United States since 1939, the availability of other dairy products and meat has increased remarkably (24). As a consequence, eggs are becoming relatively less important as a source of energy, and the negative correlation may be an expression of the excessive intake of other types of food.

A critique of the fat–cancer hypothesis has been provided by Enig and collaborators (8), who explain the increase in fat consumption in the United States as being primarily the result of an increased consumption of vegetable fat, mostly containing trans double bonds. They suggest that processed vegetable fat should be investigated as a possible etiologic agent. It should be noted that the marked increase in vegetable fat consumption has not been associated with a marked reduction in the consumption of other types of fat. This results in an excessive overall fat intake, and makes it difficult to assign etiologic roles to one particular type of fat to the exclusion of the others.

The content of cholesterol, fatty acids, and fiber in the items reported in the food consumption tables of FAO has been estimated by Liu and co-workers and utilized for correlation analysis (25). They found that the correlation of colon cancer rates with cholesterol intake remained significant when adjustments were made for other fats and fiber; adjusting for cholesterol, on the other hand, decreased most of the other correlations to nonsignificant levels.

### The Role of Fiber

Several investigators have noted a negative correlation between fat and fiber intake. Simultaneously with an increase in fat consumption, there has been a decrease in the consumption of fruits and vegetables in the United States (24). This trend is generally observed as the level of affluence of the populations under study increases. Direct correlations of cancer rates with dietary fiber have not been consistent (6), but calculation of the fiber component of diet, based on international data, is far from satisfactory. It is well known that there is a great variation in the types of vegetables consumed in different countries; for many of these, the content of fiber is either unknown or inaccurately estimated. Although the definition of "fiber" is still controversial, and the characterization of different types of fiber is under investigation, it remains true that populations with low colon cancer rates have greater amounts of bulk in the diet than those populations with high rates. Two independent studies, in Hawaii (13) and Finland (20), have shown that the daily stool weight is greater in low-risk populations. This strengthens the observation, made by Leveille, that changing the energy intake from vegetable to animal sources is a characteristic of populations at high risk for cancer of certain sites, especially breast and colon. This is well illustrated by a recent dietary survey conducted by Fajardo (10) in rural areas of Colombia with very low incidences of breast and colon cancer. In a typical village (Guaitarilla), 82.5% of the calories and 76.4% of the protein came from vegetable sources.

## Updated Correlations

To take a closer look at the role of vegetables in cancer risk, we calculated single (Pearson) and rank (Spearman) correlation coefficients for disease rates (31,32) compared to dietary information (11). The most recent available cancer rates, age-adjusted by Segi, were utilized for 1973 and matched with diet data published by FAO for 1964 to 1966. This allows an eight- to nine-year lapse between dietary data and cancer rates to accommodate partially the well-known latency period needed for the development of neoplastic processes. In a total of 41 countries, mortality data and detailed information for most dietary items were available; the only exception was the data on beans, which appeared as a separate item only in 15 countries under study. Data for the following countries were available: Australia, Austria, Belgium, Bulgaria, Canada, Costa Rica, Cuba, Czechoslovakia, Denmark, El Salvador, England, Finland, France, Greece, Hong Kong, Hungary, Iceland, Ireland, Israel, Italy, Japan, Luxembourg, Mauritius, Mexico, New Zealand, Netherlands, Nicaragua, Norway, Poland, Portugal, Romania, Singapore, Spain, Sweden, Switzerland, United States, Uruguay, Venezuela, West Germany, and Yugoslavia.

Correlation coefficients were calculated for males for the following cancer sites (1973): oral cavity, esophagus, stomach, intestines, and prostate. Rates for breast and cervical cancers were calculated for females. Additionally, rates for tuberculosis, infectious and parasitic disease, and arteriosclerotic heart disease were calculated for males (1960 to 1961). Since body size is related in part to nutrition, correlations were calculated with body height. The latter data were available for females only in 27 countries under study (27).

Table 1 shows the correlation coefficients significant at the 0.05 level. No significant correlations were found for cancer of the oral cavity, esophagus, stomach, or cervix, for tuberculosis, or for infectious diseases. The only exception was a weak (0.42) correlation between esophageal cancer and rice consumption. There were also significant correlations between the following diseases and/or cancer sites: oral cavity and esophagus (0.78), stomach and arteriosclerotic heart disease (−0.47), intestine and breast (0.90), intestine and prostate (0.73), intestine and arteriosclerotic heart disease (0.48), breast and prostate (0.77), breast and

TABLE 1. Significant (p < 0.05) Pearson's correlation coefficients: Age-adjusted mortality rates[a] vs. per capita consumption of dietary item[b] and height[c]

| | GNP | Wheat | Rice | Maize | Beans | Cattle meat | Pork | Eggs | Milk | Animal oil and fat | Beer | Animal calories | Proteins | Fat | Height (F) |
|---|---|---|---|---|---|---|---|---|---|---|---|---|---|---|---|
| Colon | 0.67 | — | −0.34 | −0.67 | −0.68 | 0.54 | 0.60 | 0.75 | 0.48 | 0.64 | 0.62 | 0.84 | 0.49 | 0.74 | 0.56 |
| Breast (F) | 0.66 | 0.34 | −0.50 | −0.66 | −0.70 | 0.58 | 0.62 | 0.75 | 0.55 | 0.64 | 0.56 | 0.84 | 0.48 | 0.75 | 0.63 |
| Prostate | 0.64 | — | −0.58 | −0.53 | −0.66 | 0.47 | 0.48 | 0.48 | 0.52 | 0.51 | 0.44 | 0.76 | 0.52 | 0.72 | 0.58 |
| Arteriosclerotic heart disease | 0.52 | — | −0.40 | — | — | 0.48 | — | — | 0.59 | 0.48 | — | 0.74 | 0.51 | 0.73 | — |
| Height | 0.70 | — | −0.42 | −0.66 | — | — | 0.71 | 0.64 | 0.48 | 0.58 | 0.47 | 0.69 | — | 0.61 | — |

[a] Reference 31.
[b] Reference 11.
[c] Reference 27.

arteriosclerotic heart disease (0.41), and prostate and arteriosclerotic heart disease (0.46).

Our findings confirmed what previous investigators have pointed out: the diseases that have a better correlation with dietary data are cancers of the intestine, breast, and prostate, and arteriosclerotic heart disease. Their correlation with total fat intake and with sources of animal protein and fat, clearly shown in Table 1, has also been extensively discussed by previous investigators. The same diseases correlate well with the physical quality of life index and with the gross national product, indicating that they are diseases of affluence. Affluence seems to bring with it dietary changes that result in excessive consumption of animal protein. Leveille has calculated that the excess protein intake is more than double the recommended dietary allowances for most age groups in the United States (24).

Table 1 emphasizes the negative correlations of the diseases under study with the consumption of rice, corn, and beans, which may suggest a protective role for these food items. As previously stated, the excessive intake of animal protein (mostly meat) in affluent societies is accompanied by a decrease in the consumption of vegetables (24). This makes it impossible, at the present time, to determine whether the "protective" effect of rice, corn, and beans is direct or whether it simply indicates less consumption of meat. The question may never be resolved, and its resolution becomes somewhat byzantine when one considers that, in the past, dietary changes in human populations have simultaneously reduced the intake of starchy vegetable foods and increased meat consumption. This may indicate that disease prevention could be accomplished by reversing both trends simultaneously. The role of starchy vegetables may be to satisfy the appetite and therefore limit the excessive meat intake. Most dietary habits are not suppressed but rather replaced.

Table 1 also shows a positive correlation between body height and cancer of the colon, breast, and prostate. This has been well described previously for breast cancer (5). The table also shows height to be correlated with affluence and with sources of animal protein and fat, as well as demonstrating a negative correlation with the consumption of rice and corn. It would be reasonable to assume that a reduction in protein intake and an increase in the consumption of starchy vegetables might, in the long run, affect the average height of the population, probably an unpopular result. On the other hand, it is hard to believe that unlimited excessive protein consumption will result in unlimited increases in the height of individuals in the community. The ideal situation should be provision of adequate energy sources to satisfy the needs of the growing body and less than excessive nutrition after full growth has been achieved. This should be a high-priority challenge for our society at this time.

## The Milk Versus Meat Controversy

Since milk, beef, pork, and eggs are the prominent sources of animal protein and fat in most wealthy societies, special attention should be given to these

TABLE 2. *Disease death rates (32,33) and consumption of milk and meat*

|  | Daily intake (gm) | | Truncated (age 35–64) death rates (per 100,000) | | |
|---|---|---|---|---|---|
|  | Milk | Meat | AHD[a] | Colon ca | Breast ca |
| Argentina | 207 | 200 | 170 | 15 | 50 |
| Finland | 878 | 56 | 385 | 6 | 39 |

[a] AHD indicates arteriosclerotic heart disease.

items. Table 1 shows positive correlations of all these food sources with the diseases under consideration. The correlation coefficient between arteriosclerotic heart disease and egg consumption in our tabulations was weakly positive (0.35) and not significant ($p = 0.08$). It should be noted, however, that the recent drop in coronary heart disease death rates in the United States has followed a decrease in the consumption of eggs and an increase in the consumption of vegetable fat. The possible causal linkage between the two events should be considered. The fact that cancer rates have not dropped simultaneously with those of heart disease may indicate differences in either pathogenesis or etiology, which should be further investigated. Most countries have similar patterns of consumption of animal fat and meat, and this accounts for the positive correlations with both items, practically impossible to separate in tabulations of data from all countries. A few countries have definite preferences for their source of animal protein, and this provides some opportunity for limited discriminatory analysis (2). One such contrasting pattern is provided by Argentina and Finland. Table 2 shows data on daily (1964 to 1966) per capita consumption of milk and meat (11), as well as the truncated (age 35 to 64) annual death rates (Finland, 1960 to 1961; Argentina, 1962 to 1964) for coronary disease and cancer of the colon and breast (29,33). The high milk intake of the Finnish is better reflected in their high heart disease rates, whereas the high beef intake of the Argentines is better reflected in their high colon cancer rate. The rates of breast cancer, however, are high in both countries, probably indicating that either source of animal protein and fat may influence its development. A similar situation seems to exist for prostatic carcinoma: truncated rates for ages 35 to 74 are 24.7 for Argentina and 17.7 for Finland.

## CONCLUSIONS

International studies have unanimously agreed that there is a strong positive correlation between the consumption of total fat and animal protein and death rates for cancer of the breast and colon, and for sclerotic heart disease. Similar but less strong correlations are seen for cancer of the prostate, ovary, and endometrium.

The separate and independent role of fat versus animal protein cannot be definitely resolved with the present human data, because consumption of both items is similarly high in wealthy societies and similarly low in poor societies.

The data suggest, but do not prove, that fat intake correlates better with arteriosclerotic heart disease and beef intake correlates better with colon cancer.

Correlation studies in humans have not resolved the question of the role of fiber in cancer development. Adequate estimates of the amount and quality of fiber in most populations are lacking.

Available data support the concept that low colon cancer rates are associated with a diet rich in vegetables, which is conducive to greater stool weight.

The present levels of consumption of animal proteins in the United States, especially meat, are probably excessive. This rise in meat consumption has been simultaneous with a decrease in the consumption of vegetables.

## ACKNOWLEDGMENT

This work is supported by contract #N01-CP-53521, National Cancer Institute.

## REFERENCES

1. Armstrong, B., and Doll, R. (1975): Environmental factors and cancer incidence in different countries, with special reference to dietary practices. *Int. J. Cancer,* 15:617–631.
2. Berg, J. W., Haenszel, W., and Devesa, S. S. (1973): Epidemiology of gastrointestinal cancer. In: *Proceedings of the Seventh National Cancer Conference,* p. 459–464. J. B. Lippincott, Philadelphia.
3. Burkitt, D. P. (1971): Epidemiology of cancer of the colon and rectum. *Cancer,* 28:3–13.
4. Carroll, K. K., Gammal, E. B., and Plunkett, E. R. (1968): Dietary fat and mammary cancer. *Can. Med. Assoc. J.,* 23:590–594.
5. DeWaard, F. (1975): Breast cancer incidence and nutritional status with particular reference to body weight and height. *Cancer Res.,* 35:3351–3356.
6. Drasar, B. S., and Irving, D. (1973): Environmental factors and cancer of the colon and breast. *Br. J. Cancer,* 27:167–172.
7. Dunn, J. E., and Buell, P. (1966): Gastrointestinal cancer among ethnic groups in California. Third World Congress of Gastroenterology, Tokyo, Japan.
8. Enig, M. G., Munn, R. J., and Keeney, M. (1978): Dietary fat and cancer trends—a critique. *Fed. Proc.,* 37:2215–2220.
9. Enstrom, J. E. (1975): Colorectal cancer and consumption of beef and fat. *Br. J. Cancer,* 32:432–439.
10. Fajardo, L. (1979): *Colombia Dietary Surveys.* Universidad del Valle, Cali, Colombia.
11. Food and Agriculture Organization (1971): *Food Balance Sheets 1964–1966.* FAO, Rome, Italy.
12. Gaskill, S. P., McGuire, W. L., Osborne, C. K., and Stern, M. (1979): Breast cancer mortality in the United States. *Cancer Res.,* 39:3628–3637.
13. Glober, G. A., Klein, K. L., Moore, J. O., and Abba, B. C. (1974): Bowel transit times in two populations experiencing similar colon cancer risks. *Lancet,* 2:80–81.
14. Gregor, O., Toman, R., and Frusova, F. (1969): Gastrointestinal cancer and nutrition. *Gut,* 10:1031–1034.
15. Haenszel, W., Berg, J. W., Segi, M., Kurihara, M., and Locke, F. B. (1973): Large bowel cancer in Hawaiian Japanese. *J. Natl. Cancer Inst.,* 51:1765–1779.
16. Hems, G. (1970): Epidemiological characteristics of breast cancer in middle and late age. *Br. J. Cancer,* 24:226–234.
17. Hems, G. (1978): The contribution of diet and childbearing to breast cancer rates. *Br. J. Cancer,* 37:974–982.

18. Howell, M. A. (1974): Factor analysis of international cancer mortality data and per capita food consumption. *Br. J. Cancer,* 29:328–336.
19. Howell, M. A. (1975): Diet as an etiological factor in the development of cancers of the colon and rectum. *J. Chronic Dis.,* 28:67–80.
20. International Agency for Research on Cancer (1977): Dietary fiber, transit time, fecal bacteria, steroids and colon cancer in two Scandinavian populations. *Lancet,* 2:207–211.
21. Jolliffe, N., and Archer, M. (1959): Statistical association between international heart disease death rates and certain environmental factors. *J. Chronic Dis.,* 9:636–652.
22. Kritchevsky, D., and Story, J. (1977): Dietary fiber and cancer. *Curr. Concepts Nutr.,* 6:41–54.
23. Lea, A. J. (1967): Neoplasms and environmental factors. *Ann. R. Coll. Surg. Engl.,* 41:432–438.
24. Leveille, G. A. (1975): Issues in human nutrition and their probable impact on foods of animal origin. *J. Anim. Sci.,* 41:723–731.
25. Liu, K., Stamler, J., Moss, D., Garside, D., Persky, V., and Soltero, I. (1979): Dietary cholesterol, fat and fiber, and colon cancer mortality. *Lancet,* 2:782–785.
26. MacMahon, B., Cole, P., Liu, T. M., Lowe, C. R., Mirra, A. P., Ravnihar, B., Salber, E. J., Valaores, V. G., and Yuasa, S. (1970): Age at first birth and breast cancer risk. *Bull. WHO,* 43:209.
27. Meredith, H. V. (1971): Worldwide somatic comparisons among contemporary human groups of adult females. *Am. J. Phys. Anthropol.,* 34:89–132.
28. Mirra, A. P., Cole, P., and MacMahon, B. (1971): Breast cancer in an area of high parity: São Paulo, Brazil. *Cancer Res.,* 31:77–83.
29. Puffer, R., and Griffith, W. (1967): *Patterns of Urban Mortality.* Pan American Health Organization, Washington, D.C.
30. Ravnihar, B., MacMahon, B., and Lindtner, J. (1971): Epidemiologic features of breast cancer in Slovenia. *Eur. J. Cancer,* 7:295–306.
31. Segi, M. (1978): *Age-adjusted Death Rates for Cancer for Selected Sites (A-classification) in 52 Countries in 1973.* Segi Institute of Cancer Epidemiology, Nagoya, Japan.
32. Segi, M., and Kurihara, M. (1966): *Cancer Mortality for Selected Sites in 24 Countries (1962–1963).* Tohoku University, Sendai, Japan.
33. Segi, M., Kurihara, M., and Tsukaham, Y. (1966): *Mortality for Selected Cancer in 30 Countries (1950–1961).* Tohoku University, Sendai, Japan.
34. Tannenbaum, A. (1940): Relationship of body weight to cancer incidence. *Arch. Pathol.,* 30:509–517.
35. Tannenbaum, A., and Silverstone, H. (1957): Nutrition and the genesis of tumors. In: *Cancer, Vol. I,* edited by R. W. Raven, pp. 306–334. Butterworth and Co., London.
36. U.S. Department of Agriculture, Agriculture Research Service (1974): *Household Food Consumption Survey 1965–1966, Report No. 18.* U.S. Government Printing Office, Washington, D.C.
37. Valaoras, V. G., MacMahon, B., Trichopoulus, D., and Polychronopoulus, A. (1969): Lactation and reproductive histories of breast cancer patients in greater Athens. *Int. J. Cancer,* 4:350–363.
38. Waterhouse, J., Muir, C., Correa, P., and Powell, J. editors (1976): *Cancer Incidence in Five Continents, Vol. III.* International Agency for Research on Cancer, Lyons, France.
39. Wynder, E. L., and Shigematsu, T. (1967): Environmental factors of cancer of the colon and rectum. *Cancer,* 20:1520–1561.
40. Wynder, E. L., Kajitani, T., Dodo, H., and Takano, A. (1969): Environmental factors of cancer of the colon and rectum: II. Japanese epidemiologic data. *Cancer,* 23:1210–1220.

*Nutrition and Cancer: Etiology and Treatment,*
edited by G. R. Newell and N. M. Ellison.
Raven Press, New York © 1981.

# Nutrition and Metabolic Epidemiology of Cancers of the Oral Cavity, Esophagus, Colon, Breast, Prostate, and Stomach

E. L. Wynder, G. D. McCoy, B. S. Reddy, L. Cohen, P. Hill, N. E. Spingarn, and J. H. Weisburger

*American Health Foundation, Naylor Dana Institute for Disease Prevention, Valhalla, New York 10595*

Detailed research in a number of laboratories, including our institute, has provided evidence that certain kinds of cancer are associated with nutrition in general and specific dietary items in particular (117). Such research in man, reliable animal models, and in cell and organ culture systems has begun to provide leads to the underlying mechanisms. These efforts have led to the evolution of working hypotheses concerning the presence and operation of etiologic factors which can be further tested through a combined approach of different research modalities.

Cancer is a set of diseases, rather than a single disease. The sole common characteristic of neoplastic diseases is that the mechanisms of growth control and differentiation of normal cell systems have been altered; either they do not operate in neoplastic cells, or else they have different quantitative operating parameters. Thus, cancer represents uncontrolled growth of cells derived from a specific organ or tissue. However, the causes and modifying elements for diverse cancers can be and, in fact, are different.

The current view is that several types of cancer in man may be associated, directly or indirectly, with nutrition, including cancers of the upper gastrointestinal tract, stomach, large bowel, pancreas, liver, breast, ovary, uterus, cervix, prostate, kidney, and urinary bladder. For a number of these target organs, nutrition and nutritional status are not the only etiologic factors. For this reason, we will discuss in this chapter only those types of cancer in which nutritional elements appear to be of primary importance—oral cavity and esophagus, stomach, large bowel, breast, and prostate.

What is the basis for the conclusion that nutrition plays a major role in the types of cancer discussed?

A. *Consideration of the time trends for each type of cancer in various parts of the world.* Figures 1 and 2 show that cancers of the stomach and the uterus have decreased appreciably in the United States over the last 50 years. On

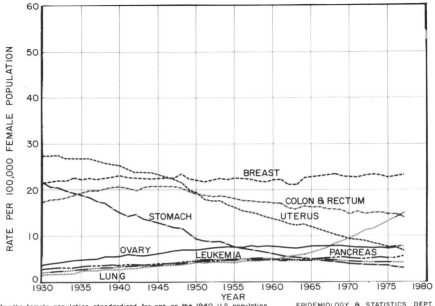

**FIG. 1.** Age-adjusted cancer death rates[a] for selected sites, females, United States, 1930–1975. Sources of data: U.S. National Center for Health Statistics and U.S. Bureau of the Census. ([a]Standardized on the age distribution of the 1940 U.S. census population.) From the American Cancer Society, ref. 2, with permission.

the other hand, cancers of the large bowel, breast, and prostate have exhibited rather stable mortalities, and have shown only a slight increase in incidence in the last 50 years. This suggests that environmental factors affecting these cancers have increased only slightly.

B. *International comparisons in mortality and incidence.* It is quite apparent that, given equal proficiency in medical analysis and record-keeping, there remain very sizable differences between countries with the highest or lowest incidences of cancers. In some cases, the difference factor is as great as 8:1 (Table 1).

C. *Changes in incidence reflecting migration from regions of high risk to regions of low risk and vice versa.* Within the same generation, or certainly within two generations, the migrant acquires the risk of the area of residence (Fig. 3).

D. *Carefully conducted studies in laboratory models, and associated experimental research efforts.*

Table 2 summarizes the key findings documenting the nutritional links and specific risk factors developed thus far. It shows only those elements specifically related through the modes of inquiry, listed above, to the type of cancer noted. There have been studies in which an association was attempted but was not productive; for example, the level of protein in the diet in relation to the occur-

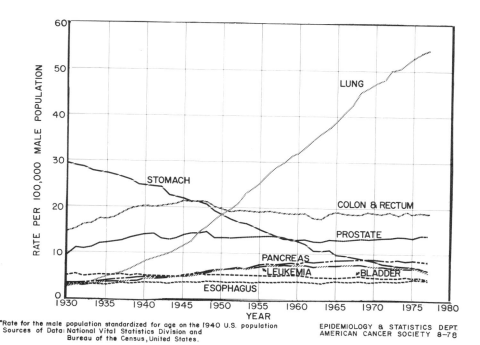

Rate for the male population standardized for age on the 1940 U.S. population
Sources of Data: National Vital Statistics Division and
Bureau of the Census, United States.

EPIDEMIOLOGY & STATISTICS DEPT.
AMERICAN CANCER SOCIETY 8–78

**FIG. 2.** Age-adjusted cancer death rates[a] for selected sites, males, United States, 1930–1975. Sources of data: U.S. National Center for Health Statistics and U.S. Bureau of the Census. ([a]Standardized on the age distribution of the 1940 U.S. census population.) From the American Cancer Society, ref. 2, with permission.

rence of breast or large bowel cancer. It must be noted that, in addition to the main risk factors delineated, there may be more subtle secondary modifying factors which require further research, or, indeed, which remain to be discovered. It is possible that such modifying factors may not necessarily be important in the human setting, if the *major* risk factors, already pinpointed, are controlled with a view to reduction of the risk for a specific type of cancer.

Within this chapter, it would be possible to discuss each kind of cancer in sequence; however, since current evidence suggests that several types of cancer may have in common a specific key risk factor operating, possibly through separate and distinct mechanisms (although a common pathway might also exist), we have elected to record the current status of the epidemiology of nutritionally associated cancers by examining the risk factors concerned.

## DIETARY FACTORS AND CANCERS OF THE UPPER ALIMENTARY AND RESPIRATORY TRACTS

Extensive epidemiologic evidence has been available for some time which indicates a strong association between chronic alcohol and tobacco use and

TABLE 1. *Range of incidence and ratio of highest to lowest[a] recorded age-adjusted incidence rate for cancers of selected sites[b]*

| | | Males | | | Females | |
|---|---|---|---|---|---|---|
| | | Range of incidence | | | Range of incidence | |
| Site | Ratio | High | Low | Ratio | High | Low |
| Esophagus | 176 | Bulawayo | Vas | 29 | South Africa (Bantu) | Katowice |
| | | 75.6 | 0.6 | | 14.3 | 0.5 |
| Colon | 30 | Hawaii (Chinese) | Ibadan | 60 | Saskatchewan | Bulawayo |
| | | 35.9 | 1.2 | | 30.0 | 0.5 |
| Rectum | 44 | Saskatchewan | Ibadan | 9 | Saskatchewan | Israel (Non-Jews) |
| | | 22.2 | 0.5 | | 13.6 | 1.6 |
| Breast | | | | 8 | Hawaii (Caucasians) | Israel (Non-Jews) |
| | | | | | 62.9 | 8.1 |
| Prostate | 21 | Alameda (Negro) | Israel (Non-Jews) | | | |
| | | 65.3 | 3.1 | | | |
| Stomach | 12 | Miyagi | Ibadan | 11 | Natal (Indians) | Nevada |
| | | 95.3 | 8.0 | | 30.0 | 2.7 |

[a] Rates based on less than five cases are excluded.
[b] From Muir, ref. 103, with permission.

cancers of the head and neck area, specifically, of the oral cavity (79,163,164). This association is further supported by the low incidence of these types of cancers in populations such as the Seventh-Day Adventists, who are known to consume less alcohol than does the general population (113).

Because of the interaction of the smoking and drinking variables, it is difficult to assess the two independently, since heavy drinkers are frequently also heavy smokers. Although some increased risk for cancer related solely to alcohol consumption is suggested by the data of Rothman and Keller (128), a marked synergy is observed when tobacco use is combined with chronic alcohol consumption. With the possible exception of esophageal cancer in France (147,148), the nature of the beverage consumed seems to be important only in terms of its ethanol content (160,173).

The respective roles played by alcohol and tobacco consumption in the etiology of head and neck cancer have yet to be rigorously defined; however, it seems reasonable to assume that tobacco and/or tobacco smoke is the source of the initiating carcinogenic stimuli, and that ethanol facilitates the reactivity of tobacco-associated initiators.

We have recently reviewed the experimental evidence and identified four possible mechanisms by which alcohol could increase the risk for cancer: alcohol as a solvent, alcohol-associated increases or decreases in liver metabolism, and alcohol-involved alterations in the metabolism of target tissues (95).

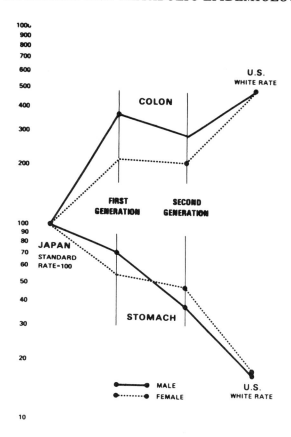

**FIG. 3.** Mortality trends of Japanese migrants to the United States. Note the relatively rapid increase of the risk of colon cancer even in the first generation, and progressive decrease of the risk for stomach cancer. The data are derived from the basic data of Haenszel and Kurihara (55).

TABLE 2. *Types of cancer associated with nutrition*

| Type | Nutritional element | Other |
|------|--------------------|-------|
| Esophagus | Vitamins? | Alcohol, smoking |
| Stomach | Vitamins C, E | Salt, pickling |
| Colon | Fat, fiber, fried food | Vitamins A, C, E? |
| Breast, prostate | Fat (fried food?) | Hormones? |
| Endometrium | Fat | Hormones |
| Pancreas | Fat | Smoking |

The possibility that nutrition might play a role in the etiology of esophageal cancer was first suggested by consideration of the association of the Plummer–Vinson (Paterson–Kelly) syndrome with cancer of the upper alimentary tract. This disease, once prevalent among Swedish women, was shown to be associated with chronic iron and vitamin deficiencies. High rates of upper alimentary tract cancer were observed, in the absence of exposure to tobacco or any other obvious carcinogen (167). Since the introduction in Sweden of a national program of iron and vitamin supplementation of essential foods, such as bread, in the early 1950s, a significant reduction in the number of cases of Plummer–Vinson syndrome and a subsequent reduction of the incidence of upper alimentary tract cancer have occurred (86).

Thus, one way in which alcohol could increase the risk for cancer would be through the nutritional deficiencies commonly associated with alcoholism (87). Since alcoholics often consume 900 or more calories a day from alcohol alone (31), it is not difficult to imagine that the rest of their dietary intake is insufficient to provide essential micronutrients. Cancers of the head and neck also seem to occur most commonly in those individuals who do not eat nutritionally balanced diets (33). Alcohol consumption can also lead to impaired absorption of nutrients and vitamins (150). That ethanol is capable of decreasing vitamin A levels is noteworthy, in view of the participation of this vitamin in regulation of epithelial cell differentiation (32,149).

Animal studies have provided evidence suggesting that nutrient deficiencies and dietary composition may play a role in esophageal carcinogenesis. Lipotrope-deficient rats fed N-nitrosodiethylamine showed increased esophageal carcinogenesis by comparison with rats fed a control diet (126). The tumors induced in these investigations were invasive squamous cell carcinomas, morphologically similar to those in man.

Mice fed a diet deficient in riboflavin develop morphologic alterations in skin and upper alimentary tract epithelium, similar to those observed in patients suffering from Plummer–Vinson disease (170). As the deficiency progresses, epithelial morphology changes progressively from atrophy to hyperkeratosis to, in several instances, hyperplasia. The experiments of Chan and Wynder (165) have shown that, following initiation with benzo*(a)*pyrene and promotion with croton oil, riboflavin-deficient mice develop tumors more rapidly than do control mice receiving a nutritionally adequate diet. In parallel studies, Chan et al. (22) have shown that basal levels of skin arylhydrocarbon hydroxylase were slightly reduced in riboflavin-deficient mice; however, skin activity in riboflavin-deficient animals was reduced to a much greater extent following a single application of dimethylbenz*(a)*anthracene (DMBA).

The work of Gerson and Meyer (51) has shown that feeding rats diets deficient in zinc causes similar changes in the morphology of the buccal mucosa. Lower levels of zinc have been observed in hair and tissue samples from esophageal cancer patients (88). In animals made deficient for vitamin A, the tracheobronchial epithelium undergoes atrophic degenerative changes (58,129), which are quite similar to the changes observed in animals exposed to tobacco smoke (38,85). Vitamin A-deficient animals have been shown to be more susceptible to polycyclic aromatic hydrocarbon (PAH) carcinogenesis (138). The recent demonstration by Meade et al. (96) that serum and liver vitamin A stores are lower in hamsters chronically exposed to tobacco smoke is consistent with the view that lowered levels of this vitamin may be associated with increased risk for cancer.

Currently available evidence thus suggests that experimental deficiencies arising from undernutrition and/or alcohol intake (impaired absorption or enhanced elimination) could play a role in the etiology of head and neck cancer. Alternatively, chronic ethanol consumption could alter intracellular metabolism of the epithelial cells at the target sites, resulting in enhanced metabolic activation of tobacco-associated carcinogens (94). Some of the more relevant features of this metabolic mechanism are that (a) the cancers associated with the head and neck are epithelial in origin; (b) these surface epithelial cells are most frequently exposed to tobacco-associated carcinogens; and (c) site-specificity of the carcinogen need not be invoked, since all sites, by virtue of their anatomic location, will be exposed to tobacco smoke. This is an important point, because no class of carcinogen need be initially excluded from consideration, since we cannot as yet say with any degree of certainty which of the many potential carcinogens in tobacco smoke are actually involved in the initiation of carcinogenesis.

Although there is a strong association between alcohol and tobacco use and cancers of the head and neck, the mechanism(s) by which these two risk factors increase cancer incidence is as yet unknown. The independent association of nutritional deficiencies with cancer of the esophagus requires that serious attention be given to the effect of chronic alcohol consumption on nutritional status, particularly on those micronutrients whose levels are shown to be decreased in populations at high risk.

## DIETARY FACTORS AND BREAST CANCER

In 1979, an estimated 100,000 new cases of breast cancer were diagnosed. More than 35,000 deaths were attributed to this disease (2), making breast cancer the primary cause of cancer deaths in women in the United States. Although the etiology of breast cancer is poorly understood, evidence from laboratory animal studies and epidemiologic investigations suggests that environmental factors play a major role in the development of this disease, and that dietary fat, in particular, is an important environmental determinant of breast cancer risk.

### Epidemiologic Evidence

The evidence that dietary fat (as an etiologic factor distinct from chemical contaminants of the diet and from genetic or other environmental factors) is a key determinant of risk is reinforced by a variety of epidemiologic studies. These include correlations between incidence and mortality and dietary fat consumption in various countries (5,16,39,52,61,91,168), the changing incidence in breast cancer in migrants from low-risk to high-risk countries (13), analysis of trends in cancer incidence in low-risk countries as they undergo "westernization" of their diets (71), and case-control studies linking increased risk for breast cancer with excessive fat intake (99,111) (see Fig. 4). Although some exceptions have been noted (44), the consensus of these studies is that total fat intake is an accurate index of breast cancer risk, particularly in the postmenopausal age groups, in which incidence rates are highest (172).

## Experimental Evidence

Because it is possible to control variables such as age, sex, time of exposure, dose of carcinogen, and diet, experimental model systems are uniquely suited to analysis of the effects of nutrition on breast carcinogenesis. The disadvantages of nutritional studies in rodents are equally certain (60), particularly with regard to their applicability to the human disease.

Some of the first studies suggesting a dietary role in breast carcinogenesis in mice were reported in the early 1940s by Tannenbaum and co-workers (134,143,145). In these studies, it was demonstrated that increased fat consumption led to increased incidence of certain types of murine cancers, such as skin and breast, but not of others, such as leukemia and liver cancer. It was also shown that obesity increased and caloric insufficiency decreased the incidence of spontaneous mouse mammary carcinoma. Increased fat intake, in the absence

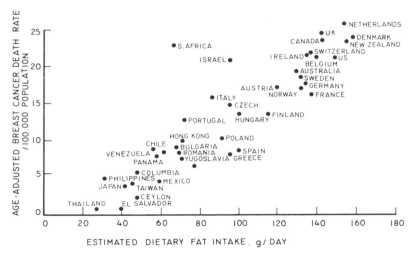

**FIG. 4.** Positive correlation between per capita consumption of dietary fat and age-adjusted mortality from breast cancer. From Wynder et al., ref. 166, with permission.

of obesity, also induced a greater frequency of mammary cancer, suggesting that dietary fat per se enhanced mammary carcinogenesis. Other macronutrients, such as protein and carbohydrate, did not demonstrate marked effects on tumor incidence.

In recent years, the most commonly used models have been those based on the induction of breast cancer in rats by specific chemicals, such as DMBA (76) and N-nitrosomethylurea (NMU) (53). In such models, a distinction can be made between the influence of diet prior to and after carcinogen administration. Using the DMBA model, Carroll and co-workers (17) demonstrated that diets with a fat content between 10% to 20% (by weight) significantly increased the frequency of breast cancer, as compared to diets containing 0.5% to 5% fat. (These values roughly mimic the proportion of calories present as fat in the Japanese [15%] and U.S. [40%] diets, in the years 1957 to 1959. The current Japanese diet consists of 20% of calories as fat, whereas total fat content of the U.S. diet has changed little over the past 20 years [70].) In addition, it was found that the effect of fat was exerted primarily on the promotion phase of breast cancer development, and that diets rich in polyunsaturated fats were more effective tumor promoters than were diets rich in saturated fats (17,50,73). Recently, we (21) have confirmed Carroll's findings in the NMU model with features that mimic human breast cancer more closely than does the DMBA tumor. A summary of laboratory studies on breast cancer and fat is shown in Table 3 (8,21,40,43,50,134,143).

Evidence from experimental and epidemiologic investigations in breast cancer has reached sufficient proportions to warrant more systematic explorations into mechanisms. Postulated mechanisms by which dietary fat may influence breast cancer fall into two basic categories: those involving direct effects of fat on tumor development, and those involving indirect effects on host metabolism. Direct effects involve changes in (a) the lipid content of the cell membrane and (b) the synthesis of prostaglandins (biologically active derivatives of the essential fatty acids [arachidonic and linoleic]). Indirect mechanisms involve subversion of the immune system, stimulation of mixed-function oxidase systems involved in carcinogen activation, alterations in fecal flora and bile acid metabolism, and alterations in the endocrine milieu of the host (see reviews by Hopkins and West [74]; Hankin and Rawlings [57]; Armstrong [4]).

In our laboratory, we have focused on the possibility that dietary fat elicits its tumor-enhancing effects by altering host endocrine metabolism—in particular, that component of the endocrine system that regulates prolactin secretion. Our interest in a fat–prolactin–breast cancer relationship was prompted by two facts: (a) prolactin is a known classic promoter substance in a number of murine breast tumor systems (159); and (b) prolactin is a liporegulatory hormone in birds and lower mammals (97), rodents (41), and possibly man (47).

For initial studies, estrogen and prolactin (30), the two most essential hormones in breast cancer development, were chosen. Using specific hormone antagonists (63), bromoergocryptine and nafoxidine, which selectively result in

TABLE 3. *Summary chart: enhancement of mammary tumor incidence in mice and rats by dietary fat[c]*

| Type of fat | Level in diet (% by weight) | Carcinogenic agent | Duration of study (mos) | Strain | Tumor incidence (%) Low fat[a] | High fat | Reference |
|---|---|---|---|---|---|---|---|
| | | | | *Mice* | | | |
| 1. Kremit[b] | 12 | None | 18 | dba | 16/50 (32) | 32/50 (64) | (143) |
| 2. Kremax[b] | 16 | None | 21 | C311 | 40/54 (74) | 48/54 (89) | (134) |
| | | | | *Rats* | | | |
| 3. Crisco[b] | 46 | Stilbestrol | 13 | AxC line 9935 | 9/12 (75) | 11/12 (92) | (40) |
| 4. Lard | 16–30 | 2-Acetylaminofluorene | 7 | AES | 2/31 (6) | 55/71 (78) | (43) |
| 5. Olive Oil | 20 | None | 10 | Sprague-Dawley | 3/25 (12) | 5/13 (39) | (8) |
| 6. Corn Oil | 20 | 7,12-Dimethylbenz (a) anthracene | 4 | Sprague-Dawley | 12/21 (57) | 21/22 (96) | (50) |
| 7. Lard | 20 | N-Nitrosomethylurea | 5 | F-344 (Fischer) | 8/20 (40) | 18/20 (90) | (22) |

[a] The low fat diets contained from 0.5 to 3% fat, except in the experiments of Dunning et al., where the level was 6.5%, and Chan et al., where the level was 5%.

[b] Partially hydrogenated cottonseed or cottonseed–soybean oil.

1. $p < 0.005$      Chi square (corrected)
2. $0.05 < p > 0.10$      Chi square (corrected)
3. $p \doteq 0.217$      Fishers exact test* (two-tailed)
4. $p < 0.001$      Chi square
5. $p \doteq 0.0941$      Fishers exact test (two-tailed)
6. $p < 0.01$      Chi square (corrected)
7. $p \doteq 0.0225$      Fishers exact test (two-tailed)

[c] Modified from Carroll, ref. 16.

"chemical hypophysectomy" and "chemical ovariectomy," we found that, in the absence of estrogenic stimulation, tumor incidence was decreased in animals fed high-fat (HF) or low-fat (LF) diets, as compared to untreated controls; however, the HF group exhibited significantly higher tumor yields than did the LF group. Animals fed HF and LF diets and treated with bromoergocryptine also exhibited decreased tumor incidence compared to controls; however, in this case, no difference in tumor incidence could be observed between the two experimental groups (18) (Table 4).

These results are consistent with the hypothesis that HF diets exert their tumor-enhancing effects by increasing circulating prolactin concentrations relative to estrogen levels. In the presence of bromoergocryptine, prolactin levels are depressed in both HF- and LF-diet animals relative to estrogen levels, which remain normal (131). As a result, although decreased compared to untreated controls, tumor incidence in the two experimental groups would be similar. Animals treated with nafoxidine are, in a physiological sense, estrogen-depleted. Based on the assumption that an HF diet stimulates prolactin secretion to a greater extent than does an LF diet, the biologically effective prolactin–estrogen ratio in the HF group would be greater than that of the LF group, and, as a consequence, tumor frequency would be greater in the HF group. Since prolactin secretion is regulated to a large extent by circulating estrogens, which interact with specific receptors in the pituitary and hypothalamus (82), animals treated with nafoxidine would be expected to display lower serum prolactin concentrations than do control animals (63). Accordingly, the lower overall tumor frequency in nafoxidine-treated animals, as compared to untreated controls, can be accounted for on the basis of a low prolactin–estrogen ratio.

These conjectures concerning the interaction between fat intake and prolactin secretion were borne out by radioimmunoassay of serum prolactin concentrations in animals fed HF and LF diets (20) (Fig. 5). Animals fed HF diets for two and five months exhibit significantly higher prolactin concentrations than does a similar group of animals fed LF diets. This effect was observed only during the proestrus–estrus peak.

The relatively greater importance of prolactin in the fat effect, in comparison to estrogen, was further suggested by studies in ovariectomized (Ovx) animals, in which it was found that Ovx animals fed an HF diet exhibited significantly higher tumor incidence than did similarly treated animals fed an LF diet (Fig. 6). Moreover, HF–Ovx animals exhibited elevated prolactin concentrations compared to LF–Ovx animals (25). Whether this was the result of a direct stimulating effect of fat on the hypothalamic–pituitary axis, or was caused by an indirect mechanism involving estrogen-produced prolactin stimulation by extraovarian mechanisms, remains to be determined. Such findings may have important ramifications on the use of LF diets as an adjunct to endocrine ablative therapy in advanced human breast cancer, and on understanding of the role of dietary fat in the development of postmenopausal breast cancer.

Results consistent with a prolactin–estrogen hypothesis were also noted when

TABLE 4. Effect of hormone antagonists on mammary tumor incidence in DMBA-treated rats[a] fed HF and LF Diets[a]

| | Diet[d] | Palpable tumor-bearing rats[a]/Total no. rats[e] | (%) | Total no. adenocarcinomas | | Mean ± SEM palpable tumors/Rat |
| --- | --- | --- | --- | --- | --- | --- |
| | | | | Palpable | Nonpalpable | |
| Control | HF | 18/22 | 82[g] | 39 (2)[f] | 12 (6) | 1.77 ± .30 |
| Control | LF | 10/19 | 52 | 15 (1) | 7 (3) | 0.78 ± .19 |
| Anti-estrogen[b] | HF | 7/18 | 39[g] | 7 (9) | 0 (7) | 0.38 ± .12 |
| Anti-estrogen | LF | 1/13 | 8 | 1 (5) | 2 (6) | 0.08 ± .001 |
| Anti-prolactin[c] | HF | 9/21 | 42 | 15 (3) | 9 (12) | 0.70 ± .19 |
| Anti-prolactin | LF | 8/22 | 36 | 12 (6) | 7 (18) | 0.54 ± .09 |

[a] DMBA 10 mgs/kg body weight administered i.g. on day 50.
[b] Nafoxidine hydrochloride (1 mg/kg body weight) administered S.C. 3x/week.
[c] 2-bromo-α-ergocryptine (3 mg/kg body weight) administered S.C. 3x/week.
[d] HF diet, 20% corn oil; LF diet, 5% corn oil.
[e] Experiment terminated at 20 weeks.
[f] Numbers in parentheses indicate fibroadenomas.
[g] Difference between HF and LF, $p < 0.05$.
Modified from Chan and Cohen, ref. 18.

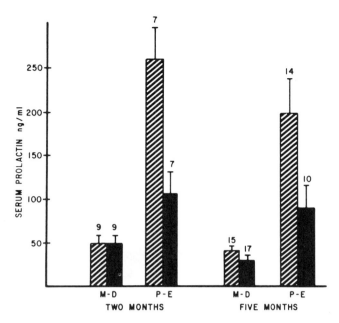

**FIG. 5.** Serum prolactin concentrations in female Sprague–Dawley rats fed high-fat (HF) (20% lard, indicated by hatched bars) and low-fat (LF) (5% lard, indicated by solid black bars) diet for two to five months. Etherized rats were bled between 2 and 4 P.M. by tail vein. Height of bars represents mean; vertical lines above each bar, SEM. Numbers above bars designate the number of individual rats assayed at metestrus–diestrus (M–D) and proestrus–estrus (P–E), as determined by vaginal smears. The difference between mean prolactin values in the HF group and LF group at P–E was significant ($p < 0.05$). Adapted from Chan et al., ref. 20.

serum hormone levels and tumor incidence were measured in NMU-treated animals fed HF and LF diets. HF-diet animals exhibited higher absolute levels of prolactin, higher prolactin–estrogen ratios, and increased tumor incidence compared to animals fed LF diets (21).

Although the molecular mechanism by which prolactin and estrogen regulate mammary tumor growth is unknown, demonstration of a direct antagonism between these two hormones has been reported by Chan et al. (23). Using established cultures of epithelial cells derived from DMBA-induced mammary adenocarcinoma, they found that estradiol inhibited cell growth in a dose-related manner, from 5 to 20 µg/ml; prolactin alone at 100 µg/ml had no effect, but could antagonize the inhibitory effects of estradiol. Further discussion of the interactions between fat intake, prolactin, and breast cancer can be found in a review by Chan and Cohen (19).

### Human Studies

Three important studies on the influence of dietary fat on blood prolactin concentrations in premenopausal women have recently been reported by Hill

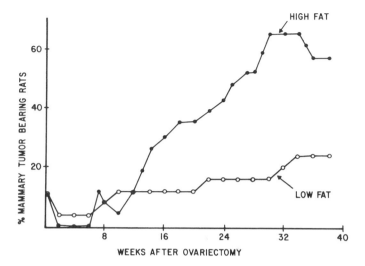

**FIG. 6.** Effect of high-fat (HF) and low-fat (LF) diet on mammary tumor incidence in ovariectomized rats. Curves represent cumulative tumor incidence. DMBA (5 mg/kg) administered on day 50 of age. Ovariectomy performed on day 130 of age, and animals were then placed on either HF (20% lard) or LF (5% lard) diet ($n = 25$). Experiment terminated nine months after ovariectomy. Numbers in parentheses represent serum prolactin concentrations (mean ± SEM). Adapted from Cohen et al., ref. 25.

et al. (65,67,69). In the first of these, sequential assays of prolactin over a 24-hr period were performed in four women after 2 months on a standard western diet (HF), and again after 2 months on a vegetarian diet (LF). Marked increases were observed in serum prolactin concentrations during periods of peak secretion (early morning hours) in three of four subjects on the western diet, as compared to the period when they were on the vegetarian diet (67). Similar results were reported in a second study of eight women following the same dietary sequence, but in whom single morning prolactin levels were measured every other day throughout one complete menstrual cycle (65).

In the third study, prolactin profiles from a low-risk population were compared to those of a high-risk population. Bantus and whites in South Africa exhibit markedly different breast cancer rates and dietary habits. The Bantu have a breast cancer mortality rate of 5/100,000 compared to 23/100,000 for South African whites (125). Moreover, the Bantu diet consists of approximately 15% of total calories as fat, whereas the fat intake of South African whites comprises 40% of calories (92). Comparison of plasma prolactin concentrations in Bantu and white South African women revealed that prolactin levels over the length of the menstrual cycle of the latter women were significantly higher than those of the former group (Fig. 7).

Recently, Armstrong (5) published the results of a study in which hormone profiles in a group of postmenopausal vegetarian women were compared with

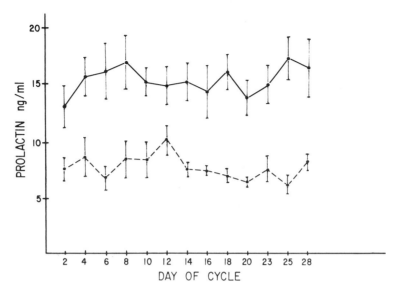

**FIG. 7.** Plasma prolactin levels in North American white women (•——•, $n = 9$) are significantly greater than in South African black (•-----•, $n = 18$) women throughout the menstrual cycle. Blood samples taken between 9–9:30 A.M. every other day of a menstrual cycle. White women maintaining the customary Western diet containing 40% fat calories and black women maintaining a strict vegetarian diet containing less than 20% fat calories. Result given as mean ± SEM. Adapted from Hill et al., ref. 69.

those of a group of postmenopausal nonvegetarian women. Plasma prolactin levels determined at a single time-point were significantly higher in nonvegetarians as compared to vegetarians.

These studies in women reinforce the concept, derived from laboratory animal studies, that both HF intake and elevated prolactin concentrations are positively correlated with increased risk for breast cancer. However, since the role of prolactin in human breast cancer is uncertain (106), it is premature, at present, to postulate a direct causal link between excessive fat intake, elevated prolactin concentrations, and increased risk for human breast cancer.

The foregoing discussion illustrates the point that continued progress in understanding the etiology of breast cancer, and its eventual prevention, will require increasingly close cooperation among a variety of different disciplines—epidemiology, endocrinology, nutrition, and cell biology. Taken independently, evidence from any one discipline may prove fragmentary and, at times, inconsistent, as Enig et al. (44) recently pointed out in an analysis of changing trends in fat consumption patterns and breast cancer incidence in the United States. When one considers the aggregate data, however, there can be little doubt that dietary fat plays an important role in breast cancer development. The questions that remain unresolved are the extent of the role played by fat and the mechanisms by which fat exerts its effect.

Of particular importance will be future studies delineating (a) the specific roles played by polyunsaturated and saturated fats in breast carcinogenesis; (b) the influence of diet on the secretion of different molecular (functional) forms of prolactin; (c) the nature of the prolactin receptor and the influence of diet on its induction; (d) the precise role of estrogens in the fat effect (estrogens generated by extragonadal mechanisms, for example, could play an indirect role via a positive feedback effect on prolactin secretion) (42); (e) the influence of varying ratios of prolactin and estrogens on the proliferative capacity of mammary tumor cells *in vitro;* and (f) the role played by prolactin in human breast cancer. Also of importance will be prospective studies comparing the effect of dietary fat on the occurrence of breast cancer in specific human populations, together with the development of more precise methods of measuring food intake in human populations.

Clearly, our understanding of the role played by nutrition in breast cancer development is still in its infancy. Considerably more work will be required before we can untangle the physiological mechanisms underlying the enhancing effect of dietary fat in rodent breast cancer, and before their relevance to breast cancer in humans can be assessed.

## DIETARY FACTORS AND PROSTATE CANCER

Cancer of the prostate occurs more often in Western countries than in Asia and Africa (37) (Fig. 8). In the United States, the mortality is higher in black men than in white men; however, white men of Scandinavian descent also have higher mortalities (10,171). Although the differences in mortality from prostatic

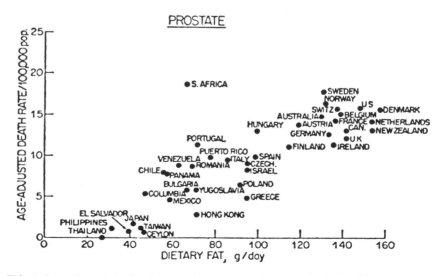

**FIG. 8.** Age-adjusted death rate plotted against the dietary fat intake in different countries.

cancer could be related to genetic and/or environmental factors, a large body of data from migrant (55,139) and descriptive–analytic studies (127) suggests that environmental and hormonal factors are primarily associated with the etiology of this disease. Thus, men migrating from Poland or Japan (low-risk areas), to the United States, a high-risk area, are at increased risk for this disease. The migrant is subject to changes in physical lifestyle and diet, which can influence hormonal status (62,102,142). Blair and Fraumeni (10) reported that urbanization increased the rate of mortality in North American black men, although differences in socioeconomic status or sanitary habits were not associated with this disease (133,171).

When dietary factors are considered, one marked difference between diets in Western societies, as opposed to Asian or African diets, is the higher total fat intake, in the form of meat and fat, in Western societies. Blair and Fraumeni (10), in a comparison of the consumption of high-fat foods in various regions of the United States, reported that a higher consumption of beef and milk products paralleled the mortality from prostatic cancer among white men.

In a comparison of North American and South African black men, Hill et al. (68) reported a lower urinary excretion of estrogens and androgens in South African black men. Interestingly, when South African black men (40 to 55 years old) were fed a Western diet, supplying 40% of the daily calories as fat derived from meat and dairy products, the urinary excretion of estrogens and androgens increased. When the study was repeated in South African black men over 60 years of age, two major differences were apparent. First, older South African men excreted more estrogens; second, a Western diet significantly decreased the urinary excretion of androgens and estrogens (Fig. 9). Thus, diet modification altered estrogen and androgen metabolism in low-risk South African black men who normally eat strict vegetarian diets. Can this difference in response, according to age and diet–hormone interaction, be related to the development of prostatic cancer?

In man, steroid hormones are derived from the testes and adrenals, testosterone and estradiol being synthesized in both glands (35,36,107,132). Studies of clearance rates and interconversion of steroid hormones in men indicate that estradiol is also derived from testosterone, and estrone from androstenedione. With age, plasma testosterone decreases (83) and estradiol increases (115), while there is a concomitant increase in plasma gonadotropins. Since prostatic cancer occurs predominantly after 60 years of age, it appears to coincide with the greatest change in hormonal activity. Consequently, as suggested by our data, dietary modification in older men may be associated with a different hormonal change from that occurring in young men.

Concerning the relationship of these diet–hormone studies to the development of prostatic lesions, several years ago, Akazaki (1) postulated that environmental factors activated latent lesions in the prostate, and that such factors were more prevalent in Western men, since these small, latent lesions occurred with constant frequency not only in Japanese and American men (12) but also in African

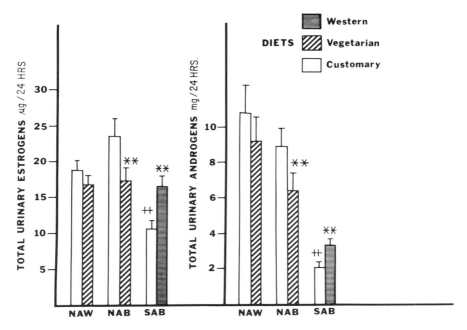

**FIG. 9.** Total urinary estrogen and androgen levels in North American white (*n* = 18) and black (*n* = 16) men and South African black (*n* = 21) men eating customary diets or fed a vegetarian diet, respectively.
$^{++}p \leq 0.01$ in South African black versus North American black men when eating customary diets.
$^{**}p \leq 0.01$ when transferred to a vegetarian or Western diet respectively. Adapted from Hill et al., ref. 68.

men (7). Since prostatic cancer is an endocrine-dependent disease (46), Wynder et al. (171) have postulated that dietary factors activate these latent lesions by means of changes in hormonal activity. However, this final link remains to be established.

Sufficient evidence is available to suggest that environmental factors, lifestyle, and diet modify hormonal status, and that these environmental factors are strongly associated with increased mortality from prostatic cancer in Western societies. To date, however, sufficient data are not available to compare the hormonal status in patients from high- and low-risk populations, or to determine the effects of diet modification on hormonal status in patients with prostatic cancer. Further metabolic epidemiologic studies are required to uncover the key endocrine factors bearing on the etiology of prostatic cancer.

### Diet and Prolactin in Male rats

The results of recent studies in male rats indicate that the influence of dietary fat on circulating prolactin concentrations is not a function of gender. Male rats fed HF diets exhibited significantly higher levels of prolactin than did male rats fed an LF diet (24). These results suggest that prolactin may be involved in cancer of the prostate, in which dietary factors appear to play an important role (4).

## DIETARY FACTORS AND COLON CANCER

Cancer of the large bowel has been the subject of several epidemiologic reviews (14,27,153,156,162,169) and the major differences of intercountry and intracountry distribution of this cancer have been detailed in recent publications (27, 153,156). The highest incidence rates are found in North America, New Zealand, and western Europe, with the exception of Finland. Intermediate rates are found in eastern Europe, and the lowest incidences are found in Africa, Asia, and Latin America (the exceptions being Uruguay and Argentina, where the mortality rates are similar to those found in North America).

Studies have shown that diets particularly high in total fat and low in certain fibers are associated with an increased incidence of large bowel cancer in man. Secondary modifiers, such as micronutrients, selenium salt, vitamin E, or vitamin A, require more research to determine whether they play a role in the etiology of colon cancer. Results of these studies include the following: (a) Logical reasoning suggests that tumorigenic compounds are contained in the colonic contents. These contents are affected by dietary patterns. (b) Epidemiologic studies have compared dietary patterns and colon cancer incidence in various parts of the world (5,15,169). Comparison of dietary patterns among U.S. (high-risk) and Japanese (low-risk) populations indicate that about 40% of the total caloric intake in the United States is from fat, whereas the Japanese derive only about 10% to 20% of their caloric intake from fat (168). (c) Migrant studies have demonstrated that migrants from low-risk to high-risk countries increase their risk for colon cancer as they accept the dietary habits of their new homeland (54,55). (d) Examination of many factors has indicated that industrialization appears to be unassociated with disease risk. For example, highly industrialized Japan has a low risk for colon cancer, but relatively rural Denmark and rural Nebraska have a high risk. (e) Time trends of colon cancer incidence in various populations have demonstrated an increased incidence of colon cancer consistent with the increase of total fat intake by a given population. (f) Population studies in Copenhagen, the metropolitan New York area, and rural Finland indicated that dietary fiber might be an important protective factor in colon cancer (77, 118). (g) Studies of specific populations within a given country, such as Seventh-Day Adventists, show that different dietary habits lead to different colon cancer rates (113). (h) A recent case-control study among U.S. blacks indicated that significantly more colon cancer patients than controls reported a high saturated fat, low-fiber eating pattern, as opposed to a low saturated fat, high-fiber diet (29).

Among the current concepts of the etiology of colon cancer is the hypothesis that bile acids of the lumen of the large bowel help to modify large bowel carcinogenesis, and that these compounds, directly or indirectly, are derived from dietary factors and are subsequently modified by the gut bacteria (66,123). The carcinogens for colon cancer may be related to the mode of cooking, particularly to frying and broiling (157). The extent of the carcinogenic stress thus produced is probably rather weak. For that reason, whether a given individual is at high risk for colon cancer may depend more on the important promoting stimulus for bile acids, which are themselves dependent on the amount of fat.

It has been postulated that the protective effect of dietary fiber may be due to adsorption, dilution, and/or metabolism of co-carcinogens, promoters, and as yet unidentified carcinogens, by the components of the fiber. There is evidence that the different types of nonnutritive fibers possess specific binding properties (140). Dietary fiber could also affect the enterohepatic circulation of bile salts (84). Fiber not only influences bile acid metabolism, thereby reducing the formation of potential tumor-promoters in colon carcinogenesis, but also exerts a solvent-like action, in that it dilutes potential carcinogens and/or co-carcinogens by its bulking effect and ability to bind water, sterols, bile acids, and fat.

## Metabolic Epidemiology

Investigations in man have been carried out in several laboratories to determine whether there are differences in fecal constituents between high-risk and low-risk populations for colon cancer, and whether changes in the diet can alter the concentration of fecal bile acids and the activity of fecal microflora.

A number of laboratory studies have provided insight into the mechanisms by which dietary fat and cholesterol become associated with high risk (66, 122,124). Examination of the components of stool as products of cholesterol and fat in the diet show that some persons in the United States and Great Britain excrete greater amounts of total bile acids and secondary bile acids than do Japanese, American Seventh-Day Adventists, or American vegetarians who eat low-fat diets. Similar findings were made when groups of volunteers were switched from an HF Western diet to an LF vegetarian-type diet (122). Patients with colon cancer had higher levels of fecal bile acids than did normal controls (123). Consideration of all these data indicate that a high-risk individual has higher levels of neutral sterols and bile acids than does a low-risk individual (124).

Finland is an interesting country in the geographic pathology of colon cancer. In virtually all other parts of the world, there is a direct parallel between the incidence of coronary heart disease and that of colon cancer. The Finnish, however, differ in having a very high risk for heart disease but a low risk for colon cancer. Investigations by two independent groups indicated that the rural Finnish consumed the same amount of total fat as did the Danish and New Yorkers, who are a high risk for colon cancer (77,118). This nutritional habit may account for the equally high risk for heart disease in all three countries.

On the other hand, the rural Finnish also consume a greater amount of total dietary fiber, mostly as whole wheat and rye bread, as compared to the Danish or metropolitan New Yorkers. The stool bulk per day of the Finnish approached three times that of New Yorkers; thus, the concentrations of luminal bile acids were three times lower, although the total amount excreted in the stool per day was identical (Fig. 10). The classic studies in experimental carcinogenesis demonstrate that promoters must be present in large amounts for a long time. The colonic mucosa of the Finnish population is obviously exposed to smaller concentrations, which, from the pharmacokinetic standpoint, would mean a less effective dosage at the point of action.

### Studies in Animal Models

Research on the mechanisms of cancer causation in the large bowel has been assisted by the discovery over the last 20 years of several animal models that induce the type of lesions seen in man (11), for example, large bowel cancer induced in rats and mice through the use of 1,2-dimethylhydrazine (DMH), azoxymethane (AOM), methylazoxymethanol (MAM) acetate, 3,2'-dimethyl-

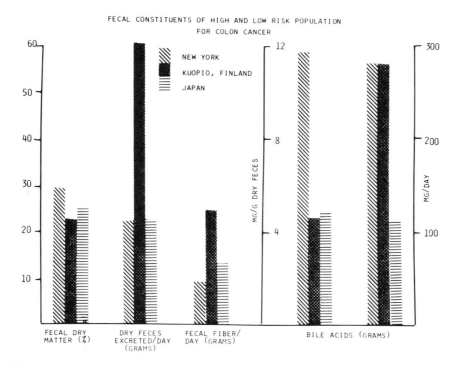

**FIG. 10.** Fecal constituents of high- and low-risk populations for colon cancer. Adapted from Reddy et al., ref. 118.

4-aminobiphenyl (DMAB), and methylnitrosourea (MNU). We, and subsequently a number of other investigators, have clearly shown, in reliable animal models for colon cancer, that animals on the HF diet had a higher incidence of DMH-, AOM-, MAM acetate-, or MNU-induced colon cancer, a higher multiplicity of adenomas and carcinomas, and occasionally, depending on the specific protocol, a shift from adenoma to carcinoma (110,121). Several lines of evidence, including our studies in conventional animals, show that dietary fat stimulates production of bile acid levels proportional to the fat levels (119). With few exceptions, at high dietary fat levels corresponding to levels consumed by man in high-risk countries, whether the fat was saturated (tallow, lard) or unsaturated (corn oil) appeared to be unimportant (120).

It was further demonstrated that the effect of high fat as a promoting stimulus was associated with the increase in bile acids (123). Nigro et al. (108) and Asano et al. (6) observed that an increase in bile salts in the colon of rats, induced by feeding cholestyramine, enhanced colon tumor formation.

The relationship between dietary fiber consumption and colon cancer has also been studied in animal models. Sprague–Dawley rats fed a diet containing 20% corn oil or beef fat and 20% wheat bran had fewer DMH-induced colon tumors than did those on the control diet containing 20% fat and no bran (161). No differences in the incidence of colon cancer were found between rats fed corn oil and those fed beef fat. Recently, Freeman et al. (49) compared DMH-induced colon tumor incidence in Sprague–Dawley rats fed either a fiber-free diet or a 4.5% purified cellulose diet. Cellulose ingestion was associated with fewer animals developing colonic neoplasia, as well as with a reduction in the total number of colon tumors.

In another study, Cruse et al. (28) reported that a diet containing 20% wheat bran had no effect on DMH-induced colon carcinogenesis in rats; however, the DMH dose levels in this experiment were so high that any protective effect of bran might not have been observable. One important concern in a study of the effect of diet on chemical carcinogenesis is to avoid too high a level of carcinogen for a prolonged period of time, as this may obscure more subtle changes induced by certain dietary modifications. In fact, the data presented by Cruse et al. (28) suggest that a high-fiber diet reduces the number of DMH-induced early deaths in rats.

The effect of dietary alfalfa, pectin, and wheat bran at 15% levels on AOM-induced colon carcinogenesis was studied in F344 rats by Watanabe et al. (152). Such carcinogenesis was lower in rats fed pectin or wheat bran diets than in rats fed the control or alfalfa diet. The effect of alfalfa, wheat bran, and cellulose on AOM-induced intestinal tumor incidence was further studied in Sprague–Dawley rats fed diets containing 10% fiber and 30% beef fat, or 20% or 30% fiber and about 6% beef fat (109). The addition of 10% fiber to an HF diet did not reduce tumor frequency. Apparently, the challenge of AOM with the high dietary fat was too great to be affected by the dietary fiber. The addition of 20% bran or cellulose, or 30% of any fiber to the 6% fat diet, significantly reduced tumor frequency. All dietary groups, except the 20% alfalfa group, showed a reduction in frequency of tumors in the proximal half of the large bowel, as compared to the fiber-free groups. The concentration, but not the total daily excretion, of fecal steroids was significantly lowered in the groups with reduced tumor frequencies.

These results indicate that the protective effect of dietary fiber in colon carcinogenesis depends on the source of fiber. The inhibition of tumor formation by certain dietary fibers may be caused by the dilution of promoters in the lumen of the large intestine by the additional bulk. The protective effect of various fibers also depends on their capacity to bind bile acids in the intestinal tract, their effect on colonic mucosa, and their indirect effect on the metabolism of carcinogens. Although additional studies will be required to elucidate the protective effects of various fibers in colon carcinogenesis, the human data and animal experiments suggest that increased intake of cereal fibers would, at least in part, reduce the risk for large bowel cancer.

Current concepts in the etiology of cancer suggest that promotion is highly dose-dependent and is also a reversible phenomenon. Thus, lowering of the concentration of bile acids by decreasing dietary fat and cholesterol and increasing dietary fibers would be almost immediately beneficial in reducing the risk of colon cancer development. This is true not only of the general public but particularly of individuals with demonstrated risk of colon cancer, such as patients who have undergone successful surgical intervention but who often have a high risk of recurrence.

Additional research is needed into the involvement of micronutrients, such as vitamin C, vitamin E plus selenium, and vitamin A, as well as their analogues, in the carcinogenic process. Certain of these elements can be envisioned to affect the production of bile acids, and thus play a direct role in promotion. Other mechanisms may involve the metabolism of putative colon carcinogens. Still other mechanisms may influence the maintenance of differentiation of colonic cells, exerting a protective effect through such action.

Current research attempts to account for the virtually unchanged mortality rate of colon cancer during the last 50 years by demonstrating that the dietary conditions leading to this disease have also remained virtually unchanged. This includes research on the carcinogens that may possibly contribute to colon cancer risk. It is postulated that such carcinogens can be produced by frying food, particularly meat. It has been shown that frying meat yields mutagens which are as yet unidentified and whose association with colon cancer remains to be demonstrated. That this lead may be a useful indicator is already apparent from the fact that vegetarian populations have a lower risk of colon cancer, although such populations usually also have lower fat and higher fiber intakes. Indeed, if frying meat can be associated with the carcinogenic process for colon cancer, it may be possible to develop inhibitors of the formation of such mutagens/carcinogens as an effective means of preventing this form of cancer, which is so prevalent in the Western world.

## POSSIBLE ORIGINS OF CARCINOGENS FOR COLON, BREAST, AND PROSTATE CANCER

Research into the etiology of colon, breast, and prostate cancers has identified several risk factors that act in concert rather than independently. These factors include the level of dietary fat and the daily intake of cholesterol, both of which control the effective total flow of bile acids through the gut. Independently, it has been demonstrated in animal models that total bile acids, and probably specific bile acids but not neutral sterols, promote large bowel cancer development. One role of fiber is considered to be its effect on the concentration of bile acids in the gut through an alteration of stool bulk. This concentration of bile acids is the key parameter in enhancement of the development of colon cancer.

The above processes all have to do with promotion of an initiated tumor cell. The question arises as to the nature of the carcinogens involved in initiation of colon tumor cells. Considering the lack of correlation between the occurrence of colon cancer in man and local industrial (especially chemical) activities, another source must be sought. Until recently, industrial Japan had a low incidence of colon cancer, but rural Nebraska and Texas, as well as urban Geneva, Switzerland, Scotland, and New Zealand, had high incidences.

An important clue to the nature of colon carcinogens came from the demonstration that charcoal broiling of meat or fish yielded mutagenic activity for *Salmonella typhimurium* TA98 (26,137,141). This required activation with a postmitochondrial fraction from induced rat liver, which suggested that the activity might relate to materials such as arylamines or certain polycyclic aromatic hydrocarbons, but not alkylnitrosamines.

A key finding in a model experiment was that a product from the pyrolysis of tryptophan was y-carboline derivative, an o-methylarylamine type of compound (11,141). Some arylamines induce liver or urinary bladder cancer in rodent models, but the corresponding o-methylarylamines often cause colon cancer in male rats and breast and colon cancer in female rats (11,154,158).

Typical, realistic conditions are used to study the development of mutagenic activity as a function of mode and temperature of cooking (137). When ground meat is placed in a preheated frying pan, the temperature curve shows a plateau at 100°C, while the water is boiled off and initial browning occurs. During that period, virtually no mutagenic activity is seen. Subsequently, the temperature rises and mutagenic activity develops. Appreciable mutagenic activity is seen upon frying to a degree such that the product is perfectly edible (112). The temperature curve in broiling in an electric oven has a somewhat different shape, since the heat output is mainly in the form of infrared radiation. Under these conditions, mutagenic activity does not develop for about 15 to 20 min, when the temperature of the meat begins to rise above 100°C and mutagenic activity develops (Figs. 11 and 12).

The structure of the mutagens to be outlined may not stem from the pyrolysis

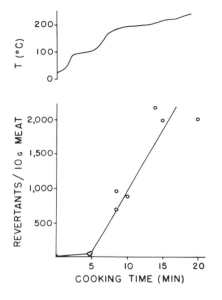

**FIG. 11.** Mutagenic activity on TA 98 with S-9 mix of the basic organic extract of fried beef patties. The ordinate shows nonspontaneous His+ revertants per initial 10 g of meat. Each point is calculated from the slope of the linear portion of a dose–response curve. Temperature was recorded at the surface of the patty and frying pan. Average beef patty weight was 92 ± 3 g. Adapted from Spingarn and Weisburger, ref. 137.

of amino acids or peptides, but rather from the formation of heterocyclic compounds from starches and amino acids. Indeed, it was shown by Spingarn and Garvie (136) that, when several kinds of simple sugars were refluxed with ammonium ions, mutagenic activity was obtained with mobilities, on high-pressure liquid chromatography systems, similar to those mutagens obtained from an

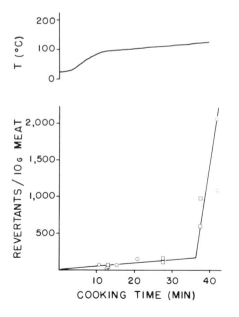

**FIG. 12.** Mutagenic activity on TA 98 with S-9 mix of the basic organic extract of charcoal broiled (□) or electrically broiled (o) beef patties. The ordinate is as described in Fig. 11. The temperature was recorded at the surface of the patty nearest the heat source. Adapted from Spingarn and Weisburger, ref. 137.

extract of fried meat, but different from the $\gamma$-carbolines (81) (N. E. Spingarn et al., *unpublished data*). Thus, the reactions are akin to those that take place during the browning reactions.

Current research is concerned with the isolation, identification, and bioassay of active mutagenic principles as a function of the mode of cooking.

## DIETARY FACTORS AND STOMACH CANCER

In the early part of the century, gastric cancer was one of the more common neoplastic diseases in the United States, but its incidence and mortality have since decreased considerably. In other parts of the world, such as Japan, the mountainous, interior regions of central and western Latin America, northern and eastern Europe, and Iceland, gastric cancer remains one of the most common types of cancer. Even in some of these areas, a decreased incidence has begun to be noted (72,78,168). This disease exhibits a north–south gradient (or south–north in the southern hemisphere), with greater incidence in more temperate or frigid zones. The risk factors for diffuse gastric cancer may be different (blood group A [56,103,104,105] and pernicious anemia and suspected associated elements) and are not considered here.

The problem of precise causative factors for cancer of the glandular stomach has been a topic of intense interest for decades (3,9,34,45,48,59,64,75,89, 114,144,155,172,174). Epidemiologic and migrant studies have demonstrated that habitual intake of specific dietary factors is associated with a high risk for gastric cancer. The intake of dried and salted fish or pickled or smoked foods also seems to be important. Also relevant are local customs and food availability, which result in a variable intake of fresh fruits and vegetables. Typically, there is a low consumption of such foods during winter and spring. Furthermore, the prevailing geochemistry may involve high levels of soil nitrate and, thus, foods and water rich in nitrate.

The reliable animal model for glandular gastric cancer, discovered by Sugimura, involves the oral administration of alkylnitrosourea compounds (89). There are antecedent lesions (intestinalization, hypoacidity, etc.) comparable to those in man with stomach cancer. We have proposed that such an alkylnitrosourea compound may also be the type of chemical responsible for stomach cancer in man (155). Sander (130) found that certain substrates could be nitrosated to carcinogenic nitrosamines and nitrosamides in the stomach, and also, we believe, during pickling in the presence of weak acids, such as acetic (vinegar) or lactic acid. Sources of the required nitrite might be (a) the reduction of nitrate in foods stored at room temperature after cooking, (b) the consumption of pickled or smoked foods, and (c) the reduction of nitrate (secreted by the salivary glands) by oral microbiologic flora (101,135,146). Mirvish et al. (100) observed that vitamin C could inhibit these nitrosation reactions. This interaction has been used to minimize the presence of nitrosamines and nitrosamides in the environment, and more so in foods (151).

We have studied the relationship between high levels of nitrite from various sources, including pickling as a potentiating element, and vitamin C as a protective and inhibitory element in gastric cancer (116). It is germane to note that vitamin E also can inhibit nitrosation reactions, perhaps through somewhat different mechanisms than those operating for vitamin C (80,98). Vitamin C is water-soluble and vitamin E lipid-soluble, and since some of the substrates nitrosated are lipid-soluble, vitamin E as an inhibitor may complement and extend the effect of vitamin C.

In our study, Sanma hiraki, a fish commonly eaten in a Japanese region at high risk for gastric cancer, was used as an experimental model. Homogenates of this fish treated with nitrite at pH 3 yielded direct-acting mutagens for *typhimurium* TA-1535 bioassay. The formation of these mutagens could be inhibited by vitamin C (90). This behavior is analogous to that found for the inhibition of the formation of nitrosamines and nitrosamides, noted above. Thus, there is support for the concept that the mutagens from nitrite-treated fish may have a nitrosamide type of functional group.

Sanma, aji, and iwashi fish yielded more mutagenic activity than did other types of fish or other foods. In the context of current practices of meat preservation with amounts of about 100 ppm nitrite, it is important to note that several types of meat failed to produce such direct-acting mutagens when treated with as much as 5,000 ppm nitrite (90).

Not all mutagens in *typhimurium* are carcinogenic (93), but we have demonstrated that the mutagenic activity created by the reaction of nitrite and Sanma hiraki fish was actually carcinogenic, and led to the production of glandular stomach cancer in rats. Since formation of the mutagens can be blocked by vitamin C, the conclusion is justified that the induction of glandular stomach cancer could also be inhibited by vitamin C.

The reader can find a detailed description elsewhere (155), but basically, nitrite-treated extracts of Sanma hiraki fish were fed to an experimental group of rats in amounts equivalent to a weekly oral dose of N-methyl-N'-nitro-N-nitrosoguanidine, used to induce adenocarcinomas of the glandular stomach in rats (89). A control group of the same rats received fish extracts without nitrite. Incidence and types of neoplastic changes in each group are given in Tables 5 and 6. For the first time, it was demonstrated that reaction of fish with nitrite at pH 3 yielded not only an extract with mutagenic activity, but one that induced cancer in the glandular stomach. The experimental design mimicked the conditions of migrants living in a high-risk region in the early part of their lives and spending the rest of their lives in a low-risk region. These rats received the extract with mutagenic activity for only six months and were then held on a control diet without further exposure to known carcinogens. Had the treatment been more prolonged, as would be the case for a model in a high-risk region, the cancer incidence might have been higher.

The nature of the mutagens responsible for carcinogenesis is not known and is being investigated. Because the formation of the mutagens was inhibited by

TABLE 5. *Incidence of stomach epithelium hyperplasia and intestinal metaplasia* [a]

| Group and treatment | Effective no. of rats | Forestomach Squamous cell hyperplasia | Glandular Stomach | |
|---|---|---|---|---|
| | | | Glandular hyperplasia | Intestinal metaplasia |
| I Fish Extract Alone | 8 | 0 | 1 [b] | 1 |
| II Fish Extract + NaNO₂ | 12 | 5 [c] | 6 [d] | 6 [e] |

[a] From Weisburger et al., ref. 155, with permission
[b] One rat had both lesions.
[c] One rat had only forestomach hyperplasia; three also had glandular hyperplasia; and one had intestinal metaplasia.
[d] One rat had only glandular hyperplasia; three also had forestomach hyperplasia; and two had intestinal metaplasia.
[e] One rat had only intestinal metaplasia; one also had only forestomach hyperplasia; two also had only glandular hyperplasia; and two had all three lesions.

vitamin C, and, like alklynitrosourea compounds, it led to glandular stomach cancer, it seems clear we are dealing with this kind of compound. In contrast to methylnitrosourea, the mutagenic activity was rather stable at pH 3 and even at higher pH values. Dilution studies with labeled methylnitrosourea showed that the mutagen is different from this compound (J. H. Weisburger, H. Marquardt, and H. F. Mower, *unpublished observations*). Nonetheless, the formation of methylnitrosourea can be blocked by vitamin C (Table 7). In this respect, the unknown mutagens and the model compound methylnitrosourea are similar.

Studies in migrants who maintained their risk for gastric cancer, when moving from a region of high risk to one of low risk, clearly demonstrated that the nature of the carcinogens operating in man are probably quite similar to what we have identified through mutagen and carcinogen bioassays. Exposure to such compounds throughout life is not required to eventually produce stomach cancer; in fact, the protocols used in this test series were designed to mimic a move from a high-risk to a low-risk situation. Thus, it seems logical to conclude that, if gastric cancer were to be prevented, exposure to agents causing this disease must be minimized or avoided from infancy onward. This means, in turn, that foods providing the necessary vitamin C, or supplementary vitamin C, should be consumed with every meal from childhood onward.

Evidence to support this concept is apparent in the case of the United States, where gastric cancer has decreased sharply for reasons unclear until now. Our approach may provide the necessary explanation. The decline may be caused by the fact that because of better distribution of food by rail, truck, and air transport during the past 50 to 75 years, fresh food sources of vitamin C have become increasingly available at an affordable cost on a year-round basis everywhere in the United States and Canada. Gastric cancer is rare in southern

TABLE 6. Sites and incidence of tumors in rats given extract of fish treated with nitrite or fish alone.[a]

| Group and treatment | Effective no. of rats | Forestomach | | Glandular Stomach | | | Pancreas | | Small intestine Adenocarcinoma |
|---|---|---|---|---|---|---|---|---|---|
| | | Papilloma | Squamous cell carcinoma | Adenoma | Adeno-carcinoma | Adeno-squamous carcinoma | Adenoma | Adeno-carcinoma | |
| I Fish extract alone | 8[b] | 0 | 0 | 0 | 0 | 0 | 0 | 0 | 0 |
| II Fish extract + NaNO₂ | 12[c] | 0 | 2[d] | 2[e] | 2[f] | 1[g] | 2 | 1 | 1[g] |

[a] From Weisburger et al., ref. 155, with permission.
[b] Three rats had interstitial cell adenoma of testis; one, renal nephroblastoma; and one, rhabdomyosarcoma.
[c] Eight rats had at least one of the tumors tabulated here. In addition, miscellaneous tumors included: one rat had cortical adenoma of adrenal gland; one, follicular adenoma of thyroid gland; and one, pulmonary adenoma.
[d] One of these rats also had a pancreatic adenoma and the other an adenocarcinoma.
[e] One rat had only an adenoma, while the other also had an adenocarcinoma.
[f] One rat also had an adenocortical adenoma and the other a gastric adenoma and a thyroid adenoma.
[g] The only tumor in one rat.

TABLE 7. *Effect of ascorbic acid on the formation of methylnitrosourea in potato incubated at pH 1.5[a,b]*

| 1 μCi Methyl-[14]C-Urea (100 ppm Methylurea) | Nitrite (100 ppm) | [Ascorbate] : [Nitrite] | Methylnitrosurea Formed[c] ±S.E. (ppm) | % Inhibition |
|---|---|---|---|---|
| + | − | − | 0.0 ± 0.0 | — |
| + | + | 0 | 19 ± 1.1 | 0 |
| + | + | 1 | 12 ± 0.8 | 37 |
| + | + | 2 | 5.0 ± 0.4 | 74 |
| + | + | 4 | 1.4 ± 0.2 | 93 |

[a] From Raineri et al., ref. 116, with permission.
[b] Five-gram samples of homogenized boiled potato (adjusted to pH 1.5) were incubated in triplicate at 37° for 10 minutes.
[c] Recovery of methylnitrosourea was 35%.

regions of the United States and in other countries where there are few seasonal variations in the availability of such vitamin C-containing foods.

In the light of the material presented here, it appears that gastric cancer is a preventable disease in areas of the world where it is still at a high level. It would be appropriate to ensure that foods containing an adequate and optimal amount of vitamin C, and perhaps vitamin E, be served with every meal.

Specific risk factors have been associated with those types of cancer discussed in this chapter, namely, cancers of the oral cavity and esophagus, stomach, colon, breast, prostate, and endometrium (Table 8). It appears that we are dealing with three quite different areas. Head and neck cancers are usually seen in people who smoke and drink heavily, and the nutritional involvement in this instance derives from the malnutrition associated with high intake of alcoholic beverages. The second type of risk factor is that associated with gastric cancer (and perhaps, in former years, with primary liver cancer, through slightly altered mechanisms), namely, the intake of foods containing vitamins C and E. The third overall scheme relates to cancers of the colon, breast, prostate, and perhaps of the ovary and endometrium, where a key element is the total

TABLE 8. *Conceptual outline of the involvement of nutritional factors in certain human cancers*

| Carcinogens in | Modifiers | Organs Affected | Preventive Measures |
|---|---|---|---|
| Tobacco smoke | Alcohol | Oral cavity, Esophagus | Less smoking and drinking Vitamins (?) |
| Nitrite + specific foods (fish, beans, *not* meats) | Salt | Stomach | Regular intake of foods with vitamin C, vitamin E; lower intake of pickled and salted foods |
| Fried foods | Fat | Colon, Breast, Prostate, Pancreas | Increase cereal fiber; lower fat and fried food intake; vitamins (?) |

daily intake of dietary fat, which is a measure of risk for which the underlying mechanisms have been partially documented. For example, in colon cancer, dietary fat increases cholesterol biosynthesis, leading to higher levels of bile acids in the gut, which exert a promoting action. Fiber from grains has an inhibiting effect, in part as the result of lowering the concentration of bile acids in the gut through increased stool bulk. For the endocrine-sensitive tissues, fat appears to control endocrine balances, but the precise balances characteristic of high-risk populations have not yet been fully delineated. In any case, for each of these diseases, the role of dietary fat and cholesterol appears to be provision of a promoting stimulus for the development of the disease.

Current active research is concerned with a fourth area, the question of the relevant carcinogens thought to stem from the mode of cooking, and, in particular, from frying foods, especially fish or meats. There is laboratory evidence to support this premise. There are also studies in humans demonstrating that vegetarians usually have a considerably lower risk for all of these diseases as compared to nonvegetarians. Experimentation in this area is concerned with the validation of these concepts and the provision of harmless inhibitors to the formation of such carcinogens during the frying of foods. It is hoped that additional research in the next few years will provide sound, reliable bases for actually reducing the risk for these cancers through prevention.

## ACKNOWLEDGMENTS

The research reported here was supported in part by Contracts CP-33208, CP-65818, CP-85659, and CP-95604, and Grants CA-17613, CA-12376, and CA-16382, awarded by the National Cancer Institute, and by National Cancer Institute Grants CA-15400 and CA-24217 through the National Large Bowel Cancer Project.

We wish to thank Mrs. Clara Horn for coordination, editorial assistance, and preparation of the manuscript.

## REFERENCES

1. Akazaki, K. (1973): Comparative histological studies on the latent carcinoma of the prostate under different environmental circumstances. In: *Host Environment Interactions in the Etiology of Cancer in Man*, edited by R. Doll and I. Vodopija, pp. 89–98. International Agency for Research on Cancer, Lyon, France.
2. American Cancer Society (1978): *1979 Cancer Facts and Figures.* American Cancer Society, New York.
3. Armijo, R., and Coulson, A. H. (1975): Epidemiology of stomach cancer in Chile: The role of nitrogen fertilizers. *Int. J. Epidemiol.,* 4:301–309.
4. Armstrong, B. K. (1979): Diet and hormones in the epidemiology of breast and endometrial cancers. *Nutr. Cancer,* 1:90–95.
5. Armstrong, B., and Doll, R. (1975): Environmental factors and cancer incidence and mortality in different countries, with special reference to dietary factors. *Int. J. Cancer,* 15:617–631.
6. Asano, T., Pollard, M., and Madsen, D. C. (1975): Effects of cholestyramine on DMH-induced enteric carcinoma in germfree rats. *Proc. Soc. Exp. Biol. Med.,* 150:780–785.
7. Barnetson, J. (1954): L'epitheliome latent de la prostate. *Semaine des Hospitaux,* 30:129–132

8. Benson, T., Lev, M., and Grand, C. G. (1956): The enhancement of mammary fibroadenomas in the female rat by a high-fat diet. *Cancer Res.,* 16:135–137.
9. Bjelke, E. (1974): Epidemiologic studies of cancers of the stomach, colon, and rectum, with special emphasis on the role of diet. *Scand. J. Gastroenterol.,* 9 (Suppl. 31):1–235.
10. Blair, A., and Fraumeni, J. F. (1978): Geographic patterns of prostatic cancer in the United States. *J. Natl. Cancer Inst.,* 61:1379–1384.
11. Bralow, S. P., and Weisburger, J. H. (1976): Experimental carcinogenesis. *Clin. Gastroenterol.,* 5:527–542.
12. Breslow, N., Chan, C. W., Dhom, G., Drury, R. A. B., Franks, L. M., Gellei, B., Lee, Y. S., Lundberg, L., Sparke, B., Sternby, N. H., and Tulinius, H. (1977): Latent carcinoma of prostate at autopsy in seven areas. *Int. J. Cancer,* 20:680–688.
13. Buell, P. (1973): Changing incidence of breast cancer in Japanese-American women. *J. Natl. Cancer Inst.,* 51:1479–1483.
14. Burkitt, D. P. (1971): Epidemiology of cancer of the colon and rectum. *Cancer,* 26:3–13.
15. Burkitt, D. P. (1975): Large bowel carcinogenesis: An epidemiologic jigsaw puzzle. *J. Natl. Cancer Inst.,* 54:3–6.
16. Carroll, K. K. (1975): Experimental evidence of dietary factors and hormone-dependent cancers. *Cancer Res.,* 35:3374–3383.
17. Carroll, K. K., and Khor, H. T. (1971): Effects of level and type of dietary fat on incidence of mammary tumors induced in female Sprague–Dawley rats by 7,12-dimethylbenz(a)anthracene. *Lipids,* 6:415–420.
18. Chan, P. C., and Cohen, L. A. (1974): Effect of dietary fat, antiestrogen and antiprolactin on the development of mammary tumors in rats. *J. Natl. Cancer Inst.,* 52:25–30.
19. Chan, P. C., and Cohen, L. A. (1975): Dietary fat and growth promotion of rat and mammary tumors. *Cancer Res.,* 35:3384–3386.
20. Chan, P. C., Didato, F., and Cohen, L. A. (1975): High dietary fat, elevation of rat serum prolactin and mammary cancer. *Proc. Soc. Exp. Biol. Med.,* 149:133–135.
21. Chan, P. C., Head, J. F., Cohen, L. A., and Wynder, E. L. (1977): Influence of dietary fat on the induction of rat mammary tumors by N-nitrosomethylurea: Associated hormone changes and differences between Sprague–Dawley and F344 rats. *J. Natl. Cancer Inst.,* 59:1279–1283.
22. Chan, P. C., Okamoto, T., and Wynder, E. L. (1972): Possible role of riboflavin deficiency in epithelial neoplasia: III. Induction of aryl carbon hydroxylase. *J. Natl. Cancer Inst.,* 48:1341–1345.
23. Chan, P. C., Tsuang, J., Head, J., and Cohen, L. A. (1976): Effects of estradiol and prolactin on growth of rat mammary adenocarcinoma cells in monolayer cultures (39210). *Proc. Soc. Exp. Biol. Med.,* 151:362–365.
24. Cohen, L. A. (1979): The influence of dietary fat on plasma and pituitary prolactin in male rats. 61st Annual Meeting of the Endocrine Society, Anaheim, Cal, p. 291.
25. Cohen, L. A., Chan, P. C., and Wynder, E. L. (1981): A high fat diet enhances the development of mammary tumors in ovariectomized rats. *Cancer* (in press).
26. Commoner, B., Vithayathil, A. J., Dolara, P., Nair, S., Madyastha, P., and Cuca, G. C. (1978): Formation of mutagens in beef and beef extract during cooking. *Science* 201:913–916.
27. Correa, P., and Haenszel, W. (1978): The epidemiology of large-bowel cancer. *Adv. Cancer Res.,* 26:1–141.
28. Cruse, J. P., Lewin, M. R., and Clark, C. G. (1978): Failure of bran to protect against experimental colon cancer in rats. *Lancet,* 2:1278–1280.
29. Dales, L. G., Friedman, G. D., Wry, H. K., Grossman, S., and Williams, S. R. (1979): A case control study of relationships of diet and other traits to colorectal cancer in American blacks. *Am. J. Epidemiol.,* 109:132–144.
30. Dao, T. L. (1969): Studies on mechanism of carcinogenesis in the mammary gland. *Prog. Exp. Tumor Res.,* 11:235–261.
31. DeLint, J. (1974): The prevention of alcoholism. *Prev. Med.,* 3:24–35.
32. DeLuca, L., Little, E. P., and Wolf, G. (1969): Vitamin A and protein synthesis by rat intestinal mucosa. *J. Biol. Chem.,* 244:701–708.
33. Department of Health, Education and Welfare (1974): *Second Special Report to the U.S. Congress on Health: New Knowledge from the Secretary of Health, Education, and Welfare,* pp. 74–124. U.S. Government Printing Office, Washington, D.C.

34. Devesa, S. S., and Silverman, D. T. (1978): Cancer incidence and mortality trends in the United States: 1935–1974. *J. Natl. Cancer Inst.*, 60:545–571.
35. Doerr, P., and Pirke, K. M. (1974): Regulation of plasma estrogens in normal adult males, I. *Acta Endocrinol.*, 75:617–624.
36. Doerr, P., and Pirke, K. M. (1975): Regulation of plasma estrogens in adult males, II. *Acta Endocrinol.*, 78:531–538.
37. Doll, R., Muir, C., and Waterhouse, J., editors (1970): *Cancer Incidence in Five Continents, Vol. II.* International Union Against Cancer, Geneva.
38. Dontenwill, W., Chevalier, H. J., Harke, H. P., LaFrenz, U., Reckzeh, G., and Schneider, B. (1973): Investigations on the effect of chronic cigarette smoke inhalation on Syrian golden hamsters. *J. Natl. Cancer Inst.*, 51:1781–1832.
39. Drasar, B. A., and Irving, D. (1973): Environmental factors and cancer of the colon and breast. *Br. J. Cancer*, 27:167–172.
40. Dunning, W. F., Curtis, M. R., and Maun, M. E. (1949): The effect of dietary fat and carbohydrate on diethylstilbestrol-induced mammary cancer in rats. *Cancer Res.*, 9:354–361.
41. Editorial (1975): The effect of prolactin on lipoprotein lipase activity. *Nutr. Rev.*, 33:341–343.
42. Edman, D. C., Aiman, E. J., Porter, J. C., and Macdonald, P. C. (1978): Identification of the estrogen product of extraglandular aromatization of plasma androstenedione. *Am. J. Obstet. Gynecol.*, 130:439–447.
43. Engel, R. W., and Copeland, D. H. (1951): Influence of diet on the relative incidence of eye, mammary, ear-duct, and liver tumors in rats fed 2-acetylaminofluorene. *Cancer. Res.*, 11:180–183.
44. Enig, M. G., Munn, R. J., and Keeney, M. (1978): Dietary fat and cancer trends: A critique. *Fed. Proc.*, 37:2215–2220.
45. Farber, E., Kawachi, T., Nagayo, T., Sugano, H., Sugano, T., Sugimura, T., and Weisburger, J., editors (1976): *Pathophysiology of Carcinogenesis in Digestive Organs.* University of Tokyo Press, Tokyo, Japan, and University Park Press, Baltimore, Maryland.
46. Fergusson, J. O. (1972): The basis of endocrine therapy. In: *Endocrine Therapy in Malignant Disease*, edited by B. A. Stoll, pp. 237–246. W. B. Saunders, London.
47. Fraser, W. M., and Blackard, W. G. (1977): The effect of lipids on prolactin and growth hormone secretion. *Horm. Metab. Res.*, 9:347–350.
48. Fraumeni, J. F., Jr., editor (1975): *Persons at High Risk of Cancer.* Academic Press, New York.
49. Freeman, H. J., Spiller, G. A., and Kim, Y. S. (1978): A double-blind study on the effect of purified cellulose dietary fiber on 1,2-dimethylhydrazine-induced rat colonic neoplasm. *Cancer Res.*, 38:2912–2917.
50. Gammal, E. B., Carroll, K. K., and Plunkett, E. R. (1967): Effects of dietary fat on mammary carcinogenesis by 7,12-dimethylbenz(a)anthracene in rats. *Cancer Res.*, 27:1737–1742.
51. Gerson, S. J., and Meyer, J. (1977): Increased lactate dehydrogenase activity in buccal epithelium of zinc-deficient rats. *J. Nutr.*, 107:724–729.
52. Gray, G. E., Pike, M. C., and Henderson, B. E. (1979): Breast cancer incidence and mortality rates in different countries in relation to known risk factors and dietary practices. *Br. J. Cancer*, 39:1–7.
53. Gullino, P. M., Pettigrew, H. M., and Grantham, P. H. (1975): N-nitrosomethylurea as mammary gland carcinogen in rats. *J. Natl. Cancer Inst.*, 54:401–414.
54. Haenszel, W. M., Berg, J. W., Segi, M., Kurihara, M., and Locke, F. L. (1973): Large bowel cancer in Hawaiian Japanese. *J. Natl. Cancer Inst.*, 51:1765–1779.
55. Haenszel, W., and Kurihara, M. (1968): Studies of Japanese migrants: I. Mortality from cancer and other diseases among Japanese in the United States. *J. Natl. Cancer Inst.*, 40:43–68.
56. Haenszel, W., Kurihara, M., Locke, F. B., Shimuzu, K., and Segi, M. (1976): Stomach cancer in Japan. *J. Natl. Cancer Inst.*, 56:265–274.
57. Hankin, J. H., and Rawlings, V. (1978): Diet and breast cancer: A review. *Am. J. Clin. Nutr.*, 31:2005–2016.
58. Harris, C. C., Sporn, M. B., Kaufman, D. G., Smith, J. M., Jackson, F. E., and Saffioti, U. (1972): Histogenesis of squamous metaplasia in the hamster tracheal epithelium caused by vitamin A deficiency or benzo(a)pyrene and ferric oxide. *J. Natl. Cancer Inst.*, 48:743–761.

59. Hayashi, N., Watanabe, K., Ishiwata, H., Mizushiro, H., Tanimura, A., and Kurata, H. (1978): Fate of nitrate and nitrite in saliva and blood of monkey administered orally sodium nitrate solution, and microflora of oral cavity of the monkey. *J. Food Hyg. Soc. Japan*, 19:392–400.
60. Hegsted, M. D. (1975): Relevance of animal studies to human disease. *Cancer Res.*, 35:3537–3539.
61. Hems, G. (1978): The contribution of diet and childbearing to breast cancer rates. *Br. J. Cancer*, 37:974–987.
62. Hendrixk, A., Heyns, S., and de Morr, P. (1968): Influence of a low calorie diet and fasting on the metabolism of dehydroepiandrosterone sulphate in adult obese subjects. *J. Clin. Endocrinol.*, 28:1525–1533.
63. Heuson, J. C., Waelbroeck, C., Legros, N., Gallez, G., Robyn, C., and L'Hermite, N. (1972): Inhibition of DMBA-induced mammary carcinogenesis in the rat by 2-Br-α-Ergocryptine (CB-154), an inhibitor of prolactin secretion, and by Nafoxidine (μ11,100A), an oestrogen antagonist. *Gynecol. Invest.*, 2:130.
64. Hiatt, H. H., Watson, J. D., Winsten, J. A., editors (1977): *Origins of Human Cancer*. Cold Spring Harbor Laboratory, Cold Spring Harbor, New York.
65. Hill, P., Chan, P. C., Cohen, L. A., Wynder, E. L., and Kuno, K. (1977): Diet and endocrine-related cancer. *Cancer*, 39:1890–1896.
66. Hill, M. J., Drasar, B. S., Aries, V., Crowther, J. S., Hawksworth, G. M., and Williams, R. E. O. (1971): Bacteria and etiology of cancer of large bowel. *Lancet*, I:95–100.
67. Hill, P., and Wynder, E. L. (1976): Diet and prolactin release. *Lancet*, II:806–807.
68. Hill, P., Wynder, E., Garbaczewski, L., Garnes, H., and Walker, A. R. P. (1979): Diet and urinary steroids in black and white North American men and black South African men. *Cancer Res.*, 39:5101–5105.
69. Hill, P., Garbaczewski, L., Helman, P., Huskisson, B., Sporangisa, E., and Wynder, E. L. (1980): Diet and menstrual activity. *Am. J. Clin. Nutr.*, 33:1192–1198.
70. Hirayama, T. (1975): Epidemiology of cancer of the stomach with special reference to its recent decrease in Japan. *Cancer Res.*, 35:3460–3468.
71. Hirayama, T. (1978): Epidemiology of breast cancer with special reference to the role of diet. *Prev. Med.*, 7:173–195.
72. Hirayama, T. (1979): Diet and cancer. *Nutr. Cancer* 1:67–81.
73. Hopkins, G. J., and Carroll, K. K. (1979): Relationship between amount and type of dietary fat in promotion of mammary carcinogenesis induced by 7,12-dimethylbenz(a)anthracene. *J. Natl. Cancer Inst.*, 63:1009–1012.
74. Hopkins, G. J., and West, C. E. (1976): Possible roles of dietary fats in carcinogenesis (minireview). *Life Sci.*, 19:1103–1116.
75. Hopps, H. C. (1978): Distribution of trace elements related to the occurrence of certain cancers, cardiovascular diseases, and urolithiasis. In: *Geochemistry and the Environment, Vol. III*, pp. 81–113. National Research Council, National Academy of Sciences, Washington, D.C.
76. Huggins, C., Grand, L. C., and Brillantes, F. P. (1961): Mammary cancer induced by a single feeding of polynuclear hydrocarbons, and its suppression. *Nature*, 189:204–207.
77. I.A.R.C. Intestinal Microecology Group (1977): Dietary fiber, transit time, fecal bacteria and steroids in two Scandinavian populations. *Lancet*, II:207–211.
78. Joossens, J. V., Kesteloot, H., and Amery, A. (1979): Salt intake and mortality from stroke. *N. Engl. J. Med.*, 300:1396.
79. Kamionkowski, M. D., and Fleshler, B., (1965): The role of alcoholic intake in esophageal carcinoma. *Am. J. Med. Sci.*, 249:696–699.
80. Kamm, J. J., Dashman, T., Newmark, H., and Mergens, W. J. (1977): Inhibition of amine–nitrite hepatotoxicity by α-tocopherol. *Toxicol. Appl. Pharmacol.*, 41:575–583.
81. Kasai, H., Nishimura, S., Nagao, M., Takahashi, Y., and Sugimura, T. (1979): Fractionation of a mutagenic principle from broiled fish by high-pressure liquid chromatography. *Cancer Lett.*, 7:343–348.
82. Kato, H., Velasco, M. E., and Rothchild, I. (1978): The role of the hypothalmus in the tonic secretion of prolactin induced by oestrogens in the rat. *Acta Endocrinol.*, 89:417–424.
83. Kent, J. R., and Acone, A. R. (1966): *Plasma Testosterone Levels and Aging in Males, Vol. 101*, pp. 31–35. Excerpta Medica Foundation, International Congress Series, Amsterdam.
84. Kern, J. F., Birkner, H. J., and Ostrower, V. S. (1978): Binding of bile acids by dietary fiber. *Am. J. Clin. Nutr.*, 31:S175–S179.

85. Kobayashi, N., Hoffman, D., and Wynder, E. L. (1974): A study of tobacco carcinogenesis: XII. Epithelial changes induced in the upper respiratory tract of Syrian golden hamsters by cigarette smoke. *J. Natl. Cancer Inst.,* 53:1085–1093.
86. Larsson, L. G., Sandstrom, A., and Westling, P. (1975): Relationship of Plummer–Vinson disease to cancer of the upper alimentary tract in Sweden. *Cancer Res.,* 35:3308–3316.
87. Leevy, C. M., Baker, H., tenHove, W., Frank, O., and Cherrick, G. (1965): B-complex vitamins in liver disease of the alcoholic. *Am. J. Clin. Nutr.,* 16:339–346.
88. Lin, H. J., Chan, W. C., Fong, L. Y., and Newberne, P. M. (1977): Zinc-levels in serum, hair and tumors from patients with esophageal cancer. *Nutr. Rep. Int.,* 15:635–643.
89. Lipkin, M., and Good, R. A. (1978): *Gastrointestinal Tract Cancer.* Plenum Medical Book Co., New York.
90. Marquardt, H., Rufino, R., and Weisburger, J. H. (1977): On the aetiology of gastric cancer: Mutagenicity of food extracts after incubation with nitrite. *Food Cosmet. Toxicol.,* 15:97–100.
91. Maruchi, N., Aoki, S., Tsuda, K., Tanaka, Y., and Toyokawa, H. (1977): Relation of food consumption to cancer mortality in Japan with special reference to international figures. *Gann,* 68:1–13.
92. Mauning, E. B., Mann, J. I., Sophangisa, E., and Truswell, A. S. (1974): Dietary patterns in urbanized blacks. *S.A. Med. J.,* 48:485–498.
93. McCann, J., Choi, E., Yamasaki, E., and Ames, B. N. (1975): Detection of carcinogens as mutagens in the *Salmonella*/microsome test: Assay of 300 chemicals. *Proc. Natl. Acad. Sci. USA,* 72:5135–5139.
94. McCoy, G. D. (1978): A biochemical approach to the etiology of alcohol related cancers of the head and neck. *Laryngoscope,* 88:59–62.
95. McCoy, G. D., and Wynder, E. L. (1979): Etiological and preventive implications in alcohol carcinogenesis. *Cancer Res.,* 39:2844–2850.
96. Meade, P. D., Tamashiro, S., Haradu, T., and Basrur, P. K. (1979): Influence of vitamin A on the laryngeal response of hamsters exposed to tobacco smoke. *Prog. Exp. Tumor Res.,* 24:320–329.
97. Meier, A. H. (1977): Prolactin, the liporegulatory hormone. In: *Comparative Endocrinology of Prolactin,* edited by H. D. Dellman, T. A. Johnson, and D. M. Klachko, pp. 153–191. Plenum Press, New York.
98. Mergens, W. J., Kamm, J. J., Newmark, H. L., Fiddler, W., and Pensabene, J. (1978): α-Tocopherol: Uses in preventing nitrosamine formation. In: *Environmental Aspects of N-Nitroso Compounds,* edited by E. A. Walker, L. Griciute, M. Castegnaro, R. E. Lyle, and W. Davis, pp. 199–212. International Agency for Research on Cancer, Lyon, France.
99. Miller, A. B. (1977): Role of nutrition in the etiology of breast cancer. *Cancer,* 39:2704–2708.
100. Mirvish, S. S. (1977): N-nitroso compounds: Their chemical and *in vivo* formation and possible importance as environmental carcinogens. *J. Toxicol. Environ. Health,* 2:1267–1277.
101. Mirvish, S. S., Karlowski, K., Sams, J. P., and Arnold, S. D. (1978): Studies of nitrosamide formation: Nitrosation in solvent, water and solvent systems, nitrosomethylurea formation in the rat stomach and analysis of a fish product for ureas. In: *Environmental Aspects of N-Nitroso Compounds,* edited by E. A. Walker, L. Griciute, M. Castegnaro, R. E. Lyle, and W. Davis, pp. 161–174. International Agency for Research on Cancer, Lyon, France.
102. Modlinger, R. S. Schonmuller, J. M., and Arora, S. P. (1979): Stimulation of aldosterone, renin and cortisol by tryptophan. *J. Clin. Endocrinol. Metab.,* 48:599–603.
103. Muir, C. D. (1975): International variation in high-risk populations. In: *Persons at High Risk of Cancer,* edited by J. F. Fraumeni, pp. 293–306. Academic Press, New York.
104. Muñoz, N., Asvall, J. (1971): The trends of intestinal and diffuse types of gastric cancer in Norway. *Int. J. Cancer,* 8:144–157.
105. Muñoz, N., Connelly, R. (1971): Time trends of intestinal and diffuse types of gastric cancer in the United States. *Int. J. Cancer,* 8:158–164.
106. Nagasawa, H. (1979): Prolactin and human breast cancer: A review. *Eur. J. Cancer,* 15:267–279.
107. Nieschlag, E., and Kley, H. K. (1975): Possibility of adrenal–testicular interaction as indicated by plasma androgens in response to HCG in men with normal, suppressed and impaired adrenal function. *Horm. Metab. Res.,* 7:326–330.

108. Nigro, N. D., Bhadrachari, N., and Chomchai, C. C. (1973): A rat model for studying colonic cancer—effect of cholestyramine on induced tumors. *Dis. Colon Rectum,* 16:438.
109. Nigro, N. D., Bull, A. W., Klopfer, B. A., Pak, M. S., and Campbell, R. L. (1979): Effect of dietary fiber on azoxymethane-induced intestinal carcinogenesis in rats. *J. Natl. Cancer Inst.,* 62:1097–1102.
110. Nigro, N. D., Singh, D. V., Campbell, R. L., and Pak. M. S. (1975): Effect of dietary beef fat on intestinal tumor formation by azoxymethane in rats. *J. Natl. Cancer Inst.,* 54:429–442.
111. Nomura, A., Henderson, B. E., and Lee, J. (1978): Breast cancer and diet among the Japanese in Hawaii. *Am. J. Clin. Nutr.,* 31:2020–2025.
112. Pariza, M. W., Ashoor, S. H., Chu, S. F., and Lund, D. B. (1979): Effects of temperature and time on mutagen formation in pan-fried hamburger. *Cancer Lett.,* 7:63–69.
113. Phillips, R. L. (1975): Role of life-style and dietary habit in risk of cancer among Seventh-Day Adventists. *Cancer Res.,* 35:3513–3522.
114. Piper, D. W. (1978): *Stomach Cancer, Vol. 34.* International Union Against Cancer, Geneva.
115. Pirke, K. M., and Doerr, P. (1970): Age related changes in free plasma testosterone, dihydrotestosterone and estradiol. *Acta Endrocrinol.,* 80:171–178.
116. Raineri, R., and Weisburger, J. H. (1975): Reduction of gastric carcinogens with ascorbic acid. *Ann. N. Y. Acad. Sci.,* 258:181–189.
117. Reddy, B. S., Cohen, L. A., McCoy, D., Hill, P., and Weisburger, J. H. (1980): Nutrition and its relationship to cancer. *Adv. Cancer Res.,* 32:237–245.
118. Reddy, B. S., Hedges, A. R., Laakso, K., and Wynder, E. L. (1978): Metabolic epidemiology of large bowel cancer: Fecal bulk and constituents of high-risk North American and low-risk Finnish population. *Cancer,* 42:2832–2838.
119. Reddy, B. S., Mangat, S., Sheinfil, A., Weisburger, J. H., and Wynder, E. L. (1977): Colon carcinogenesis: Effect of type and amount of dietary fat and 1,2-dimethylhydrazine on biliary bile acids and fecal bile acids and neutral sterols in rats. *Cancer Res.,* 37:2132–2137.
120. Reddy, B. S., Narisawa, T., Vukusich, D., Weisburger, J. H., and Wynder, E. L. (1976): Effect of quality and quantity of dietary fat and dimethylhydrazine in colon carcinogenesis in rats. *Proc. Soc. Exp. Biol. Med.,* 151:237–239.
121. Reddy, B. S., Watanabe, K., and Weisburger, J. H. (1977): Effect of high-fat diet on colon carcinogenesis in F344 rats treated with 1,2-dimethylhydrazine, methylazoxymethanol acetate or methylnitrosourea. *Cancer Res.,* 37:4156–4159.
122. Reddy, B. S., Weisburger, J. H., and Wynder, E. L. (1975): Effects of high-risk and low-risk diets for colon carcinogenesis on fecal microflora and steroids in man. *J. Nutr.,* 105:878–884.
123. Reddy, B. S., Weisburger, J. H., and Wynder, E. L. (1978): Colon cancer: Bile salts as tumor promoters. In: *Carcinogenesis, Vol 2,* edited by T. J. Slaga, A. Sivak, and R. K. Boutwell, pp. 453–464. Raven Press, New York.
124. Reddy, B. S., and Wynder, E. L. (1973): Large bowel carcinogenesis: Fecal constituents of populations with diverse incidence rates of colon cancer. *J. Natl. Cancer Inst.,* 50:1437–1442.
125. Robertson, M. A., Harington, J. S., and Bradshaw, E. (1971): The cancer patterns in Africans at Baragwanath Hospital, Johannesburg. *Br. J. Cancer,* 25:377–384.
126. Rogers, A. E., Sanchez, O., Feinsod, F. M., and Newberne, P. M. (1974): Dietary enhancement of nitrosamine carcinogenesis. *Cancer Res.,* 34:96–99.
127. Ross, R. K., McCurtis, J. W., Henderson, B. E., Menck, H. R., Mack, T. M., and Martin, S. P. (1979): Descriptive epidemiology of testicular and prostatic cancer in Los Angeles. *Br. J. Cancer,* 39:284–291.
128. Rothman, E., and Keller, A. Z., (1972): The effect of joint exposure to alcohol and tobacco on risk of cancer of the mouth and pharynx. *J. Chronic Dis.,* 25:711–716.
129. Salley, J., and Bryson, W. (1957): Vitamin A deficiency in the hamster. *J. Dent. Res.,* 36:935–944.
130. Sander, J., Schweinsberg, F., LaBar, J., Burkle, G., and Schweinsberg, E. (1975): Nitrite and nitrosable amino compounds in carcinogenesis. *Gann,* 17:145–160.
131. Schulz, K. D., Geiger, W., delPozo, E. and Künzig, H. J. (1978): Pattern of sexual steroids, prolactin, and gonadotropic hormones during prolactin inhibition in normal cycling women. *Am. J. Obstet. Gynecol.,* 132:561–566.
132. Sciarra, F., Sorcini, G., DiSilverio, F., and Gagliardi, V. (1973): Plasma testosterone and

androstenedione after orchidectomy in prostatic adenocarcinoma. *Clin. Endocrinol.,* 2:101–109.

133. Seidman, H. (1970): Cancer death rate by site and sex for religious and socioeconomic groups. *Environ. Res.,* 3:234–250.
134. Silverstone, H., and Tannenbaum, A. (1950): The effect of the proportion of dietary fat on the rate of formation of mammary carcinoma in mice. *Cancer Res.,* 10:448–453.
135. Spiegelhalder, B., Eisenbrand, G., and Preussman, R., (1976): Influence of dietary nitrate on nitrite content of human saliva: Possible relevance to *in vivo* formation of N-nitroso compounds. *Food Cosmet. Toxicol.,* 14:545–548.
136. Spingarn, N. E., and Garvie, C. T. (1979): Formation of mutagens in sugar–ammonia model systems. *J. Agric. Food Chem.,* 27:1319–1321.
137. Spingarn, N. E., and Weisburger, J. H. (1979): Formation of mutagens in cooked food: I. Beef. *Cancer Lett.,* 7:259–264.
138. Sporn, M. B., Dunlop, N. M., Newton, D. L., and Mith, J. M. (1976): Prevention of chemical carcinogenesis by vitamin A and its synthetic analogs (retinoids). *Fed Proc.,* 35:1332–1338.
139. Staszewski, J., and Haenszel, W. (1965): Cancer mortality among the Polish-born in the United States. *J. Natl. Cancer Inst.,* 35:291–297.
140. Story, J. A., and Kritchevsky, D. (1978): Bile acid metabolism and fiber. *Am. J. Clin. Nutr.,* 31:S175–S179.
141. Sugimura, T., Kawachi, T., Nagao, M., Yahagi, T., Seino, Y., Okamoto, T., Shudo, K., Kosuge, T., Tsuji, K., Wakabayashi, K., Iitaka, Y., and Itai, A. (1977): Mutagenic principle(s) in tryptophan and phenylalanine pyrolysis products, *Proc. Japan Acad.,* 53:58–61.
142. Sutton, J. R., Coleman, M. J., Casey, J., and Lazarus, S. (1973): Androgen responses during physical exercise. *Br. Med. J.,* 1:520–522.
143. Tannenbaum, A. (1942): The genesis and growth of tumors: III. Effect of a high fat diet. *Cancer Res.,* 2:468–475.
144. Tannenbaum, S. R., Moran, D., Rand, W., Cuello, C., and Correa, P. (1979): Gastric cancer in Colombia: IV. Nitrate and other ions in gastric contents of residents from a high-risk region. *J. Natl. Cancer Inst.,* 62:9–12.
145. Tannenbaum, A., and Silverstone, H. (1957): Nutrition and the genesis of tumors. In: *Cancer, Vol. I,* edited by R. W. Raven, pp. 306–334. Butterworth and Co., London.
146. Tannenbaum, S. R., Weisman, N., and Fett, D. (1976): The effect of nitrate intake on nitrite formation in human saliva. *Food Cosmet. Toxicol.,* 14:549–552.
147. Tuyns, A. J., and Masse, L. M. F. (1973): Mortality from cancer of the esophagus in Brittany. *Int. J. Epidemiol.,* 2:242–245.
148. Tuyns, A. J., Pequignot, G., and Jensen, O. M. (1977): Le cancer de l'oesophage en Ille-et-Ulaive en fonction des niveaux de consummation d'alcool et de tabac: Des resques qui se multiplient. *Bull. Cancer (Paris),* 64:45–60.
149. Vaughn, F. L., and Bernstein, I. A. (1976): Molecular aspects of control in epidermal differentiation. *Mol. Cell Biochem.,* 12:171–179.
150. Vitale, J. J., and Coffey, J. (1971): Alcoholism and vitamin metabolism. In: *The Biology of Alcoholism,* edited by B. Kissin and H. Begleiter, pp. 327–352. Plenum Publishers, New York.
151. Walker, E. A., Griciute, L., Castegnaro, M., Lyle, R. E., and Davis, W., editors (1978): *Environmental Aspects of N-nitroso Compounds.* International Agency for Research on Cancer, Lyon, France.
152. Watanabe, K., Reddy, B. S., Weisburger, J. H., and Kritchevsky, D. (1979): Effect of dietary alfalfa, pectin and wheat bran on azoxymethane- or methylnitrosourea-induced colon carcinogenesis in F344 rats. *J. Natl. Cancer Inst.,* 63:141–145.
153. Waterhouse, J., Muir, C., Correa, P., and Powell, J., editors (1976): *Cancer Incidence in Five Continents, Vol. III.* International Union Against Cancer, Geneva.
154. Weisburger, J. H. (1979): Mechanism of action of diet as a carcinogen. *Cancer,* 43:1987–1995.
155. Weisburger, J. H., Marquardt, H., Hirota, N., Mori, H., and Williams, G. (1980): Induction of glandular stomach cancer in rats with an extract of nitrite-treated fish. *J. Natl. Cancer Inst.,* 64:163–167.
156. Weisburger, J. H., Reddy, B. S., and Joftes, D. L., editors (1975): *Colorectal Cancer.* International Union Against Cancer, Geneva.
157. Weisburger, J. H., Reddy, B. S., Spingarn, N. E., and Wynder, E. L. (1980): Current views

on the mechanisms involved in the etiology of colorectal cancer. In: *Colorectal Cancer: Prevention, Epidemiology, and Screening,* edited by S. J. Winawer, P. Sherlock, and D. Schottenfeld, pp. 19–41. Raven Press, New York.

158. Weisburger, J. H., and Williams, G. M. (1980): Chemical carcinogenesis. In: *Cancer Medicine,* edited by J. F. Holland and E. Frei, III, 2nd edition. Lea and Febiger, Philadelphia.

159. Welsch, C. W., and Nagasawa, H. (1977): Prolactin and murine mammary tumorigenesis: A review. *Cancer Res.,* 37:951–963.

160. Williams, R. R., and Horn, J. W., (1977): Association of cancer sites with tobacco and alcohol consumption and socioeconomic status of patients. *J. Natl. Cancer Inst.,* 58:525–547.

161. Wilson, R. B., Hutcheson, D. P., and Wideman, L. (1977): Dimethylhydrazine-induced colon tumors in rats fed diets containing beef fat or corn oil with and without wheat bran. *Am. J. Clin. Nutr.,* 30:176–181.

162. Wynder, E. L. (1975): The epidemiology of large bowel cancer. *Cancer Res.,* 35:3388–3394.

163. Wynder, E. L., Bross, I. J., and Day, E. (1956): Epidemiological approach to the etiology of cancer of the larynx. *J.A.M.A.,* 160:1384–1391.

164. Wynder, E. L., Bross, I. J., and Feldman, R. M. (1957): A study of the etiological factors in cancer of the mouth. *Cancer,* 10:1300–1323.

165. Wynder, E. L., and Chan, P. C. (1970): The possible role of riboflavin deficiency in epithelial neoplasia: II. Effect of skin tumor development. *Cancer,* 26:1221–1224.

166. Wynder, E. L., Chan, P. C., Cohen, L. A., MacCornack, F., and Hill, P. (1976): Etiology and prevention of breast cancer. In: *Cancer Campaign, Early Diagnosis of Breast Cancer, Vol. 1,* edited by E. Grundmann and L. Beck, pp. 1–28. Gustav Fischer Verlag, New York.

167. Wynder, E. L., and Fryer, J. H. (1958): Etiologic considerations of Plummer–Vinson (Paterson–Kelly) syndrome. *Ann. Intern. Med.,* 49:1106–1128.

168. Wynder, E. L., and Hirayama, T. (1977): Comparative epidemiology of cancers in the United States and Japan. *Prev. Med.,* 6:567–594.

169. Wynder, E. L., Kajitani, T., Ishikawa, S., Dodo, H., and Takano, A. (1969): Environmental factors of cancer of the colon and rectum: II. Japanese epidemiological data. *Cancer,* 23:1210–1220.

170. Wynder, E. L., and Klein, V. E. (1965): The possible role of riboflavin deficiency in epithelial neoplasia: I. Epithelial changes of mice in simple deficiency. *Cancer,* 18:167–180.

171. Wynder, E. L., Mabuchi, K., and Whitmore, W. F. (1971): Epidemiology of cancer of the prostate. *Cancer,* 28:344–360.

172. Wynder, E. L., Peters, J. A., and Vivona, S. (1975): Symposium: Nutrition in the causation of cancer. *Cancer Res.,* 35:3231–3550.

173. Wynder, E. L., and Stellman, S. D. (1977): Comparative epidemiology of tobacco-related cancers. *Cancer Res.,* 37:4608–4622.

174. Zaldivar, R., and Wetterstrand, W. H. (1978): Nitrate nitrogen levels in drinking water of urban areas with high and low risk populations from stomach cancer: An environmental epidemiology study. *Z. Krebsforsch,* 92:227–234.

*Nutrition and Cancer: Etiology and Treatment,*
edited by G. R. Newell and N. M. Ellison.
Raven Press, New York © 1981.

# General Mechanisms of Carcinogenesis

## Guy R. Newell

*Professor of Epidemiology, The University of Texas System Cancer Center, M. D. Anderson
Hospital and Tumor Institute, Houston, Texas 77030*

### GENERAL MECHANISMS OF CARCINOGENESIS

Knowledge of the causes of cancer in man has been significantly enhanced in recent years by epidemiologic and laboratory studies. Cigarette smoking was shown to be associated with lung cancer long before some of the current concepts pertaining to mechanisms of action were developed. Although the mechanism by which cigarette smoke causes cancer is still unknown, its establishment as a human carcinogen is indisputable. Currently, 90% of all lung cancers in men, or 40% of all cancers in men, can be attributed to smoking tobacco. Likewise, alcohol combined with tobacco contributes to a substantial number of head, neck, and other cancers. Radiation is another well-recognized carcinogen, as are several chemicals, especially those associated with the workplace. Some viruses are almost certainly human carcinogens, and more information about drugs and physiologic substances (such as hormones) as carcinogens is becoming available. By no means should we overlook the increasing awareness and potential importance of dietary factors in carcinogenesis, as attested to in this volume by the number of chapters devoted to it. The purpose of this discussion is to summarize some current concepts of the mechanisms of carcinogenesis, many of which come from knowledge of specific etiologic agents just mentioned. A recent review of the etiology of human cancer is available (3), as is a review of the rapidly evolving concepts of mechanisms of carcinogenesis (5).

The relative importance of genetic versus environmental factors is difficult to determine in most cases. The expression of cancer is, in fact, an interaction among the functions elaborated by the genes, perhaps modulated by viruses or virally coded information, and external environmental factors. A familiar example of the interaction of environmental factors with genetic background is skin cancer and sunlight, whereby light-skinned, less-protected individuals are much more susceptible to skin cancer than are dark-skinned, better-protected individuals.

### Genetic Factors

Only a small proportion of cancers are inherited through the germ line as single-gene defects or chromosomal aberrations that predispose an individual to develop certain forms of cancer. Although more than 200 single-gene disorders have been associated with cancers, they account for less than 5% of all malignancies. In general, cancers associated with hereditary syndromes occur less frequently than do sporadic (nonhereditary) occurrences of the same cancers. They usually occur earlier in life; they tend to occur in multiple family members among several generations; they may affect bilateral organs or multiple sites within the same organ; and they may predispose to other tumor types or other somatic defects (9).

Many studies have attempted to measure cancer among family members. These studies have shown that first-degree relatives have a greater frequency of cancer of the same site, but not of cancers in general. In adults, the increased risk is about threefold for most common cancers—breast, stomach, colon, endometrium, prostate, lung, and malignant melanoma. Among children, there is a fourfold increase for the combination of leukemia, brain tumors, and soft-tissue sarcomas. It is not possible to determine how much of this increased risk is the result of genetic similarity or common environmental exposures.

Studies of migrant populations suggest that much of the racial difference in cancer frequencies is probably environmentally related, because migrants (especially Japanese) assume the prevailing rate of the country to which migration has taken place. For example, Japanese migrants to the United States assume high rates for colon and breast cancers and low rates for stomach cancer (6).

## Identification of Carcinogens

The identification of carcinogens and their removal from society and direct contact with humans is a goal of many scientists, regulators, and legislators. Carcinogens can be identified by human epidemiologic studies or by animal studies. For example, epidemiologic studies first implicated cigarette smoke as causing lung cancer and diethylstilbesterol as causing vaginal cancer in women whose mothers took the drug during pregnancy. Bioassays in animals first incriminated saccharin and reserpine as carcinogens, although there is little, if any, evidence that they cause cancer in humans. Although identification of carcinogens and their removal from human contact is a laudable goal, it is not easily accomplished. At the identification stage, both human studies and animal bioassays are fraught with difficulties. At the control stage, many individual, societal, or even political influences may prevent removal of an identified carcinogen (i.e., cigarettes).

The vast majority of substances known to be carcinogenic in humans have also been shown to cause cancer in at least one animal species. Most investigators believe that if a substance is shown to be carcinogenic in any animal species at any dose, it must be presumed to cause cancer in man. As such, this should provide sufficient warning to adopt measures to prevent human exposure. There is, however, some discussion as to the scientific validity of extrapolating directly from animal experiments to man (10). The justification for this extrapolation is based on the following considerations:

A. For several carcinogens for which there exist some quantitative human exposure data, the dose that causes cancer in humans and in laboratory animals is reasonably similar.

B. Studies of subchronic toxicity of cancer chemotherapeutic agents in laboratory animals and in man suggested that man may be up to ten times more sensitive than is the small laboratory animal.

C. Smaller animals tend to metabolize and excrete foreign organic chemicals more rapidly than do larger animals.

D. Chemically induced cancer is viewed as having the potential for originating in a single cell, and a human has hundreds of times more susceptible cells than does a mouse or rat.

E. Although the cells of a smaller animal turn over or replicate at perhaps twice the rate of human cells, man's lifespan is 35 times that of the mouse or rat, and this may render man more susceptible.

Certain repair processes and protective mechanisms do exist which may remove or neutralize some effects of carcinogenic damage; however, since 16% of deaths in the United States are caused by cancer, these repair mechanisms are essentially overwhelmed.

In the past few years, considerable research has been carried out to develop *in vitro* methods that can be used to predict the carcinogenic potential of chemical compounds. One important use of these short-term tests will be to determine which chemicals should be committed to more expensive long-term animal tests. These short-term assays can be divided into three categories:

A. Induction of neoplastic transformation of mammalian cells in culture.

B. Determination of mutagenesis or chromosomal changes in microorganisms or mammalian cells.

C. Assessment of the effects of interactions between carcinogens and target macromolecules.

The expectation is that these tests will lead to the establishment of a fast, inexpensive, and predictable matrix of tests that can serve as an effective prescreen for further carcinogenicity testing.

### Biochemical Mechanisms

Although we do not have complete understanding of the mechanisms by which chemicals cause cancer, several basic biologic facts are generally accepted:

A. Carcinogenesis is dose-dependent; that is, the larger the dose, the more tumors produced and the shorter the lag time.

B. There is a long lag time between exposure and development of tumors (in humans, between 5 and 30 years).

C. There is no evidence of a threshold dose of a carcinogen below which there is no risk of cancer.

D. Carcinogens can act transplacentally; that is, they can cross the placental barrier and cause tumors in the offspring.

E. Conversion from normal tissue to a cancer is a multistep process, such that initiating agents are enhanced by promoting agents, hormonal agents, and other cofactors.

F. Cells in a state of rapid turnover (cellular proliferation) are more susceptible to the action of carcinogens.

G. The same chemical can cause tumors that are recognized differently by immune mechanisms in different individuals (antigenic diversity).

H. The same chemical can cause different types of tumors (diversity of phenotypes).

Although compounds other than organic chemicals can cause cancer, e.g., asbestos or arsenic, one of the few unifying principles in the field is the belief that many organic chemicals must undergo metabolic activation in the body before being able to induce cancer (8). Once activated, the carcinogen becomes electron-poor (electrophilic reactant) and can then bind with electron-rich areas of the cells, such as nucleic acids (DNA and RNA) and cellular proteins (Fig. 1). The binding of the carcinogen to the cell then interferes with the structure and function of the modified molecules. This change could account for many of the physiologic properties of cancer cells, such as their impaired interaction with neighboring noncancer cells, impaired cell surface functions, increase in transport of necessary nutrients (thus giving the cancer cell an undue advantage over its neighbors), enhanced ability to multiply and proliferate at the expense of other cells, and ability to break away (metastasize) and implant in other organ sites. This metabolism of carcinogens is mediated by species- and tissue-

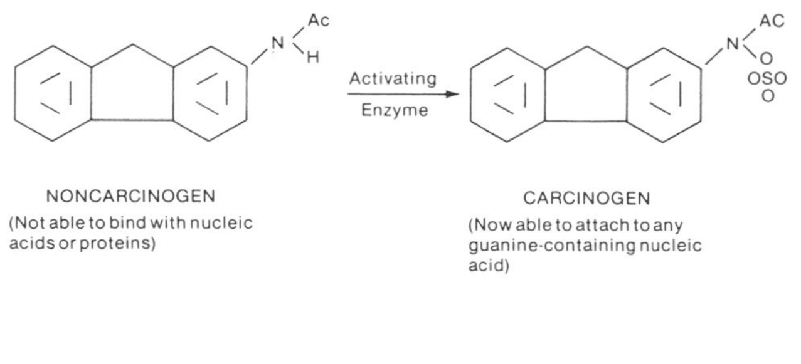

NONCARCINOGEN
(Not able to bind with nucleic acids or proteins)

CARCINOGEN
(Now able to attach to any guanine-containing nucleic acid)

**FIG. 1.** Chemical carcinogen model. AAF = N-2-acetylaminofluorene.

specific enzymes, and is the major determinant of species and tissue susceptibility to a given carcinogen. For example, there is evidence that the amount of enzyme known as AHH (aryl hydrocarbon hydroxylase), which metabolizes benzo*(a)*pyrene and related compounds in cigarette smoke, varies considerably among individuals. This variation, which appears to be hereditary, may explain why some heavy smokers do not get lung cancer.

### Initiation and Promotion

There is renewed interest in the two-stage mechanism of carcinogenesis, which suggests that an initiation phase is the result of a mutational change in a cell and is followed by a promotion phase, believed to be epigenetic in action (1). The somatic cell mutation theory of cancer accounts for (a) the irreversible nature of neoplastic transformation, (b) the almost unlimited variety of tumors, and (c) the tendency for individual tumor cells to reproduce themselves. Because a mutational change in the genome of a cell is a very rapid process, mutation as a sole mechanism could not account for the long latent period of cancer induction, which can be 30 years or more. This can be reconciled, however, by applying the mutational theory only to the initiation phase of carcinogenesis, followed by an epigenetic promotional phase. A dormant tumor cell resulting from mutation can be activated by promoting action after very long intervals. The fairly close correlation between mutagens and carcinogens adds support for involvement of a mutational change in some stage of carcinogenesis. The mechanism of promoting action is not as clear, although several mechanisms have been postulated. The most detailed information about the two-stage initiation–promotion process comes from experimental studies in mouse skin; however, there are other examples of initiation–promotion in other organs. Most believe that, in the broad sense of "external" or "environmental" factors, some kind of precipitating or modifying influences play an important role in the mechanism of carcinogenesis in animals and man.

### Chemicals

Several different classes of chemicals are known to cause cancer in humans. No common structural feature among them can be used for their identification; therefore, a variety of bioassays and other test systems is required, complicating the problems of detection and environmental surveillance, as well as the action of governmental regulatory agencies.

Of 296 chemicals reviewed by the International Agency for Research on Cancer (IARC), the experimental evidence of carcinogenicity in at least one animal species was considered to be adequate for 145. Of these 296, 21 were shown to be associated with the occurrence of cancer in man (Table 1); for 15, exposure was solely or mainly occupational; for 5, medicinal; and for 1, dietary (12).

TABLE 1. *Chemicals carcinogenic to man*

| Chemical | Type of Exposure | Target Organ(s) |
| --- | --- | --- |
| Aflatoxin | Dietary | Liver |
| 4-aminobiphenyl | Occupational | Bladder |
| Arsenic | Occupational, medicinal | Skin, ? lung |
| Asbestos | Occupational | Lung, pleural cavity, gastro-intestinal tract |
| Auramine | Occupational | Bladder |
| Benzene | Occupational | Bone marrow |
| Benzidine | Occupational | Bladder |
| Bis(chloromethyl) ether | Occupational | Lung |
| Cadmium oxide | Occupational | Prostate |
| Chromium | Occupational | Lung |
| Chloramphenicol | Medicinal | Bone marrow |
| Cyclophosphamide | Medicinal | Bone marrow |
| Diethylstilbesterol | Medicinal | Vagina, uterus |
| Hematite (mining) | Occupational | Lung |
| Melphalan | Medicinal | Bone marrow |
| Mustard gas | Occupational | Lung |
| 2-naphthylamine | Occupational | Bladder |
| N,N-bis (2-chloromethyl) 2-naphthylamine | Medicinal | Bladder |
| Nickel (refining) | Occupational | Nasal cavity, lung |
| Soot and tars | Occupational, environmental | Lung, skin |
| Vinyl chloride | Occupational | Liver, brain, lung |

## Radiation

Radiation bands of the electromagnetic spectrum for which carcinogenicity has been established include ultraviolet rays and ionizing rays (roentgen rays and gamma rays). Whether the microwave region of the spectrum is carcinogenic is unknown. Particulate radiation (alpha particles, beta particles, neutrons, and protons) is also carcinogenic. This type of radiation is used most often in cancer treatment.

Theories of radiation carcinogenesis have long invoked somatic mutation and virus activation as mechanisms (13). The multistage model for carcinogenesis would suggest that radiation acts in the initiation phase followed by a promoter phase. Radiation may act synergistically with other factors, e.g., the excess of lung cancers in United States uranium miners who are also cigarette smokers is greater than would be expected if the separate carcinogenic effects of mining alone and cigarette smoking alone were merely additive. This, along with the synergistic effect of asbestos exposure and cigarette smoking, is interpreted as evidence for a multistage mechanism of carcinogenesis, with radiation and asbestos exposure serving as an initiating agent and cigarette smoking as a promoting agent.

The types of cancer resulting from radiation exposure depend on several factors—dose and dosage, age at irradiation, sex, genetic susceptibility, and endocrine factors. In addition, many other variables have been observed to influence the carcinogenic effects of radiation, including immunologic response, biologic microflora, stress, diet, and rate of cell proliferation. After irradiation of the whole body or trunk, as occurred with exposure to the atomic bomb, the cancers occurring with increased frequency among adults within the first 25 to 30 years after exposure included leukemias (except chronic lymphocytic) and cancers of the female breast, thyroid gland, lung, stomach and other gastrointestinal organs, salivary gland, and lymphoid tissues. Conspicuously absent were tumors of the endocrine glands (other than thyroid) and cancers of the larynx, liver, genitourinary tract, skin, brain, muscle, and connective tissue. This suggests that the latter types are less susceptible to radiation induction than are those types developing among atomic bomb survivors. Among children exposed prenatally by diagnostic radiologic examination of the mother, the types of cancer that occur are similar to common childhood cancers that occur among nonirradiated children, e.g., acute leukemias, brain tumors, and sarcomas of embryonal and miscellaneous forms.

The natural background intensity of ultraviolet radiation varies with latitude and correlates with the incidence of skin cancer. For ionizing radiation, no correlation has been established between natural background levels and the incidence of cancer. Exposure to radiation from man-made sources comes primarily from the use of X-rays in medical diagnosis. Other man-made sources, as yet, contribute only minimally to the total, although their relative importance is growing. Examples of relative amounts of X-ray exposure from several sources are shown in Table 2.

From epidemiologic studies on irradiated human populations, it would appear that any increased exposure to ultraviolet or ionizing radiation in excess of natural background levels is likely to contribute to the overall risk of cancer. The amount of this contribution cannot be measured precisely; therefore, a linear, nonthreshold, dose–incidence relationship is generally accepted, so that, theoretically, any dose of ionizing radiation is potentially harmful. Nevertheless, it is essential that these presumptive risks are adequately offset by commensurate benefits.

## Viruses

Viruses can be considered as packaged genetic information. They consist of a core of DNA or RNA that contains the information necessary for virus replication and oncogenesis. Transmission occurs by two methods, "vertically" as part of the genetic inheritance passed from one generation of cells to the next (endogenous viruses), and "horizontally" in a mode similar to other infectious agents

TABLE 2. *Average amounts of X-ray exposures*

| Source | Average dose (mrem) |
|---|---|
| Natural background (per year) | 100 |
| Medical diagnosis (per year) | 75 |
| Chest X-ray (1 film) | 10 |
| Jet flight, Los Angeles–London (round trip) | 4 |
| Global fallout (per year) | 4 |
| Three-Mile Island accident (50-mile radius) | 1.5 |
| Nuclear power (per year) | 0.3 |

From A. C. Upton, *personal communication*, with permission.

(exogenous viruses). The essential aspect of viral carcinogenesis is the introduction of new genetic material into the host chromosome.

The expression of cancer-virus genes may take three forms: Virus or viral activity may be completely suppressed, partially expressed, or completely expressed, the latter process resulting in the formation of new virus particles. Evidence from animal models has shown that many viruses can cause malignant transformation without necessarily undergoing a complete cycle of multiplications as discrete entities within infected cells. Cells that have been transformed by viruses often have common properties, because the nucleic acid component directs the synthesis of a finite number of proteins that occur within the cell or at the cell surface. These reactions are predictable, and their products are directly measurable by sensitive biochemical and immunological tests.

A characteristic of RNA tumor viruses is an enzyme, commonly known as reverse transcriptase, which transcribes viral RNA into a complementary strand of DNA. DNA transcription can then integrate into the chromosome of the host cell. Thus, genetic information of the RNA virus, is transcribed into DNA, integrates into the germ cells of the host, becomes a unit of genetic inheritance, and is passed vertically to succeeding generations as an endogenous viral genome. The steps of subsequent viral multiplication do not always interfere with normal cellular processes; thus, the infected cells are not obligated to die. However, integration of only a single virus equivalent is sufficient to transform a susceptible normal cell into a cancerous one.

Animals of various species are known to carry the genome of one or more endogenous viruses, which apparently become integrated into their host's genetic machinery early in evolutionary development (11). Using probes made from viral RNA, gene products related to viruses known to cause cancers in animals have been detected in human tissues (4). Although a causal relationship between RNA-containing particles and cancer in man has not been demonstrated, involvement of these viruses in the etiology of some human cancers seems probable.

Horizontal transmission of some viruses with an RNA core is common in mice, chickens, cats, gibbons, and cattle. Transmission to other species which results in cancer can be accomplished under experimental conditions. In general, human serologic studies to identify these RNA viruses have been negative (7).

Herpes viruses, horizontally transmitted viruses with a DNA core, have been implicated on the basis of their close association with human neoplasms. The strongest laboratory and epidemiologic evidence implicates Epstein–Barr virus as a causative factor in Burkitt's lymphoma and nasopharyngeal carcinoma, and herpes simplex virus as a possible causative factor in carcinoma of the cervix (2). Several small DNA viruses possess cancer-causing properties demonstrable by inoculation into small laboratory animals, but there is little evidence that these take part in the etiology of human cancers.

### Inhibition of Carcinogens

Inhibition of carcinogens occurs by enhancement of defenses that prevent cancer-producing agents from reaching or reacting with critical target sites (14). An increasing number and diversity of such compounds is being identified with the capacity to inhibit the occurrence of cancer when administered prior to or simultaneously with cancer-causing agents. These compounds encompass a wide range of chemical structures and some synthetic chemicals, as well as naturally occurring constituents of food (Table 3). Several mechanisms for inhibiting chemical carcinogens include decreased activation and/or increased detoxifications, scavenging action to prevent carcinogens from reaching their target sites in the cell, alteration of cell membrane permeability, alteration of transport, or competitive inhibition. The chemical diversity of these compounds suggests that the ability to inhibit carcinogens does not depend on chemical characteristics per se, and that many other inhibitors exist. A fuller understanding of mechanisms of action would help in discovering other such compounds. It should be noted, however, that some of these inhibitors are toxic, or even carcinogenic. It is likely that compounds with increasing inhibitory potency and fewer side effects will be found.

TABLE 3. *Inhibiting agents*

---

Phenolic antioxidants and ethoxyquin
 (includes butylated hydroxyanisole [BHA] and butylated hydroxytoluene [BHT])
Disulfiram and related compounds
Organic isothiocyanates and organic thiocyanates
 (naturally occurring constituents of edible cruciferous plants)
Coumarins, ascorbic acid, and other lactones
Selenium and selenium salts
Inducers of increased microsomal mixed-function oxidase activity
 (includes polyclic hydrocarbons, which are themselves carcinogenic, the flavones, and phenobarbital; may also enhance carcinogenesis
Inhibitors of microsomal mixed-function oxidase activity
Physiologic trapping agents

---

## REFERENCES

1. Berenblum, I. (1979): Theoretical and practical aspects of the two-stage mechanism of carcinogenesis. In: *Carcinogens: Identification and Mechanisms of Action,* edited by A. Clark Griffin and Charles R. Shaw, pp. 25–36. Raven Press, New York.
2. de-The, G. (1977): Viruses as causes of some human tumors? Results and prospectives of the epidemiologic approach. In: *Origins of Human Cancer,* edited by H. H. Hiatt, J. D. Watson, and J. A. Winsten, pp. 1113–1132. Cold Spring Harbor Laboratory, Cold Spring Harbor, Maine.
3. Fraumeni, J. F., Jr. (1975): *Persons at High Risk of Cancer: An Approach to Cancer Etiology and Control.* Academic Press, New York.
4. Gardner, M. B., Rosheed, S., Shimizu, S., Rongey, R. W., Henderson, B. E., McAllister, R. M., Klement, V., Charman, H. P., Gilden, R. V., Heberling, R. L., and Huebner, R. J. (1977) Search for RNA tumor viruses in humans. In: *Origins of Human Cancer,* edited by H. H. Hiatt, J. D. Watson, and J. A. Winsten, pp. 1235–1252. Cold Spring Harbor Laboratory, Cold Spring Harbor, Maine.
5. Griffin, A. C., and Shaw, C. R. (1979): *Carcinogens: Identification and Mechanisms of Action.* Raven Press, New York.
6. Haenszel, W. (1975): Migrant studies. In: *Persons at High Risk of Cancer: An Approach to Cancer Etiology and Control,* edited by J. F. Fraumeni, Jr., pp. 361–372. Academic Press, New York.
7. Heath, C. W., Jr., Caldwell, G. C., and Feorino, P. C. (1975): Viruses and other microbes. In: *Persons at High Risk of Cancer: An Approach to Cancer Etiology and Control,* edited by J. F. Fraumeni, Jr., pp. 241–265. Academic Press, New York.
8. Miller, J. A., and Miller, E. C. (1977): Ultimate chemical carcinogens as reactive mutagenic electrophiles. In: *Origins of Human Cancer,* edited by H. H. Hiatt, J. D. Watson, and J. A. Winsten, pp. 605–627. Cold Spring Harbor Laboratory, Cold Spring Harbor, Maine.
9. Mulvihill, J. J. (1975): Congenital and genetic diseases. In: *Persons at High Risk of Cancer: An Approach to Cancer Etiology and Control,* edited by J. F. Fraumeni, Jr., pp. 3–38. Academic Press, New York.
10. Rall, D. P. (1977): Species differences in carcinogenesis testing. In: *Origins of Human Cancer,* edited by H. H. Hiatt, J. D. Watson, and J. A. Winsten, pp. 1383–1390. Cold Spring Harbor Laboratory, Cold Spring Harbor, Maine.
11. Todaro, G. J. (1977): RNA tumor virus genes (virogenes) and the transforming genes (oncogenes): Genetic transmission, infectious spread, and modes of expression. In: *Origins of Human Cancer,* edited by H. H. Hiatt, J. D. Watson, and J. A. Winsten, pp. 1169–1196. Cold Spring Harbor Laboratory, Cold Spring Harbor, Maine.
12. Tomatis, L. (1977): The value of long-term testing for the implementation of primary prevention. In: *Origins of Human Cancer,* edited by H. H. Hiatt, J. D. Watson, and J. A. Winsten, pp. 1339–1357. Cold Spring Harbor Laboratory, Cold Spring Harbor, Maine.
13. Upton, A. C. (1977): Radiation effects. In: *Origins of Human Cancer,* edited by H. H. Hiatt, J. D. Watson, and J. A. Winsten, pp. 477–500. Cold Spring Harbor Laboratory, Cold Spring Harbor, Maine.
14. Wattenberg, L. W. (1979): Inhibitors of carcinogenesis. In: *Carcinogens: Identification and Mechanisms of Action,* edited by A. C. Griffin and C. R. Shaw, pp. 299–316. Raven Press, New York.

Nutrition and Cancer: Etiology and Treatment,
edited by G. R. Newell and N. M. Ellison.
Raven Press, New York © 1981.

# Mutagens in Food as Causes of Cancer

Takashi Sugimura, Takashi Kawachi, Minako Nagao,
and Takie Yahagi

*National Cancer Center Research Institute, Tsukiji 5-1-1, Chuo-ku, Tokyo 104, Japan*

The carcinogenic process consists of two main steps; initiation and promotion. Initiation is a process related to mutagenesis; in which mutagens produce mutations in crucial genes in the cell nucleus. Promotion, the second step, is a process related to phenotypic expression. Mutagens can be described as mutagenic carcinogens, genotoxic carcinogens, or mutacarcinogens; the term "carcinogens" includes genotoxic carcinogens and promoters. The relation between carcinogenesis and nutrition involves both mutagenic carcinogens and nonmutagenic promoters, but this chapter is concerned primarily with mutagens in food that cause cancer.

Mutagenesis that may result in carcinogenesis occurs in somatic cells of various organs. There are two types of mutagens, direct-acting mutagens and promutagens. Direct-acting mutagens, which do not require metabolic activation and are mostly in a reactive form, may be ingested with food. Sulfhydryl compounds and antioxidants in the food can interact with and decrease the amount of direct mutagens. Other nutritional components and food constituents also change the amount of activated, ultimate mutagens through various mechanisms. Ultimate mutagens yielded by metabolic activation are eliminated by reaction with sulfhydryl compounds and antioxidants.

Promutagens (procarcinogens) may also be ingested with food. The metabolic activation of promutagens is modulated by other components in food. For instance, naturally occurring flavonoids can suppress the metabolic activation of benzo(a)pyrene (54). The metabolic detoxification process is also modulated by food constituents. It has been shown that riboflavin (vitamin $B_2$) activates azo reductase in the liver, and that this enzyme decreases the carcinogenicity of 4-dimethylaminoazobenzene in rats (25). Kinoshita's (14) report on hepatocarcinogenicity in rats was not immediately confirmed by other scientists because Kinoshita fed his rats rice mixed with vegetable oil containing azo dyes, a diet that is deficient in riboflavin, so the rats developed hepatomas rapidly and in high incidence. This hepatocarcinogenesis was very efficiently suppressed by the addition of riboflavin to the diet. Azo dyes were metabolically activated to ultimate reactive forms (ultimate mutagens), whereas azo dyes were inactivated by azo reductase. Riboflavin in the diet suppressed the carcinogenicity of azo dyes by stimulating this inactivation process.

These findings on how riboflavin is related to hepatocarcinogenesis clearly indicate the relationship between nutrition and carcinogenesis (25). However, compounds having an azo bond on each side of benzidine, such as Congo red, can be activated to exert mutagenicity by activated azo reductase in the presence of riboflavin (23,42). In this case, azo reduction yields a mutagenic compound related to benzidine.

Mutagens in food can be divided into two types on the basis of their source: industrially and naturally occurring mutagens. In theory, the former should be controllable; that is, it should be possible to eliminate contaminating industrial mutagens from food by technical improvements. For instance, if food additives are demonstrated to be mutagenic, they can be replaced by nonmutagenic compounds. In contrast, naturally occurring mutagens in food are difficult to eliminate. These can be classified into four categories. One category includes mutagens in edible plants, such as pyrrolizidine alkaloids and flavonoids (39). A second type is mutagens produced by fungi, such as aflatoxin $B_1$. A third type is mutagens produced by cooking. For instance, charred parts of proteinous food are mutagenic, and the browning process can also produce mutagens. A fourth category is comprised of the nitrosamines, which are formed from nitrites and amines. Nitrites are added to food as preservatives, and are also present in the body as a product of the reduction of nitrates in vegetables. Amines are present in various foods, especially preserved fish. Thus, when nitrites are added as a preservative to food containing amines, nitrosamines may be formed endogenously.

The purpose of food preservatives is to protect foods from spoiling and to increase their utility. However, the effects of additives in food must be carefully considered, and we will consider here the man-made food preservative AF-2. Various ways of cooking foods also yield mutagens. As mentioned above, heating proteinous food results in the formation of many mutagens. We will examine the formation of mutagens during cooking. Finally, the endogenous formation of mutagens in the body is believed to be important in the development of human cancer, so we will consider the endogenous formation of nitroso-compounds.

## THE FOOD ADDITIVE AF-2

Nitrofuran derivatives have been widely used as preservatives of foods and feeds. In Japan, nitrofurazone was used from 1952 to 1965, and nitrofurylacrylamide from 1954 to 1965. The structures of nitrofurazone and nitrofurylacrylamide are shown in Table 1. After extensive studies to obtain a more effective preservative, 2-(2-furyl)-3-(5-nitro-2-furyl)acrylamide, with the trade name AF-2, was introduced in the market in 1965. Its structure is also shown in Table 1. Use of this preservative was approved by the Japanese Ministry of Health and Welfare, since tests had indicated that it was not carcinogenic in rats and mice (28). The concentrations of AF-2 allowed were 2.5 ppm in fish cake, 5

TABLE 1. *Nitrofuran derivatives once used as food preservatives in Japan*

| Name | Structure | Dates of use in Japan | Specific mutagenic activity Revertants/$\mu g$[a] |
|------|-----------|----------------------|--------------------------------------------------|
| Nitrofurazone (5-Nitro-2-furaldehyde semicarbazone) | $O_2N-\text{furan}-CH=NN<^H_{CONH_2}$ | 1952 → 1965 | $9 \times 10^2$ |
| Nitrofurylacrylamide (3-[5-Nitro-2-furyl]-acrylamide) | $O_2N-\text{furan}-CH=C<^H_{CONH_2}$ | 1954 → 1965 | $4 \times 10^3$ |
| AF-2 (2-[2-Furyl]-3-[5-nitro-2-furyl]acrylamide) | $O_2N-\text{furan}-CH=C<^{\text{furan}}_{CONH_2}$ | 1965 → 1974 | $4 \times 10^4$ |

[a] *S. typhimurium* TA100 without S-9 mix

ppm in red bean paste, soybean curd, and fish sausage, and 20 ppm in fish-meal paste. In some areas of the world, diseases of malnutrition, such as kwash-iorkor, are still a big problem. In Japan, however, fish is a major source of protein and reasonably cheap, so preservatives in fish products are eaten in considerable quantity. When treated with AF-2, which was thought to be a good preservative, fish sausage could safely be kept at room temperature for several months.

In 1973, AF-2 was found to be mutagenic in *Escherichia coli* WP-2 and H/r30 (10,15). Many nitrofurans, some of which were carcinogenic, were also found to be mutagenic in *Salmonella typhimurium* TA100 (56), although not *S. typhimurium* TA1535 (57). Since many other nitrofuran derivatives are both mutagenic and carcinogenic, the finding that AF-2 was mutagenic suggested that it was also carcinogenic. Soon afterwards, the carcinogenicity of AF-2 was demonstrated by Ikeda et al. (6). They fed mice a diet containing 0.05%, 0.15%, and 0.45% AF-2 and observed dose-dependent production of malignant squamous cell carcinomas in the forestomach. The use of AF-2 was then promptly banned.

This is an example of how carcinogenicity can be predicted when mutagenicity is established. If another compound were similarly found to be highly mutagenic, no one would hesitate to take immediate action to ban its use in foods in these days. But in the case of AF-2, scientists were loath to ban a product before its carcinogenicity was demonstrated in long-term *in vivo* experiments.

The TD$_{50}$ value, an index proposed by Meselson and Russell (24), which was defined as the daily dose/kg body weight that, when fed over a standard lifetime, induces tumors in half of the animals tested, was calculated for AF-2 as 24 mg/kg/day (A) on the basis of data collected by Kinebuchi et al. (13). Assuming the total annual AF-2 production of three tons (based on figures from the Ministry of International Trade and Industry) was consumed by the

Japanese population, the average intake of AF-2 per capita would be 0.012 mg/kg/day (B). Ironically, the ratio of B to A is 1:2,000, which indicates that, at its actual level of intake, AF-2 is not a major risk for humans. However, in evaluating the risk of AF-2, we must consider other negative and positive factors. For instance, not all the AF-2 manufactured was eaten, since some was degraded in the food and some food containing AF-2 was not sold. About one-quarter of the Japanese population develops cancer, but the cancers develop in various sites in the body, whereas cancers largely caused by AF-2 should develop in particular organs, and the risk to these organs would be much higher. These considerations indicate that, unlike occupational exposure to chemical carcinogens, exposure to mutagen-carcinogens in food does not involve an especially large dose and, in most cases, is difficult to demonstrate from epidemiological data.

All things considered, the actual intake of AF-2 seems to have been too small to cause any appreciable risk of human cancer. However, in the future, nonmutagenic and noncarcinogenic food preservatives must be developed. In this way, it will be possible to overcome the shortage of proteinous foods in out-of-the-way places. Moreover, the problem of a slight risk of cancer, indicated by mutagenicity and carcinogenicity in experimental animals, must be weighed against the urgent need for protein to prevent severe malnutrition. This kind of minor problem is inevitable in dealing realistically with the difficult and important problem of malnutrition in the world.

## MUTAGENS PRODUCED DURING COOKING

Cooking adds flavor to many raw foods and makes them more easily digestible, thus enhancing their nutritional value. Studies on the formation of carcinogens during cooking started 20 years ago. For instance, the content of benzo(a)pyrene in beefsteak was determined in 1964 (18). Mutagens in cooked foods, especially

TABLE 2. *Mutagenic activity of cooked foods[a]*

| Food | Sample size | Cooking procedure | Cooking time (min) | Revertants per sample[b] | Revertants per m² |
|---|---|---|---|---|---|
| White bread | 1 slice | Broiling | 6 | 205 | 18,600 |
| Pumpernickel bread | 1 slice | Broiling | 12 | 945 | 96,500 |
| Biscuit | 1 each | Baking | 20 | 735 | N.C. |
| Pancake | 1 each | Frying | 4 | 2,500 | 153,000 |
| Potato | 1 small slice | Frying | 30 | 200 | 329,000 |
| Beef | 1 patty | Frying | 14 | 21,700 | 3,830,000 |

[a] From Spingarn et al., ref. 37, with permission.
[b] Mutagen level after cooking food just beyond the normal range of edibility. The basic fraction was tested on TA98 with S-9 mix.

in the charred parts of broiled dried fish and beefsteak, were first reported in 1977 (31,32,42). The charred parts of these broiled foods were mutagenic in *S. typhimurium* TA98 and TA100 in the presence of S-9 mix for metabolic activation. We found that the benzo(*a*)pyrene content of these samples could account for only about 1/100 to 1/10,000 of their mutagenicity (31), indicating that most of the mutagenicity was due to mutagens other than aromatic hydrocarbons. Moreover, since the specific mutagenicity of nitrosamine compounds is very low (58), the mutagenicity could not be due to nitrosamines. Neither could it be due to mycotoxin, because the mutagenicity was found almost exclusively in the charred parts of these foods. Experiments showed that mutagens were mainly formed by the pyrolysis of protein, but not of carbohydrates, nucleic acids, or fat (30,41). Pyrolysis of amino acids also yielded strong mutagens, tryptophan, glutamic acid, and serine having the highest mutagenic potential (16,22,32,41). Besides amino acids, compounds containing nitrogen, such as creatine, creatinine, ornithine, and N-glucosamine, also yielded mutagens upon pyrolysis (16,32). Table 2 shows data on the mutagenicity of cooked foods, which suggest that those foods must contain other mutagens (38).

It seemed difficult to identify new mutagenic principles in crude material, such as broiled foods, so attempts were first made to purify mutagens from pyrolysates of amino acids. Most of the mutagenicity in amino acid and protein pyrolysates was recovered in the basic fraction. The active principle in a basic fraction of a D,L-tryptophan pyrolysate was purified by column chromatographies on silica gel, alumina, CM-Sephadex C-25, and Sephadex LH-20, and the two crystalline materials obtained were identified as the compounds 3-amino-1,4-dimethyl-5*H*-pyrido[4,3-*b*]indole (Trp-P-1) and 3-amino-1-methyl-5*H*-pyrido[4,3-*b*]indole (Trp-P-2) (16,40). These two mutagens have higher specific mutagenic activity in TA98 than does aflatoxin $B_1$ (39,41). Similarly, two new substances were isolated from an L-glutamic acid pyrolysate and identified as 2-amino-6-methyldipyrido[1,2-*a*:3',2'-*d*]imidazole (Glu-P-1) and 2-aminodipyrido[1,2-*a*:3',2'-*d*]imidazole (Glu-P-2) (62). X-ray crystallography, nuclear magnetic resonance, and high-resolution mass spectrography were very useful in determining the structures of these new heterocyclic amine compounds. The specific mutagenicity in TA98 of Glu-P-1 is also higher than that of aflatoxin $B_1$, while that of Glu-P-2 is lower (39,41).

Trp-P-1, Trp-P-2, Glu-P-1, and Glu-P-2 were later synthesized chemically (1,46,47). 3,4-Cyclopentenopyrido[3,2-*a*]carbozole (Lys-P-1) was isolated from a pyrolysate of L-lysine (52), and 2-amino-5-phenylpyridine (Phe-P-1) from a pyrolysate of D,L-phenylalanine (16,40). Trp-P-1, Trp-P-2, Glu-P-1, and Glu-P-2 were also detected in pyrolysates of proteins (51,60). 2-Amino-α-carboline (AαC) and 2-amino-3-methyl-α-carboline (AMαC) were obtained from pyrolysates of soybean globulin by Yoshida et al. (64). Benzo(*f*)quinoline and phenanthridine were also isolated from protein pyrolysates (16). Trp-P-1 and Trp-P-2 were detected in broiled sardine (61). Of these mutagens, Trp-P-1, Trp-P-2, Glu-P-1, Glu-P-2, and Lys-P-1 are newly described compounds, and all are

TABLE 3. *Structures and specific mutagenic activity of compounds formed by pyrolysis of amino acids and proteins*

| Structure | Abbreviation or name | Specific mutagenic activity (Revertants per $\mu g$) | |
| --- | --- | --- | --- |
| | | TA98 | TA100 |
| | IQ[a] | 433,000 | 7,000 |
| | Trp-P-2[a] | 104,000 | 1,800 |
| | Glu-P-I[b] | 49,000 | 3,200 |
| | Trp-P-I[a] | 39,000 | 1,700 |
| | Methyl-IQ[a] | 18,500 | 103 |
| | Glu-P-2[b] | 1,900 | 1,200 |
| | A$\alpha$C[c] | 300 | 20 |
| | AM$\alpha$C[c] | 200 | 120 |
| | Lys-P-I[c] | 86 | 99 |
| | Phe-P-I[c] | 41 | 23 |
| | Benzo($f$)quinoline[c] | 0.69 | 7.4 |
| | Phenanthridine[c] | 0.57 | 2.9 |

[a] 10 $\mu l$ per plate of S-9 fraction from liver of rats treated with polychlorinated biphenyls.
[b] 30 $\mu l$ per plate
[c] 150 $\mu l$ per plate

mutagenic with metabolic activation. The structures of these mutagens and their specific mutagenic activities in TA98 and TA100, with the optimal amount of S-9 for each compound, are given in Table 3. All of these compounds are heterocyclic amine derivatives except Lys-P-1, benzo*(f)*quinoline, and phenanthridine.

The biological activities of Trp-P-1 and Trp-P-2 have been studied most extensively. These compounds are mutagenic in TA100 and TA98, and mutagenic (17) and clastogenic (M. Ishidate, *personal communication*) in cultured mammalian cells. They can also induce sister chromatid exchanges (49).

Trp-P-1 and Trp-P-2 caused malignant transformation of cultured hamster embryonal cells in Pienta's system (45), and the transformed cells could be successively transplantable in the cheek pouch of adult hamsters (43). Subcutaneous injections of Trp-P-1 into hamsters and rats induced malignant fibrosarcomas at the site of injection (9). Mice fed a diet containing Trp-P-1 or Trp-P-2 developed many hepatomas (*unpublished observation* in our laboratory). All these findings demonstrate the intrinsic carcinogenicity of Trp-P-1 and Trp-P-2. Although their mutagenic effects in TA98 are greater than those of aflatoxin $B_1$, results *in vivo* suggest that Trp-P-1 and Trp-P-2 are weaker carcinogens than aflatoxin $B_1$ (55). The contents of Trp-P-1 and Trp-P-2 are on the order of 10 ng/g of broiled fish (61). The intake of these two heterocyclic amines in food could not alone account for the development of human cancer. However, Trp-P-1 and Trp-P-2 are only two of many mutagenic compounds in cooked food. Various tests are now being carried out on Glu-P-1, Glu-P-2, Lys-P-1, A$\alpha$C, and AM$\alpha$C. Furthermore, long-term *in vivo* feeding experiments on these compounds are in progress, and it seems probable that these heterocyclic amines will also be found to be carcinogenic *in vivo*. Actually, Glu-P-1 has been shown to transform Chinese hamster embryonal cells (44). Thus, the integrated effects of various mutagenic heterocyclic amines in foods may well be sufficient to account for the development of human cancer. Very recently, two more strong mutagens were isolated from broiled fish in our laboratory; their structures are 2-amino-3-methylimidazo[4,5-*f*]quinoline (IQ) and 2-amino-3,5-dimethylimidazo[4,5-*f*]quinoline (Me IQ).

The presence of mutagens in cooked hamburger and beef extract was first reported by Commoner et al. (3). Studies indicated that the yield of mutagenic activity increased with the time of heating and with the temperature (35). However, the conditions under which hamburgers are normally cooked are much milder than those for charring by exposure to a naked flame. The structure of the active substance is still uncertain, but a fairly purified substance with specific mutagenic activity roughly equivalent to that of Glu-P-1 has been obtained (B. Commoner, *personal communication*).

Fried beef and Difco beef extract heated on a hot plate can be used as sources of the mutagenic material, and the basic fraction of the materials extracted with methylene chloride contains most of their mutagenic activity. Column chromatographies on silica gel, Sephadex LH-20, and HPLC are efficient procedures for obtaining pure mutagen. The substance isolated from beef extract seems to be identical to one of two newly isolated, strong mutagens from broiled fish, IQ (11,37). Tests on various biological activities of the mutagen and its carcinogenicity *in vitro* and *in vivo* should be performed after elucidating its structure and establishing a method for its organic synthesis. This type of mutagen can also be produced under milder conditions than those for pyrolysis of amino acids and proteins, and normal cooking often produces suitable conditions for its production. The mechanisms of its formation may be related to the browning reaction (36). It is also likely that there are several other mutagens in fried beef and heated beef extract, fried fish, and heated fish meat. Fried potato also has mutagenic activity in TA98 (Table 2) and TA100 with metabolic activation (38). Furthermore, a direct mutagen in TA100 is formed on pyrolysis of sugar and carbohydrate (32,41).

Charred beefsteak is known to induce drug-metabolizing systems in rats and humans (4,34). Although the significance of this induction is not yet known to be related to activation or inactivation of promutagens *in vivo,* there are several reports that P-450 catalyzes activation of Trp-P-1 and Trp-P-2 (8,33). Vegetable extracts can inactivate Trp-P-1 and Trp-P-2 (T. Kada, *personal communication*). Myeloperoxidase and hydrogen peroxide also inactivate Trp-P-1, Trp-P-2, Glu-P-1, and AαC (59). Peroxidase is known to be present in horseradish and milk. Thus, other food materials modulate the mutagenic activity of mutagens produced during cooking, so it is important to eat a variety of foods with balanced nutritional values.

### Nitrosamines: Endogenous Formation of Mutagens

Nitrites have long been used as food preservatives. Ham, sausage, and fish roe are the most common foods to which nitrites are added. Nitrosamines are readily formed in the presence of secondary amines under weakly acidic conditions (26) similar to those in the human stomach. The nitrite contents of various foods have been determined (7,12) and results have shown that there are two main sources of nitrites: pickles, in which nitrites may be formed by reduction of nitrates, and sausages and ham, which contain added nitrites as a food preservative.

Fish products are known to have high levels of secondary amines, and roasting increases that level (Table 4). For instance, raw and broiled sardines contain 0.13 and 1.05 $\mu$mole/g, respectively. The roe of cod contains as much as 3 $\mu$mole/g, whereas the amine content of beef, pork, and chicken is less than 0.02 $\mu$mole/g even after broiling (7). Some Japanese pressed ham containing fish meat contains 0.025 $\mu$g/g of dimethylnitrosamine (7). Trimethylamine oxide is a good precursor of dimethylamine, but trimethylamine is not (7).

The cycle of nitrate/nitrite metabolism has been studied extensively by Tannenbaum (48). Nitrates in vegetables are a major source of nitrites formed in saliva and in the stomach. Moreover, nitrates are excreted in the saliva and

TABLE 4. *Secondary amines in raw and roasted fish*[a]

| Fish | Raw[b] | Roasted |
|------|------|---------|
| Abalone | 0.01 | 0.04 |
| Cod | 0.18 | 0.48 |
| Cod roe | 3.40 | 3.20 |
| Crab | 0.01 | 0.04 |
| Cuttlefish | 0.01 | 0.15 |
| Herring | 0.29 | 0.68 |
| Mackerel | 0.05 | 0.54 |
| Mackerel pike | 0.07 | 1.23 |
| Oyster | 0.00 | 0.01 |
| Plaice | 0.02 | 0.50 |
| Sardine | 0.13 | 1.08 |
| Sea urchin | 0.09 | 0.23 |
| Shrimp | 0.10 | — |
| Tuna | 0.12 | 0.15 |

[a] From Ishidate et al. (7).
[b] $\mu$mole/g, calculated as dimethylamine.

reduced to nitrites by bacteria in the oral cavity and stomach. Chronic gastritis and intestinal metaplasia favor bacterial reduction of nitrates to nitrites. Nitrites are also formed from ammonia in the distal ileum. The intestinal contents of humans, obtained by ileostomy, were found to contain some nitrites, but no nitrates. Nitrites formed from ammonia may be absorbed into the circulation and react with oxyhemoglobin, resulting in stoichiometric formation of methemoglobin and nitrates. These nitrates then contribute to the pool formed by nitrates ingested with food. It has been calculated that the endogenous formation of nitrates occurs at a rate of 1 mmole/day.

Many nitrosamine derivatives are mutagenic as well as carcinogenic (29,58). These compounds must be activated metabolically to show mutagenic activity, but some nitrosamides are mutagenic without metabolic activation. The transnitrosation reaction is catalyzed by an enzyme(s) present in the intestinal flora (20). This enzyme forms direct-acting mutagens, nitrosamides, from indirect-acting mutagens, nitrosamines. The intestinal flora vary considerably with the composition of the food, so formation of nitrosamides may also depend on the composition of the food (5).

Vitamin C inhibits the formation of nitrosamines (27). In extensive studies, Bruce et al. (2) found that the level of mutagens in human feces decreased on administration of vitamin C (4 g/day). Similarly, administration of $\alpha$-tocopherol (400 mg/day) greatly diminished the mutagen content of feces.

Incubation of soy sauce with nitrites at pH 3 yielded a strong mutagen(s) that required metabolic activation (19). Although the precursor amine is not yet known, soy sauce, which is produced largely from proteinous sources and is widely used in many southeast Asian countries, could be an important source of endogenously formed nitrosamines. Weisburger et al. (53) found that oral ingestion of dried fish treated with nitrites under acidic conditions produced hyperplastic lesions in the glandular stomach of rats. It has also been reported that mutagens are formed by incubation of dried fish and nitrites under acidic conditions, and that the presence of vitamin C during incubation greatly decreases their formation (21).

However, in contrast to the claim that nitrites always increase mutagenic risk, at least one case of nitrites reducing the mutagenic risk has been found (50,63). Under weakly acidic conditions, nitrites inactivate the potent mutagens Trp-P-1, Trp-P-2, and Glu-P-1 as a result of deamination. The required concentration of nitrites is approximately 10 ppm (50).

All the above findings support the idea that nitroso-related mutagens, and possibly carcinogens, are formed endogenously in very complex ways. All the factors contributing to their formation are consistent with certain nutritional conditions. Thus, understanding the nature and mechanisms of endogenous mutagens may well be important for understanding the relationship between food and the development of human cancer.

## ACKNOWLEDGMENTS

This research was supported in part by grants-in-aid for cancer research from the Ministry of Education, Science, and Culture, the Ministry of Health and Welfare, Japan, the Princess Takamatsu Cancer Research Fund, and the Nissan Science Foundation.

## REFERENCES

1. Akimoto, H., Kawai, A., Nomura, H., Nagao, M., Kawachi, T., and Sugimura, T. (1977): Syntheses of potent mutagens in tryptophan pyrolysate. *Chem. Lett.,* 1061–1064.
2. Bruce, W. R., Varghese, A. J., Wang, S., and Dion, P. (1979): The endogenous production of nitroso compounds in the colon and cancer at that site. In: *Naturally Occurring Carcinogens-Mutagens and Modulators of Carcinogenesis,* edited by E. C. Miller, J. A. Miller, I. Hirono, T. Sugimura, and S. Takayama, pp. 221–228. University Park Press, Baltimore.
3. Commoner, B., Vithayathil, A. J., Dolara, P., Nair, S., Madyastha, P., and Cuca, G. C. (1978): Formation of mutagens in beef and beef extract during cooking. *Science,* 201:913–916.
4. Conney, A. H., Pantuck, E. J., Hsiao, K.-C., Garland, W. A., Anderson, K. E., Alvares, A. P., and Kappas, A. (1976): Enhanced phenacetin metabolism in human subjects fed charcoal-broiled beef. *Clin. Pharmacol. Ther.,* 20:633–642.
5. Hill, M. J., Drasar, B. S., Aries, V., Crowther, J. S., Hawksworth, G., and Williams, R. E. O. (1971): Bacteria and aetiology of cancer of large bowel. *Lancet,* 1:95–100.
6. Ikeda, Y., Horiuchi, S., Furuya, T., Uchida, O., Suzuki, K., and Azegami, J. (1974): *Induction of Gastric Tumors in Mice by Feeding of Furylfuramide.* Food Sanitation Study Council, Ministry of Health and Welfare, Tokyo, Japan.
7. Ishidate, M., Tanimura, A., Ito, Y., Sakai, A., Sakuta, H., Kawamura, T., Sakai, K., Miyazawa, F., and Wada, H. (1972): Secondary amines, nitrites and nitrosamines in Japanese foods. In: *Topics in Chemical Carcinogenesis,* edited by W. Nakahara, S. Takayama, T. Sugimura, and S. Odashima, pp. 313–322. University of Tokyo Press, Tokyo.
8. Ishii, K., Ando, M., Kamataki, T., Kato, R., and Nagao, M. (1980): Metabolic activation of mutagenic tryptophan pyrolysis products (Trp-P-1 and Trp-P-2) by a purified cytochrome P-450-dependent monooxygenase system. *Cancer Lett.,* 9:271–276.
9. Ishikawa, T., Takayama, S., Kitagawa, T., Kawachi, T., Kinebuchi, M., Matsukura, N., Uchida, E., and Sugimura, T. (1979): *In vivo* experiments on tryptophan pyrolysis products. In: *Naturally*

*Occurring Carcinogens-Mutagens and Modulators of Carcinogenesis,* edited by E. C. Miller, J. A. Miller, I. Hirono, T. Sugimura, and S. Takayama, pp. 159–167. University Park Press, Baltimore.

10. Kada, T. (1973): *Escherichia coli* mutagenicity of furylfuramide. *Jpn. J. Genet.,* 48:301–305.
11. Kasai, H., Yamaizumi, Z., Wakabayashi, K., Nagao, M., Sugimura, T., Yokoyama, S., Miyazawa, T., Spingarn, N. E., Weisburger, J. H., and Nishimura, S. (1980): Potent novel mutagens produced by broiling fish under normal conditions. *Proc. Jpn. Acad.* 56:278–283.
12. Kawabata, T., Ohshima, H., Uibu, J., Nakamura, M., Matsui, M., and Hamano, M. (1979): Occurrence, formation, and precursors of N-nitroso compounds in Japanese diet. In: *Naturally Occurring Carcinogens-Mutagens and Modulators of Carcinogenesis,* edited by E. C. Miller, J. A. Miller, I. Hirono, T. Sugimura, and S. Takayama, pp. 195–209. University Park Press, Baltimore.
13. Kinebuchi, M., Kawachi, T., Matsukura, N., and Sugimura, T. (1979): Further studies on the carcinogenicity of a food additive, AF-2, in hamsters. *Food Cosmet. Toxicol.,* 17:339–341.
14. Kinoshita, R. (1936): Research on the cancerogenesis of the various chemical substances. *Gann,* 30:423–426 (in Japanese).
15. Kondo, S., and Ichikawa-Ryo, H. (1973): Testing and classification of mutagenicity of furylfuramide in *Escherichia coli. Jpn. J. Genet.,* 48:295–300.
16. Kosuge, T., Tsuji, K., Wakabayashi, K., Okamoto, T., Shudo, K., Iitaka, Y., Itai, A., Sugimura, T., Kawachi, T., Nagao, M., Yahagi, T., and Seino, Y. (1978): Isolation and structure studies of mutagenic principles in amino acid pyrolysates. *Chem. Pharm. Bull. (Tokyo),* 26:611–619.
17. Kuroda, Y. (1979): Mutagenic activity of tryptophan pyrolysates on human diploid cells in culture. *Proc. Jpn. Cancer Assoc.,* 38th Ann. Meet., Tokyo, Abstract #540, p. 155. (in Japanese).
18. Lijinsky, W., and Shubik, P. (1964): Benzo(a)pyrene and other polynuclear hydrocarbons in charcoal-broiled meat. *Science,* 145:53–55.
19. Lin, J. Y., Wang, H.-I., and Yeh, Y.-C. (1979): The mutagenicity of soy bean sauce. *Food Cosmet. Toxicol.,* 17:329–331.
20. Mandel, M., Ichinotsubo, D., and Mower, H. (1977): Nitroso group exchange as a way of activation of nitrosamines by bacteria. *Nature,* 267:248–249.
21. Marquardt, H., Rufino, F., and Weisburger, J. H. (1977): On the aetiology of gastric cancer: Mutagenicity of food extracts after incubation with nitrite. *Food Cosmet. Toxicol.,* 15:97–100.
22. Matsumoto, T., Yoshida, D., Mizusaki, S., and Okamoto, H. (1977): Mutagenic activity of amino acid pyrolyzates in *Salmonella typhimurium* TA98. *Mutat. Res.,* 48:279–286.
23. Matsushima, T., Sugimura, T., Nagao, M., Yahagi, T., Shirai, A., and Sawamura, M. (1980): Factors modulating mutagenicity in microbial tests. In: *Short-term Mutagenicity Test System for Detecting Carcinogens,* edited by K. Norpoth and R. C. Garner, pp. 273–285. Springer-Verlag, Berlin.
24. Meselson, M., and Russell, K. (1977): Comparisons of carcinogenic and mutagenic potency. In: *Origins of Human Cancer,* edited by H. H. Hiatt, J. D. Watson, and J. A. Winsten, pp. 1473–1481. Cold Spring Harbor Laboratory, Cold Spring Harbor, New York.
25. Miller, J. A., and Miller, E. C. (1953): The carcinogenic aminoazo dyes. *Adv. Cancer Res.,* 1:339–396.
26. Mirvish, S. S. (1972): Studies on N-nitrosation reactions: Kinetics of nitrosation, correlation with mouse feeding experiments, and natural occurrence of nitrosatable compounds (ureides and guanidines). In: *Topics in Chemical Carcinogenesis,* edited by W. Nakahara, S. Takayama, T. Sugimura, and S. Odashima, pp. 279–295. University of Tokyo Press, Tokyo.
27. Mirvish, S. S., Wallcave, L., Eagen, M., and Shubik, P. (1972): Ascorbate nitrite reaction: Possible means of blocking the formation of carcinogenic N-nitroso compounds. *Science,* 177:65–68.
28. Miyaji, T. (1971): Acute and chronic toxicity of furylfuramide in rats and mice. *Tohoku J. Exp. Med.,* 103:331–369.
29. Montesano, R., and Bartsch, H. (1976): Mutagenic and carcinogenic N-nitroso compounds: Possible environmental hazards. *Mutat. Res.,* 32:179–228.
30. Nagao, M., Honda, M., Seino, Y., Yahagi, T., Kawachi, T., and Sugimura, T. (1977): Mutagenicities of protein pyrolysates. *Cancer Lett.,* 2:335–340.
31. Nagao, M., Honda, M., Seino, Y., Yahagi, T., and Sugimura, T. (1977): Mutagenicities of smoke condensates and the charred surface of fish and meat. *Cancer Lett.,* 2:221–226.

32. Nagao, M., Yahagi, T., Kawachi, T., Seino, Y., Honda, M., Matsukura, N., Sugimura, T., Wakabayashi, K., Tsuji, K., and Kosuge, T. (1977): Mutagens in foods, and especially pyrolysis products of protein. In: *Progress in Genetic Toxicology*, edited by D. Scott, B. A. Bridges, and F. H. Sobels, pp. 259–264. Elsevier/North-Holland Biomedical Press, Amsterdam.

33. Nebert, D. W., Bigelow, S. W., Okey, A. B., Yahagi, T., Mori, Y., Nagao, M., and Sugimura, T. (1979): Pyrolysis products from amino acids and protein: Highest mutagenicity requires cytochrome $P_1$-450. *Proc. Natl. Acad. Sci. USA*, 76:5929–5933.

34. Pantuck, E. J., Hsiao, K.-C., Kuntzman, R., and Conney, A. H. (1975): Intestinal metabolism of phenacetin in the rat: Effect of charcoal-broiled beef and rat chow. *Science*, 187:744–746.

35. Pariza, M. W., Ashoor, S. H., Chu, F. S., and Lund, D. B. (1979): Effects of temperature and time on mutagen formation in pan-fried hamburger. *Cancer Lett.*, 7:63–69.

36. Spingarn, N. E., and Garvie, C. T. (1979): Formation of mutagens in sugar–ammonia model systems. *J. Agric. Food Chem.*, 27:1319–1321.

37. Spingarn, N. E., Kasai, H., Vuolo, L. L., Nishimura, S., Yamaizumi, Z., Sugimura, T., Matsushima, T., and Weisburger, J. H. (1980): Formation of mutagens in cooked foods. III. Isolation of a potent mutagen from beef. *Cancer Lett.*, 9:177–183.

38. Spingarn, N. E., Slocum, L. A., and Weisburger, J. H. (1980): Formation of mutagens in cooked foods. II. Foods with high starch content. *Cancer Lett.*, 9:7–12.

39. Sugimura, T. (1979): Naturally occurring genotoxic carcinogens. In: *Naturally Occurring Carcinogens-Mutagens and Modulators of Carcinogenesis*, edited by E. C. Miller, J. A. Miller, I. Hirono, T. Sugimura, and S. Takayama, pp. 241–261. University Park Press, Baltimore.

40. Sugimura, T., Kawachi, T., Nagao, M., Yahagi, T., Seino, Y., Okamoto, T., Shudo, K., Kosuge, T., Tsuji, K., Wakabayashi, K., Iitaka, Y., and Itai, A. (1977): Mutagenic principle(s) in tryptophan and phenylalanine pyrolysis products. *Proc. Jpn. Acad.*, 53:58–61.

41. Sugimura, T., and Nagao, M. (1979): Mutagenic factors in cooked foods. *CRC Crit. Rev. Toxicol.*, 6:189–209.

42. Sugimura, T., Nagao, M., Kawachi, Ty, Honda, M., Yahagi, T., Seino, Y., Sato, S., Matsukura, N., Matsushima, T., Shirai, A., Sawamura, M., and Matsumoto, H. (1977): Mutagen-carcinogens in food, with special reference to highly mutagenic pyrolytic products in broiled foods. In: *Origins of Human Cancer*, edited by H. H. Hiatt, J. D. Watson, and J. A. Winsten, pp. 1561–1577. Cold Spring Harbor Laboratory, Cold Spring Harbor, New York.

43. Takayama, S., Hirakawa, T., and Sugimura, T. (1978): Malignant transformation *in vitro* by tryptophan pyrolysis products. *Proc. Jpn. Acad.*, 54B:418–422.

44. Takayama, S., Hirakawa, T., Tanaka, M., Kawachi, T., and Sugimura, T. (1979): *In vitro* transformation of hamster embryo cells with a glutamic acid pyrolysis product. *Toxicol. Lett.*, 4:281–284.

45. Takayama, S., Katoh, Y., Tanaka, M., Nagao, M., Wakabayashi, K., and Sugimura, T. (1977): *In vitro* transformation of hamster embryo cells with tryptophan pyrolysis products. *Proc. Jpn. Acad.*, 53B:126–129.

46. Takeda, K., Ohta, T., Shudo, K., Okamoto, T., Tsuji, K., and Kosuge, T. (1977): Synthesis of a mutagenic principle isolated from tryptophan pyrolysate. *Chem. Pharm. Bull. (Tokyo)*, 25:2145–2146.

47. Takeda, K., Shudo, K., Okamoto, T., and Kosuge, T. (1978): Synthesis of mutagenic principles isolated from L-glutamic acid pyrolysate. *Chem. Pharm. Bull. (Tokyo)*, 26:2924–2925.

48. Tannenbaum, S. R. (1979): Endogenous formation of nitrite and N-nitroso compounds. In: *Naturally Occurring Carcinogens-Mutagens and Modulators of Carcinogenesis*, edited by E. C. Miller, J. A. Miller, I. Hirono, T. Sugimura, and S. Takayama, pp. 211–220. University Park Press, Baltimore.

49. Tohda, H., Oikawa, A., Kawachi, T., and Sugimura, T. (1980): Induction of sister-chromatid exchanges by mutagens from amino acid and protein pyrolysates. *Mutat. Res.*, 77:65–69.

50. Tsuda, M., Takahashi, Y., Nagao, M., Hirayama, T., and Sugimura, T. (1980): Inactivation of mutagens from pyrolysates of tryptophan and glutamic acid by nitrite in acidic solution. *Mutat. Res.*, 78:331–339.

51. Uyeta, M., Kanada, T., Mazaki, M., Taue, S., and Takahashi, S. (1979): Assaying mutagenicity of food pyrolysis products using the Ames test. In: *Naturally Occurring Carcinogens-Mutagens and Modulators of Carcinogenesis*, edited by E. C. Miller, J. A. Miller, I. Hirono, T. Sugimura, and S. Takayama, pp. 169–176. University Park Press, Baltimore.

52. Wakabayashi, K., Tsuji, K., Kosuge, T., Takeda, K., Yamaguchi, K., Shudo, K., Iitaka, Y.,

Okamoto, T., Yahagi, T., Nagao, M., and Sugimura, T. (1978): Isolation and structure determination of a mutagenic substance in L-lysine pyrolysate. *Proc. Jpn. Acad.*, 54B:569–571.

53. Weisburger, J. H., Marquardt, H., Hirota, N., Mori, H., and Williams, G. M. (1980): Induction of cancer of the glandular stomach in rats by an extract of nitrite-treated fish. *J. Natl. Cancer Inst.*, 64:163–167.

54. Wiebel, F. J., Gelboin, H. V., Buu-Hoi, N. P., Stout, M. G., and Burnham, W. S. (1974): Flavones and polycyclic hydrocarbons as modulators of aryl hydrocarbon [benzo*(a)*pyrene] hydroxylase. In: *The Biochemistry of Disease (Vol. 4), Chemical Carcinogenesis,* edited by P. O. P. Ts'o and J. A. DiPaolo, Part A, pp. 249–270. Marcel Dekker, Inc., New York.

55. Wogan, G. N. (1973): Aflatoxin carcinogenesis. *Methods Cancer Res.*, 7:309–344.

56. Yahagi, T., Matsushima, T., Nagao, M., Seino, Y., Sugimura, T., and Bryan, G. T. (1976): Mutagenicities of nitrofuran derivatives on a bacterial tester strain with an R factor plasmid. *Mutat. Res.*, 40:9–14.

57. Yahagi, T., Nagao, M., Hara, K., Matsushima, T., Sugimura, T., and Bryan, G. T. (1974): Relationships between the carcinogenic and mutagenic or DNA-modifying effects of nitrofuran derivatives, including 2-(2-furyl)-3-(5-nitro-2-furyl)acrylamide, a food additive. *Cancer Res.*, 34:2266–2273.

58. Yahagi, T., Nagao, M., Seino, Y., Matsushima, T., Sugimura, T., and Okada, M. (1977): Mutagenicities of *N*-nitrosamines on *Salmonella*. *Mutat. Res.*, 48:121–130.

59. Yamada, M., Tsuda, M., Nagao, M., Mori, M., and Sugimura, T. (1979): Degradation of mutagens from pyrolysates of tryptophan, glutamic acid and globulin by myeloperoxidase. *Biochem. Biophys. Res. Commun.*, 90:769–776.

60. Yamaguchi, K., Zenda, H., Shudo, K., Kosuge, T., Okamoto, T., and Sugimura, T. (1979): Presence of 2-aminodipyrido[1,2-*a*:3',2'-*d*]imidazole in casein pyrolysate. *Gann*, 70:849–850.

61. Yamaizumi, Z., Shiomi, T., Kasai, H., Nishimura, S., Takahashi, Y., Nagao, M., and Sugimura, T. (1980): Detection of potent mutagens, Trp-P-1 and Trp-P-2, in broiled fish. *Cancer Lett.*, 9:75–83.

62. Yamamoto, T., Tsuji, K., Kosuge, T., Okamoto, T., Shudo, K., Takeda, K., Iitaka, Y., Yamaguchi, K., Seino, Y., Yahagi, T., Nagao, M., and Sugimura, T. (1978): Isolation and structure determination of mutagenic substances in L-glutamic acid pyrolysate. *Proc. Jpn. Acad.*, 54B:248–250.

63. Yoshida, D., and Matsumoto, T. (1978): Changes in mutagenicity of protein pyrolyzates by reaction with nitrite. *Mutat. Res.*, 58:25–40.

64. Yoshida, D., Matsumoto, T., Yoshimura, R., and Matsuzaki, T. (1978): Mutagenicity of amino-α-carbolines in pyrolysis products of soybean globulin. *Biochem. Biophys. Res. Commun.*, 83:915–920.

*Nutrition and Cancer: Etiology and Treatment,*
edited by G. R. Newell and N. M. Ellison.
Raven Press, New York © 1981.

# Relationship of Nutrition to Immunology and Cancer

## Laurie Hoffman-Goetz and George L. Blackburn

*Nutrition Support Service and Nutrition/Metabolism Laboratory, Cancer Research Institute, New England Deaconess Hospital, Harvard Medical School, Boston, Massachusetts 02215*

Nutrition, immunology, and cancer are three broad areas whose interrelationships were not systematically investigated until recently. Nutritional support of the cancer patient, primarily through the process of arresting weight loss, improves the patient's sense of well-being, increases the likelihood of a positive response to tumor therapy, and decreases the morbidity associated with cancer treatment and/or secondary infections (57,36). Nutritional support can be a significant component in the implementation of effective antitumor therapies.

Cancer-induced cachexia and anorexia are major factors in the development of malnutrition, which commonly leads to attenuation of optimal immune functions, an increase in morbidity associated with secondary infections, and an increase in mortality arising from infection-related complications (6,8,9,16,73). Cancer-related malnutrition is exacerbated by surgery, chemotherapy, and radiotherapy, and can preclude the necessary radical treatment of the tumor. In certain tumor groups, nutritional intervention can improve the host's nutritional and immunological status, with a consequent improvement in response rate to cancer therapy.

## THE IMMUNE SYSTEM

To the clinician and biologist, immunity implies resistance to infectious agents, foreign particles, toxins, living cells, and cancer. Immunologic competence is based on the individual's ability to recognize foreign molecules (antigens) and to react to such substances with specific responses. Although the immune system involves the complex interactions of lymphocytes, phagocytes, the vascular system, immunoglobulins, complement, endogenous protein mediators, lymphokines, and other factors, for simplicity, three major types of leukocyte-mediated reactions can be elucidated: (a) the thymus-derived (T) lymphocyte, which stimulates the cellular immune response; (b) the bursal equivalent, immunoglobulin-synthesizing (B) lymphocyte; and (c) the heterogenous population of accessory cells, including macrophages, monocytes, Kupffer cells, and a variety of other

73

mobile and fixed-tissue phagocytes which participate in the induction of the immune response. These three populations of leukocytes (T, B, and A) can be further subdivided into groups of specialized cells on the basis of their specific and restricted immunologic functions and unique identifying surface markers or receptor sites (63,83).

The T-lymphocyte population can be classified as suppressors, helpers, and killers (41), and each of these subpopulations is functionally and biophysically distinct from the others. The accessory cell population has received considerable attention in recent years, largely because of the pivotal nature of the macrophage in the regulation and induction of many immune responses (7,25,28).

Host immunologic mechanisms are, at the same time, local and systemic, specific and nonspecific, humoral and cellular. It is difficult to identify any specific antigen that fails to elicit multiple leukocyte responses. Indeed, the concept of overlapping host defenses, or "immunologic redundancy," is crucial to the understanding of susceptibility to disease. Most cooperative immune interactions and activities depend on protein synthesis. Nutritional deprivation or depletion, caused by dietary inadequacies, increased protein catabolism after injury, or cancer, may result in altered immune competence.

There is a variety of techniques for measuring the impact of nutritional status on immune function. These diagnostic methods range from a simple white blood cell count to the skin-test antigen reactions (23). The more complex the cell-to-cell interactions in producing the responses being measured, the more likely it is that extraneous factors will be introduced into the results. On the other hand, the techniques that measure simple cell activity parameters may provide very little clinically significant information about the actual immune mechanisms and functions.

### T-Cell-Dependent Immunity

Cellular immunity, including the so-called "delayed hypersensitivity reactions," is of profound importance in host defense against microbial diseases, autoimmune disorders, some acquired allergies, and cancer. Cellular immunity is primarily T-lymphocyte dependent, although B-cell and A-cell populations also have regulatory and modulating effects on cell-mediated immunity (70).

Prior to entering the circulation or lymphoid tissue, T-cells differentiate into small lymphocytes with specific antigen receptor sites on their cell surfaces. The specific antigen receptor sites on the surface of T-lymphocytes form the basis of cell-mediated immunity. Induction and amplification of cellular immunity occurs when immunologically reactive T-lymphocytes, bearing the appropriate surface receptor sites, combine with a specific antigen. Whether the T-cell differentiates into an immunologically reactive cell, becomes specifically tolerant, or ignores the antigen depends on a variety of factors, including the concentration of antigen and the interaction with other specialized T-cells (e.g., helper cells), lymphokines, and accessory macrophages (39).

Delayed hypersensitivity skin reactions characterize the immunologic alterations that accompany cellular immune responses. If tuberculin or some other appropriate stimulatory antigen is injected intradermally in a sensitized individual, an erythematous, indurated lesion develops, reaching its maximum size 48 to 72 hours after injection. Microscopic examination of the lesion area reveals a mild inflammatory response, with only a few lymphocytes initially present. During the subsequent 48 to 72 hours, the site becomes densely infiltrated with lymphocytes and accessory cells (primarily macrophages). The binding of the T-lymphocyte receptor sites to the specific antigen provides the stimulus for the elaboration of substances known as lymphokines, which mediate various nonspecific and accessory cell immune responses.

Interferon, migration inhibitory factor (MIF), and macrophage activation factor (MAF) are only a few of the lymphokines that actively affect immunocompetence (19). Interferons are a heterogenous group of proteins elaborated by T-lymphocytes which induce an antiviral state in noninfected cells (31). Migration inhibitory factor, a lymphokine produced by activated T-lymphocytes, retards the migration of macrophages (and monocytes) from the microcirculation into the interstitial spaces and the tissues. Changes in the surface properties of the macrophages, resulting in greater adherence or "stickiness" to the lesion site, occur in the presence of MIF (70). Macrophage activation factor enhances the bactericidal and phagocytic aggressiveness of target macrophages. Other lymphokines elaborated by activated lymphocytes act as mitogens, stimulating differentiation and proliferation of uncommitted lymphocytes. In addition to lymphokines secreted by activated lymphocytes that have as their target cells monocytes and macrophages, macrophages and monocytes produce prostaglandins ($E_1$ and $E_2$) which appear to have certain regulatory effects on lymphocyte proliferation (44). A feedback loop with A-, T-, and B-cells participating in cellular immunity and delayed hypersensitivity responses supports the concept of a complex, cooperative immunologic system (Fig. 1).

## B-Cell-Dependent Immunity

The induction of immunoglobulin-synthesizing cells (plasma cells) from B-lymphocytes is a complex endpoint reaction. Cooperation between T-, B-, and A-cell populations is necessary for the mediation of this reaction. Synthesis of the five immunoglobulin classes (IgG, IgM, IgE, IgD, and IgA) requires T-, B-, and A-cell interactions (33). Defects in A- or T-cell action would decrease or inhibit immunoglobulin responses; conversely, defects in immunoglobulin production influence the activation of complement factors, the degree of phagocytosis, and the appearance of certain types of delayed hypersensitivity reactions (28,35).

Of the major classes of immunoglobulins, IgG is the most abundant and perhaps the most important in man, insofar as it includes antibodies to most bacteria, virus-neutralizing antibodies, precipitating antibodies, hemagglutinins,

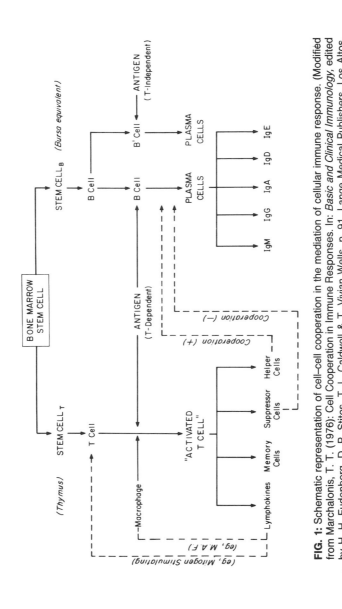

**FIG. 1:** Schematic representation of cell–cell cooperation in the mediation of cellular immune response. (Modified from Marchalonis, T. T. (1976): Cell Cooperation in Immune Responses. In: *Basic and Clinical Immunology*, edited by H. H. Fudenberg, D. P. Stites, T. L. Caldwell & T. Vivian Wells, p. 91. Lange Medical Publishers, Los Altos, California.)

and incomplete hemolysins. IgM is a powerful activator of the complement system in man and is the predominant immunoglobulin formed in response to Gram-negative bacteria. IgE represents an important class of immunoglobulin which includes reagins that cause many allergic reactions. Although the function of IgD is not clear at this time, it is usually associated with IgM-synthesizing cells, suggesting that it is involved in antigen recognition or functions as a precursor of IgM. IgA ("secretory IgA") is found predominantly in the submucosal surfaces of the respiratory and gastrointestinal tracts and secretory glands. Secretory IgA serves as a first-line defense against invasion of microorganisms across mucosal surfaces.

Transplantation of certain organs is now a common clinical procedure, although a large percentage of such transplants are eventually rejected by the host. The rejection response has both humoral and cellular components. Circulating immunoglobulins in the serum of the recipient can react with donor (foreign) cells. This is associated with hyperacute graft rejection (accelerated or immediate graft rejection), deposition of platelets and fibrin in the graft vessels, and invasion of the neighboring tissues by granulocytes. A more delayed and slowly progressive rejection is accompanied by invasion and infiltration of the graft tissue by host monocytes.

One of the principal "functions" of immunoglobulin is its specific attachment to antigen and the activation of the complement cascade. Activation and fixation of the complement cascade ($C'1q,r,s:C'2-4,C'3,C'5-6,C'7,C'8,C'9$) initiates bacteriolysis. Split products of $C'3$ are pivotal mediators of the primary immune response. C3a has anaphylatoxic, chemotactic, and leukocyte-mobilizing properties, whereas C3b promotes opsonization through immune adherence (17,58).

The complement system is involved in the elimination of foreign cells, the initiation and control of the inflammatory response, and the circulation of blood vis-á-vis its potent kinin influences on vascular reactivity (58). The complement system stands at the center of effector processes of specific host immune reactions, and near the center for nonspecific host defenses.

## Accessory Cell-Dependent Immunity

Natural resistance to potential antigens, which forms the basis of nonspecific immunity, is mediated primarily through the accessory cell population; however, nonspecific immunity also includes the combined effects of anatomic barriers, lymphokines, and various endogenous effector–mediator substances that are products of activated lymphocytes and phagocytes.

The phagocytic, chemotactic, and bactericidal activities of the A-cell populations are critical to the maintenance of immune competence. The A-cell phagocytes remove foreign particles and pathogens in the processes of chemotaxis, opsonization, ingestion, and killing. The action of chemotactic substances on A-cells is presumably on the surface receptor sites, resulting in a change in their direction of movement.

Opsonization, the process by which antigens are prepared for ingestion by phagocytes, is pivotal in the immune reactions of A-cells. Serum opsonins prepare the antigen for digestion by acting as receptor site "bridges" on the surface of the phagocyte, amplifying the contact and adherence with the antigen. Ingestion or encapsulation of the antigen within a phagosome and the destruction of the particle occurs in association with degranulation and release of the granule contents into the phagosomic vacuole. Such granules contain abundant hydrolytic enzymes, such as myeloperoxidase, lysosyme, catalase, and bacteriostatic proteins, such as lactoferrin. Although the mechanisms by which pathogens are killed within the phagosome are not well understood, two systems of bacteriolysis are present: oxidative and nonoxidative (25).

Endogenous mediators synthesized by A-cells also interact in nonspecific immunity. For example, endogenous pyrogen (also known as leukocytic endogenous mediator), which may be synthesized or cleaved from an inactive precursor in tissue and in mobile phagocytes, stimulates a variety of metabolic alterations during acute infection and inflammation, including the development of fever and the alteration in plasma trace mineral levels. These responses have a particularly important role in Gram-negative bacteriostasis (43,88).

## TESTS FOR IMMUNOCOMPETENCY

One of the major challenges of modern medicine is the translation of basic knowledge in immunology to clinically useful diagnostic and therapeutic agents. Assays of immune function vary from the simple counting of peripheral lymphocyte populations to the extremely sophisticated radioimmunoassay of immunoglobulin. No one test of immune function delineates all the endpoint reactions among A-, T-, and B-cells, synthesis of complement, production of lymphokines, or endogenous mediator products of phagocytes. Perhaps the most valuable information gained by these immunodiagnostic procedures is that of the enormous complexity and cooperation that exist among the leukocyte populations.

### Measurements of Peripheral Blood T-, B-, and A-cells

Enumeration of total lymphocytes in peripheral circulation has been used as a rough index of immune function; for example, patients with "classic" kwashiorkor have a mild leukopenia that may be correlated with depressed synthesis of visceral proteins and depressed immune functions (42). However, the interpretation of reduced lymphocyte counts is complicated by many variables. The presence of a large wound may transiently decrease blood lymphocytes as a result of the lymphocytes' migration into the lesion site (86). This trapping of lymphocytes out of the circulation is probably important in explaining the rapid changes in total lymphocyte counts. The normal number of peripheral blood lymphocytes varies from individual to individual. It is not altogether clear at what point a decrease in peripheral blood lymphocyte number affects or reflects immunocompetency. It may be that moderate decreases in the total lymphocyte number are functionally irrelevant to immune competence.

It is therefore obvious that an evaluation of possible defects in lymphocytes cannot be based solely on peripheral blood counts. Tests that quantitate subpopulations of lymphocytes and measure the functional activities of these cells are often required for full evaluation of the immune defense system. For example, although a total peripheral lymphocyte count may be normal, the proportion of functional subpopulations (T-cell versus B-cell; killer cell versus helper cell) may be profoundly altered. Such alterations in the proportion or percentage of specific functional types of lymphocytes can be evaluated by tests of morphology and function, i.e., enumeration of T-cells by sheep cell rosettes (E rosettes), enumeration of B-cells by immunofluorescence with anti-immunoglobulin serum, and/or rosette formation with red cells coated with complement.

## Mitogen-Induced Lymphocyte Proliferation

A variety of substances can stimulate the proliferative expansion of specific T- and B-lymphocytes. The functional ability of lymphocytes to proliferate or undergo blastogenesis can be measured *in vitro* by assessing mitogen-induced proliferation. Plant lectins, such as phytohemagglutinin (PHA), concanavalin A (ConA), and pokeweed mitogen (PWM) stimulate lymphocyte receptors, triggering cell division. PHA and ConA stimulate T-cell proliferation (72) in the presence of macrophages (65). PWM will stimulate B-cell blastogenesis only when both T- and A-cell interactions are present (39).

Although mitogen-induced proliferative assays can indicate immune dysfunction of T-, B-, and A-cells, these assays fail to measure the more subtle changes in immune function, such as the failure to secrete lymphokines. In addition, patients with known immune deficits, such as those characterized by myasthenia gravis, may have normal or even elevated mitogen responses (9). Consequently, a decreased mitogen-induced response probably indicates defective immune competence, but a normal mitogen response may not always indicate normal immune function.

The primary difficulty in the utilization of mitogen assays is the exacting technical methodology required, which can greatly modify the results. (Mitogen assays are performed by measuring the uptake of tritiated thymidine [$^3$H-TdR] by lymphocytes after *in vitro* culture with mitogen [82].) The commercially available mitogen preparations, such as PHA, have differential stimulatory effects on lymphocyte proliferation. Contamination and impurities in PHA preparations can cause the agglutination of cells, with a resultant decrease in the response observed (56). Patients do not represent a homogeneous population of normal proliferative responses. Each patient must be used as his/her own control, and the data cannot be averaged. In addition, such factors as the concentration of lymphocytes, incubation time, geometry of the culture vessel, dose of mitogen, and dose–response kinetics of mitogen-stimulated cultures can greatly affect the results of this test.

Despite the inherent difficulties in evaluating radioisotope-treated cultures, such as $^3$H-TdR mitogen preparations, one study by Reilly and associates (69) has produced some provocative results in the *in vivo* metabolic interaction between the host liver tissue, tumor, and nutritional status. These investigators found that starvation in tumor-bearing rats resulted in an increase in DNA synthesis, as measured by $^3$H-TdR incorporation into tumor DNA, when compared with normally fed tumor-bearing control rats. Reilly et al. suggested that acute fasting may result in increased tumor growth, as measured by the uptake of the radioactive DNA precursor.

### Delayed Hypersensitivity Reactions to Skin-Test Antigens

Measurement of the response to an intradermal injection of antigen, such as purified protein derivative (PPD), histoplasmin, *Candida* antigen, streptokinase–streptodornase (SK–SD), and mumps antigen, is one of the most widely utilized assays for analysis of immune competency. This assay has the advantage of measuring aggregate or comprehensive *in vivo* reactions. The induration measured at the site of the intradermal antigen is the endpoint reaction of a complex series of cell-to-cell interactions and lymphokine mediation. In delayed hypersensitivity responses, the antigen stimulates A- and then T-cells to effect the sensitization of T-lymphocytes. When the antigen is reinjected at the site, the sensitized T-lymphocytes are mobilized to the injection area. Lymphokines are secreted by the sensitized or activated T-lymphocytes, which chemotactically stimulate A-cells into the area and activate them via monocyte chemotactic factor (MCF) and leukocyte chemotactic factor (LCF).

The maximal positive skin-test response requires the interaction of macrophages (53). In addition, adequate lymphokine production, effective monocyte chemotaxis, and fully functional A-, T-, and B-cells are needed to effect the delayed hypersensitivity skin-test response.

The limitation of skin-antigen tests is that there are both physiological and technical problems inherent in the interpretation of delayed hypersensitivity responses; for example, capillary obstruction and vascular reactivity can greatly modify the response. Technical difficulties, such as variations in the strength of commercial antigen preparations, can influence the actual manifestations of the response (62). The etiologic mechanisms of immune deficiency also cannot be determined by this test; however, immune surveillance and assessment of health risk are greatly benefited.

### Immunoglobulin Synthesis

As with all other immune responses, the induction of mature immunoglobulin-synthesizing plasma cells involves the cooperative interaction of A-, T-, and B-cells (33). The problems associated with the measurement of the *de novo* synthesis of nonspecific antibody and the *de novo* stimulation of plasma cells require that highly sophisticated laboratory procedures be used.

### Accessory Cell Functions

Immunologic competence of A-cell functions may provide the optimal test for the evaluation of nutritional and oncologic influences on host defense mechanisms. Accessory cell functions are highly sensitive to alterations in substrate availability (24).

One of the most widely used tests for A-cell function is nitroblue tetrazolium dye (NTD) reduction. NTD is a clear, yellowish water-soluble dye that forms a dark blue dye, formazan, when it is reduced. Polymorphonuclear leukocytes assayed *in vitro* first ingest and then reduce the dye. Extraction of the polymorphonuclear leukocytes and spectrophotometric measurement of the reduced dye are useful means of assaying overall metabolic integrity of A-cells.

In light of the pivotal role of accessory cells (e.g., macrophages) in mediation of many immune responses, certain A-cell functions and their relation to nutritional and oncologic parameters should be more fully investigated. The response of monocytes to migration inhibitory factor (MIF) and the ability of A-cells to produce endogenous mediators (endogenous pyrogens), as well as their role in T-cell proliferation, also require investigation.

### Complement Levels

Radioimmunodiffusion is the most common technique for assaying complement levels (78). This assay is, however, dependent on the quality of the antiserum used. Moreover, nontechnical problems affecting the tests must be evaluated; for example, infection is known to dramatically decrease complement levels by activating and then catabolizing complement proteins. It also appears that in all but the most severe nutritional stresses, complement synthesis and functional integrity are protected (67).

In summary, tests of immune function measure a variety of different cell types, activities, and interactions. The basic cooperation among A-, B-, and T-cells in proliferation and recruitment, antibody production, and cellular immunity probably has a high metabolic priority (35). These parameters are, however, reduced by malnutrition and immunosuppressive drug therapy in the cancer patient.

## IMPACT OF NUTRITION ON IMMUNITY

Any nutrient deficiency or excess that adversely affects DNA synthesis, cell division and replication, differentiation of immunologically reactive cells, synthesis of complement, lymphokines, and endogenous mediator proteins, or the processes of normal cellular metabolism would be expected to affect immune function. The association of malnutrition and increased susceptibility to infection has been the subject of many epidemiologic, clinical, and experimental manipulations. It is clinically well known that infections tend to be more severe in malnourished patients. Infection from any cause can put the patient in a catabolic state, resulting in negative nitrogen balance, elevation in catecholamines, hyperglycemia, and further compromise of nutritional status. However, there is no cause–effect relationship between malnutrition and infection; rather, the data presented in the current literature show a strong correlation between nutritional status and susceptibility to infection, probably as a result of altered immune competency (2,8,9,16,17,23,24,29,35,37,40,45,47).

Of the two recognized extreme variants of protein–calorie malnutrition, kwashiorkor and marasmus, the former is characterized by an impairment in protein synthesis, as manifest by depressed serum protein levels, and the latter is characterized by better-protected serum levels, with a depression in standard anthropometric measurements.

Many patients in the United States, in the course of hospital therapy, consume a moderate-carbohydrate, low-protein diet, either enterally or parenterally. Often, the patient is given only intravenous glucose and electrolytes, but in the presence of severe catabolic stress caused by illness, trauma, or neoplasm, this type of nutritional support is inadequate and the patient may develop some form of malnutrition, often with a concomitant decline in immune responsiveness. Bistrian et al. (8) have shown that, in acute adult protein malnutrition found among hospitalized patients, cellular immunity is significantly depressed, as measured by contact sensitization to dinitrochlorobenzene (DNCB) and skin-test Candida antigen. The mechanism of the depressed cellular immunity in such patients is related, in part, to a significant leukopenia. The failure to develop a normal inflammatory reaction to DNCB is similar to the failure in classic pediatric kwashiorkor. The underlying mechanism for the depression in lymphocyte number and function was thought to be a depletion of amino acids available for protein synthesis by the combined effects of catabolic stress and infused dextrose.

To evaluate the effects of marasmic depletion on immune function, Bistrian et al. (9) studied 12 hospitalized patients with histories of recent illness and weight loss but without histories of primary immunodeficient disease or concurrent stress that may have activated differential immune functions. Immune function was assessed by a variety of techniques including delayed hypersensitivity (SK–SD and Candida allergic extract), total peripheral lymphocyte count, T- and B-cell quantification, and lymphocyte transformation in vitro. These investigations revealed that skin-test reactivity to antigens was reduced in adult marasmus; unlike adult hypoalbuminemic malnutrition, total lymphocyte counts were normal, the proportion of T-cells was not changed, and lymphocyte transformation was not significantly affected by adult marasmus. The authors suggested that the reasons the in vivo skin tests showed defective immune function and the in vitro tests did not may be related to the provision of amino acids in the culture media. The availability of amino acids in the culture media may have restored the immune function if the lymphocytes were still functional. Failure to achieve normal in vitro function by optimizing conditions with culture media in adult-type kwashiorkor (hypoalbuminemic malnutrition) may be the result of a deficit in the lymphocyte function per se.

Harvey et al. (36) nutritionally assessed 161 cancer patients prior to institution of oncologic therapy and found significant correlations between nutritional therapy, immune status, and patient outcome (mortality rate). Eighty-four percent of the initially anergic cancer patients who became immune competent with nutritional support had a significantly lower mortality rate compared with those cancer patients who remained anergic throughout their hospital stays. Patients who were initially immune competent and later became anergic had a higher mortality rate than did patients whose immune function was preserved.

A schematic diagram depicting the role of nutrition in cancer/immunologic interactions is given in Fig. 2. Major components in assessing the impact of nutritional support in anticancer therapies are tumor type, tumor size, and specific antineoplastic therapy required.

### Effect of Protein on Immune Function

Protein intake can markedly influence immune function. "Pure" protein deficiency, however, rarely occurs; more common is a multiple deficiency syndrome (characterized by a decrease in protein as well as calories).

Patients with mild to moderate hypoalbuminemia ($<3$ g/100 ml serum) may present with defects in cellular and hormonal immunity, delayed killing of phagocytosed antigens, and defects in tissue integrity (e.g., atrophy of the thymus gland) (74,79). Delayed hypersensitivity skin-test reactions may be absent, and leukopenia, particularly of T-lymphocytes, is evident.

Adult-hypoalbuminemia and pediatric kwashiorkor are usually associated with normal or high levels of immunoglobulins. The abundance of plasma cells in various tissues and extracellular fluids suggests that the patients may be attempting to mount an appropriate immune response (59). Some investigators have found that these patients are unable to respond to certain antigens with appropriate antibody production (45). Experimental investigations have also shown that protein depletion attenuates the production of endogenous mediator substances, such as endogenous pyrogen, from host A-cell populations (37).

Although there is abundant experimental, clinical, and epidemiologic evidence that correlates malnutrition with deficient immune function, the results of these studies are difficult to interpret, since many of the observed data are highly variable for three reasons. First, the antigens (e.g., skin test, humoral inducing) may not be standardized or specific. Second, certain antigens (e.g., polio) differ from other bacterial toxoids in the way they affect B-cells or involve T-helper or T-killer cells. Third, blood complement factors, macrophages, lymphokines, and endogenous pyrogen amplify and modulate the biological effects of T- and B-cells and of immunoglobulin. The status of these components must be evaluated before defective antibody or cellular immune function can be implicated with certainty in malnourished patients.

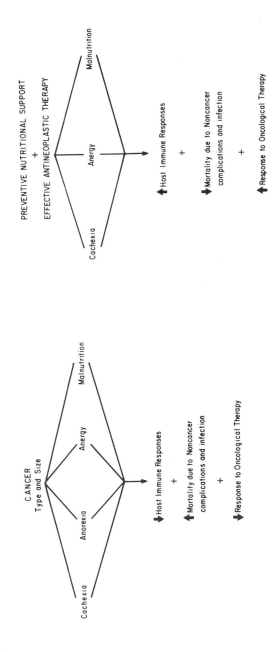

**FIG. 2:** Support and adjuvant role of nutrition in oncologic and immunologic interactions.

## Effect of Calories on Immune Function

Moderate calorie restriction does not appear to impair immune function as long as nutrient intake is adequate. Indeed, moderate calorie restriction throughout life may be beneficial. Experimental studies have shown that animals fed adequate but calorie-restricted diets lived 30% to 40% longer, their "optimal" immune function peaked later, and they had fewer spontaneous tumors, than did animals fed *ad libitum* (50,84,90).

## Effect of Fat on Immune Function

In several studies (52,54), the administration of polyunsaturated fatty acids resulted in the depression of T-cell function. Animals lost their ability to reject skin allografts when fed diets high in polyunsaturated fatty acids (54). Such animals also exhibit diminished T-cell responses to mitogen (13). Polyunsaturated fatty acids have been used as an adjuvant to immunosuppression in renal transplant patients (52). The mechanisms by which polyunsaturated fatty acids affect immune function are not known.

On the other hand, investigations by Ota and associates (61) have shown that esterified essential fatty acids increase the mitogenic response of human T-lymphocytes and the antigenic response of human lymphocytes *in vitro*. The addition of Intralipid (10% soybean oil emulsion–high linoleic acid) to culture media enhanced both PHA and Varidase lymphocyte transformation. The investigators suggested that, based on the *in vitro* results, the addition of Intralipid to a nutritional regimen for feeding malnourished patients may enhance their immunologic responses. Since patient survival or tumor response to chemotherapy, surgery, and radiotherapy has been related to the maintenance of host immunocompetence, intravenous hyperalimentation with essential fatty acids may improve the immunologic response during conventional oncologic therapies.

## Effect of Iron on Immune Function

Iron-deficiency anemia is a serious nutritional problem worldwide. Iron deficiency can exist without anemia and depletion of iron stores without any changes in the blood values; this type of deficiency can be associated with defects in DNA synthesis and cell proliferation, with tissue changes and enzyme aberrations. Iron deficiency can render a phagocyte (A-cell) immunoincompetent (47); for example, myeloperoxidase, an iron-based bactericidal enzyme localized within phagocytic granules, has a reduced concentration during iron-deficiency anemia. Iron deficiency probably affects all phagocytic cells, both fixed and mobile, in their ability to kill bacteria (4).

On the other hand, iron overload, hyperferremia, and/or hypotransferrinemia have been implicated in increased susceptibility to infections, particularly those of Gram-negative bacterial origin (88). The incidence of bacterial infections is enhanced in kwashiorkor/hypoalbuminemic malnutrition (51), sickle cell anemia (48), leukemia (14), and in all diseases in which iron saturation of transferrin is close to 100% (15). Procedures that reduce the percentage saturation of transferrin, lactoferrin, and other iron-binding proteins may enhance resistance to bacterial infections. Patients with iron deficiency and dimorphic anemias had low frequencies of bacterial infections (48,49). Mice fed iron-deficient diets had increased survivorship as compared with control mice when challenged with *Salmonella typhimurium* (66). There is extensive literature describing the effects of iron overload (dietary, hyperferremia due to hemolytic diseases, hyperferremia due to hypotransferrinemia) on host defense mechanisms. An excess of iron facilitates bacterial growth in biological fluids; however, although the experimental data are clear, their extrapolation into clinical situations is not as sharply defined. Because of multiple factors operating in the malnourished, cachectic, and/or acutely infected patient, it is still difficult to partition the role of a single factor, such as iron, in host immunologic function and susceptibility to infection.

## IMPACT OF CANCER ON NUTRITION STATUS

### Nutritional Consequences of Carcinoma

Cancer cachexia is a widely recognized but poorly understood clinical syndrome. The manifestations of cancer cachexia include anorexia, anergy, and alteration of metabolic integrity. Weight loss is a common finding in the patient with cachexia, probably as a result of anorexia, altered metabolism, and decreased absorption of food. Mullen and Hobbs (57) report that 10% weight loss is not uncommon in cancer cachexia.

Although the pathogenesis of cachexia is unclear and is probably complex, anorexia is considered to be the single major contributory factor. Other factors have been implicated, including altered taste perception (20,21), elevated blood lactate levels (5), increased thermogenic expenditures (3), and various psychological factors (64). Whatever the etiology of anorexia and cancer cachexia, the consequent nutritional deficits lead to a reduction in body fat, visceral protein, and skeletal muscle.

There are a few studies on the energy metabolism and nutritional requirements of cancer patients. Gold (34) found an increase in lactate production and Cori cycle activity. Increased conversion of lactate to glucose in the Cori cycle of cancer patients was correlated with weight loss and energy expenditure estimated at 10% of the patient's basal metabolic rate. Sims (77) found that cancer patients tend to convert glucose to fat before oxidation, rather than to oxidize glucose directly, and that this resulted in an increased energy expenditure of 20%. Additional studies are needed to ascertain the metabolic and nutritional requirements of cancer patients; however, from the limited number of studies currently available in the literature, it seems clear that cancer patients require higher energy intake to maintain homeostatic energy balance (87).

Alterations in electrolyte and mineral balance occur in certain cancer patients (11). Hypokalemia often accompanies adenocarcinomas of the colon. Elevated serum copper levels characteristically occur in patients with Hodgkin's disease (38). Correction of micronutrient deficiencies is essential for restoration of lean body mass and various immunologic functions.

A recent epidemiologic/nutritional survey of cancer patients in an acute care hospital showed that such patients had a mean weight loss of 10%, decreased fat stores, decreased serum albumin and transferrin levels, decreased lymphocyte counts, and impaired cellular immunity as measured by delayed hypersensitivity skin-test reactions (10). The picture that emerges from this type of study is of prevalent malnutrition, particularly of a combined adult marasmus/hypoalbuminemic malnutrition in adult cancer patients.

Cancer therapy, including surgery, chemotherapy, and radiotherapy, can alter the nutritional status of the cancer patient. For example, carcinomas of the gastrointestinal tract are usually managed by surgical resection. Since the gastrointestinal tract is the primary access route for nutrients, the problem of nutritional impairment is particularly significant. Induction of nutritional imbalances occurs as the result of decreased reservoir and emptying functions, decreased concentrations of digestive enzymes normally activated by gastric acid (85), decreased stimulation of secretin secretion (85), and decreased calorie intake. Perhaps the primary causative factor in nutritional depletion and weight loss in the gastrectomy patient is the decreased intake of calories. This is further complicated by inappropriate and/or inadequate nutritional support following surgical resection.

The nutritional consequences of small bowel carcinomas and subsequent surgical resection can be quite significant in terms of nutrient wastage. Massive small bowel resection results in gastric hypersecretion, leading to diarrhea and nutrient loss (32). In patients with massive small bowel resection, the appearance of dysfunctionalized segments ("blind loop syndrome") is linked to stasis, infection, diarrhea, steatorrhea, and weight loss (46).

Hepatic metastatic disease is often associated with nutritional problems both preoperatively and postoperatively. Prior to hepatic surgery, patients can become nutritionally compromised, and primary corrective surgery may be delayed. Postoperatively, cachexia and stress may further aggravate protein–calorie malnutrition at a time when adequate protein and calories are necessary for tissue regeneration and wound healing.

Cancer chemotherapy can produce deleterious side effects that alter the nutritional status of the cancer patient, such as nausea, vomiting, oral pain, and diarrhea, which can result in decreased appetite and decreased body weight. Chemotherapy-related malnutrition exacerbates the problems of an already nutritionally compromised patient. Diarrhea induced by chemotherapeutic agents is associated with dehydration, electrolyte imbalances, and nutritional depletion.

Radiotherapy given in high curative doses may also exacerbate a nutritionally compromised state. Radiotherapy to the head and neck can result in radiomucositis, with sore throat, dry mouth, pain on swallowing, decreased appetite, and decreased ability to taste (22). Small-bowel radiotherapy can produce nausea, diarrhea, weight loss, and consequent malnutrition; radiation enteritis is a frequent side effect of radiotherapeutic treatments (22).

Both the clinical and experimental data indicate that cancer produces malnutrition, and that surgery, chemotherapy, and/or radiotherapy are often synergistic to the initial condition of inadequate nutritional status. Regardless of the type of therapy used or the specific type of carcinoma present, the nutritional consequences of cancer and cancer therapy are profound and cumulative.

## CONCLUSIONS

Nutritional support of the cancer patient that improves immunologic integrity, concomitant with reduction of tumor size by appropriate antineoplastic therapy, decreases morbidity and mortality rates. The goal of the oncologic nutritionist is to provide maximum nutritional support of cancer patients as early in therapy as possible. An integral component of the patient's treatment and follow-up is nutritional assessment and support. Nutritional deterioration leading to malnutrition, anergy, and cachexia, and subsequent noncancer deaths and complications, may be avoided by early integrated, prevention-oriented nutritional support programs.

Early characterization of immune competency, with subsequent serial immune testing, is an important surveillance method. Development of malnutrition, together with changes in immune function, should alert the oncologist to the need for prompt nutritional support. Such nutritional intervention programs help preserve the patient's fitness and quality of life, as well as contribute to the efficacy of antineoplastic therapies.

## ACKNOWLEDGMENTS

This investigation was supported in part by grant number GM 22401-02 from the National Institutes of General Medical Sciences, NIH, and NO1-CP-65870 from the National Cancer Institute.

## REFERENCES

1. Abramsky, O., Aharonou, A., Webb, C., and Fuchs, S. (1975): Cellular immune response to acetylcholine receptor-rich fraction in patients with myasthenia gravis. *Clin. Exp. Immunol.,* 19:11–16.
2. Alvarado, J., and Luthringer, D. G. (1971): Serum immunoglobulins in edematous protein–calorie malnourished children. *Clin. Pediatr.,* 10:174–179.
3. Andersson, B., and Larsson, B. (1961): Influence of local temperature changes in the preoptic area and rostral hypothalamus on the regulation of food and water intake. *Acta Physiol. Scand.,* 52:75–89.
4. Baggs, R. B., and Miller, S. A. (1975): Defect in resistance to *Salmonella typhimurium* in iron deficient rats. *J. Infect. Dis.,* 130:409–411.
5. Baile, C. A., Zinn, W. M., and Mayer, J. (1970): Effects of lactate and other metabolites on food intake of monkeys. *Am. J. Physiol.,* 219:1606–1613.

6. Beisel, W. R. (1977): Malnutrition as a consequence of stress. In: *Malnutrition and the Immune Response,* edited by R. M. Suskind, pp. 21–26. Raven Press, New York.
7. Berlinger, N. T., Lopez, C., and Good, R. A. (1976): Facilitation or attenuation of mixed leukocyte culture responsiveness by adherent cells. *Nature,* 260:145–146.
8. Bistrian, B. R., Blackburn, G. L., Scrimshaw, N. S., and Flatt, J. P. (1975): Cellular immunity in semi-starved states in hospitalized adults. *Am. J. Clin. Nutr.,* 28:1148–1155.
9. Bistrian, B. R., Sherman, M., Blackburn, G. L., Marshall, R., and Shaw, C. (1977): Cellular immunity in adult marasmus. *Arch. Intern. Med.,* 137:1408–1411.
10. Blackburn, G. L., and Bistrian, B. R. (1977): Nutritional support resources in hospital practice. In: *Nutritional Support of Medical Practice,* edited by H. A. Schneider, C. E. Anderson, and D. B. Courrsin, pp. 139–151. Harper & Row Publishers, Hagerstown, New Jersey.
11. Blackburn, G. L., Maini, B., Bistrian, B. R., and McDermott, W. V., Jr. (1977): The effect of cancer on nitrogen, electrolytes and mineral metabolism. *Cancer Res.,* 37:2348–2353.
12. Brady, J. A., Overfield, T., and Hammes, L. M. (1966): Depression of the tuberculin reaction by viral vaccines. *N. Engl. J. Med.,* 274:67–72.
13. Broitman, S. A., Vitale, J. J., Vavrousek-Jakuba, E., and Gottlieb, L. S. (1977): Polyunsaturated fat, cholesterol and large bowel tumorigenesis. *Cancer Res.,* 40:2455–2463.
14. Caroline, L., Rosner, F., and Kozinn, P. (1969): Elevated serum iron, low unbound transferrin and candidiasis in acute leukemia. *Blood,* 34:441–451.
15. Caroline, L., Taschdjian, C. L., Kozinn, P. J., and Schade, A. L. (1964): Reversal of serum fungistasis by addition of iron. *J. Invest. Dermatol.,* 42:415–419.
16. Chandra, R. K. (1977): Cell-mediated immunity in fetally and postnatally malnourished children from India and Newfoundland. In: *Malnutrition and the Immune Response,* edited by R. M. Suskind, pp. 111–116. Raven Press, New York.
17. Cooper, F. C., Good, R. A., and Mariani, T. (1974): Effects of protein insufficiency on immune responsiveness. *Am. J. Clin. Nutr.,* 27:647–664.
18. Copeland, E. M., Daly, J. M., and Dudrick, S. J. (1977): Nutrition as an adjunct to cancer treatment in the adult. *Cancer Res.,* 37:2451–2456.
19. David, J. R., and David, R. A. (1972): Cellular hypersensitivity and immunity: Inhibition of macrophage migration and the lymphocyte mediators. *Prog. Allergy,* 16:300–449.
20. DeWys, W. D. (1974): A spectrum of organ systems that respond to the presence of cancer: Abnormalities of taste as a remote effect of a neoplasm. *Ann. N.Y. Acad. Sci.,* 230:427–434.
21. DeWys, W. D. (1977): Anorexia in cancer patients. *Cancer Res.,* 37:2354–2358.
22. Donaldson, S. S. (1977): Nutritional consequences of radiotherapy. *Cancer Res.,* 37:2407–2413.
23. Douglas, S. D., and Schopfer, K. (1976): Analytical review: Host defense mechanisms in protein–energy malnutrition. *Clin. Immunol. Immunopathol.,* 5:1–5.
24. Douglas, S. D., amd Schopfer, K. (1977): The phagocyte in protein–calorie malnutrition: A review. In: *Malnutrition and the Immune Response,* edited by R. M. Suskind, pp. 231–244. Raven Press, New York.
25. Drutz, D. J. (1976): Immunity and infection. In: *Basic and Clinical Immunology,* edited by H. H. Fudenberg, D. P. Stites, J. Caldwell, and J. V. Wells, pp. 182–184. Lange Medical Publishers, Los Altos, California.
26. Dudrick, S. J., and Long, J. M. (1977): Applications and hazards of intravenous hyperalimentation. *Annu. Rev. Med.,* 28:517–528.
27. Dudrick, S. J., Wilmore, D. W., Vars, H. M., and Rhoads, J. E. (1969): Can intravenous feeding as the sole means of nutrition support growth in the child and restore weight loss in an adult? *Ann. Surg.,* 169:974–984.
28. Eisen, H. N. (1974): *Immunology: An Introduction to Molecular and Cellular Principles of the Immune Response.* Harper & Row Publishers, Hagerstown, New Jersey.
29. Faulk, W. P., Demaeyer, E. M., and Davies, A. J. S. (1974): Some effects of malnutrition on the immune response in man. *Am. J. Clin. Nutr.,* 27:638–646.
30. Feigin, R. D. (1977): Interaction of nutrition and infection: Plans for future research. *Am. J. Clin. Nutr.,* 30:1553–1563.
31. Finter, N. D., editor (1973): *Interferons and Interferon Inducers.* North Holland/American Elsevier Publishers, New York.
32. Frederick, P. L., Sizer, J. S., and Osborne, M. P. (1965): Relation of massive bowel resection in gastric secretion. *N. Engl. J. Med.,* 272:509–514.
33. Gershon, R. K. (1976): The role of the T cell in the immune response. *Adv. Exp. Med. Biol.,* 73(Pt. B):3–13.

34. Gold J. (1974): Cancer cachexia and gluconeogenesis. *Ann. N.Y. Acad. Sci.,* 230:103–110.
35. Good, R. A., Jose, D., Copper, W. E., Fernandez, G., Kramer, T., and Yunis, E. (1977): Influence of nutrition and antibody production and cellular immune response in man, rats, mice and guinea pigs. In: *Malnutrition and the Immune Response,* edited by R. M. Suskind, pp. 169–183. Raven Press, New York.
36. Harvey, K. B., Bothe, A., Jr., and Blackburn, G. L. (1979): Nutritional assessment and patient outcome during oncological therapy. *Cancer,* 43:2065–2069.
37. Hoffman-Goetz, L., and Kluger, M. J. (1979): Protein deficiency: Its effects on body temperature in health and disease states. *Am. J. Clin. Nutr.,* 32:1423–1427.
38. Hrgovcic, M., Tessmer, C., Thomas, F., Fuller, L., Gamble, J., and Shullenberger, C. (1973): Significance of serum copper levels in adult patients with Hodgkin's disease. *Cancer,* 31:1337–1345.
39. Insel, R. A., and Merler, E. (1977): The necessity for T cell help for human tonsil B cell responses to pokeweed mitogen: Induction of DNA synthesis, immunoglobulin, and specific antibody production with a T cell helper factor produced with pokeweed mitogen. *J. Immunol.,* 118:2007–2014.
40. Irvin, T. T. (1978): Effects of malnutrition and hyperalimentation on wound healing. *Surg. Gynecol. Obstet.,* 146:33–37.
41. Jandinski, J., Cantor, H., Tadakuma, T., Peavy, D. L., and Pierce, C. W. (1976): Separation of helper T cells from suppressor T cells expressing different Ly components: I. Polyclonal activation: Suppressor and helper activities are inherent properties of distinct T cell subclasses. *J. Exp. Med.,* 143:1382–1390.
42. Keusch, G. T., Urrutia, J. J., Guerrero, O., Casteneda, G., and Douglas, S. D. (1977): Rosette-forming lymphocytes in Guatemalan children with protein–calorie malnutrition. In: *Malnutrition and the Immune Response,* edited by R. M. Suskind, pp. 117–122. Raven Press, New York.
43. Kluger, M. J., and Rothenberg, B. A. (1979): Fever and reduced iron: Their interaction as a host defense response to bacterial infection. *Science,* 203:374–376.
44. Kurland, J. I., Kincade, P. W., and Moore, M. A. S. (1977): Regulation of B-lymphocyte clonal proliferation by stimulatory and inhibitory macrophage-derived factors. *J. Exp. Med.,* 146:1420–1434.
45. Law, D. K., Dudrick, S. J., and Abdou, N. I. (1973): Immunocompetence of patients with protein–calorie malnutrition. *Ann. Intern. Med.,* 79:545–550.
46. Lawrence, W. (1977): Nutritional consequences of surgical resection of the gastrointestinal tract for cancer. *Cancer Res.,* 37:2379–2386.
47. MacDougall, L. G., Anderson, R., and Katz, J. (1975): The immune response of iron deficient children: Impaired cellular defense mechanisms with altered humoral components. *J. Pediatr.,* 86:833–843.
48. Masawe, A. E., and Msazumuhire, H. (1973): Growth of bacteria *in vitro* in blood from patients with severe iron deficiency anemia and from patients with sickle cell anemia. *Am. J. Clin. Pathol.,* 59:706–711.
49. Masawe, A. E., Munindi, U., and Swai, G. (1974): Infections in iron deficiency and other types of anemia in the tropics. *Lancet,* II:314–317.
50. McCay, C. M., Crowell, M. F., and Maynard, L. A. (1935): The effect of retarded growth upon the length of life span and upon the ultimate body size. *J. Nutr.,* 10:63–75.
51. McFarlane, H., Reddy, S., Adcock, K., Adeshina, H., Cooke, A. R., and Akene, J. (1970): Immunity, transferrin and survival in kwashiorkor. *Br. Med. J.,* 4:268–270.
52. McHugh, M. I., Wilkinson, R., Elliott, R. W., Field, E. J., Dewar, P., Hall, R. R., Taylor, R. M. R., and Uldall, P. R. (1977): Immunosuppression with polyunsaturated fatty acids in renal transplantation. *Transplantation,* 24:263–267.
53. Meakins, J. L., McLean, A. P. H., Kelly, R., Bubenik, O., Pietsch, J. B., and MacLean, L. D. (1978): Delayed hypersensitivity and neutrophil chemotaxis: Effect of trauma. *J. Trauma,* 18:240–247.
54. Mertin, J., and Hunt, R. (1976): Influence of polyunsaturated fatty acids on survival of skin allografts and tumor incidence in mice. *Proc. Natl. Acad. Sci. U.S.A.,* 73:928–931.
55. Miller, C. L. (1978): Immunological assays as measurements of nutritional status: A review. *J. Parenteral Enteral Nutr.,* 2:554–566.
56. Miller, J. D. B., Blackburn, G. L., Bistrian, B. R., Rienhoff, H. Y. and Trerice, M. (1977): Effect of deep surgical sepsis on protein sparing therapies and nitrogen balance. *Am. J. Clin. Nutr.,* 30:1528–1532.

57. Mullen, J. L., and Hobbs, C. L. (1979): Nutritional management. In: *The Cancer Patient*, edited by B. R. Cassileth, pp. 149–168. Lea & Febiger Publishers, Philadelphia.
58. Muller-Eberhard, H. J. (1968): The serum complement system. In: *Textbook of Immunobiology*, edited by P. A. Miescher and H. J. Muller-Eberhard, pp. 33–47. Grune and Stratton, New York.
59. Munson, D., Franco, D., Arbeter, A., Velez, H., and Vitale, J. J. (1974): Serum levels of immunoglobulins, cell mediated immunity and phagocytosis in protein calorie malnutrition. *Am. J. Clin. Nutr.*, 27:625–628.
60. Oppenheim, J. T., and Schecter, B. (1976): Lymphocyte transformation. In: *Manual of Clinical Immunology*, edited by N. R. Rose and H. Friedman, pp. 81–94. American Society for Microbiology, Washington, D.C.
61. Ota, D. M., Copeland, E. M., Corriere, J. N., Jr., Richie, E. R., Jacobson, K., and Dudrick, S. J. (1978): The effects of a 10% soybean oil emulsion on lymphocyte transformation. *J. Parental Enteral Nutr.*, 2:112–115.
62. Palmer, D. L., and Roed, W. O. (1974): Delayed hypersensitivity skin testing: I. Response rates in a hospitalized population. *J. Infect. Dis.*, 130:132–137.
63. Parish, C. R. (1975): Separation and functional analysis of subpopulations of lymphocytes bearing complement and Fc receptors. *Transplant. Rev.*, 25:98–120.
64. Plumb, M. M., Holland, J., Park, S. K., Dykstra, L., and Holmes, J. (1974): Depressive symptoms in patients with advanced cancer: A controlled assessment (abstract). *Psychosom. Med.*, 36:459.
65. Potter, M. R., and Moore, M. (1977): The effect of adherent and phagocytic cells on human lymphocyte PHA responsiveness. *Clin. Exp. Immunol.*, 27:159–164.
66. Puschman, M., and Ganzoni, A. M. (1977): Increased resistance of iron-deficient mice to *Salmonella* infection. *Infect. Immun.*, 17:663–664.
67. Raffi, M., Hashemi, S., Nahani, J., and Mohagheghpair, N. (1977): Immune responses in malnourished children. *Clin. Immunol. Immunopathol.*, 8:1–6.
68. Randel, H. T. (1958): Alterations in gastrointestinal tract function following surgery. *Surg. Clin. North Am.*, 38:585–602.
69. Reilly, J. J., Goodgame, J. T., Jones, D. C., and Brennan, M. F. (1977): DNA synthesis in rat sarcoma and liver: The effect of starvation. *J. Surg. Res.*, 22:281–286.
70. Rockland, R. E. (1976): Mediators of cellular immunity. In: *Basic and Clinical Immunology*, edited by H. H. Fudenberg, D. P. Stites, J. L. Caldwell, and J. V. Wells, pp. 102–113. Lange Medical Publishers, Los Altos, California.
71. Rosenthal, A. S., and Shevach, E. M. (1974): The function of macrophages in T lymphocytes antigen recognition. In: *Contemporary Topics in Immunobiology*, edited by W. Weigle, p. 147. Plenum Press, New York.
72. Schmidtke, J. R., and Hatfield, S. (1976): Activation of purified human thymus-derived (T) cells by mitogens: II. Monocyte–macrophage potentiation of mitogen-induced DNA synthesis. *J. Immunol.*, 116:357–362.
73. Scrimshaw, N. S., Taylor, C. E., and Gordon, J. E. (1968): *Interactions of Nutrition and Infection*. World Health Organization Monograph #57, Geneva.
74. Sellmeyer, E., Bhettay, E., Truswell, A., Meyers, O., and Hansen, J. (1972): Lymphocyte transformation in malnourished children. *Arch. Dis. Child.*, 47:429–435.
75. Shils, M. E. (1977): Nutritional problems associated with gastrointestinal and genitourinary cancer. *Cancer Res.*, 37:2366–2372.
76. Sibbit, W. L., Bankhurst, A. D., and Williams, R. C. (1978): Studies of cell subpopulations mediating mitogen hyperresponsiveness in patients with Hodgkin's disease. *J. Clin. Invest.*, 61:55–64.
77. Sims, E. A. H. (1976): Experimental obesity, dietary induced thermogenesis and their clinical implications. *J. Clin. Endocrinol. Metab.*, 5:377–395.
78. Sirisinha, S., Suskind, R. M., Edelman, R., Kulapongs, P., and Olson, R. E. (1977): The complement system in protein calorie malnutrition: A review. In: *Malnutrition and the Immune Response*, edited by R. M. Suskind, pp. 309–320. Raven Press, New York.
79. Smythe, P. M., Brereton-Stiles, G. G., Coovadia, H. M., Grace, H. J., Loening, W. E. K., Mafoyane, A., Parent, H. A., and Vos, G. H. (1971): Thymolymphatic deficiency and depression of cell-mediated immunity in protein–calorie malnutrition. *Lancet* II:939–943.
80. Soderberg, L. S. F., and Coons, A. H. (1978): Complement dependent stimulation of normal lymphocytes by immune complexes. *J. Immunol.*, 120:806–811.
81. Stiehm, E. R. (1977): Biology of immunoglobulins: Humoral and secretory: A review. In: *Malnu-*

*trition and the Immune Response*, edited by R. M. Suskind, pp. 141–183. Raven Press, New York.

82. Stites, D. P. (1976): Laboratory methods for detecting cellular immune function. In: *Basic and Clinical Immunology*, edited by H. H. Fudenberg, D. P. Stites, J. L. Caldwell, and J. V. Wells, pp. 316–330. Lange Medical Publishers, Los Altos, California.

83. Stobo, J. D., Paul, W. E., and Henney, C. S. (1973): Functional heterogeneity of murine lymphoid cells: IV. Allogeneic mixed lymphocyte reactivity and cytolytic activity as functions of distinct T cell subsets. *J. Immunol.*, 110:652–674.

84. Stutman, O. (1974): Cell mediated immunity and aging (abstract). *Fed. Proc.*, 33:2028.

85. Vanamee P., Lawrence, W., Jr., Levin, S., Peterson, A., and Randall, H. (1959): Further observations on postgastrectomy steatorrhea: The effect of high carbohydrate intake and of hydrochloric acid administration on fat absorption. *Ann Surg.*, 150:517–528.

86. Waithe, W. E., and Kirschow, K. (1978): Lymphocyte response to activators. In: *Handbook of Experimental Immunology*, edited by D. M. Weir, Chapter 26. Blackwell Scientific Publications, Oxford.

87. Waterhouse, C., Fenninger, L. D., and Keutmann, E. H. (1951): Nitrogen exchange and calorie expenditure in patients with malignant neoplasms. *Cancer*, 4:500–514.

88. Weinberg, E. D. (1978): Iron and infection. *Microbiol. Rev.*, 42:45–66.

89. Winchester, R. J., and Ross, G. (1976): Methods for enumerating lymphocyte populations. In: *Manual of Clinical Immunology*, edited by N. R. Rose and H. Friedman, pp. 64–76. American Society for Microbiology, Washington, D.C.

90. Yunis, E. J., and Greenberg, L. J. (1974): Immunopathology of aging. *Human Pathol.*, 5:122–125.

*Nutrition and Cancer: Etiology and Treatment,*
edited by G. R. Newell and N. M. Ellison.
Raven Press, New York © 1981.

# The Relationship of Diet to Cancer and Hormones

*,†,‡Suresh Mohla and *,**Wayne E. Criss

*Departments of Oncology, **Biochemistry, †Pharmacology, and ‡Physiology and
Biophysics, Howard University Cancer Center, Washington, D.C. 20059*

In this review, attention will focus on the relationships among diet, hormones, and cancer, especially the influence of dietary fluctuations on hormone-dependent cancers. Efforts will be made to delineate the interrelationships among nutritional factors and hormones that may eventually lead to the development or enhancement of a malignancy in certain tissues. The endocrine-dependent cancers to be considered include cancers of the ovary, prostate, breast, thyroid, and uterine endometrium.

## DIET AS AN ENVIRONMENTAL FACTOR

In evaluating the etiology of endocrine-dependent cancers, one must inquire into the role of environmental factors. Are environmental factors primarily carcinogens, such as the polycyclic hydrocarbons or nitrosamines, are they factors that serve generally to lower or raise biological thresholds and thus permit subsequent action by ubiquitous carcinogens, or do they serve to promote a preneoplastic state? Epidemiological evidence clearly indicates that the incidence of certain hormone-dependent cancers (e.g., breast cancer) varies among population groups and is affected by many environmental factors. Diet is one environmental factor that plays a prominent role in the causation of certain major forms of cancer (10,78,133,144,159,168). Studies of migrants from low- to high-cancer-risk countries suggest that diet is a key factor associated with increased risk of breast cancer (68,152). Studies by Carroll and Khor (30) have drawn attention to the high intake of fat and associated increased incidence of breast cancer in Western countries (30,168). The incidence of breast cancer in white women, is greater at all ages than that in Japanese women. The differences are especially evident in postmenopausal women. The well-established correlations between breast cancer rates and increased age and a recent report of increased rates of breast cancer in younger white women suggest a continued and perhaps increased influence of environmental factors in cancer causation (78).

## Dietary Fat

One of the most suspicious etiological agents in the diet of animals and humans is dietary fat. Studies of both pre- and postmenopausal Canadian women have shown an association between increased fat intake and an increased incidence of breast cancer (124). In addition, a report from California has demonstrated an association between a high level of dietary fat and a higher incidence of prostatic cancer (142). These associations between cancer incidences and fat intake have been confirmed experimentally in animals. For example, high-fat diets have been shown to enhance the development of spontaneous as well as chemically induced tumors (30,83). Other dietary factors, such as high levels of protein (30,83,120,141), amino acids (141), and dairy products (57), have also been implicated in tumorigenesis.

Evidence concerning the possible effects of fat intake on neoplasms in humans comes from a variety of epidemiological studies. Wynder and co-workers (167,169) have noted an association between "Westernization" of diet and an increased incidence of cancers of the digestive organs and the hormone-related cancers of the breast, ovary, endometrium, and prostate. In the adolescent Western girl, the age of menarche has been steadily decreasing over the last century (157). In addition, changing diets and life-styles have led to increased numbers of obese girls in Western societies (37,56). Since obesity precipitates an earlier initiation of puberty, which in turn confers a higher risk of breast cancer (154), the importance of nutritional factors affecting adolescent growth becomes very evident. "Westernization" by migration (48,99), dietary modification, or obesity per se (46,160) may increase the risk of breast cancer in women.

Recent studies indicate that the hormone levels of Japanese and Bantu women (who are at low risk) are different from those of white women (who are at high risk). Serum lipid levels are higher in postpubertal white girls. It has also been shown that dietary factors can shorten the menstrual cycle in white women (78).

## Diet, Hormones, and Breast Cancer

Ovarian dysfunction occurs in many premenopausal women with breast cancer (155). As several characteristically different types of menstrual cycle patterns occur (149) and as estrogen therapy produces ovarian dysfunction, changes in estrogen levels may be associated with the development of the breast disease. MacFayden et al. (114) have reported a reduction in estrogen levels in breast cancer patients, while Hill et al. (78,80) have reported a fall in estradiol levels in premenopausal Bantu and Japanese women with breast cancer. The question of whether estrogens are a boon or a culprit is unresolved (170). Much of the problem stems from lack of knowledge of the hormonal status of perimenopausal woman and the erroneous assumption that postmenopausal or castrated women have little or no circulating estrogen. In fact, estradiol and estrone are present in the ovarian veins of postmenopausal women (94) and in castrated women (16,95,139). In this regard, Hill et al. (79) have shown that subgroups of white women with different risks for breast cancer have different estrogen levels.

The extent to which dietary factors can explain different incidences of breast cancer in menopausal Japanese and white women remains unknown. On the basis of epidemiological and cytological data in Dutch women, DeWaard and Baanders-van Holewijn (47) have suggested a bimodal incidence of breast cancer, the early phase being related to ovarian activity and the later phase, occurring at or after menopause, being related to adrenal activity. Although the relative activity of ovaries and adrenals in postmenopausal white women has been studied (161), no comparable data on Asian women are available. Consequently, if adrenal activity is subject to dietary control and estradiol is a promotional factor (other factors being equal), it should be possible to decrease the incidence of menopausal breast cancer with dietary manipulation. The incidence of breast cancer in postmenopausal white vegetarians should be less than in postmenopausal meat-eaters. These suppositions have yet to be confirmed.

In attempts to understand the relationships among environmental factors, hormone levels, and breast disease, attention should be focused on studies of women in high-risk groups who are in their prepuberal and puberal years. Although data are available on the effect of hormone levels on growth characteristics during puberty, no explanation of the mechanism initiating progressively earlier menarche or establishing the length of the period between menarche and the onset of regular menses is available. Should differing endocrine status in women correlate with different incidences of breast cancer, then androgen and estrogen activity should be simultaneously evaluated.

Dietary factors influence tumor incidences and hormone profiles in laboratory animals, as well as hormone profiles in women. Additional studies on the quantity and quality of dietary intake are required to define the specific relationships of diet to hormone levels and the development of hormone-dependent cancers. Data from epidemiological studies in humans and from laboratory studies in animals indicate that the modifying effects of diet may also be exerted through specific effects on the adrenal gland and other complex endocrine systems of the host.

The dietary state can influence the rate of steroid hormone metabolism; e.g., the production rate of putative cancer-promoting factors, such as estrogens, may be altered (110). Diet can also alter the route or pattern of urinary steroid metabolism.

## HORMONE PRODUCTION RATES IN HUMAN BREAST AND ENDOMETRIAL CANCERS

There is circumstantial evidence linking estrogens to breast and uterine cancers. Estrogens are necessary for the induction of breast tumors in animals. Furthermore, women who have undergone early oophorectomy are at a diminished risk for breast cancer, thus indicating a supportive or permissive role for estrogens (106). It has been known for over a century that there is a relationship between breast cancer and the endocrine glands (18,38,84,136). The endocrine cycles of the body modify the size and activity of the female tissue; e.g., female breast tissue is 100 times more susceptible to neoplastic change than male tissue (20).

Oophorectomy-induced regression of breast cancer was reported by Beatson (18) as early as 1896. It has now been demonstrated that estrogen treatment can reactivate tumor growth. However, the notion that women who receive diethylstilbestrol therapy during pregnancy are likely to have an increased incidence of breast cancer, has not been supported in a recent study (22). In addition to estrogens (12,44,74,75,89–92,119,136,137,156), progesterone, androgens, glucocorticoids (75,77,126), prolactin and insulin (77,121,136,166), and thyroxine (21,25,55) have been implicated in the etiology of breast cancer.

Similarly, there is ample evidence to implicate estrogenic hormones in the formation of carcinoma of the endometrium. Endometrial carcinoma does not occur in women with gonadal dysgenesis, unless they have received estrogen replacement therapy, and the studies of Gusberg (66) suggest that estrogens play a crucial role in the progression from endometrial hyperplasia to endometrial carcinoma. A considerable number of patients with endometrial carcinoma have polycystic ovaries or estrogen-producing ovarian tumors. Endometrial carcinoma is extremely rare in patients with no estrogen secretion, e.g., those with Turner's syndrome (61), but these patients can develop endometrial carcinoma when exposed to estrogen therapy (41,118,151). Endometrial cancer is also known to occur in breast cancer patients who receive estrogen therapy (82,97,115). Epidemiological data suggest that women with endometrial or breast cancer tend to have had a late menopause, and thus longer period of stimulation by ovarian hormones (81,116,158). Therefore, a major issue to be examined is the association between nutrition and estrogen production and the resulting effects on the menstrual cycle and formation of breast cancer.

The dominant plasma estrogen in postmenopausal women is estrone (109,139), most of which is produced by conversion of androstenedione to estrone in the peripheral tissues (108,110). Only a small fraction of estrone is secreted by the adrenal gland (108). Androstenedione is produced in the ovary (94) and the adrenal cortex (164). Therefore, both the production rate and the plasma level of estrone depend on the secretion rate of androstenedione and its rate of conversion to estrone.

Androstenedione is converted to estrone in the liver (23), brain (130), and fat tissue (146). Although it is difficult to assess the relative contributions of each tissue, fat plays an important role in the aromatization of androstenedione to estrone (106). Estrogen stimulation is positively correlated with obesity in postmenopausal women (47). This may be because the extent of conversion of androstenedione to estrone is positively correlated with body weight (113). The latter finding strongly suggests that extraglandular conversion of androstenedione to estrone occurs in the adipose tissue. Obesity and aging appear to act in concert to potentiate the conversion of plasma androstenedione to estrone in extraglandular sites; the conversion is higher in obese postmenopausal women than in obese premenopausal women (111).

These biochemical phenomena can be related to breast cancer and endometrial cancers through observations that obesity is associated with an increased risk of breast and endometrial cancer. Obese women appear to have a two- to fourfold greater risk of endometrial cancer than nonobese women (116). DeWaard and Baanders-van Holewijn have postulated that obesity, or possibly high body weight, is associated with an increased risk of breast cancer in women over 50 years of age (47).

The characteristic features in postmenopausal women that are associated with increased extraglandular estrone formation also place women at an increased risk of developing endometrial cancer (111). Grodin et al. (64,65) have reported increased estrone production rates in women with endometrial hyperplasia, a probable early stage of endometrial cancer. The rate of conversion of androstenedione to estrone has been shown to be higher in women with endometrial cancer than in controls (69). This increased estrone formation (as a result of increased aromatization of androstenedione) occurs during aging (73) and in hepatic disease (59,113). Both of these conditions also place women at an increased risk of endometrial cancer (50,88,153). Increased synthesis (extraglandular) of estrone also occurs if the plasma levels of androstenedione are increased, e.g., in patients with polycystic ovarian disease, hyperthecosis, and endocrine and nonendocrine tumors of the ovary (7,66,106,112). With each of these conditions, the risk of development of endometrial carcinoma is increased. From these considerations, MacDonald et al. (111) have concluded that "the constitutional features of women that are associated with increased extraglandular estrone formation are similar to those observed in women who are at increased risk of developing endometrial cancer." Thus, there is considerable circumstantial evidence that estrogens play a crucial role in the development of endometrial cancer.

It has been proposed that anovulatory cycles are related to the development of uterine cancer, "the endocrine correlate being a continued unopposed estrogen effect" (106). A similar suggestion has been made with respect to breast cancer (149). In addition, this phenomenon may provide a link in the association between breast and uterine cancers. Grattorola (60) provided data showing an association between breast cancer and anovulation. There are several indications that a history of infertility is more common in women with breast cancer than in other women (106). Many reports have directed attention to the association of obesity and infertility with endometrial cancer. Dunn and Bradbury (50) found a high incidence of obesity and infertility in women with endometrial cancer.

Therefore, factors tending to produce more estrone and unopposed estrogen effects can be related to endometrial and breast cancer on one hand and to nutritional status on the other (105,106). Thus, a credible link exists among

nutritional excess, obesity, increased production of estrone during the perimenopausal years, and increased risk of endometrial cancer (36). The same mechanism
may operate in breast cancer. However, it is certainly premature to conclude
that this mechanism accounts for all breast or endometrial cancers.

### Effect of Diet on Hormone Levels and Mammary Cancer in Animals

Evidence that dietary factors (especially fat) have a mammary tumor-promoting effect that is based on alterations in the hormonal milieu has also been
observed in experimental animals. In laboratory animals, diets high in fats have
been shown to enhance the development of both spontaneous and chemically
induced tumors (30,83). A marked effect of obesity on the induction of mammary
carcinoma in both normal and castrated C3H mice has also been reported (163).

Anti-estrogens or estrogen antagonists have been shown to block the growth-
promoting effect of estrogens in normal tissues (29,49,128,129) and cause regression in breast cancer (44,74,156). The antiestrogenic effect is probably achieved
by preventing the association of estrogen with specific receptors (54,91,134);
therefore, it is reasonable to assume that anti-estrogens could effectively counter
any endogenous estrogenic stimulation of breast cancer growth.

Although anti-estrogens decrease the extent of and shorten the length of
time required for tumor development, the incidence of tumors in rats fed a
high-fat diet remains higher than that in rats fed a low-fat diet (31). Antiestrogens
partially counteract the estrogen-induced increase in prolactin levels (76), but
not so effectively as ergocryptine, an inhibitor of prolactin secretion. Since the
general effects of antiestrogen and prolactin inhibition differ markedly, it is
apparent that the anti-estrogens cannot be acting simply as prolactin inhibitors,
although reduction of an estrogen-induced increase in serum prolactin may
contribute to the overall results seen when an anti-estrogen is used *in vivo*. In
contrast, antiprolactin drugs (e.g., CB-154) have been shown to suppress completely the formation of all palpable tumors induced by dimethylbenzanthracene
and also to abolish the differential induction response seen with high- and low-
fat diets. These data suggest that the enhancement of mammary tumor growth
by high dietary fat may be mediated through alterations in circulating prolactin
levels (31). Studies on levels of circulating hormones have revealed higher prolactin and estrogen levels in tumor-bearing rats fed a high-fat diet than in tumor-
bearing rats fed a low-fat diet. The high-fat-diet group with palpable tumors
also showed a higher prolactin-to-estrogen ratio than the high-fat-diet group
without tumors (33). On the basis of these observations, it has been postulated
that mammary tumor cell proliferation is stimulated when the prolactin-to-estrogen ratio is high and is inhibited when the ratio is low. Chronic high fat intake
elevates serum prolactin levels, thus raising the prolactin-to-estrogen ratio and
thereby promoting mammary tumor cell growth (32,33). Inasmuch as prolactin
secretion is regulated in part by circulating estrogens (35), high dietary fat
may conceivably affect estrogen levels first, which in turn influence prolactin

secretion. However, at least two reports indicate no correlation between estrogen and prolactin concentrations in blood samples from healthy or tumor-bearing animals (33,71). Caution must be exercised in evaluating results from experiments in which blood for prolactin measurements is collected by cardiac puncture under light ether anesthesia, a condition that has been shown to stimulate prolactin secretion (19). The changes observed by Chan et al. (33) may therefore be the result of changes in the basal level or triggering mechanisms for the release of prolactin, which could be caused by anesthesia and might thus account for the differences found in the high-fat- versus low-fat-diet groups.

Although the roles of estrogen and prolactin in mammary tumorigenesis have not been fully elucidated, synergism between estrogen and prolactin presumably regulates transformation of the breast nodule into a malignant tumor, as well as tumor maintenance or progression (24,40,45,165,166). The ovarian hormones and prolactin, or at least their residual effects, are critical in the chemical transformation of the rat mammary gland epithelium, but pituitary hormones alone can promote the growth of these transformed cells (166). Although physiological doses of estrogen may enhance the action of prolactin, larger doses may inhibit the direct stimulatory effect of prolactin on normal and neoplastic mammary tissue (122,131,132). Recent evidence has also indicated that prolactin may increase the number of estrogen receptors (14,104,162) and prolactin receptors (39). It is then conceivable that elevated levels of serum prolactin, especially in patients with a high prolactin-to-estrogen ratio, restore the prolactin receptors. Prolactin receptors, in turn, restore cytoplasmic estrogen receptors so that normal estrogen receptor translocation and resumption of tumor growth are achieved.

### Diet and Androgen Metabolism in Breast Cancers

Diet can alter the metabolism of the adrenal C-19 steroids (72,87,145). Adrenal activity can be increased by a high-protein diet (51). As most (80%) of the dehydroepiandrosterone (DHEA) arises from the adrenal gland, the plasma DHEA level is an indicator of adrenal activity. Hill et al. (78) have reported increased plasma androgen levels in postmenopausal white women compared to their Japanese counterparts. Bulbrook, et al. (28) have reported higher rates of excretion of androgens in healthy white women than in Japanese. In older Japanese and Polish patients with breast cancer, a decrease in plasma DHEA and increased urinary excretion of DHEA have also been observed (78,152).

The metabolism of testosterone to $5\alpha$-dihydrotestosterone ($5\alpha$-DHT) and androstenedione (A-dione) is different in patients with benign disease than in patients with malignant disease. While fibroadenomas show the conversion of testosterone to both $5\alpha$-DHT and A-dione, adenocarcinomas show conversion only to A-dione (140), which in turn can be converted to estrone. Thus, there is a difference in the ability of benign and malignant breast tissue to metabolize androgens. Collectively, these data imply a change in adrenal synthesis or metabolism of DHEA as a result of diet or the presence of cancer.

Another important aspect of the role of hormones is the ability of human breast cancer tissue to sulfurylate steroids into physiologically active metabolites (3,6). For example, human breast tumors have been shown to produce estrogens via such a mechanism (1,5,6,93,125). Dao and Libby (42,43) have demonstrated that sulfurylation of steroids by human mammary carcinoma is highly correlated with the response of these patients to endocrine-ablative procedures, such as adrenalectomy, and their ultimate prognosis. The failure of tumor preparations to sulfurylate steroid hormones *in vitro,* has been related to a complete lack of response to adrenalectomy and a particularly grave prognosis. When DHEA and 17$\beta$-estradiol were compared as substrates for tumor sulfotransferases, a lack of response to adrenalectomy and poor prognosis were observed in patients whose ratios of DHEA sulfate to 17$\beta$-estradiol sulfate were less than 1:1. The group with the best response and prognosis showed a DHEA sulfate-to-17B-estradiol sulfate ratio greater than 1 (42,43). Similarly, in studies on primary breast cancer performed at the time of mastectomy, these ratios were found to be correlated with prognosis, as determined by the presence or absence of metastases or early recurrence (43). Further evidence has indicated that low levels of DHEA sulfotransferases are responsible for patients' having a less than 1:1 ratio of DHEA sulfate to 17$\beta$-estradiol sulfate (4). It has been suggested that DHEA sulfate formation in the breast tumor is controlled mainly by sulfotransferases. These enzymes act as a shunt, regulating the level of free DHEA and related compounds that are available for metabolism to steroids, and thus influence the growth of mammary tissue (4). In addition, DHEA can serve as a precursor for androstenedione and testosterone in mammary carcinoma tissue (6), and these in turn can be converted to estrogens (1,4).

Estrogen sulfotransferases have been shown to be under hormonal control in uterine tissue and, in conjunction with 17$\beta$-estradiol dehydrogenase, serve to regulate the concentration of free estradiol in the uterus during the estrous and menstrual cycles (26,135). Therefore, an imbalance in the levels of the two types of sulfotransferase in the tumor could disturb the hormonal milieu and increase the growth rate of the tumors (4). The activity of 17$\beta$-dehydrogenase in converting estradiol to estrone was studied in patients with estrogen receptor-positive and estrogen receptor-negative breast cancers. An inverse relationship between the presence of estrogen receptors and 17$\beta$-dehydrogenase activity was observed; in all estrogen receptor-negative patients estradiol was transformed to estrone, while very few estrogen receptor-positive patients displayed 17$\beta$-dehydrogenase activity. Further, the 17$\beta$-dehydrogenase activity in receptor-negative patients steadily decreased in premenopausal patients as they approached menopause, whereas the activity steadily increased in postmenopausal patients with the duration of menopause (2).

Alterations in androgen metabolism have been postulated to be a criterion in identifying patients with advanced breast carcinoma who might respond favorably to adrenalectomy. Bulbrook and co-workers (15,27) have proposed that the excretion of androgen metabolites (etiocholanolone and androsterone) could allow prediction of response to adrenalectomy or hypophysectomy in breast cancer patients. However, nonspecific factors associated with illness, starvation, or fasting have also been shown to alter androgen metabolism (73,123,171). Therefore, unless patient groups are matched carefully by age, weight, caloric intake, drugs taken, extent of disease, and hepatic function, meaningful comparisons of androgen metabolites in cancer patients cannot be made (106).

### Estrogen Metabolites in Breast Cancer

Urinary metabolites of estrogen have been used to predict response to therapy in breast cancer patients (99). However, since hepatic metabolism determines the steroid excretion pattern, factors that influence liver enzyme activities may also alter urinary steroids independent of secretion rates. Consequently, it may be hazardous to infer differences in the endocrine milieu of patients on the basis of apparently consistent alterations in urinary steroids without considering a host of environmental dietary factors (106,107). It has been noted that more estriol is secreted by obese women than by normal controls (25). Thyroid hormones have been shown to alter estrogen and prolactin metabolism (21,25,55). It is necessary, therefore, also to consider thyroid status carefully. Attempts have been made to link the presence or absence of estriol conjugates with relative risks of breast cancer development (102,103). However, factors (e.g., nutrition) that influence alterations in estrogen metabolism must be understood and considered before assigning other than empirical value to urinary estriol excretion in cancer patients (106). It should be emphasized that estriol, under physiological conditions, has been shown to be an active estrogen (11) that can also induce mammary tumorigenesis in mice (143).

## DIET, HORMONES, AND PROSTATIC CANCER

Cancer of the prostate tends to be a disease of old age; very few men under the age of 40 have prostatic carcinoma. It is possible that the causative factors for prostate cancer do not operate until about age 40 or later (63). Prostatic tissue is endocrine responsive and its growth is regulated by hormones. Consequently, hormones play a vital role in the growth, development, differentiation, and maintenance of prostatic tissue. The therapy for prostatic cancer is based on the hypothesis that the neoplasm is also hormone dependent. The classic studies of Huggins and Hodges (85), in which they reported regression of metastatic prostatic carcinoma after estrogen treatment, heralded a new era in the hormonal management of neoplastic disorders.

Although prostatic tissue is stimulated by circulating androgens, it has not been possible to relate the appearance of prostatic disease to plasma levels of androgen (96). Patients with prostatic carcinoma have the same plasma concentrations of testosterone, dihydrotestosterone, and A-dione as patients with benign prostatic hypertrophy (67). The probability that estrogens also contribute to the hormonal regulation of prostatic function has been considered for years; estrogens are capable of producing two direct effects on the sex accessory organs, squamous metaplasia of the epithelium and growth of the fibromuscular stroma (53,117).

Epidemiological data (142) have suggested a positive correlation between high levels of dietary fat and prostatic cancer. The incidence of prostatic cancer is higher in blacks than in whites (148). It is six times higher in American black men than in Nigerian black men (100). Further, in one study, circulating levels of plasma testosterone were found to be nearly twice as high in Americans as in Nigerians; it is interesting to note that there was no difference in the incidence of latent carcinoma between American and Nigerian men (86). In a similar study, the incidence of latent carcinoma of the prostate in Japanese men living in Hawaii was the same as that in Japanese living in Japan, even though the Hawaiian Japanese had a higher rate of invasive prostatic cancer (8). Therefore, "it is worth suggesting that nutritional status and hormonal milieu may be altered in such a way as to promote the transition of latent to clinical carcinoma of the prostate" (107).

Obese men have been shown to have lower testosterone levels than men of ideal body weight; the mean sex hormone–binding globulin is also lower in obese men (58). Further, total serum testosterone and free testosterone levels correlate negatively with total body weight. Massive obesity in some men may cause a defect in the hypothalamic–pituitary axis, as evidenced by a low free testosterone level in the absence of elevated gonadotropins or by an increased response to luteinizing hormone releasing hormone (58). On the other hand, Schneider et al. (147) have reported that, although serum testosterone concentrations were reduced in obese men compared to lean controls, the dialyzable testosterone fractions were elevated. Thus, the calculated free testosterone concentrations were normal in obese men. In contrast, peripheral conversion of testosterone to estradiol and of A-dione to estrone is increased in obese men in proportion to the percentage above ideal weight, even though there are no signs of feminization (147). What effect this continued elevation of estradiol and estrone has on prostatic morphology is an area for future research. It is especially relevant because estrogens have been shown to cause squamous cell metaplasia of the epithelium and to promote growth of the fibromuscular stroma (53,117).

Other important aspects in the study of prostatic carcinoma are the 5 α-DHT and estrogen receptors (high-affinity, low-capacity, heat-labile, cytosol-binding proteins present in prostatic tissue). These receptor proteins have been identified in patients with benign prostatic hypertrophy (BPH) and prostatic carcinoma (52,70,127). Further, receptor affinity has been shown to be higher in patients with carcinoma of the prostate than in those with BPH (101). Studies using tissue measurements of DHT have revealed lower concentrations of tissue DHT in carcinoma patients than in patients with BPH (9). A recent report (98) has examined this phenomenon of DHT concentrations in primary versus metastatic prostatic cancer patients. The results demonstrate a major impairment in the formation of DHT by metastatic prostatic cancer patients compared to primary site cancer or BPH patients, and a similar but less evident alteration in primary site cancer patients compared to BPH patients. This abnormality in testosterone metabolism is of major importance in attempts to achieve effective hormonal control of prostatic cancer. Mohla et al. (127) have recently demonstrated specific estrogen receptors in patients with BPH and prostatic carcinoma. It is quite likely that estrogens, by binding with their cytoplasmic receptors and translocating these receptors to the nucleus, may act on the prostate directly, in addition to acting via the central nervous system.

Prolactin has also been shown to control growth of prostatic tissue; prostatic atrophy following hypophysectomy is greater than that following castration (62,150). Hypophysectomy results in objective tumor regression in about one third of patients, while 50% to 75% demonstrate subjective remission, as evidenced by lack of bone pain or increase in appetite. Prolactin has also been shown to synergize with testosterone in increasing prostatic growth (138). There are prolactin-specific receptors in the rat ventral prostate (13,17), and binding of prolactin is androgen dependent (34).

These biochemical results suggest the importance of hormones in the control of prostatic growth. Nutritional parameters may alter these factors, thereby changing the critical hormonal milieu. Any alteration of this milieu could result in abnormal growth. Only a limited number of epidemiologic studies (86,142) have addressed the relationship among hormones, diet, and carcinogenesis. Additional studies should be an important feature of subsequent clinical investigations, and should yield valuable information on the etiology, diagnosis, and therapeutic management of prostatic neoplasms.

## ACKNOWLEDGMENTS

The excellent clerical assistance of Yvonne Prince and Selma Eatmon and the technical assistance of Blaine Hunter are gratefully acknowledged. This research was supported in part by NIH-NCI-CA-14718.

## REFERENCES

1. Abul-Hajj, Y. J. (1975): Metabolism of dehydroepiandrosterone by hormone-dependent and hormone-independent human breast carcinoma. *Steroids,* 26:488–500.
2. Abul-Hajj, Y. J., Iverson, R., and Kiang, D. T. (1979): Estradiol 17β-dehydrogenase and estradiol binding in human mammary tumors. *Steroids,* 33:477–484.
3. Adams, J. B. (1964): Enzymic synthesis of steroid sulphates. II. Presence of steroid sulphokinase in human mammary carcinoma extract. *J. Clin. Endocrinol. Metab.,* 24:988–996.
4. Adams, J. B., and Chandra, D. P. (1977): Dehydroepiandrosterone sulfotransferase as a possible shunt for the control of steroid metabolism in human mammary carcinoma. *Cancer Res.,* 37:278–284.
5. Adams, J. B., and Li, K. (1975): Biosynthesis of 17β-oestradiol in human breast carcinoma tissue and a novel method for its characterization. *Br. J. Cancer,* 31:429–433.
6. Adams, J. B., and Wong, M. S. F. (1968): Paraendocrine behavior of human breast carcinoma:

*In vitro* transformation of steroids to physiologically active hormones. *J. Endocrinol.,* 41: 41–52.

7. Aiman, J., Nalick, R. H., Jacobs, A., Porter, J. C., Edman, C. D., Vellios, F., and MacDonald, P. C. (1977): The origin of androgen and estrogen in a virilized postmenopausal woman with bilateral benign cystic teratomas. *Obstet. Gynecol.,* 49:695–704.

8. Akazaki, K., and Stennerman, G. N. (1973): Comparative study of latent carcinoma of the prostate among Japanese in Japan and Hawaii. *J. Natl. Cancer Inst.,* 50:1137–1144.

9. Albert, J., Geller, J., Geller, S., and Lopez, D. (1976): Prostate concentrations of endogenous androgens by radioimmunoassay. *J. Steroid Biochem.,* 7:301–307.

10. Alcantara, E. N., and Speckman, E. W. (1976): Diet, nutrition and cancer. *Am. J. Clin. Nutr.,* 29:1035–1047.

11. Anderson, J. N., Peck, E. J., Jr., and Clark, J. H. (1975): Estrogen-induced uterine responses and growth: Relationship to estrogen receptor binding by uterine nuclei. *Endocrinology,* 96:160–167.

12. Antunnes, C. M. F., and Stolley, P. D. (1977): Cancer induction by exogenous hormones. *Cancer,* 39:1896–1898.

13. Aragona, C., Bohnet, H. G., and Friesen, H. G. (1977): Localization of prolactin binding in prostate and testis: The role of serum prolactin concentration of the testicular LH receptor. *Acta Endocrinol.,* 84:402–409.

14. Asselin, J., Kelly, P. A., Caron, M. C., and Labrie, F. (1977): Control of hormone receptor levels and growth of 7,12-dimethylbenz(a)anthracene-induced mammary tumors by estrogens, progesterone and prolactin. *Endocrinology,* 101:666–671.

15. Atkins, H., Bulbrook, R. D., and Flaconer, M. A. (1968): Urinary steroids in the production of response to adrenalectomy or hypophysectomy. *Lancet,* 2:1263–1264.

16. Baird, D. T., and Guevara, A. (1969): Concentration of unconjugated estrone and estradiol in peripheral plasma in non-pregnant women throughout the menstrual cycle, castrate and post-menopausal women and in men. *J. Clin. Endocrinol. Metab.,* 29:149–156.

17. Barkey, R. J., Shani, J., Amit, T., and Barzikai, D. (1977): Specific binding of prolactin to seminal vesicle, prostate and testicular homogenates of immature, mature and aged rats. *J. Endocrinol.,* 174:163–173.

18. Beatson, G. T. (1896): On treatment of inoperable cases of carcinoma of mamma: Suggestion for new method of treatment with illustrative cases. *Lancet,* 2:104–107, 162–165.

19. Bellinger, L. L., and Mendel, V. E. (1975): Hormone and glucose responses to serial cardiac puncture in rats. *Proc. Soc. Exp. Biol. Med.,* 148:5–8.

20. Bernstein, T. C. (1977): What are my chances of getting breast cancer? *J.A.M.A.,* 238:345–346.

21. Bhattacharya, A., and Vonderhaar, B. K. (1979): Thyroid hormone regulation of prolactin binding to mouse mammary gland. *Biochem. Biophys. Res. Commun.,* 88:1405–1411.

22. Bibbo, M., Haenszel, W. M., Wied, G. L., Hubby, M., and Herbst, A. L. (1978): A twenty-five year follow-up study of women exposed to diethylstilbestrol during pregnancy. *N. Engl. J. Med.,* 298:763–766.

23. Bolt, W., Ritzl, F., and Bolt, H. M. (1966): Uber die periphere unwandlung von androgens hormone in oestrogen beim menschen. *Verh. Dtsch. Ges. Inn. Med.,* 72:461–465.

24. Bradley, C. J., Kledzik, G. S., and Meites, J. (1976): Prolactin and estrogen dependency of rat mammary cancers at early and late stages of development. *Cancer Res.,* 36:319–324.

25. Brown, J. B., and Strong, J. A. (1965): The effect of nutritional status and thyroid function on the metabolism of estradiol. *J. Endocrinol.,* 32:107–117.

26. Buirchell, B. J., and Hahnel, R. (1975): Metabolism of estradiol-17β in human endometrium during the menstrual cycle. *J. Steroid Biochem.,* 6:1489–1494.

27. Bulbrook, R. D. (1972): Urinary androgen excretion and the etiology of breast cancer. *J. Natl. Cancer Inst.,* 46:1039–1042.

28. Bulbrook, R. D., Thomas, B. S., Utsonomiya, J., and Hamaguchi, E. (1967): The urinary excretion of 11-deoxy-17-oxosteroids and 17-hydroxy-corticoids by normal Japanese and British women. *J. Endocrinol.,* 37:401–406.

29. Callentine, M. R., Humphrey, R. R., Lee, L. L., Windsor, B. L., Schottin, N. H., and O'Brien, O. P. (1966): Action of an estrogen antagonist on reproductive mechanism in the rat. *Endocrinology,* 79:153–167.

30. Carroll, K. K., and Khor, H. T. (1975): Dietary fat in relation to tumorigenesis. *Prog. Biochem. Pharmacol.,* 10:308–353.

31. Chan, P. C., and Cohen, L. A., (1974): Effect of dietary fat, antiestrogen, antiprolactin on the development of mammary tumors in rats. *J. Natl. Cancer Inst.,* 52:25–30.
32. Chan, P. C., and Cohen, L. A. (1975): Dietary fat and growth promotion of rat mammary tumors. *Cancer Res.,* 36:3384–3386.
33. Chan, P. C., Head, J. F., Cohen, L. A., and Wynder, E. L. (1977): Influence of dietary fat on the induction of mammary tumors by N-Nitrosomethylurea: associated hormone changes and differences between Sprague-Dawley and F344 rats. *J. Natl. Cancer Inst.,* 59:1279–1283.
34. Charreau, E. H., Attramadal, A., Torjesen, P. A., Calandra, R., Purvis, K., and Hansson, V. (1977): Androgen stimulation of prolactin receptors in rat prostate. *Mol. Cell. Endocrinol.,* 7:1–7.
35. Chen, C. L., and Meites, J. (1970): Effects of estrogen and progesterone on serum and pituitary prolactin levels in ovariectomized rats. *Endocrinology,* 86:503–505.
36. Cole, P., and Cramer, D. (1977): Diet and cancer of endocrine target organs. *Cancer,* 40:434–437.
37. Colley, J. R. D. (1974): Obesity in school children. *Br. J. Prev. Soc. Med.,* 28:221–225.
38. Cooper, A. P. (1836): *The Principles and Practice of Surgery: Founded on the Most Extensive Hospital and Private Practice, During a Period of Nearly 50 Years; with Numerous Plates, Illustrative Both of Healthy and Diseased Structures, Vol. 1.* E. Cox, London.
39. Costlow, M. E., Buschow, R. A., and McGuire, W. L. (1975): Prolactin stimulation of prolactin receptors in rat liver. *Life Sci.,* 17:1457–1466.
40. Costlow, M. E., Buschow, R. A., and McGuire, W. L. (1976): Prolactin receptors in 7,12-dimethylbenz(a)anthracene-induced mammary tumors following endocrine ablation. *Cancer Res.,* 36:3941–3943.
41. Cutler, S. B., Forbes, A. P., Ingersol, F. M., and Schully, R. E. (1972): Endometrial carcinoma after stilbestrol therapy. *N. Engl. J. Med.,* 287:628–631.
42. Dao, T. L., and Libby, P. R. (1971): Enzymic synthesis of steroid sulfate by mammary cancer and its clinical implications. *Natl. Cancer Inst. Monog.,* 34:205–210.
43. Dao, T. L., and Libby, P. R. (1972): Steroid sulfate formation in human breast tumors and hormone dependency. In: *Estrogen Target Tissues and Neoplasia,* edited by T. L. Dao, pp. 181–200. University of Chicago Press, Chicago.
44. DeSombre, E. R., and Arbogast, L. Y. (1974): Effect of the antiestrogen CI628 on the growth of rat mammary tumors. *Cancer Res.,* 34:1971-1976.
45. DeSombre, E. R., Kledzik, G., Marshall, S., and Meites, J. (1976): Estrogen and prolactin receptor concentrations in rat mammary tumors and response to endocrine ablation. *Cancer Res.,* 36:354–358.
46. DeWaard, F. (1975): Breast cancer incidence and nutritional status with particular reference to body weight and height. *Cancer Res.,* 35:3351–3356.
47. DeWaard, F., and Baanders-van Halewijn, E. A. (1969): Cross-sectional data on estrogenic smears in a post-menopausal population. *Acta Cytol.,* 13:675–678.
48. Dickinson, L. E., MacMahon, B., Cole, P., and Brown, J. P. (1974): Estrogen profiles of Oriental and Caucasian women in Hawaii. *N. Engl. J. Med.,* 291:1211–1213.
49. Duncan, G. W., Lyster, S. C., Clark, J. J., and Lednicer, D. (1963): Antifertility activities of two diphenyl-dihydro-naphthalene derivatives. *Proc. Soc. Exp. Biol. Med.,* 112:439–442.
50. Dunn, L. J., and Bradbury, J. T. (1967): Endocrine factors in endometrial carcinoma. *Am. J. Obstet. Gynecol.,* 97:465–471.
51. Edozien, J. C. (1971): Biochemical normals in Nigerians: Urinary 17-oxosteroids and 17-oxogenic steroids. *Lancet,* 1:258–259.
52. Ekman, P., Snochowski, M., Zetterberg, A., Hogberg, B., and Gustafsson, J. A. (1979): Steroid receptor content in human prostatic carcinoma and response to endocrine therapy. *Cancer,* 44:1173–1181.
53. Emmens, C. W., and Parkes, A. S. (1947): Effects of exogenous estrogens on the male mammal. *Vitam. Horm.,* 5:233.
54. Ferguson, E. R., and Katzenellenbogen, B. S. (1977): A comparative study of antiestrogen action: Temporal patterns of antagonism of estrogen stimulated uterine growth and effects on estrogen receptor levels. *Endocrinology,* 100:1252–1259.
55. Fishman, J., Hellman, L., Zumoff, B., and Gallagher, T. F. (1965): Effect of thyroid on hydroxylation of estrogen in man. *J. Clin. Endocrinol.,* 25:365–368.
56. Frisch, R. E., and Revelle, R. (1971): The height and weight of girls and boys at the time

of initiation of adolescent growth spurt in height and weight and the relationship to menarche. *Hum. Biol.,* 43:140–159.

57. Gaskill, S. P., McGuire, W. L., Osborne, C. K., and Stern, M. P. (1979): Breast cancer mortality and diet in the United States. *Cancer Res.,* 39:3628–3637.

58. Glass, A. R., Swerdloff, R. S., Bray, G. A., Dahms, W. T., and Atkinson, R. L. (1977): Low serum testosterone and sex-hormone-binding-globulin in massively obese men. *J. Clin. Endocrinol. Metab.,* 45:1211–1219.

59. Gordon, G. G., Olivo, J., Rafii, F., and Southern, A. L. (1975): Conversion of androgens to estrogens in cirrhosis of the liver. *J. Clin. Endocrinol. Metab.,* 40:1018–1026.

60. Grattorola, R. (1964): The premenstrual endometrial pattern of women with breast cancer. *Cancer,* 17:1119–1122.

61. Gray, P. H., Anderson, C. T., and Munnel, F. W. (1970): Endometrial adenocarcinoma and ovarian agenesis: Report of a case. *Obstet. Gynecol.,* 35:513–518.

62. Grayhack, J. T. (1963): Pituitary factors influencing growth of the prostate. *J. Natl. Cancer Inst. Monog.,* 12:189–199.

63. Greenwald, P., Kirmss, V., and Burnett, W. S. (1979): Prostate cancer epidemiology: Widowerhood and cancer in spouses. *J. Natl. Cancer Inst.,* 62:1131–1136.

64. Grodin, J. M., McDonald, P. C., and Siiterin, P. K. (1971): *Dynamics of Androgen and Oestrogen Secretion in Control of Gonadol Steroid Secretion,* edited by D. T. Baird and J. A. Strong, pp. 158–168. Edinburgh University Press, Edinburgh.

65. Grodin, J. M., Siiterin, P. K., and McDonald, P. C. (1973): Sources of estrone production in post-menopausal women. *J. Clin. Endocrinol. Metab.,* 36:207–214.

66. Gusberg, S. A. (1967): Hormone dependence of endometrial carcinoma. *Obstet. Gynecol.,* 30:287–293.

67. Habib, F. K., Lee, I. R., Stitch, S. R., and Smith, P. H. (1976): Androgen levels in the plasma and prostatic tissues of patients with benign hypertrophy and carcinoma of the prostate. *J. Endocrinol.,* 71:99–107.

68. Haenszel, W., and Kurihara, M. (1968): Studies of Japanese migrants. I. Mortality from cancer and other diseases among Japanese in the United States. *J. Natl. Cancer Inst.,* 40: 43–68.

69. Hausknecht, R. W., and Gusberg, S. A. (1973): Estrogen metabolism in patients at high risk for endometrial carcinoma. *Am. J. Obstet. Gynecol.,* 116:981–984.

70. Hawkins, E. F., Nijs, M., and Brassine, C. (1977): Steroid receptors in human prostate: Detection of tissue-specific androgen binding in prostate cancer. *Clin. Chim. Acta,* 75:303–312.

71. Hawkins, R. A., Freedman, B., and Marshall, A. (1975): Oestradiol-17β and prolactin levels in rat peripheral plasma. *Br. J. Cancer,* 32:179–185.

72. Hendrix, A., Heyns, W., and DeMoor, P. (1968): Influence of low calorie diet and fasting on the metabolism of dehydroepiandrosterone sulfate in adult obese subjects. *J. Clin. Endocrinol.,* 28:1525–1533.

73. Hernsell, D. L., Grodin, J. M., Brenner, P. F., Siiterin, P. K., and McDonald, P. C. (1974): Plasma precursors of estrogen. II. Correlation of the extent of conversion of plasma androstenedione to estrone with age. *J. Clin. Endocrinol. Metab.,* 38:476–479.

74. Heuson, J. C., Coune, A., and Staquet, M. (1972): Clinical trial of nafoxidine, an estrogen antagonist in advanced breast cancer. *Eur. J. Cancer,* 8:387–389.

75. Heuson, J. C., Mattheiem, W. H., and Rozencweig, M. editors (1976): *Breast Cancer: Trends in Research and Treatment.* Raven Press, New York.

76. Heuson, J. C., Waelbroechk, C., Legros, N., Gallez, G., Robyn, C., and L'Hermit, N. (1972): Inhibition of DMBA-induced mammary carcinogenesis in the rat by 2-Br-ergocryptine (CB154), an inhibitor of prolactin secretion, and by nafoxidine (U11100), an estrogen antagonist. *Gynecol. Invest.,* 2:130–137.

77. Hilf, R., Harmon, J. T., Matusik, R. J., and Ringler, M. B. (1976): Hormonal control of mammary cancer. In: *Control Mechanisms in Cancer,* edited by W. E. Criss, T. Ono, and J. R. Sabine, pp. 1–24. Raven Press, New York.

78. Hill, P., Chan, P., Cohen, L., Wynder, E., and Kuno, K. (1977): Diet and endocrine related cancer. *Cancer,* 39:1820–1826.

79. Hill, P., Wynder, E. L., and Helman, P. (1978): Nutrition and hormone levels in relation to breast cancer and coronary heart disease. *Clin. Oncol.,* 4:35–45.

80. Hill, P., Wynder, E. L., Helman, P., Hickman, R., Rona, G., and Kuno, K. (1976): Plasma hormone levels in different ethnic populations of women. *Cancer Res.,* 36:2297–2301.
81. Hirayama, T., and Wynder, E. L. (1962): A study of the epidemiology of cancer of the breast. II. The influence of hysterectomy. *Cancer,* 15:28–38.
82. Hoover, R., Fraumeni, J. F., Jr., Everson, R., and Meyers, M. E. (1976): Cancer of the uterine corpus after hormone treatment for breast cancer. *Lancet,* 1:885–887.
83. Hopkins, G. J., and Carroll, K. K. (1979): Relationship between amount and type of dietary fat in promotion of mammary carcinogenesis induced by 7,12-dimethyl-benz(a)anthracene. *J. Natl. Cancer Inst.,* 62:1009–1012.
84. Huggins, C., and Bergenstal, D. M. (1952): Inhibition of human mammary and prostatic cancers by adrenalectomy. *Cancer Res.,* 12:134.
85. Huggins, C., and Hodges, C. B. (1941): Studies on prostatic cancer. I. The effect of castration, of estrogen and of androgen injection on serum phosphatases in metastatic carcinoma of the prostate. *Cancer Res.,* 1:293–297.
86. Jackson, M. A., Ahluwalia, B. S., Herson, J., Heshmat, M. Y., Jackson, A. G., Jones, G. W., Kapoor, S. K., Kennedy, J., Kovi, J., Lucas, A. O., Nkposong, E. O., Olisa, E., and Williams, A. O. (1977): Characterization of prostatic carcinoma among blacks: A continuation report. *Cancer Treat. Rev.,* 61:167–172.
87. Jacobson, G., Seltzer, C. C., Bondy, P. K., and Mayer, J. (1964): Importance of body characteristics in the excretion of 17-ketosteroids and 17-ketogenic steroids in obesity. *N. Engl. J. Med.,* 271:651–656.
88. Javert, C. T., and Renning, E. L. (1963): Endometrial cancer survey of 610 cases treated at Women's Hospital (1919–1960). *Cancer,* 16:1057–1064.
89. Jensen, E. V., Block, G. E., Smith, S., and DeSombre, E. R. (1973): Hormonal dependency of breast cancer. In: *Breast Cancer: A Challenging Problem,* edited by M. L. Griem, E. V. Jensen, J. E. Ultmann, and R. W. Wisler, pp. 55–62. Springer-Verlag, Berlin.
90. Jensen, E. V., Block, G. E., Smith, S., Kyser, K., and DeSombre, E. R. (1971): Estrogen receptors and breast cancer response to adrenalectomy. *Natl. Cancer Inst. Monog.,* 34:55–70.
91. Jensen, E. V., Jacobson, H. I., Smith, S., Jungblut, P. W., and DeSombre, E. R. (1972): The use of estrogen antagonist in hormone receptor studies. *Gynecol. Invest.,* 3:108–122.
92. Jensen, E. V., Polley, T. Z., Smith, S., Block, G. E., Ferguson, D. J., and DeSombre, E. R. (1975): Prediction of hormone dependency in human breast cancer. In: *Estrogen Receptors in Human Breast Cancer,* edited by W. L. McGuire, P. O. Carbone, and E. P. Vollmer, pp. 37–56. Raven Press, New York.
93. Jones, D., Cameron, E. H. D., Griffiths, K., Gleave, E. N., and Forrest, A. P. M. (1970): Steroid metabolism by human breast tumors. *Biochem. J.,* 116:919–921.
94. Judd, H. L., Judd, G. E., Lucas, W. E., and Yen, S. S. C. (1974): Endocrine function of the postmenopausal ovary: Concentration of androgens and estrogens in ovarian and peripheral vein blood. *J. Clin. Endocrinol.,* 30:1020–1023.
95. Judd, H. L., Lucas, W. E., and Yen, S. S. C. (1974): Effect of oophorectomy on circulating testosterone and androstenedione levels in patients with endometrial cancer. *Am. J. Obstet. Gynecol.,* 118:793–797.
96. Kent, J. R., and Acone, A. S. (1966): Plasma testosterone and aging in males. In: *Androgen in Hormonal and Pathological Conditions,* edited by A. Vermeulen and D. Exley. Proceedings of the Second Symposium on Steroid Hormones, Ghent, June, 1965. Inter. Congr. Series No. 101, pp. 31–35. Excerpta Medica Foundation, Amsterdam.
97. Khandekar, J. D., Victor, T. A., and Mukhopadhyaya, P. (1978): Endometrial carcinoma following estrogen therapy for breast cancer. *Arch. Intern. Med.,* 138:539–541.
98. Kliman, B., Prout, G. R., Jr., MacLaughlin, R. A., Daly, J. J., and Griffin, P. P. (1978): Altered androgen metabolism in metastatic prostate cancer. *J. Urol.,* 119:623–626.
99. Kodama, M., Kodama, T., Yoshida, M., Totania, R., and Aoki, K. (1975): Hormonal status of breast cancer. II. Abnormal urinary steroid excretion. *J. Natl. Cancer Inst.,* 54:1275–1282.
100. Kovi, J., and Heshmat, M. Y. (1972): Incidence of cancer in Negroes in Washington, D.C. and selected African cities. *Am. J. Epidemiol.,* 96:401–413.
101. Kreig, M., Grobe, I., Voigt, K. D., Altenahr, E., and Klosterhalpen, H. (1978): Human prostatic carcinoma: Significant differences in its androgen binding and metabolism compared to the human benign prostatic hypertrophy. *Acta Endocrinol.,* 88:397–407.

102. Lemon, H. M. (1969): Endocrine influences on human mammary cancer formation. *Cancer,* 23:781–790.
103. Lemon, H. M., Wotiz, H. H., and Parson, L. (1966): Reduced estriol excretion in patients with breast cancer prior to endocrine therapy. *J.A.M.A.,* 196:1128–1136.
104. Leung, B. S., and Sasaki, G. H. (1975): On the mechanism of prolactin and estrogen action in 7,12-dimethyl-benzanthracene-induced mammary carcinoma in the rat. II. In vivo tumor responses and estrogen receptor. *Endocrinology,* 97:564–572.
105. Lipsett, M. B. (1974): Endocrine responsive cancers in man. In: *Textbook of Endocrinology,* edited by R. H. Williams, pp. 1071–1083. W. B. Saunders Co., Philadelphia.
106. Lipsett, M. B. (1975): Hormones, nutrition and cancer. *Cancer Res.,* 35:3359–3361.
107. Lipsett, M. B. (1979): Interaction of drugs, hormones, and nutrition in the causes of cancer. *Cancer,* 43:1967–1981.
108. Longcope, C. (1971): Metabolic clearance and production rates of estrogens in postmenopausal women. *Am. J. Obstet. Gynecol.,* 111:778–781.
109. Longcope, C., Kato, T., and Horton, R. (1969): Conversion of blood androgens to estrogens in normal adult men and women. *J. Clin. Invest.,* 48:2191–2201.
110. MacDonald, P. C., and Siiteri, P. K. (1974): The relationship between the extraglandular production of estrone and the occurrence of endometrial neoplasia. *Gynecol. Oncol.,* 2:2159–2163.
111. MacDonald, P. C., Edman, C. D., Hemsell, D. L., Porter, J. C., and Siiterin, P. K. (1975): Effect of obesity on conversion of plasma andro-stenedione to estrone in postmenopausal women with and without endometrial cancer. *Am. J. Obstet. Gynecol.,* 130:448–455.
112. MacDonald, P. C., Grodin, J. M., Edman, C. D., Vellios, F., and Siiterin, P. K. (1976): Origin of estrogen in a postmenopausal woman with a nonendocrine tumor of the ovary and endometrial hyperplasia. *Obstet. Gynecol.,* 47:644–650.
113. MacDonald, P. C., and Siiterin, P. K. (1974): The relationship between the extraglandular production of estrone and the occurrence of endometrial neoplasia. *Gynecol. Oncol.,* 2:2159–2163.
114. MacFayden, I. J., Prescott, R. F., Groom, G. V., Forrest, A. P. M., Golder, M. P., Fahmy, D. R., and Griffiths, N. (1976): Circulating hormone concentrations in women with breast cancer. *Lancet,* 1:1100–1102.
115. MacMahon, B. (1969): Association of carcinomas of the breast and corpus uteri. *Cancer,* 23:275–280.
116. MacMahon, B. (1974): Risk factors for endometrial cancer. *Gynecol. Oncol.,* 2:122–129.
117. Mawhinney, M. G., and Belis, J. A. (1976): Androgens and estrogens in prostatic neoplasia. In: *Advances in Sex Hormone Research, Vol. 2,* edited by R. L. Singhal and J. A. Thomas, pp. 141–148. University Park Press, Baltimore.
118. McCarroll, A. M., Montgomery, D. A. D., Harley, J. Mcd. G., McKeown, E. F., and Mac-Henry, J. C. (1975): Endometrial carcinoma after cyclical oestrogen–progestogen therapy for Turner's syndrome. *Br. J. Obstet. Gynaecol.,* 82:421–425.
119. McGuire, W. L., Carbone, P. P., and Vollmer, E. P., editors (1975): *Estrogen Receptors in Human Breast Cancer.* Raven Press, New York.
120. McSheheey, T. W. (1974): The onset of mammary adenocarcinoma in mice: A possible correlation with nutrition. *Ecol. Food Nutr.,* 3:147.
121. Meites, J. (1972): The relation of estrogen and prolactin to mammary tumorigenesis in the rat. In: *Estrogen Target Tissue and Neoplasia,* edited by T. L. Dao, pp. 275–286. University of Chicago Press, Chicago.
122. Meites, J., Cassel, E., and Clark, J. (1971): Estrogen inhibition of mammary tumor growth in rats: Counteraction by prolactin. *Proc. Soc. Exp. Biol. Med.,* 137:1225–1227.
123. Metcalf, M. G. (1974): The breast cancer discriminant: Effect of age, obesity, hirsuitism, starvation and changes in adrenocortical and gonadal activity. *J. Endocrinol.,* 63:263–272.
124. Miller, A. B., Kelly, A., Choi, N. W., Matthews, V., Morgan, R. W., Munan, L., Burch, J. D., Feather, J., Howe, G. R., and Jain, M. (1978): A study of diet and breast cancer. *Am. J. Epidemiol.,* 107:499–509.
125. Miller, W. R., and Forrest, A. P. M. (1974): Oestradiol synthesis by a human breast carcinoma. *Lancet,* 2:866–868.
126. Mohla, S., and Anderson, W. A. (1978): Role of steroid hormones in mammary cancer. In:

*Endocrine Control in Neoplasia,* edited by R. K. Sharma and W. E. Criss, pp. 315–332. Raven Press, New York.

127. Mohla, S., Davis, J. L., Jackson, A. G., and Jones, G. (1979): Androgen and estrogen receptors in human prostatic carcinoma and benign, prostatic hypertrophy (abstract #18). Seventh Annual Meeting of Southeastern Cancer Research Association, Atlanta, Georgia.

128. Mohla, S., and Prasad, M. R. N. (1968): Inhibition of oestrogen-induced glycogen synthesis in the rat by clomiphene. *Steroids,* 11:571–578.

129. Mohla, S., and Prasaad, M. R. N. (1969): Estrogen–antiestrogen interaction: Effect of U1100A, MRL-41, and U1155A on estrogen-induced glycogen synthesis in the rat during delayed implantation. *Acta Endocrinol (Kbh.),* 62:489–497.

130. Naftolin, F., Ryan, K. J., and Petro, Z. (1972): Aromatization of androstenedione by the hypothalamus of adult male and female rats. *Endocrinology,* 90:295–298.

131. Nagasawa, H., and Yanai, R. (1971): Reduction by pituitary isograft of inhibitory effect of large doses of estrogen on incidence of mammary tumors induced by carcinogen in ovariectomized rats. *Intl. J. Cancer,* 8:463–467.

132. Nagasawa, H., and Yanai, R. (1974): Effect of estrogen and/or pituitary isograft on nucleic acid synthesis of carcinogen-induced mammary tumors in rats. *J. Natl. Cancer Inst.,* 52:1219–1222.

133. Newell, G. R., editor (1978): *Status report: Diet, Nutrition and Cancer Program.* National Cancer Institute, National Institutes of Health, Bethesda.

134. Nicholson, R. I., Davies, P., and Griffiths, K. (1977): Effects of oestradiol-17β and tamoxifen on nuclear oestradiol-17β receptors in DMBA-induced rat mammary tumours. *Eur. J. Cancer,* 13:201–208.

135. Pack, B. A., and Brooks, S. C. (1974): Cyclic activity of estrogen sulfotransferases in the gilt uterus. *Endocrinology,* 95:1680–1690.

136. Pearson, O. H., Molina, A., Butler, T. P., Uerena, L., and Nasr, H. (1972): Estrogens and prolactin in mammary cancer. In: *Estrogen Target Tissue and Neoplasia,* edited by T. L. Dao, pp. 287–305. University of Chicago Press, Chicago.

137. Pearson, O. H., West, C. D., Hollander, V., and Treves, N. L. (1954): Evaluation of endocrine therapy for advanced breast cancer. *J.A.M.A.,* 154:234.

138. Peyre, A., Revault, J. P., and Laporte, P. (1968): Potentiating effect of endogenous prolactin on male mouse sexual accessory glands with testosterone. *C. R. Soc. Biol. (Paris),* 162:1592–1595.

139. Rader, M. D., Flickinger, G. L., DeVilla, G. O., Mikuta, J. J., and Mikhail, G. (1973): Plasma estrogens in post-menopausal women. *Am. J. Obstet. Gynecol.,* 116:1069–1073.

140. Rose, L. I., Underwood, R. E., Dunning, M. T., Williams, G. E., and Pinkus, G. S. (1975): Testosterone metabolism in benign and malignant breast lesions. *Cancer,* 36:399–403.

141. Ross, M. H., and Bras, G. (1973): Influence of protein under- and overnutrition on spontaneous tumor prevalence in the rat. *J. Nutr.,* 103:944.

142. Rotkin, I. D. (1977): Studies in the epidemiology of prostatic cancer: Expanded sampling. *Cancer Treat. Rev.,* 61:173–180.

143. Rudali, G., Apion, F., and Muel, B. (1975): Mammary cancer produced in mice with estriol. *Eur. J. Cancer,* 11:39–41.

144. Saracci, R., and Repetto, F. (1978): Epidemiology of breast cancer. *Semin. Oncol.,* 5:342–350.

145. Savage, D. G. L., Forsythe, C. C., and Cameron, J. (1975): Excretion of individual adrenocortical steroids in obese children. *Arch. Dis. Child.,* 49:946–954.

146. Schindler, A. E., Ebert, A., and Friedrich, E. (1972): Conversion of androstenedione to estrone by human fat tissue. *J. Clin. Endocrinol. Metab.,* 35:627–630.

147. Schneider, G., Kirschner, M. A., Berkowitz, R., and Ertel, N. W. (1979): Increased estrogen production in obese men. *J. Clin. Endocrinol. Metab.,* 48:633–638.

148. Seidman, E., Silverberg, F., and Holleb, A. I. (1976): Cancer statistics 1976: A comparison of black and white populations. *Cancer,* 26:2–30.

149. Sherman, B. M., and Korenman, S. G. (1974): Inadequate corpus luteum function: A pathophysiological interpretation of human breast cancer epidemiology. *Cancer,* 33:1306–1311.

150. Silverberg, G. D. (1977): Hypophysectomy in the treatment of disseminated prostatic carcinoma. *Cancer,* 39:1727–1731.

151. Sirota, D. K., and Marinoff, S. C. (1975): Endometrial carcinoma in Turner's syndrome following prolonged treatment with diethylstilbestrol. *Mt. Sinai J. Med.,* 42:586–590.
152. Sonka, J., Vitkova, M., Gregorova, I., Tomsova, Z., Hilgertova, J., and Stas, J. (1973): Plasma and urinary dehydroepiandrosterone in cancer. *Endokrinologie,* 62:61–68.
153. Speert, H. (1949): Endometrial cancer and hepatic cirrhosis. *Cancer,* 2:597.
154. Staszewski, J. (1971): Age of menarche and breast cancer. *J. Natl. Cancer Inst.,* 47:935–940.
155. Swain, M. C., and Bulbrook, R. D. (1974): Ovulatory failures in the normal population and in patients with breast cancer. *J. Obstet. Gynecol. Br. Commonw.,* 81:640–643.
156. Tagnon, H. J. (1977): Antiestrogens in treatment of breast cancer. *Cancer,* 39:2959–2964.
157. Tanner, J. M. (1973): Trends towards earlier menarche in London, Oslo, Copenhagen, The Netherlands and Hungary. *Nature,* 243:95–96.
158. Trichopoulous, D., MacMahon, B., and Cole, P. (1972): Menopause and breast cancer risk. *J. Natl. Cancer Inst.,* 48:605–613.
159. Vakil, D. V., and Morgan, R. W. (1973): Etiology of breast cancer. II. Epidemiological aspects. *Can. Med. Assoc. J.,* 109:201–206.
160. Valaros, V. G., MacMahon, B., Trichopoulous, D., and Polychronopoulou, A. (1969): Lactation and reproductive histories of breast cancer patients in Greater Athens. *Intl. J. Cancer,* 4:350–363.
161. Vermeullen, A. (1976): The hormonal activity of the postmenopausal ovary. *J. Clin. Endocrinol. Metab.,* 42:247–253.
162. Vignon, F., and Rochefort, H. (1976): Regulation of estrogen receptors in ovarian-dependent rat mammary tumors. I. Effects of castration and prolactin. *Endocrinology,* 98:722–729.
163. Waxler, S. H., and Leef, M. F. (1966): Augmentation of mammary tumors in castrated obese C3H mice. *Cancer Res.,* 26:860–862.
164. Weinheimer, B., Oertel, G. W., Leppla, W., Blaise, H., and Bette, L. (1965): Plasma steroid concentrations of adrenal venous blood from women with and without hirsutism. In: *Second International Symposium on Steroid Hormones,* pp. 36–40, Ghent, Belgium.
165. Welsch, C. W. (1972): Effect of brain lesions on mammary tumorigenesis. In: *Estrogen Target Tissue and Neoplasia,* edited by T. L. Dao, pp. 317–331. University of Chicago Press, Chicago.
166. Welsch, C. W., and Nagasawa, H. (1977): Prolactin and murine tumorigenesis: A review. *Cancer Res.,* 37:951–963.
167. Wynder, E. L. (1979): Dietary habits and cancer epidemiology. *Cancer,* 43:1955–1961.
168. Wynder, E. L., Bross, I. J., and Hirayama, T. (1960): A study of the epidemiology of cancer of the breast. *Cancer,* 13:599–601.
169. Wynder, E. L., Kajitani, T., Ishikawa, S., Dodo, H., and Takano, A. (1969): Environmental factors in cancer of the colon and rectum. II. Japanese epidemiological data. *Cancer,* 23:1210–1220.
170. Wynder, E. L., and Schneiderman, M. A. (1973): Exogenous hormones, boon or culprit. *J. Natl. Cancer Inst.,* 51:729–731.
171. Zumoff, B., Bradlow, H. L., Gallagher, T. F., and Hellman, L. (1971): Decreased conversion of androgens to normal 17-ketosteroid metabolites: A nonspecific consequence of illness. *J. Clin. Endocrinol.,* 32:824–832.

*Nutrition and Cancer: Etiology and Treatment,*
edited by G. R. Newell and N. M. Ellison.
Raven Press, New York © 1981.

# Dietary Diaries and Histories

## O. M. Jensen

*Danish Cancer Registry, Strandboulevarden 49, DK 2100 Copenhagen, Denmark*

Food is composed of chemicals, and it is the purpose of dietary surveys in the study of cancer causation to measure human exposure to food components, alone or in combination. However, as Marr observes (16), "there is no generally accepted method of measuring the dietary intake of free-living individuals."

Various dietary constituents, such as fat, fiber, and alcohol, have been suggested as risk factors for cancer of different sites. Some etiological hypotheses have been supported by correlation studies in which the information on diet is obtained from food balance sheets (1), i.e., information derived from statistics on production, import, and exports. Such studies are hampered by inaccuracies in determining food consumption, since information on food wastage and distribution patterns is not included, and systematic differences may exist among various countries in reports of food supplies (14). Food balance sheets and household surveys clearly give an inadequate description of the relationship between diet and cancer in individuals.

Recent comprehensive reviews have described and compared in depth the survey methods used in nutritional research (16,18,19,26), and readers are referred to these papers for details. The present chapter briefly outlines the various survey methods used to determine individuals' food consumption, and reviews the application of the various methods in studies of diet in cancer causation.

## DIET AS AN EPIDEMIOLOGICAL VARIABLE

A number of problems pertaining to diet as an epidemiological variable make it difficult to study the impact of food on the development of human cancer. First, food, sufficient or insufficient, is ubiquitously available and all human beings are exposed to its nutrient and nonnutrient components. Thus, for most major food components, a "nonexposed" group does not exist in developed societies, and as the basis for comparative epidemiology, it is necessary to categorize persons by consumption levels within an often rather limited range. This requires tools that permit a precise classification of individuals. For want of such tools, differences in dietary patterns may empirically be suspected to be obscured, and studies associating diet and cancer in individuals have, under such conditions, generally been of limited persuasiveness.

Second, food consists of many components, including carbohydrates, fats, and proteins, as well as minerals and other micronutrients. The presence of food preservatives and the influences of processing, preparation, and storage are also important determinants of food composition (15). Food as an environmental agent is thus composed of a number of variables, some or all of which it may be important to study alone or in combination. Such complexity requires precise tools for disentanglement, which is necessary for evaluating associations between diet and cancer.

Finally, the long latency period in cancer development presents a common difficulty in etiological studies of these diseases. As long as 20 to 30 years may be required for some cancers to develop following initial exposure to an environmental carcinogen. For this reason, if diet can act as a carcinogenic risk factor after short-term exposure, it may be important to relate cancer occurrence in an individual to his or her diet during a limited period of time some 20 to 30 years earlier. The consumption of certain foods over a prolonged period of time (even life-long) is also important. In both cases, fallibility of human memory and changes in individuals' dietary patterns add to the epidemiologist's difficulties in determining the role of diet in human cancer development.

Such features of food as an environmental variable must be kept in mind when devising tools for its measurement. Records of food consumption and interview methods have been developed to characterize individuals' food intake. Such methods must be adapted to the special problems posed by cancer epidemiological research, and the method chosen depends on the problem to be studied. The objective of any study for which dietary information is desired must thus be clearly defined (28).

## DIETARY INQUIRY METHODS

Inquiry methods for collecting information on individuals' food consumption are listed in Fig. 1. Some are based on "dietary keeping," or determining current food intake by recording weights or household measures of foods actually consumed. Another set is based on recalling past intake, either as food eaten during a specified period of time or as food usually consumed, i.e., "dietary history." The level of detail may vary. In the shortcut methods, which are modifications of the two principal methodologies, the amount of information obtained to assess an individual's food intake is limited.

### Food Record Methods

The precise weighing method involves weighing all ingredients used to prepare dishes and subtracting the weights of inedible wastage. The cooked weight of the individual's portions and the table waste are also recorded. The weighing is carried out by a trained nutritionist in the home of the person under study. Analysis of the individual's nutrient intake is carried out by applying food

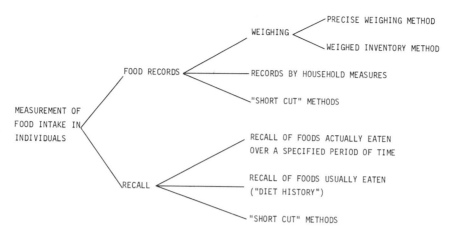

**FIG. 1.** Methods of measuring food consumption in individuals.

table values or by determining the chemical composition of ingredients from aliquot samples of the food.

The precise weighing method provides the most accurate estimate of an individual's nutrient intake. However, it requires such close supervision and such a high degree of long-term cooperation by the person studied that it is unsuitable for investigations that include large numbers of individuals. This method had not been used in population-based studies of food and cancer etiology, and its main use would seem to be as a reference for the indirect validation of simpler methods.

The weighed inventory method consists of recording the weights of prepared food immediately before consumption; plate waste is subtracted after weighing at the end of the meal. The method is simple enough to be carried out by the subjects themselves, but appropriate instructions and supervision are needed. Analysis is normally based on food table values.

The results of the weighed inventory method are probably slightly less accurate than those obtained by precise weighing. The weighed inventory method has been used to study the relation between cancer and the dietary habits of general population samples (12), but it is too complicated to be useful in larger population-based studies. It provides an excellent reference for the indirect validation of simpler methods.

With the household measures method, the types of food eaten are recorded and the amounts consumed are estimated on the basis of everyday measures (e.g., number of helpings, teaspoonsful). The conversion to weights and cubic measures is based on standard recipes and measures or on values obtained from earlier surveys of weighed food intake. The accuracy of the quantitative estimates may be improved by carefully checking the recorded information with the subject at the end of the survey. The nutrient analysis is normally based on food table values.

The omission of weights automatically introduces an additional degree of uncertainty about quantitative estimates of food consumption compared to the weighing methods described above. Recording in household measures is simpler than weighing, and can be carried out by the persons surveyed. Less supervision is required than with the weighing methods, so it may be useful in studies of large population samples if the validity of the estimated food intakes can be assured. No studies have been reported in which this method has been used on a large scale to associate individual food habits with the risk of cancer.

Attempts have been made to develop a shortcut diary-keeping method by limiting the recording of current food intake to meals eaten in a given period (16). Such a method provides only food intake frequencies, which may be combined to give so-called food scores. In a further step, food scores may be converted to nutrient scores in an attempt to determine an individual's nutrient intake.

The development of such simple methods is clearly desirable for use in prospective and certain types of retrospective epidemiological investigations in which the aim is to categorize a large number of individuals into high and low extremes with regard to the consumption of various food components. The crux of the matter is whether such categorization is feasible and valid. Marr (16) found that the feasibility and validity depend on the food under study, and shortcut methods require careful evaluation before they are implemented.

## Dietary Recall

With the first form of dietary recall, the subject is asked to list what he or she has eaten during a specified period of time (e.g., 24 hours) prior to the inquiry. Quantification of the foods eaten is attempted by asking amounts in household measures or by using visual aids in the form of two- or three-dimensional food models (20,21) or photographs that show different sizes of helpings (10). The recall method may be administered by an interviewer or take the form of a mailed questionnaire. Analysis of nutrient intake is normally based on food tables.

Recall of foods eaten over various periods of time prior to the interview has been attempted, but the 24-hour recall is most commonly used. However, it is used little in cancer epidemiological studies of individuals because the menu of the day recalled might be highly atypical. This method is nevertheless believed to provide a good estimate of current food consumption by groups, for individual day-to-day deviations from the normal diet will cancel each other out.

On the assumption that human growth and development are influenced by long-term food habits, the "dietary history" method was developed to obtain information on a respondent's usual dietary pattern. This method, originally developed by Burke (5), consists of three parts. First, what a person usually eats at a given meal is recorded. Second, information is obtained on the dietary habits by means of a pre-recorded, detailed list of foods. Third, the subject keeps a three-day food record from which estimates are made of the amounts of food usually eaten.

Modified versions of the original dietary history method have been extensively used in studies of the relation between diet and cancer development (23,24,27). The main modification consists of omitting the three-day food record and obtaining quantitative estimates of food intake by using visual aids (21) or by recording amounts in household measures. Conversion to nutrient intake is obtained by means of food table values. This method can be applied in large epidemiological studies of individuals, but it must be administered by trained nutritionists with a thorough knowledge of the dietary patterns prevalent in the population under study.

As with food record keeping, shortcut recall methods have been developed in an attempt to meet the epidemiologist's need to investigate large numbers of persons. Such methods may consist of asking subjects to recall the frequency with which they eat various foods per day, week, or month, or they may be limited to inquiring about the consumption of special foods under study. Analysis of the data is undertaken on a food frequency basis alone or by computing food scores on the basis of various conversion factors. As with the shortcut recall methods, nutrient scores may be obtained from the food scores.

Such shortcut methods have been widely used in studies of diet and cancer (3,7–9,11,17). Since they are relatively simple, they can be applied in studies involving large numbers of individuals, but, as with any of the methods mentioned above, their usefulness depends on the ability to classify persons correctly into various consumption strata with a minimum of overlap.

## SOURCES OF ERROR IN DIETARY INQUIRIES

The fact that, as Marr (16) observes, no method of measuring the dietary intake of free-living individuals is generally accepted may in part be the result of the different sources of error working to varying degrees in dietary inquiries. Bias may be introduced at a number of levels when a person is surveyed or when information on food consumption is transformed into estimates of nutrient intake.

### Human Memory

The fallibility of human memory poses a problem in all methods based on the recall of foods eaten. A person may forget to report food eaten or may provide an inaccurate estimate of the quantity. Such omissions or errors are generally not believed to be random, but may be more common with certain foods. Thus, foods eaten less frequently or not so recently would tend not to be remembered, and foods believed to be socially acceptable might be reported in larger quantities than foods the individual feels he or she should not be eating. Memory as a source of error in dietary surveys seems to depend on the age and sex of the individual; younger women remember food better than older men (6). Although generally recognized as important, this source of error in dietary surveys needs further investigation.

## Change of Dietary Habits

Suppression of information about "unacceptable" foods may also occur in a survey employing the diary method. This may take the form of deliberate omissions when the individual keeps the record himself, or changes in eating habits may be introduced by the mere act of being surveyed. As with the memory bias mentioned above, such suppression probably tends to obscure true differences in individuals' dietary patterns. Although it is difficult to measure the magnitude of this source of error in the food recording methods, the generally good correspondence between recall and record methods suggests that its importance has been overestimated.

## Use of Food Tables

Tables listing the composition of foods are used extensively to derive estimates of nutrient intake, and they often provide the only practical means of obtaining such information from records or questionnaires on food consumption. Certain limitations of food tables, however, represent potential sources of error in the results obtained from dietary surveys.

First, food table values are based on chemical analyses that may be inexact. This lack of precision may be caused by difficulties in separation of closely related substances (e.g., chemical analyses may overestimate the vitamin C content of certain foods). It may also be the result of inadequate analytical methods, such as measures of dietary fiber content based on treatment of the fiber with acids and alkalis; the introduction of Southgate's enzymatic method provided completely new fiber values (22). Also, food table figures generally represent average values, which in cases of regional or seasonal extremes may provide an incorrect estimate of the nutrient content of the food actually consumed. Food table values adjusted as closely as possible to the population under survey would minimize the error from this source (19).

Second, food tables may be incomplete by not listing all the foods consumed by the individuals surveyed. This is particularly true with mixed dishes, which are often analyzed in terms of their components as determined by the use of standard recipes.

Third, food table values are applied to recorded information by nutritionists, leaving room for the introduction of human error, particularly when judgment or interpretation on the part of the nutritionist is required. Rigid training and standardization in the use of food tables may reduce this source of error.

Finally, information on bioavailability is not included in food tables. Thus, the presence of a given amount of a nutrient does not necessarily mean that the amount is physiologically available, since absorption may be hindered by other substances in the food, as when calcium binds to phytates in the intestines.

The justification for the use of food tables in a given survey situation can only be based on a comparison of nutrient intakes derived from food table and chemical analyses of duplicate portions or aliquot samples of foods eaten. In her review, Marr (16) found that "absolute agreement for every individual is not achieved" and that "agreement is better for some nutrients than others. However, because there is a close association between the calculated and analysed values, it is possible to compare individuals' intakes relative to each other and to compare groups of individuals both in terms of means and at the extremes of the distribution for calories and some nutrients."

## QUALITY OF DIETARY INQUIRY METHODS

Standardization and quality control are essential in epidemiological surveys, and dietary studies are no exception. Evaluating methods used to measure food intake requires assessing their repeatability and validity.

### Repeatability

Repeatability is the level of agreement between replicate measurements (2). Its components are random and systematic subject variation and within- and between-observer variation; these can also be referred to as biological (subject) and measurement (observer) variations. Thus, if replicate surveys show differences in a subject's diet for different days or periods, these differences may result from the well-known biological day-to-day or seasonal variation. Day-to-day variations tend to be random and thus to cancel each other out when large groups of persons are surveyed, whereas seasonal variations may be systematic, leading to bias in the results that cannot be measured.

Similarly, the same observer may obtain different results in measuring a person's food consumption even when no true differences exist, for example, in two interviews on the same day. Such within-observer variations tend to be random and thus cancel each other out in larger groups, whereas between-observer variations—different observers obtaining different estimates of a subject's food consumption—tend to be systematic and thus more serious.

Subject variation should be reduced as far as possible to estimate observer variation. Every effort should be made to locate and minimize systematic error by rigorous standardization and testing of the questionnaires or records developed to obtain information on food consumption. Standardization of techniques, including constant monitoring of observers involved in a given survey, is a remedy for systematic variation, which is so undesirable in epidemiological surveys.

Estimating the repeatability of food consumption measures obtained by a given method is thus an essential part of the pilot phase of a dietary survey. Such estimates are obtained by determining the correlation between two measurements on the same individual or by calculating the proportion of agreed-upon positives out of total positives for either time on repeated measures. A high degree of repeatability between replicate measurements of food intake has been shown to exist for the precise weighing, weighed inventory, and dietary history methods (16).

## Validity

Validity is the extent to which a method measures what it purports to measure (2). Although poor repeatability implies poor validity, a repeatable method is not necessarily valid, as it may be systematically wrong. Determining the validity of dietary inquiries is hindered by the lack of an objective reference measure of food consumption, making estimates of sensitivity and specificity impossible. Indirect validation of dietary inquiry methods has been attempted by comparing the results obtained from studying the same group of persons by different methods.

Highly valid methods for determining a person's dietary pattern are desirable, but not essential, in studies aimed at comparing food intake by various groups of persons. Provided a method introduces the same degree of systematic error for all persons surveyed and has a high degree of repeatability, it may serve to classify adequately the dietary patterns of the individuals under study. Lack of knowledge about validity may thus be compensated for in part by other measures of quality, and should not impede studies of diet and cancer.

## COMPARISON OF DIETARY METHODS

In the absence of possibilities for direct validation of dietary inquiry methods, investigators have resorted to comparing recall and record methods, on the assumption that the weighing methods described above provide the best estimate of a person's food intake.

The results of various investigations are often conflicting, as described extensively by Marr (16) and van der Haar and Kromhout (26). In general, however, both the 24-hour recall method and the dietary history method result in slightly higher estimates of total energy, fat, protein, and carbohydrate intake than the food record methods. Shortcut record and recall methods have shown a good correlation between derived food scores and measured intakes obtained by weighing. Difficulties arise, however, when an individual's nutrient intake is assessed on the basis of the scores obtained by the shortcut methods. If a method validly measures one nutrient, one cannot simply assume it measures other nutrients with equal validity.

### Cooperation, Supervision, and Response Rate

The degree of supervision and the cooperation required vary with the inquiry method, and in turn influence the response rate in dietary surveys. Thus, such items should be considered in choosing a method for a study.

Food record methods require a very high degree of cooperation for a prolonged period of time (minimum of four to seven days), and when food is weighed, close supervision is necessary. Both factors tend to reduce the response rate in weighed intake surveys, and biased results may be obtained if only motivated persons capable of cooperating are enrolled. Supposed difficulties should, however, not preclude the use of these methods. A four-day survey using the weighed inventory method had a response rate of 70% to 75% in random samples of Danish and Finnish men aged 50 to 59 years; this was similar to the rate for a previous four-day study using descriptive estimates of food recorded as actually consumed (13), a method that requires less supervision and cooperation.

Dietary recall methods do not call for supervision if the food record part of the dietary history is omitted. Cooperation is limited to the time needed for interviewing, usually about one hour. Response rates are thus generally higher than with food record methods; e.g., 83% of a randomly selected French population agreed to a dietary history interview (25).

Thus, the response rate in dietary surveys tends to be inversely related to the complexity of the method used and, unfortunately, to the probable validity of the estimate of an individual's food consumption. In any study, one must decide whether a high response rate, and thus a highly representative sample of the group under study, outweighs the disadvantage of a less valid method. There is also the practical consideration of lower costs of obtaining information by the dietary recall and shortcut methods than by food record and weighing methods in particular.

## CONCLUSIONS

The cancer epidemiologist has at his disposal a number of methods for estimating individual dietary patterns. The method chosen should meet the general objective of classifying correctly large numbers of individuals with regard to their dietary patterns or consumption of various food components. The consumption of specific food additives may be investigated by asking questions about the consumption of certain foods, whereas an estimate of protein intake would require information on the intake of virtually all foods. The investigator must ask himself whether a correct classification of individuals with regard to the intake of the food under study (in quartiles, for example) can be obtained by shortcut methods or will need more complex food record or recall methods. Furthermore, there is frequently a need for large numbers of subjects, which often imposes a certain degree of simplicity and consideration of costs.

Close collaboration between the nutritionist and the epidemiologist is necessary. As the cancer epidemiologist should be aware of the various methods mentioned above and their advantages and disadvantages, so the nutritionist should be familiar with the needs of the cancer epidemiologist attempting to relate dietary patterns and cancer occurrence in the same individual with an interval of a decade or more between exposure and possible effect. It is hoped that such collaboration will lead to the further development of simple dietary inquiry methods and improvements in validation techniques, such as the use of urinary nitrogens as an indicator of protein intake (4).

An adequate description of the methods employed, as well as information on their validity and repeatability, is a prerequisite for the interpretation of results emerging from dietary studies. Such studies require careful planning and execution. Often representatives of several disciplines must be called on to overcome the difficulties outlined above and to advance the knowledge of the etiological role of food in cancer development.

## REFERENCES

1. Armstrong, B., and Doll, R. (1975): Environmental factors and cancer incidence and mortality in different countries, with special reference to dietary practices. *Int. J. Cancer,* 15:617–631.
2. Barker, D. J. P., and Rose, G., editors (1976): *Epidemiology in Medical Practice.* Churchill Livingstone, Edinburgh, London, and New York.
3. Bjelke, E. (1973): *Epidemiologic Studies of Cancer of the Stomach, Colon and Rectum, With Special Emphasis on the Role of Diet, Vols. I–IV.* Thesis submitted to the Graduate School Faculty of the University of Minnesota. Xerox University Microfilms, Ann Arbor, Michigan.
4. Borgström, B., Dencker, I., Krabisch, L., Nordén, Å., and Åkeson, B. (1975): Assessment of food consumption. *Scand. J. Soc. Med.,* Suppl. 10:14–25.
5. Burke, B. S. (1947): The dietary history as a tool in research. *J. Am. Diet. Assoc.,* 23:1041–1046.
6. Campbell, V. A., and Dodds, M. L. (1967): Collecting dietary information from groups of older people. *J. Am. Diet. Assoc.,* 51:29–33.
7. Dales, L. G., Friedman, G. D., Ury, H. K., Grossman, S., and Williams, S. R. (1979): A case-control study of relationships of diet and other traits to colorectal cancer in American Blacks. *Am. J. Epidemiol.,* 109:132–144.
8. Graham, D., Scholtz, W., and Martino, P. (1972): Alimentary factors in the epidemiology of gastric cancer. *Cancer,* 30:927–938.
9. Haenszel, W., Kurihara, M., Segi, M., and Lee, R. C. K. (1972): Stomach cancer among Japanese in Hawaii. *J. Natl. Cancer Inst.,* 49:969–985.
10. Hankin, J. H., Rhoads, G. G., and Glober, G. A. (1975): A dietary method for an epidemiologic study of gastrointestinal cancer. *Am. J. Clin. Nutr.,* 28:1055–1061.
11. Higginson, J. (1966): Etiological factors in gastrointestinal cancer in man. *J. Natl. Cancer Inst.,* 37:527–545.
12. *IARC Annual Report* (1978). International Agency for Research on Cancer, Lyons, France.
13. IARC Microecology Group (1977): Dietary fiber, transit time, fecal bacteria, steroids and colon cancer in two Scandinavian populations. *Lancet,* 2:207–211.
14. James, W. P. T. (1978): Introductory remarks. *Nutrition and Cancer,* 1:89–91.
15. MacLaren, D. S., editor (1976): *Nutrition and Its Disorders.* Churchill Livingstone, Edinburgh, London, and New York.
16. Marr, J. W., editor (1971): Individual dietary surveys: Purposes and methods. In: *World Review of Nutrition and Dietetics, Vol. 13,* pp. 105–164. Karger, Basel.
17. Modan, B., Lubin, F., Barrell, V., Greenberg, R. A., Modan, M., and Graham, S. (1974): The role of starches in the etiology of gastric cancer. *Cancer,* 34:2087–2092.
18. Morgan, R. W., Jain, M., Miller, A. B., Choi, N. W., Matthews, V., Munan, L., Burch, J. D., Feather, J., Howe, G. R., and Kelly, A. (1978): A comparison of dietary methods in epidemiologic studies. *Am. J. Epidemiol.,* 107:488–498.
19. Pekkarinen, M. (1967): Chemical analysis in connection with dietary surveys in Finland. *Voeding,* 28:1–8.
20. Pekkarinen, M. (1970): Methodology in the collection of food consumption data. *World Rev. Nutr. Diet.,* 12:145–171.
21. Péquignot, G., and Cubeau, J. (1973): Enquêtes méthodologiques comparant chez les mêmes

sujets la consommation alimentaire appréciée par interrogatoire à la consommation mesurée par pesée. *Rev. Epidémiol. Santé Publique,* 21:585–608.
22. Southgate, D. A. (1969): Determination of carbohydrates in foods. II. Unavailable carbohydrates. *J. Sci. Food Agric.,* 20:331.
23. Tuyns, A. J., Péquignot, G., and Jensen, O. M. (1977): Le cancer de l'oesophage en Ille-et-Vilaine en fonction des niveaux de consommation d'alcool et de tabac: Des risques qui se multiplient. *Bull. Cancer,* 64:45–60.
24. Tuyns, A. J., Péquignot, G., and Jensen, O. M. (1979): Role of diet, alcohol and tobacco in oesophageal cancer, as illustrated by two contrasting high-incidence areas in the North of Iran and West of France. *Front. Gastrointest. Res.,* 4:101–110.
25. Tuyns, A. J., Péquignot, G., Jensen, O., and Pomeau, Y. (1975): La consommation individuelle de boissons alcoolisées et de tabac dans un échantillon de la population en Ille-et-Vilaine. *Revue Alcoolisme,* 21:105–150.
26. van der Haar, F., and Kromhout, D. (1978): Food intake, nutritional anthropometry and blood chemical parameters in 3 selected Dutch schoolchildren populations. *Mededelingen Landbouwhogeschool Wageningen,* Nederland, 78–9, pp. 4–28.
27. Wynder, E., and Shigematsu, T. (1967): Environmental factors of cancer of the colon and rectum. *Cancer,* 20:1520–1561.
28. Young, C. M. (1965): Comparison of results of dietary surveys made by different methods. In: *Proc. Fourth Int. Congr. Dietet., Stockholm, 1965,* pp. 119–126. Ivar Haeggströms Tryckeri AB.

*Nutrition and Cancer: Etiology and Treatment,*
edited by G. R. Newell and N. M. Ellison.
Raven Press, New York © 1981.

# Anthropometric Measurements

## Jere D. Haas and Katherine M. Flegal

*Division of Nutritional Sciences, Cornell University, Ithaca, New York 14853*

Anthropometric measurements are useful tools for evaluating the health of an individual and of the population as a whole. Height and weight are measures routinely used for clinical diagnosis and public health evaluation. The nutritional sciences rely heavily on anthropometric techniques to measure the functional morphological changes that accompany the development and treatment of nutritional diseases. These methods can be very valuable in assessing nutritional status in children and adults. They have been used to evaluate the nutritional status of cancer patients, as well as in epidemiological and clinical research in cancer. However, these anthropometric methods should not be used uncritically. In this chapter, we shall present a critique of several common applications of these methods. Our critique will not be restricted to evaluating the nutritional status of cancer patients, but will deal broadly with the evaluation of nutritional status in clinical, research, and survey situations.

First, we shall discuss some conceptual and statistical problems with the use of simple measures of height and weight. Next, we shall consider the use of anthropometry in assessing body composition, as well as some limitations in using formulas to estimate total body composition from anthropometric measures. Finally, we shall present data to demonstrate the major sources of measurement error in skinfold measurements of adiposity.

To appreciate an evaluation of nutritional anthropometric methods and techniques, the reader must be familiar with the rationale behind anthropometry and the techniques commonly employed. The most common anthropometric measurements used in nutritional assessment are weight, height (or recumbent length), head, limb and trunk circumferences, and skinfold thickness at various sites. Measurements less commonly used, but potentially informative, include sitting height, lower limb length, and biacromial and biiliocristal diameters. Although the rationale for some of these measurements can be briefly presented here, it is recommended that the reader consult one of the numerous publications that deal with measurement techniques (5,12,18,29,35).

Anthropometry is based on the concept that an appropriate measurement should reflect morphological variation in response to a functionally significant physiological change. For example, skinfold calipers can be used to measure the thickness of the adipose layer. In most cases, a significant reduction in adipose tissue thickness reflects a shift in the individual's energy balance. Although this specificity is desirable, much of the anthropometry employed in nutritional status assessment is not specific for a particular nutritional imbalance. This is not necessarily bad, if one keeps in mind the purpose for which anthropometry is used. As a first-order indicator of nutritional compromise, rapid weight loss is a good indicator of a potential health problem. To understand the exact nature of the problem, more extensive examination of body composition or biochemical testing would be required. But as a screening procedure, anthropometry is a useful tool for the nutritionist or clinician.

Specificity can be improved by the imaginative use of a battery of anthropometric techniques. A good example is the use of weight, height, and age to classify a child as acutely or chronically malnourished in terms of protein and energy intake (24,28). A child who is short relative to healthy children the same age could be considered chronically malnourished. A child who is light for his age may be suffering from acute malnutrition. If weight and height are both substandard but weight-for-height is normal, the diagnosis of chronic malnutrition is strengthened. If weight is very low compared to that of healthy children of the same age, and height and weight-for-height are also reduced, the child would be diagnosed as suffering from severe acute malnutrition superimposed on chronic undernutrition. The diagnoses are based on the simple understanding that growth in body mass is much more labile than skeletal growth. The former is rapidly affected by short-term changes in nutrition, while the latter requires longer nutritional insult.

## PROBLEMS IN THE USE OF WEIGHT AND HEIGHT INDICES

Weight relative to height is the most widely used indicator of nutritional status in adults. The ponderal index (height/weight$^{1/3}$), Quetelet's index (weight/height$^2$), and percent of standard weight adjusted for height are all measures commonly used to assess the degree to which an individual is overweight or underweight. However, weight and height measurements are surprisingly difficult to use and interpret, particularly when comparing one individual or group of individuals with others. It is also difficult to translate the general concepts of overweight and underweight into precise and accurate measures. Two specific problems arise. First, although weight alone means little apart from height, it is not clear how to incorporate information about height into comparisons of weight. Second, it is not clear how to identify a normal, ideal, or desirable weight to use as a standard in assessing relative overweight and underweight.

The methods proposed to deal with these problems are rather unsatisfactory. A common practice is to choose some standard set of weights and to express an individual's weight as a percentage of the standard weight for the appropriate sex, height, and in some cases age. Two advantages of this method are that the weights of persons of different heights can be compared because they are translated into percentages and that relative overweight or underweight is expressed directly as a percentage of standard weight.

The disadvantage of this method is that it is based on use of a standard weight, and there is no well-developed theoretical basis for defining standard weights. Proposed standards range from simply using the average weight for a specific sex–age–height group in the same population to using tabulated values based on mortality experience for persons of different weights taken from life insurance company data. These standards are often quite different, and when different practitioners or investigators use different standards their results cannot be directly compared.

The idea of defining an index that is a function of height and weight alone and does not depend on use of any standard weight is thus quite attractive. Many such indices have been developed and several are in common use today.

The index most commonly used is probably Quetelet's index, weight divided by the square of height $(W/H^2)$; the next most commonly used is $W/H$. Both of these indices are often referred to as the body mass index. The ponderal index, $H/W^{1/3}$, was once in vogue, partly because of its association with somatotyping, but has fallen into some disfavor recently as its undesirable properties have become better known. Keys and his associates (14) describe several indices and illustrate their properties using data from different populations.

Indices of these types are commonly used in epidemiological studies to compare groups within populations and to compare populations with one another. Examples of the use of such indices in studies of breast cancer can be found in articles by de Waard (2) and by Hakama and his associates (8). More recently, it has been suggested that Quetelet's index, in conjunction with specific cutoff points, should be used to classify individuals as overweight or underweight (20).

These indices possess an appealing simplicity, which masks some of the complications associated with their use. Several assumptions are incorporated into their construction and evaluation, not all of which are obvious. Some are questionable even in the populations in which the indices have been developed and tested, and it is not clear when they hold true in other populations. Two assumptions appear to be mutually contradictory.

Khosla and Lowe (15) established criteria for an acceptable weight and height index. They consider that the index of the general form $W/H^n$ that best satisfies their criteria is one that is most nearly a constant along a line described by the linear regression of weight on height in a population. The value $n$ in this index is simply an algebraic function of the intercept and slope parameters of the regression. This makes it apparent that the best index by their criteria is highly population-specific. The regression line, which is derived from the average weight-for-heights in a population, is used to define a kind of standard weight-for-height. Thus, the best index depends both on the average weights-for-heights in a population and on the average increase in weight associated with an increase in height. In effect, this index is standardized for the weight-for-height characteristics of a specific population.

The use of a linear regression of weight on height presumes that weight can be described adequately as a linear function of height and that the variance of weight is the same at different heights. These particular assumptions are unlikely to be met in many populations. Should one test these assumptions for the population under study? And if these assumptions are not met, should a different procedure be used? These questions have not been systematically addressed.

One of the criteria for the "best" index is that it be independent of height. It seems reasonable that the proportions of overweight and underweight people should not differ at different heights. However, in any population there could be some empirical association between height and degree of overweight or underweight, mediated, for example, through genetic differences affecting both stature and weight or through environmental conditions affecting both. Such differences are defined out of existence by this procedure.

In practice, $n$ is usually rounded to the nearest integer, which is generally either 1 or 2. This introduces an arbitrary, nonlinear dependence on height. Thus, the procedure usually followed to define a "best" index involves first trying to eliminate all dependence on height and then introducing a new dependence on height.

As discussed above, these indices are based on the average weights in a population, and evaluated by how they express these weights. Little attention has been given to the question of how appropriately or consistently these indices express deviations from the norm. In fact, algebraically, to the extent that they are independent of height, as defined previously, they have the property that they express the same percent deviation from the mean at different heights with the same numerical value of the index. Thus, a man who is 6 feet tall and 20% over the expected mean weight for his height, as predicted by the regression equation, will have the same numerical value of the index as will a man who is 5 feet tall and 20% over the predicted mean weight for his height. This is tantamount to saying that the normal variation in weight is not constant, but increases with height. It also contradicts the assumption that the variance of weight is constant at different heights, on which the original regression equation was based. Thus, the use of these indices involves two contradictory assumptions simultaneously.

In general, weight-for-height indices have few of the advantages that are often claimed. In particular, they do not provide an objective, standard-free assessment of weight-for-height, as is often asserted. Although these indices can indeed be computed without using any tables of standard weights, the criteria for defining the "best" index for a population are highly population-specific and require knowledge of the average weight-for-height in that population.

These indices do not appear to offer any advantages when they are used to compare individuals within a population. Percentages of standard weights contain as much information as any index, and the use of percentages requires fewer and more explicit assumptions than the use of indices. Moreover, it does not appear that these indices can validly be used to compare individuals or groups from different populations. If the "best" index is the same in both populations, then a comparison based on percentages of average or standard weights will again be as informative as comparisons using an index, and will again require fewer assumptions. On the other hand, if the "best" index is not the same in the two populations, then it is not clear what index should be used to compare them.

Finally, it is inappropriate to use these indices as indicators of fatness or leanness. Even though weight and fatness are strongly associated, these indices do not measure fatness accurately enough to be useful (14,31).

## BODY COMPOSITION

Both height and weight are composite measures of gross morphology. If the components of weight and height are understood, these measures can be more clearly interpreted in various situations. Total body weight is a composite of all body constituents, including water, minerals, fat, and protein. Each of these components varies with specific aspects of nutriture. The ability to measure these individual components would greatly improve the specificity of assessment of nutritional status. Various models of body composition have been developed employing biochemical, isotopic, densitometric, radiographic, and anthropometric techniques. Anthropometric methods are generally used to identify two components, muscle and fat.

Anthropometric assessment of body fat is done with skinfold calipers that measure the double thickness of the subcutaneous layer of fat plus skin. This adipose layer is deposited over most of the body surface and its thickness at various sites on the body has been shown to be correlated with other measures of body fat determined by densitometry, radiography, ultrasonography, and autopsy. In measuring skinfold thickness, it is important to recognize that considerable individual variation in adiposity exists as a function of age, sex, race, and site on the body (13,16,17). As will be explained in more detail below, errors in measurements of skinfold thickness vary considerably along the same lines. In addition, fat distribution in and around the body varies with sex, age, race, and nutritional and health status (16), and this variation severely limits the interpretation of a skinfold measurement from a single measuring site, such as the triceps. This is particularly true when one uses formulas for estimating total body fat based on skinfold and other anthropometric measurements.

Anthropometric techniques to estimate muscle size use measures of limb circumference and skinfold thickness. The mid-upper arm is the most commonly measured site for this purpose (5,6,9,12). Muscle circumference is estimated by correcting the total arm circumference by the thickness of the overlying adipose layer. The corrections are based on the assumptions that the cross-section of the mid-upper arm approximates a circle, that the adipose layer is evenly distributed around the arm, and that the bone (humerus) contribution to the arm composition is constant across subjects. The fact that these assumptions are rarely met is a major source of error in the quantification of actual mid-upper arm muscle dimensions, especially among obese subjects (9).

One can also criticize the use of an estimate of muscle development at one measuring site as a reflection of the total body protein reserve. For example, the relationship between mid-upper arm muscle circumference and plasma proteins in surgical patients has been shown to be weak (34). Clearly, more research is needed to validate these measurements of protein nutritional status in clinical populations.

Height can also be divided into components that reflect linear dimensions of the lower extremities, trunk, and head. These measurements are often used in indices or as ratios to indicate body proportions. Linear measurements can be combined with breadth, circumference, and weight to categorize a person's body shape (26).

Measures of body composition, proportion and shape have a different significance in adults than in growing children. The skeletal dimensions of adults are fixed and linear proportions are therefore unchanging (except for postural effects of aging). For this reason, anthropometric measures of soft-tissue body composition and body shape are useful in evaluating current nutritional status in an adult. However, since linear growth is continuous in infants, children, and adolescents, measures of body proportion are particularly useful in evaluating growth processes that may be affected by nutritional compromise. The differential growth rates of various linear segments of the body at different ages (26) provide a useful criterion for evaluating whether previous nutritional stress may have affected the growth of a child. Short stature in an adult may reflect general nutritional stunting during growth. The additional knowledge that the person has a disproportionately short trunk would suggest that this stunting was prepubertal, based on the knowledge that the legs normally grow proportionately faster than the trunk during childhood, while the reverse is true during puberty (26). Therefore, chronic undernutrition only during childhood would have presumably affected growth of the legs, while trunk and leg growth would have proceeded normally during the pubertal phase, when nutritional problems were reduced.

The dynamics of change in the soft components of muscle and fat during growth can be analyzed in a similar fashion, but over a shorter period of change in nutriture. The relationships between changes in fat thickness and muscle growth are different in infancy, childhood, adolescence, and adulthood (17, 19,26). Because of the close association between fatness and caloric reserves and between muscularity and protein status, the relationship between measures of these two types of tissue provides a useful tool for assessing the gross nutritional status of a person at specific stages of the life cycle.

## THE USE OF ANTHROPOMETRY TO PREDICT TOTAL BODY FAT

Although the thickness of the subcutaneous layer of adipose tissue at specific sites can be inferred directly from measurements of skinfold thickness, it is common to estimate the total amount of body fat from formulas that use skinfold thickness combined with anthropometric measurements, such as diameters and circumferences. Many such formulas have been published, and some idea of the wide variety of anthropometric measurements that have been used in such formulas can be gathered from Young's presentation (33). Durnin and Womersley (3), Sloan and co-workers (25), and Jackson and Pollock (11) describe some commonly used formulas. The investigator who considers using one of these formulas should have a good understanding of how they were developed and what their limitations are.

Such formulas are derived by essentially the same method. The investigators assemble a group of individuals, make a wide variety of anthropometric measurements on each person, and estimate each person's fatness by a standard method for determining body composition, often by underwater weighing. They then seek to develop an equation that describes some dependent variable, such as percent body fat, as a linear function of a subset of the anthropometric measurements. Stepwise regression or some other multiple regression variable selection procedure is generally used to choose what anthropometric variables enter into the final equation. The final equation can then be used as a formula to predict body fat from anthropometric measurements.

The objective of this procedure is quite narrowly defined. It is to find the linear combination of the available independent variables that best describes the dependent variable in the sample examined. There are many reasons why such a formula should not satisfactorily predict body fat in other individuals, particularly those who differ markedly from the individuals in the original sample.

Many anthropometric measurements are correlated with body fat, and thus might appear to be good candidates for use in predicting body fat. However, a major problem is that they are also often strongly correlated with each other (this phenomenon is known as multicollinearity). As a consequence, the numerical coefficients associated with each measurement tend to be variable and unstable. The variance of the coefficients is quite high. They are unstable in the sense that, depending on what other variables are included in the equation, their numerical value may change quite strikingly—for example, from a large positive number to a large negative number. As a result, the choice of variables to include in the final equation is largely arbitrary and the estimates of the coefficients associated with these variables are quite imprecise. Minor random fluctuations within the sample may have unduly strong effects on the final formula. This explains in part why combinations of measurements in different formulas are so varied.

The underlying relationship between a given anthropometric measurement and percent body fat is often not linear. Few of these equations include any transformations of the variables that might reflect this nonlinearity. For example, it is well known that most skinfold measurements are not normally distributed in a healthy population (11,13,27). Log transformations should be used to normalize these distributions for use in regression models. However, this is rarely done.

In short, the numbers in a formula may not indicate anything about the underlying biological relationship of a particular anthropometric measurement to percent body fat, even in the sample, but only something about the linear aspect of that relationship in conjunction with the other measurements included in the formula.

The sources of biological variation that may affect the relationships between anthropometric measurements and body fat are many. In general, differences in fat distribution patterns (subcutaneous versus visceral and central versus peripheral), muscle development, and skeletal form all affect these relationships. These sources of variation can be minimized, although not eliminated, by choosing a group of individuals who are relatively homogeneous with regard to age, sex, race, and social and environmental background. Within such a group, body composition tends to be relatively uniform. Furthermore, associations between anthropometric measurements and body fatness are relatively constant within such a group. As a consequence, a formula for predicting body fat will usually be population specific, and will tend to give fairly good results when applied to a population that is similar to the original sample.

However, in a different group, the results will often not be as good. One reason is that the relationships between the anthropometric variables and body fatness are likely to be different. Another reason is that such a formula is likely to predict well only within the range of combinations represented in the original sample. For example, if the original group consisted of people with a similar degree of muscularity, no characteristic that distinguishes people with different degrees of muscularity is likely to appear in the formula derived from that group. Consequently, the formula will tend not to distinguish large muscular people from large obese people.

These methods include an implicit assumption that the dependent variable measures body fat more precisely than the independent variables. However, the generally accepted methods of determining body composition, such as measurements of body density, total body potassium, or total body water, are fairly imprecise. These methods are still indirect assessments of body composition, and each is based on a set of standard assumptions. The validity of these assumptions varies with age, sex, diet, exercise, and heredity (4,22,23,32).

Thus, not only do the relationships between anthropometric measurements and measurements of body fat differ in different subpopulations, but the relationships between actual body fatness and measurements of body fat also differ. This introduces further uncertainty into the problem of using an equation derived from one group to predict body fatness in another group.

It is questionable whether any of these formulas give sufficiently accurate predictions to be useful in practical applications. Typically, the standard deviation of percent body weight as fat is around 5% to 10% of body weight within a relatively uniform group. The standard error of percent body weight as fat, adjusted for the effects of anthropometric measurements, is typically around 2.5% to 5% of body weight. It is not clear whether a reduction in variability of this magnitude is useful, and little attention has been paid to this question.

These formulas often have not been validated on a different sample from that used to develop them. When they are tested on a second sample, they typically do not perform as well. Unfortunately, many of the formulas that appear to do quite well in predicting fatness in a new sample share a certain property, on closer inspection, that makes them less useful. Rather than predicting percent body fat from anthropometric measurements, they are predicting the weight of body fat from total body weight. This is tantamount to asserting that percent body fat is a constant. Such formulas crop up surprisingly often in forms that are frequently hard to recognize. However, any formula in which the predicted variable is neither body density nor percent body fat, and which includes actual body weight or lean body weight as one of the independent variables, is probably of this type. (See, for example, the studies of Weltman and Katch [30] and Noppa et al. [21].) Although these formulas are not invalid, they do not provide much new information, and although they predict the weight of body fat quite well, they do not predict the actual percent of body weight as fat any better than other formulas.

Before deciding to use one of these formulas, one should take into account a number of considerations. These formulas work best with individuals who are similar to those from whom the formula was originally developed and who fall within the range of variability of the original group. Thus, a formula that was developed with overweight people will probably not be suitable for thin individuals, and vice versa. The validity of the formula should be assessed for each new population in which it is to be used, as it cannot be assumed to be appropriate. The purpose of using such a formula should be examined, and it should be decided what level of predictive accuracy is needed and whether it can be achieved using a particular formula.

## SOURCES OF ERROR IN SKINFOLD MEASUREMENT

Often in clinical practice insufficient thought is given to sources of measurement error in anthropometric assessment. In many clinical evaluations, anthropometric measurements have been made by inexperienced or improperly trained personnel. Moreover, there is often little regard for proper training and quality control measures to insure the reduction of measurement error.

Habicht et al. (7) have addressed this problem in relation to the selection of anthropometric indicators of nutritional status in children. They identify three sources of error that can affect the sensitivity of an indicator of nutritional status, and call these sources imprecision, undependability, and inaccuracy. Imprecision is the error associated with reproducibility of a measurement by the same observer (intraobserver) and by different observers (interobserver). Undependability is the error associated with reproducibility of a measurement influenced by changes in nonnutritional factors. For example, daily changes in body water content or stomach contents will influence the day-to-day reproducibility of body weight and thus reduce the dependability of body weight as an indicator of protein–energy malnutrition. Inaccuracy is the error associated with a poor correlation between the indicator of nutritional status and the underlying nutriture it is designed to reflect.

It is essential to understand how these sources of error affect various anthropometric indicators of nutritional status. To illustrate this point, we will refer to preliminary data analysis of skinfold measures in which these sources of measurement error have been estimated.

The reader is advised to consult Cameron (2) or Habicht et al. (7) for detailed explanation of how to compute and interpret the estimates of measurement error. Only a brief summary of the formulas will be given here.

Skinfold measurements are indicators of fat thickness but they do not measure fat directly. There are potential sources of error in the use of skinfolds to measure fatness and indicate energy balance. One can view these sources of error systematically in relation to the total variance observed in a sample, as expressed in the following equation:

$$V_T = V_N + V_E$$

where $V_T$ is total sample variance, $V_N$ is variance due to the effect of nutrition (in the case of skinfolds, this is usually energy status), and $V_E$ is variance due to all the combined sources of error. If $V_N/V_T$ is high, i.e., close to unity, then the indicator can be considered a sensitive indicator of nutriture. The closer the value is to zero, the less sensitive and more error-prone is the measure. Therefore, efforts should be made to quantify $V_E$ and to identify its components. These components or sources of error variance can be expressed as

$$V_E = V_P + V_D + V_A$$

where $V_P$ is error due to imprecision, $V_D$ is error due to undependability, and $V_A$ is error due to inaccuracy.

$V_P$ and $V_D$ are relatively easy to compute, while $V_A$ is nearly impossible to estimate. Imprecision and undependability (also referred to collectively as unreliability) are both estimated by standard test–retest procedures. Unbiased replicate measurements are taken on the same subject, and the variance around the mean of the replicates is estimated. The test–retest protocol is organized slightly differently, depending on whether $V_P$ or $V_D$ is to be computed. Since error caused by imprecision usually includes both interobserver error ($V_B$) and intraobserver error ($V_W$), i.e.,

$$V_P = V_B + V_W,$$

it is necessary to identify both these sources of error. However, if there is no intention of having more than one examiner throughout the course of a study and the data are not to be compared to data obtained by another examiner or study, it is not necessary to estimate $V_B$, and $V_P$ will equal $V_W$. To estimate $V_W$, the same examiner measures skinfolds on the same subject twice, with the second measurements not biased by the first. This bias is eliminated by using easily removable adhesive markers to identify measuring sites at each measuring trial and by performing the reexamination about one hour after the first examination. $V_B$ is estimated using two examiners who measure the same subject. The second examiner should not be biased by the measurements taken by the first examiner.

Since dependability of skinfold measurements relates to nonnutritional factors that may influence the reproducibility of a measurement, it is necessary to use a test–retest protocol that takes this variation into account. The major source of error due to undependability probably relates to periodic changes in the hydration of the adipose layer, which affects compressibility of the skinfold. This variation in hydration may be related to diurnal fluctuations or, in women, to fluctuations during the menstrual cycle. Therefore, a retest for dependability should be done about two weeks after the first examination and at a different time of the day.

Depending on the population to be studied, different sources of undependability error may be identified (10) and different test–retest schedules required. If the energy balance of a subject is unstable and might lead to a change in body fat over the period of time required to estimate $V_D$, the subject should not be included in the validation procedure.

The reliability of skinfold measurements may be related to other nonnutritional factors such as sex, age, genetic background, muscle tone, disease state, amount of fat measured, and measuring site. These factors should also be considered when selecting and validating skinfold measurements.

The results of these calculations can be presented in various ways. Since one is usually interested in knowing how much of the total sample variance is due to measurement (unreliability) error, the results can be expressed as

$$\text{Percent error} = \frac{V_B + V_W + V_D}{V_T} \times 100$$

The preliminary results of such an analysis are presented in Table 1 for skinfold measurements. Validation procedures were applied to seven skinfold measurements in 99 healthy subjects (52 men, 47 women) who ranged in age from 19 to 92 years. The subjects also ranged from lean to overweight, so the error in measurement could be evaluated relative to the amount of fat measured. As can be seen in Table 1 and Fig. 1, there is considerable variation in the total error among skinfold sites. The least error-prone is the triceps site, with 3.6% of the total variance (45.9) resulting from the unreliability of the technique. The most error-prone site is the suprailiac site, with 16.1% error. It is also evident that more of the error is interobserver ($V_B$) than intraobserver ($V_W$) for nearly all of the sites. Compared to a commonly used anthropometric measurement, mid-upper arm circumference, skinfolds are more prone to measurement error. Only 2% of the variance in arm circumference is measurement error, while all but one skinfold site have a higher degree of measurement error by twofold or more. Calculations of total error due to unreliability of data reported by Habicht et al. (7) yield slightly higher values for skinfolds in

TABLE 1. Components of unreliability in measurements of skinfold thickness (mm) at 7 sites (sexes combined, N = 99)

| Skinfold site | Sample mean | Sample variance[a] $V_T$ | Error variances[b] | | | Total[c] | Error as percent of $V_T$ | | |
|---|---|---|---|---|---|---|---|---|---|
| | | | $V_W$ | $V_B$ | $V_D$ | | Within[d] | Between[e] | Dependability[f] |
| Triceps | 14.0 | 45.9 | .32 | .96 | .36 | 3.6 | 0.7 | 2.1 | 0.8 |
| Biceps | 5.4 | 19.1 | .34 | .74 | .81 | 9.8 | 1.7 | 3.8 | 4.2 |
| Subscapular | 12.2 | 25.9 | .27 | 1.49 | .56 | 8.9 | 1.0 | 5.7 | 2.2 |
| Abdominal | 16.1 | 77.8 | .77 | 2.13 | 1.04 | 5.1 | 1.0 | 2.7 | 1.3 |
| Suprailiac | 9.4 | 29.2 | .43 | 2.82 | 1.46 | 16.1 | 1.5 | 9.6 | 5.0 |
| Medial calf | 10.8 | 34.5 | .35 | .88 | .37 | 4.6 | 1.0 | 2.5 | 1.1 |
| Anterior thigh | 18.8 | 88.5 | .48 | 2.13 | 1.02 | 4.1 | 0.5 | 2.4 | 1.2 |
| Arm circumference | 28.8 | 15.7 | .10 | .14 | .07 | 2.0 | 0.6 | 0.9 | 0.5 |

[a] Often expressed as standard deviations (S.D.) of the mean where S.D. = $V_T^{-2}$.

[b] $V_W$ = Within-examiner or intraobserver error. $V_B$ = Between-examiner or interobserver error corrected for within-examiner error. $V_B + V_W$ = error due to imprecision = $V_P$. $V_D$ = error due to undependability corrected for between- and within-examiner error.

[c] Percent of total variance $V_T$ that is due to all estimates of unreliability = $\{[V_W + V_B + V_D]/V_T\} \times 100$.

[d] Percent of total variance that is due to intraobserver error = $(V_W/V_T) \times 100$.

[e] Percent of total variance that is due to interobserver error = $(V_B/V_T) \times 100$.

[f] Percent of total variance that is due to undependability $(V_D/V_T) \times 100$.

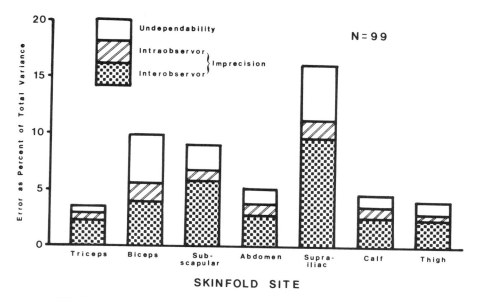

FIG. 1. Components of unreliability in skinfold measurements at seven sites.

malnourished children than those reported in Table 1 for healthy adults. Those authors also report reliability error estimates for the same children in height (1%) and weight (5%), as well as for other measurements.

It is clear that there is considerable variation in measurement error from site to site. There is also variation between men and women, as shown in Fig. 2. Generally, there is more error in measuring skinfolds in women than in men. This observation, however, seems to be related to sex differences in the amount of adipose tissue at any site. When an analysis of variance is run to examine the sources of variation in measurement reliability (Table 2), it is clear that most of the variation within our sample is due to the thickness of tissue. When covariation in tissue thickness is statistically controlled, sex differences have virtually no effect on intraobserver, interobserver, or undependability error. Age variation in the sample also has very little effect on measurement error. However, the covariate, tissue thickness, is significantly related to each of the three sources of unreliability error at nearly all skinfold sites. The exceptions are dependability ($V_D$) at the triceps and thigh sites.

The relationship between measurement error and thickness of the adipose layer is demonstrated graphically in Fig. 3 for the triceps and subscapular sites. From these graphs, it is clear that interobserver error increases most rapidly as tissue thickness increases, while intraobserver error and undependability change relatively little. The relationship between tissue thickness and dependability error at the subscapular site is actually curvilinear, with the greatest dependability (least error due to undependability) found at about 10 to 20 mm of tissue thickness and the least dependable measurements taken at the extremes.

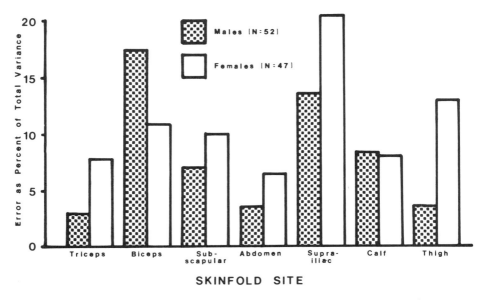

**FIG. 2.** Sex differences in unreliability of skinfold measurements at seven sites.

While this preliminary examination of the sources of measurement unreliability in skinfolds is informative, it does not tell the whole story. It is still necessary to evaluate the accuracy with which skinfolds actually measure adipose tissue thickness and reflect energy nutritional status. Although there may be no technique that can be used to measure adipose tissue or energy nutritional status *in vivo* with absolute accuracy, there are indirect techniques that are more accurate than skinfold measurements. Correlations between various skinfold measurements and estimates of body density are fairly high (r = −.7 to −.9), which suggests a strong degree of association between these two techniques of body fat determination (4). A high correlation (r = .92) has also been reported for the relationship between skinfold thickness and measurements of adipose tissue from soft tissue radiographs (1).

To insure the best use and valid interpretation of nutritional anthropometry, it is essential that proper training and quality control be maintained, following a procedure similar to that described above. There is no reason why a research team or clinical nutrition support unit should not require the same degree of quality control for anthropometric procedures as they expect for clinical chemistry studies.

## CONCLUSIONS

From this critique of commonly used anthropometric techniques, several conclusions can be drawn.

TABLE 2. *Summary of analysis of variance for the effects of age, sex, and tissue thickness on measurement error in skinfolds*

| Skinfold site | Tissue thickness[a] | Main effects | | Sex x age interaction |
|---|---|---|---|---|
| | | Sex | Age | |
| Intraobserver error ($V_W$) | | | | |
| Triceps | .001[b] | ns | ns | .034 |
| Biceps | <.001 | ns | ns | ns |
| Subscapular | <.001 | .012 | ns | ns |
| Abdomen | <.001 | ns | ns | .010 |
| Suprailiac | <.001 | ns | ns | ns |
| Calf | <.001 | ns | ns | .018 |
| Thigh | .003 | ns | ns | ns |
| Interobserver error ($V_B$) | | | | |
| Triceps | .001 | ns | ns | .003 |
| Biceps | <.001 | ns | ns | ns |
| Subscapular | <.001 | ns | .012 | ns |
| Abdomen | <.001 | ns | ns | ns |
| Suprailiac | <.001 | ns | ns | ns |
| Calf | <.001 | ns | ns | ns |
| Thigh | <.002 | ns | ns | ns |
| Undependability ($V_D$) | | | | |
| Triceps | ns | ns | ns | .037 |
| Biceps | <.001 | ns | .002 | ns |
| Subscapular | .002 | ns | ns | ns |
| Abdomen | .002 | ns | ns | ns |
| Suprailiac | .005 | ns | ns | .003 |
| Calf | .003 | ns | ns | ns |
| Thigh | ns | ns | ns | ns |

[a] Tissue thickness is a covariate that enters the regression model first, followed by the main effects and interaction.

[b] Values reported in the table are significance levels for the F-ratio; ns = not significant ($P < .05$).

A. Although weight and height are the most commonly used anthropometric indicators of nutritional status, weight-for-height indices are of little use as indicators of overweight and underweight or of fatness and leanness. A more acceptable way of expressing weight relative to height is through the use of weight as a percentage of some standard weight-for-height. This contains as much information as a weight-for-height index, but requires fewer assumptions.

B. Considerably more information regarding nutritional status can be obtained by measuring body composition. Skinfold thickness and body circumference are commonly used anthropometric measurements that indirectly indicate body composition at specific sites. Major difficulties arise when one attempts to estimate total body composition from such anthropometric measurements with commonly used formulas. Comparisons of body composition among individuals and populations are better accomplished by direct comparisons of anthropometric

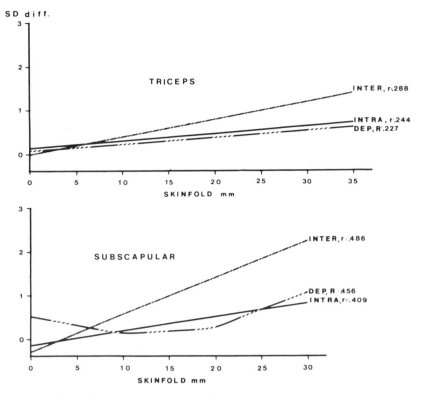

**FIG. 3.** The relationship between skinfold thickness and measurement error at the triceps and subscapular sites. Measurement error is expressed as the square root of the variance (S.D. diff.) and presented separately for intraobserver (intra), interobserver (inter), and dependability (dep) components of error. The r and R values are simple and multiple correlation coefficients, respectively. N = 99.

indicators. This requires a broad consensus on the number and type of measurements to be used.

C. The selection of appropriate anthropometric indicators of nutritional status should be made with proper consideration for the sources of measurement error inherent in the method. It should be recognized that components of error (precision, dependability, accuracy) may vary with such factors as the subject's age, sex, clinical state, nutritional status, and genetic background, and the level of examiner training. A properly designed training and quality control program should be an essential part of any research protocol and nutrition support service that uses anthropometry to assess nutritional status. One who recognizes the limitations of nutritional anthropometry discussed in this chapter will have a better understanding of the research and diagnostic potential of nutritional assessment techniques.

## ACKNOWLEDGMENTS

We would like to thank the following colleagues for their assistance in the preparation of this chapter: Kim Andrup, Linda Buttel, Ed Frongillo, Jean-Pierre Habicht, Maria Irisarri, Kusum Mainigi, John Spitzer, and Daphne A. Roe. The research on skinfold measurement error was conducted under a contract (NO1-CP-85652) from the Diet, Nutrition, and Cancer Program of the National Cancer Institute. This is a report from the Agricultural Experiment Station of Cornell University, Division of Nutritional Sciences.

## REFERENCES

1. Baker, P. T., Hunt, E. E., and Sen, T. (1958): The growth and interrelations of skinfolds and brachial tissues in man. *Am. J. Phys. Anthropol.*, 16:39–58.
2. Cameron, N. (1978): Methods of auxological analysis. In: *Human Growth, Vol. 2. Postnatal Growth*, edited by F. Falkner and J. M. Tanner, pp. 31–91. Plenum Press, New York.
3. de Waard, F. (1975): Breast cancer incidence and nutritional status with particular reference to body weight and height. *Cancer Res.*, 35:3351–3356.
4. Durnin, J. V. G. A., and Womersley, J. (1974): Body fat assessed from total body density and its estimation from skin fold thickness: Measurements on 481 men and women aged from 16 to 72 years. *Br. J. Nutr.*, 32:77–97.
5. Fomon, S. J. (1976): *Nutritional Disorders of Children: Prevention, Screening and Follow-Up.* DHEW Publ. (NSA) 76-5612, Washington, D.C.
6. Frisancho, A. R. (1974): Triceps skinfold and upper arm muscle size norms for assessment of nutritional status. *Am. J. Clin. Nutr.*, 27:1052–1058.
7. Habicht, J. P., Yarbrough, C., and Martorell, R. (1979): Anthropometric field methods: Criteria for selection. In: *Nutrition and Growth*, edited by D. B. Jelliffe and E. F. P. Jelliffe, pp. 365–387. Plenum Press, New York.
8. Hakama, M., Soini, I., Kuosma, E., Lehtonen, M., and Aromaa, A. (1979): Breast cancer incidence: Geographical correlations in Finland. *Int. J. Epidemiol.*, 8:33–40.
9. Heymsfield, S. B., Olafson, R. P., Kutner, M. H., and Nixon, D. W. (1979): A radiographic method of quantifying protein–calorie undernutrition. *Am. J. Clin. Nutr.*, 32:693–702.
10. Himes, J. H., Roche, A. F., and Siervogel, R. M. (1979): Compressibility of skinfolds and the measurement of subcutaneous fatness. *Am. J. Clin. Nutr.*, 32:1734–1740.
11. Jackson, A. S., and Pollock, M. L. (1978): Generalized equations for predicting body density of men. *Br. J. Nutr.*, 40:497–504.
12. Jelliffe, D. B. (1966): *The Assessment of the Nutritional Status of the Community.* World Health Organization Monograph No. 53, Geneva.
13. Johnston, F. E., Hamill, P. V. V., and Lemeshow, S. (1974): Skinfold thickness in a national probability sample of U.S. males and females aged 6 through 17 years. *Am. J. Phys. Anthropol.*, 40:321–324.
14. Keys, A., Fidanza, F., Karvonen, M. J., Kimura, N., and Taylor, H. L. (1972): Indices of relative weight and obesity. *J. Chron. Dis.*, 25:329–343.
15. Khosla, T., and Lowe, C. R. (1967): Indices of obesity derived from body weight and height. *Br. J. Prev. Soc. Med.*, 21:122–128.
16. Malina, R. M. (1966): Patterns of development in skinfolds of Negro and white Philadelphia children. *Hum. Biol.*, 38:89–103.
17. Malina, R. M. (1969): Quantification of fat, muscle and bone in man. *Clin. Orthop.*, 65:9–38.
18. Malina, R. M., Hamill, P. V. V., and Lemeshow, S. (1976): *Selected body measurements of children 6–11 years, U.S. Vital and Health Statistics*, Ser. 11, No. 104. DHEW Publ. (HSM)13-1601, Washington, D.C.
19. Maresh, M. M. (1966): Changes in tissue widths during growth. *Am. J. Dis. Child.*, 111:142–155.
20. National Diabetes Data Group (1979): Classification and diagnosis of diabetes mellitus and other categories of glucose intolerance. *Diabetes*, 28:1039–1057.

21. Noppa, H., Anderson, M., Bengtsson, C., Bruce, A., and Isaksson, B. (1979): Body composition in middle-aged women with special reference to the correlation between body fat mass and anthropometric data. *Am. J. Clin. Nutr.,* 32:1388–1395.
22. Pierson, R. N., Jr., Lin, D. H. Y., and Phillips, R. A. (1974): Total-body potassium in health: Effects of age, sex, height and fat. *Am. J. Physiol.,* 226:206–212.
23. Robson, J. R. K., Buzin, M., and Soderstrom, R. (1971): Ethnic differences in skinfold thickness. *Am. J. Clin. Nutr.,* 24:864–868.
24. Seoane, N., and Latham, M. C. (1971): Nutritional anthropometry in the identification of malnutrition in children. *J. Trop. Pediatr.,* 17:98–104.
25. Sloan, A. W., Burt, J. J., and Blyth, C. A. (1962): Estimation of body fat in young women. *J. Appl. Physiol.,* 17:967–970.
26. Tanner, J. M. (1962): *Growth at Adolescence,* 2nd ed. Blackwell Scientific Publ., Oxford.
27. Tanner, J. M., and Whitehouse, R. H. (1962): Standards for subcutaneous fat in British children. *Br. Med. J.,* 1:446–450.
28. Waterlow, J. C. (1972): Classification and definition of protein–calorie malnutrition. *Br. Med. J.,* 3:566–569.
29. Weiner, J. S., and Lourie, J. A. (1969): *Human Biology: A Guide to Field Methods.* F. A. Davis, Philadelphia.
30. Weltman, A., and Katch, V. L. (1978): A non-population-specific method for predicting total body volume and percent fat. *Hum. Biol.,* 50:151–158.
31. Womersley, J. A., and Durnin, J. V. G. A. (1977): A comparison of the skinfold method with extent of "overweight" and various weight–height relationships in the assessment of obesity. *Br. J. Nutr.,* 38:271–284.
32. Womersley, J., Durnin, J. V. G. A., Boddy, K., and Mahaffey, M. (1976): Influence of muscular development, obesity and age on the fat-free mass of adults. *J. Appl. Physiol.,* 41:223–229.
33. Young, C. M. (1965): Body composition and body weight: Criteria of overnutrition. *Can. Med. Assoc. J.,* 93:900–910.
34. Young, G. A., and Hill, G. L. (1978): Assessment of protein–calorie malnutrition in surgical patients from plasma proteins and anthropometric measurements. *Am. J. Clin. Nutr.,* 31:429–435.
35. Zerfas, A. J. (1979): Anthropometric field methods: General. In: *Nutrition and Growth,* edited by D. B. Jelliffe and E. F. P. Jelliffe, pp. 339–364. Plenum Press, New York.

*Nutrition and Cancer: Etiology and Treatment,*
edited by G. R. Newell and N. M. Ellison.
Raven Press, New York © 1981.

# Biochemical Testing in Nutritional Assessment

## James L. Mullen and Michael H. Torosian

*Department of Surgery, University of Pennsylvania School of Medicine,
Philadelphia, Pennsylvania 19104*

The prevalence of protein–calorie malnutrition in hospitalized cancer patients is now widely recognized and documented. The frequency of malnutrition in the medical and surgical electively hospitalized population has been as high as 50%, depending on the criteria. The clinical relevance of malnutrition has been demonstrated by many studies which document an increased morbidity and mortality associated with the malnourished state (1).

Despite the multitude of biochemical, immunologic, anthropometric, and body compositional parameters used for nutritional assessment, no single test has emerged as the sole accurate indicator of nutritional status. The more difficult goal is to identify patients with subclinical nutritional abnormalities amenable to nutritional therapy before clinically obvious malnutrition ensues, with its attendant complications. This review of biochemical nutritional assessment factors will provide the necessary background for such assessment of the cancer patient.

## SERUM PROTEINS

### Total Proteins

The serum protein level was one of the first biochemical tests included in nutrition surveys. It soon became apparent that this index was neither sensitive nor specific for assessment of nutritional status. In severe cases of kwashiorkor, the total protein level was often below normal. In marasmus, however, and in some instances of advanced kwashiorkor, the total protein level was within the normal range (6).

Marasmus is caused by insufficient energy intake and is primarily associated with cannibalism of the body's energy stores (muscle and fat), with resultant abnormal anthropometrics. It is characteristic for patients with severe degrees of marasmus to have normal serum total protein and albumin levels. Kwashiorkor, on the other hand, is a consequence of protein deficiency and is clinically characterized by edema and by low serum albumin levels (95). Despite a low albumin fraction, the serum total protein level is variable, largely because of the unpredictable level of immunoglobulins. An increase in the immunoglobulin level occurs in response to secondary infections or parasite infestations, and is quite common in malnourished patients in tropical and subtropical areas. This immunoglobulin response is of sufficient magnitude to reverse the serum albumin/globulin ratio and to significantly alter the serum total protein levels (15). This occurs despite the fact that radioisotopic tracer techniques consistently reveal decreased protein synthesis and degradation in malnourished patients.

Thus, the serum total protein level is affected by both nutritional factors and infection. Because important nonnutritional stimuli affect immunoglobulin levels in kwashiorkor and because little change in total proteins is observed in marasmus, the serum total protein level is of little value in assessing an individual's nutritional status.

## Albumin

Albumin is a protein with a molecular weight of 65,000 daltons, and is composed of 575 amino acid residues. It functions to maintain plasma oncotic pressure and as a transport carrier of metals, fatty acids, amino acids, metabolites, enzymes, drugs, and hormones. Albumin is the major protein synthesized by the liver, and, with the exception of hepatomas, is the only site of albumin synthesis. Albumin is normally present in the serum at a concentration between 3.5 to 5.0 g per 100 ml (62).

The serum albumin level is characteristically below normal in patients with kwashiorkor but is maintained within the normal range even in advanced cases of marasmus. Albumin levels in patients with kwashiorkor have been found in the range of 1.5 to 2.0 g/100 ml in many different parts of the world. Whitehead et al. (1971) suggested that serum albumin levels below 3.0 g/100 ml were associated with early signs of edema before clinically evident malnutrition developed (95). This study was performed in Uganda, a community prone to kwashiorkor, and cannot be extrapolated to areas predominantly affected by marasmus.

Cohen et al., in 1962, studied [131]I-labeled albumin distribution in patients with kwashiorkor before and after repletion (15). In the malnourished state, total body albumin decreased to 50% of normal, with the circulating fraction at 60% of normal and the extravascular component at 30% of normal. This study demonstrated that depressed serum albumin levels were not simply the result of redistribution from the intravascular to the extravascular space.

The initial studies of albumin metabolism in malnourished patients were designed to evaluate the contribution of decreased synthesis and/or increased degradation. Radioisotopic dilution techniques employing [125]I- and [131]I-labeled albumin were used by several investigators initially, but were conducted or interpreted incorrectly, leading to erroneous conclusions.

Albumin has a half-life of approximately 20 days in normal humans. In the first study utilizing [131]I-albumin in malnourished subjects, Gitlin et al., in 1958, found no change in the rate of albumin catabolism in malnourished children

(22). However, this study was initiated after therapy had begun, and incorrectly concluded that low serum albumin levels were the result of decreased albumin synthesis. In 1962, Picou et al. and Cohen et al. demonstrated that the rate of catabolism of [131]I-albumin was decreased to approximately one-third to one-half of normal values in malnourished patients (15,55). Numerous animal and human studies have subsequently confirmed these results. However, the radioisotopic dilution technique was unable to measure the rate of albumin synthesis directly. Only when performed under steady-state conditions could the rate of synthesis be inferred.

McFarlane et al. developed a technique capable of measuring albumin synthesis directly which involved [14]C-carbonate labeling of the hepatic arginine pool. The three assumptions for valid interpretation of this test included: (1) [14]C-carbonate is a flash label; (2) the synthetic rates of albumin and urea remain stable during the study period; and (3) albumin and urea are synthesized from the same precursor arginine pool (37,59). Relatively few studies using this technique have been conducted in malnourished humans. In 1972, Kelman et al. studied albumin synthesis using the [14]C-carbonate technique in eight patients on both normal and low-protein diets (29). The rate of albumin synthesis fell from 245 mg/kg per day on a 70-gram protein diet to 85 mg/kg per day after four to six weeks on a isocaloric 10-gram protein diet. Albumin catabolism was studied at the same time using [125]I-labeled albumin. The catabolic rate fell from 173 mg/kg per day on the normal diet to 111 mg/kg per day on the low-protein diet.

Many animal studies, utilizing [14]C-labeled leucine in a manner similar to the [14]C-carbonate technique, have further elucidated the factors controlling albumin synthesis. Kirsch et al. studied the synthetic and catabolic rates of albumin in rats during protein depletion and after resumption of normal diets (30). The rate of albumin synthesis gradually declined during the 12 days of protein-free intake and was paralleled by a decline in serum albumin concentrations. The catabolic rate remained within the normal range for six to seven days before falling abruptly. With the initiation of protein repletion in the same group of animals, the serum albumin concentration and catabolic rate responded gradually. The rate of synthesis, however, responded immediately and became normal within 24 hours after starting protein intake. Morgan et al. demonstrated an increase in the rate of albumin synthesis as early as 30 minutes after refeeding protein-depleted rats (45). Because of the inability of actinomycin D to inhibit this dramatic response, the increased rate of albumin synthesis appears to be directly mediated by amino acid availability. Kirsch et al. and Rothschild et al., in 1969, directly demonstrated rapid changes in albumin synthetic rates in isolated liver systems in response to amino acid concentration (31,61). Tryptophan appears to be especially important and may stabilize the ribosomal messenger RNA complex involved with albumin synthesis.

In summary, the serum albumin concentration is a reliable index for objective assessment of clinically evident forms of kwashiorkor. The relatively long half-life of albumin (20 days) and the results of many animal studies have shown that intravascular albumin levels change gradually in response to nutritional alterations. The rate of albumin synthesis falls gradually during protein depletion and increases almost immediately after return to a normal diet. The catabolic rate is subject to a delayed, abrupt decline during protein depletion, and responds gradually after refeeding. Serial synthetic and catabolic rates have not been studied systematically in malnourished human populations. From the available evidence, however, it appears that neither the serum albumin concentration nor the rates of albumin synthesis or catabolism are able to accurately detect early stages of malnutrition.

### Transferrin

Transferrin is a $\beta$-globulin with a molecular weight of approximately 76,000 daltons. It is a glycoprotein synthesized mainly in human liver and, in insignificant amounts, by peripheral lymphocytes. Transferrin transports iron in the plasma and may aid in the defense against bacterial infection by binding iron. Each molecule of transferrin has two specific iron-binding sites, each of which can chelate one atom of iron. The affinity constant for each of these iron-binding sites is approximately $10^{30}$ (44).

Transferrin levels were not measured directly in the initial studies of protein–calorie malnutrition. Total iron-binding capacity (TIBC) was assayed instead and was assumed to be equivalent to the amount of iron required to saturate plasma transferrin completely. TIBC was found to be consistently below normal in patients with kwashiorkor in many different parts of the world, including Central America, Africa, and Egypt (1,18,33). As with albumin, patients with marasmus exhibited normal serum TIBC levels.

Direct measurement of serum transferrin levels was not practically possible until the development of the radial immunodiffusion technique by Mancini in 1965 (35). In normal and iron-deficient subjects, transferrin levels were found to correlate well with TIBC. However, in patients with kwashiorkor, cirrhosis, or hemachromatosis, the transferrin levels determined by immunologic methods were significantly lower than those calculated from the TIBC (44). The existence of additional iron-containing compounds, such as ferritin, was postulated in these individuals.

The serum transferrin concentration under normal conditions ranges from 180 to 260 mg/100 ml. Antia et al. found that the serum transferrin concentration fell to approximately one-fifth the normal value in a group of Nigerian children with kwashiorkor (5). The response of these patients to treatment correlated much more closely with the transferrin level than with clinical grading of the severity of the disease. The transferrin level rose within the first week in response to a high-protein diet and was an accurate measure of the efficacy of treatment.

McFarlane et al., in 1970, noted similar results in a study of 40 Nigerian children with kwashiorkor (38). Patients who eventually died had significantly lower serum transferrin levels before, during, and after initiation of therapy than those who recovered. Gabr et al., in 1971, also demonstrated in an Egyptian population with kwashiorkor that transferrin levels were related to the prognosis and severity of disease (19). In contrast to the serum transferrin concentration, serum albumin levels had no prognostic value in this study. This finding was probably due to the difference in half-lives of the two proteins. Albumin has a half-life of 20 days under normal conditions. This is markedly prolonged by the decreased catabolic rate in protein–calorie malnutrition. Transferrin has a significantly shorter half-life of approximately eight days and responds more quickly to nutritional changes (44).

Thus, the serum transferrin level is an important prognostic index in cases of advanced kwashiorkor. Serial transferrin measurements are also reliable indicators of therapeutic responsiveness. Both areas of clinical usefulness have been amply documented in outcome studies in hospitalized cancer and noncancer populations. In an attempt to identify earlier nutritional changes, proteins with even shorter half-lives, such as retinol-binding protein and prealbumin, have been investigated.

### Retinol-binding Protein and Prealbumin

Retinol-binding protein is an $\alpha_1$-globulin with a molecular weight of approximately 21,000 daltons. This protein is synthesized by the liver and transports retinol, the circulating form of vitamin A, in the plasma. Retinol-binding protein is normally present in the serum at a concentration of 40 to 50 $\mu g/ml$ and circulates in $1:1$ molar ratio with prealbumin. Prealbumin is thyroxine-binding protein and exists as a tetramer of identical or nearly identical subunits. It has a molecular weight of 54,000 daltons and a normal serum concentration of 200 to 300 $\mu g/ml$ (23). Retinol-binding protein and prealbumin have significantly short half-lives of 10 hours and 24 hours, respectively (96). For this reason, it was believed that changes in the serum concentration of these two proteins might herald relatively early changes in liver protein synthesis and nutritional status. Both animal and human studies have been conducted in an attempt to test this hypothesis.

Muhilal et al. and Peterson et al., in 1974, demonstrated that serum retinol-binding protein levels were decreased in protein-depleted rats (2,5,46). The half-life of retinol-binding protein was increased by 50% and the rate of synthesis decreased to approximately 40% of normal during dietary protein depletion. During subsequent protein repletion, the synthesis of retinol-binding protein was stimulated and increasing serum levels were noted within hours, with normal serum concentrations present within three days.

Another confounding factor that influences serum retinol-binding protein levels is vitamin A intake. Vitamin A deficiency induces a low retinol-binding protein concentration regardless of dietary protein consumption. This effect appears to be mediated by interference with hepatic secretion rather than with synthesis. Normal levels of both retinol-binding protein and retinol in this situation can be produced by administration of vitamin A alone (50).

Nutritional status and vitamin A intake were also found to be important regulators of retinol-binding protein levels in humans. Ingenbleek et al., in 1975, discovered that retinol-binding protein levels were 81% of normal in 39 Sengalese children with protein–calorie malnutrition (27). Upon repletion, the retinol-binding protein concentration doubled after one week and reached normal levels by the twenty-second day of treatment. However, prealbumin and retinol concentrations paralleled the response of retinol-binding protein despite the lack of administration of vitamin A. Smith et al. found significantly decreased levels of retinol-binding protein, prealbumin, and retinol in 21 Egyptian children with kwashiorkor (73). All levels were significantly increased after the second week of treatment with a high-protein diet. No differences were discovered in the retinol-binding protein or retinol concentrations in those with marasmus. Similar results have been noted in other parts of the world, including Thailand, Jordan, India, and Central America.

Venkataswamy et al., in 1977, studied a subgroup of malnourished Indian children who were xerophthalmic secondary to vitamin A deficiency (84). Administration of vitamin A alone did not increase retinol-binding protein levels to the normal range. However, vitamin A therapy, in combination with high protein intake, brought the retinol-binding protein and prealbumin levels to normal within one week. This study substantiated the regulatory effects of both vitamin A and dietary protein intake on retinol-binding protein levels in humans.

Smith et al. compared the temporal relationships of several biochemical changes following therapy of malnourished patients in Central America and Thailand (72,74). The response of retinol-binding protein, prealbumin, and retinol levels preceded corresponding changes in albumin and total protein levels. These experiments, as well as those discussed previously, however, have been conducted on severely malnourished patients. Mild and moderate degrees of protein–calorie malnutrition still require investigation, although similar findings can be expected.

The detection of mild or subclinical malnutrition remains an important goal in the field of nutritional assessment. Retinol-binding protein and prealbumin are promising biochemical markers because of their relatively short biological half-lives and their rapid response to nutritional therapy. Additional clinical research is required in this area, especially in regard to a prospective analysis in the clinical arena.

### Complement

The complement system is comprised of a series of proteins which interact in sequential fashion to produce a multitude of effects. Complement proteins have been synthesized *in vitro* by cultures of human liver, lymph nodes, bone marrow, and intestinal epithelial cells. The macrophage is believed to be the major source of complement protein in these sites (79). Activation of this complex group of proteins is important in host defense against bacterial infections. The complement system has been investigated in malnourished patients because of the increased susceptibility of such individuals to infection.

Sirisinha et al., in 1973, measured the levels of nine different components of complement in 20 malnourished Thai children (70). Eight out of nine proteins (the exception being C-4) were significantly decreased in patients with kwashiorkor, as compared to controls. Only three of nine components (C-5, C-6, and C-3-proactivator) were below normal in those with marasmus. The levels of all complement proteins increased with protein repletion.

Infection may also adversely affect complement levels and must be considered an etiologic factor in addition to nutritional status. Chandra, in 1975, demonstrated decreased C-3 and serum hemolytic complement activity in 35 malnourished Indian children (14). Twelve of these patients, who had concomitant infections, exhibited more pronounced decreases in C-3 and serum hemolytic complement activities.

Several other studies have also demonstrated similar results with regard to C-3 levels and serum hemolytic complement activities in protein–calorie malnutrition. Nutritional repletion and treatment of infection can reverse these abnormalities. Liver dysfunction may also affect serum complement levels. Decreased complement components have been demonstrated in patients with cirrhosis, hepatitis, chronic passive congestion, and schistosomiasis (63). Increased levels of complement have been reported with various types of cancer. Verhaegen et al. demonstrated increased complement levels in patients with locally recurrent or metastatic disease and nearly normal levels in patients in remission (85). Other studies, however, reveal no significant difference in complement activity between cancer patients and controls.

Thus, abnormalities in complement levels are present in a number of pathological states. As with the question of delayed hypersensitivity, the usefulness of complement proteins in nutritional assessment requires further study.

## Proteinase Inhibitors

The proteinase inhibitors are serum proteins. They include $\alpha_1$-antitrypsin, $\alpha_1$-antichymotrypsin, and $\alpha_2$-macroglobulin. These proteinase inhibitors function to prevent tissue damage caused by proteases released during phagocytosis. The serum concentrations of $\alpha_1$-antitrypsin and $\alpha_1$-antichymotrypsin vary in response to tissue injury or inflammation. It has been suggested that proteinase inhibitors might interrupt the mobilization of endogenous protein in malnourished patients with infection. Such changes could interfere with the adaptive responses to protein–calorie malnutrition, with subsequent disturbances in homeostasis (65).

Razaban et al., in 1975, reported decreased levels of $\alpha_1$-antitrypsin and $\alpha_2$-macroglobulin in 75 Nigerian children with protein–calorie malnutrition (58). Schelp et al., in 1978, found normal $\alpha_1$-antitrypsin, decreased $\alpha_2$-macroglobulin, and increased $\alpha_1$-antichymotrypsin levels in malnourished patients from Thailand (65). The same investigators, in 1979, demonstrated decreased $\alpha_1$-antitrypsin and $\alpha_2$-macroglobulin concentrations in both kwashiorkor and marasmus (66). The patients with kwashiorkor in this subsequent study had normal levels of $\alpha_1$-antichymotrypsin, while those with marasmus exhibited increased levels. In cases of protein–calorie malnutrition complicated by infection, the levels of $\alpha_1$-antitrypsin, $\alpha_1$-antichymotrypsin, and $\alpha_2$-macroglobulin have been shown to be increased. The increase in these proteinase inhibitors may exacerbate the metabolic abnormalities induced by malnutrition. Further clinical investigation is required in this area.

### Ribonuclease Activity

Plasma ribonuclease activity is elevated in chronic renal and hepatic disease (25). Although previous studies have reported elevations in patients with myelomatosis and/or breast carcinoma, these changes appear to be correlated with abnormalities in renal function (68). Albanese et al., in 1972, discovered an inverse relationship between nitrogen balance and plasma ribonuclease levels in patients receiving anabolic and catabolic steroids (2). Sigulem et al. revealed increased ribonuclease concentrations in patients with protein–calorie malnutrition, with return to normal levels after two weeks of dietary therapy (69). Shenkin et al., in 1976, also demonstrated increased ribonuclease levels in malnourished patients (42). However, ribonuclease levels in these patients were correlated to a certain extent with renal function, making interpretation of this study difficult. The value of serum ribonuclease levels remains unproven in the field of nutritional assessment.

## AMINO ACID AND ENZYME LEVELS

### Serum Amino Acid Levels

Abnormalities in plasma amino acid levels in kwashiorkor have been identified by many investigators. In general, decreased levels of essential amino acids with normal or increased levels of nonessential amino acids are present. Whitehead, in 1964, proposed a ratio of several nonessential amino acids including glycine, serine, glutamine, and taurine to methionine and the branched chain amino acids: leucine, isoleucine, and valine (91). He suggested that subclinical degrees of kwashiorkor could be detected by this ratio and that the aminogram of patients with marasmus was normal.

Studies conducted in various parts of the world revealed similar results. Holt et al. demonstrated decreased concentrations of the essential amino acids tyrosine and arginine in patients with kwashiorkor in nine different countries (24). McLaren et al., in 1965, revealed an increased ratio of nonessential to essential amino acids in Jordanian children with kwashiorkor, but no change in those with marasmus (40). Arroyave, in 1970, and Smith et al., in 1974, discovered similar changes in malnourished children from Guatamala and India, respectively (7,77).

Other investigators, however, were unable to confirm these findings. Truswell et al., in 1966, found an elevated ratio of nonessential to essential amino acids in only 50% of patients with kwashiorkor (83). The remainder of these patients exhibited normal ratios. Anasuya et al., in 1968, concluded that the amino acid ratio showed great variation in kwashiorkor and was not a reliable index of malnutrition (4). No correlation has been demonstrated between the magnitude of the ratio of nonessential to essential amino acids and the serum albumin concentration or the clinical severity of protein–calorie malnutrition.

In addition, the previously suggested difference in plasma aminograms between patients with kwashiorkor and marasmus has not been universally demonstrated. Arroyave et al. found levels of essential amino acids in marasmus that were intermediate between those seen in kwashiorkor and those observed in normal subjects (8). Saunders et al., in 1967, found no difference in the plasma amino-grams between patients with kwashiorkor and marasmus (64). They reported decreased concentrations of all amino acids except glycine and histidine, with the greatest reduction in the branched-chain amino acids.

Other factors have been shown to affect plasma amino acid concentrations. Dietary protein intake produces a dramatic change in the aminogram of patients with kwashiorkor. Saunders et al. demonstrated increased concentrations of all amino acids except glycine within 24 hours of dietary repletion of patients with kwashiorkor (64). Whitehead et al. noted significant changes in the ratio of nonessential to essential amino acids in patients with kwashiorkor after only one protein meal (94). Thus, dietary history and sampling time are important determinants of the plasma amino acid pattern.

Hormonal influences also affect the fluctuation of amino acids throughout the body and are believed to be important in the pathophysiology of kwashiorkor and marasmus. Whitehead et al. proposed that insulin stimulation in response to dietary carbohydrates in patients with kwashiorkor was important in the development of abnormal plasma aminograms (93). The calorie deprivation char-acteristic of marasmus was thought to inhibit insulin release without distortion of plasma amino acid concentrations. Several studies conducted on human volun-teers indicate that insulin is one of several important factors affecting plasma amino acid composition (67).

In conclusion, the plasma aminogram is not a consistently reliable index of nutritional status. There is no relationship between amino acid concentrations or ratios and the serum albumin concentration or the clinical course of malnutri-tion. The plasma amino acid pattern appears to reflect recent dietary intake more accurately than it reflects chronic nutritional status. Hormonal mechanisms are an additional confounding variable.

## Enzyme Levels

Inconsistent results have been reported in studies of serum enzyme levels in protein–calorie malnutrition. Several investigators have demonstrated increased transaminase levels in malnourished patients. McLean et al., in 1966, correlated elevated serum glutamic pyruvic transaminase and bilirubin levels with increased mortality, but this relationship has not been confirmed by others (41). Even greater serum concentrations of glutamic pyruvic transaminase and isocitric dehydrogenase were reported in patients recovering from malnutrition, and it was suggested that this was caused by increased enzyme synthesis (42). Other studies found no changes in serum transaminase levels with malnutrition or during the recovery phase. Liver biopsy in patients with malnutrition has generally revealed fatty infiltration, which is unrelated to serum enzyme activity (88).

Balmer et al., in 1968, observed low levels of creatine kinase in patients with kwashiorkor in Uganda (9). However, those with marasmus and with severe cases of kwashiorkor often exhibited normal or elevated creatine kinase levels. They concluded that creatine kinase concentration was a fair index of muscle mass except during periods of active muscle breakdown in severe cases of malnutrition. Reindorp reported decreased creatine kinase levels in malnutrition but noted similar effects in infection (60). Serum choline esterase activity was also shown to be decreased in malnourished patients (88). Aryl sulfatase, a lysosomal enzyme, was reported to be elevated in malnourished patients (28). This elevation was thought to result from lysosomal membrane fragility secondary to vitamin A deficiency. The activities of creatine kinase, cholinesterase, and aryl sulfatase all returned to normal following nutritional therapy.

Various hepatic enzyme concentrations have also been analyzed. Stephen et al., in 1968, demonstrated adaptive enzyme changes in liver biopsy specimens from malnourished Jamaican infants (80). An increase in the hepatic amino acid synthetase activity, with a concomitant decrease in the urea cycle enzyme argininosuccinase, was detected. This modification allows more efficient utilization of the available amino acid pool for the synthesis of protein instead of urea (89). Similar enzyme changes have been reproduced in protein-depleted rats and have reverted to normal following protein therapy.

In summary, serum enzyme levels have not been shown to vary consistently with protein–calorie malnutrition. Enzyme changes may occur in the liver and may represent an important adaptive mechanism in malnutrition. Neither serum nor hepatic enzyme levels have been clinically useful in the field of nutritional assessment.

## URINARY TESTS OF PROTEIN CATABOLISM/GROWTH

### Urinary 3-Methylhistidine Excretion

Certain histidine residues in actin and myosin molecules are methylated, after synthesis of these peptide chains, to produce 3-methylhistidine. There is no other endogenous or exogenous source of this methylated amino acid. Upon proteolysis, 3-methylhistidine is not modified or reutilized, but is excreted unchanged in the urine. Only trace amounts are excreted in the feces. As a result of these unique properties, the urinary 3-methylhistidine level is a direct measure of muscle catabolism (49).

Rao et al., in 1973, demonstrated that the urinary 3-methylhistidine concentration was decreased in children from India with kwashiorkor and marasmus (57). Both the absolute concentration and the amount of 3-methylhistidine excreted per kilogram of body weight were reduced and reverted to normal levels following treatment. Munro et al., in 1978, found similar results in children with advanced degrees of malnutrition (49).

Studies have also been conducted during periods of fasting in humans. It has been consistently shown that the urinary 3-methylhistidine level is decreased in human subjects after prolonged fasting (34,36). Long et al., however, noted increased urinary concentrations during the acute phase of starvation (34). This has not been confirmed by other investigators.

Urinary 3-methylhistidine concentration can serve as a valid index of skeletal and visceral muscle catabolism. This area requires further investigation in the study of protein–calorie malnutrition.

### Urinary Hydroxyproline Excretion

Urinary hydroxyproline is derived almost entirely from collagen catabolism and is therefore markedly influenced by growth rate. Picou et al., in 1965, demonstrated decreased hydroxyproline and creatinine excretion in malnourished Jamaican infants (53). In order to distinguish changes in the hydroxyproline excretion from changes in body weight alone, Whitehead proposed the hydroxyproline index (92):

$$\frac{mM\ OH\text{–proline/liter urine}}{mM\ creatinine/liter\ urine/kg\ body\ weight}$$

Whitehead, in 1965, found decreased values of the hydroxyproline index in patients with kwashiorkor and marasmus (92). This index returned to normal in patients who exhibited weight gain following treatment. Similar results have been obtained by others. A decreased hydroxyproline index was also seen in underweight children who showed no other obvious signs of protein calorie malnutrition (26,92).

However, the hydroxyproline index appears to have little predictive value in assessing nutritional status. McLaren et al., in 1970, found no correlation between the initial body weight of malnourished patients and urinary hydroxyproline excretion (39). Furthermore, there was no relationship between this index and the rate of height increase following malnutrition. This study concluded that anthropometric parameters were more reliable than urinary hydroxyproline excretion as a measure of nutritional status.

Other factors, such as age and malaria infestation, were also shown to affect urinary hydroxyproline excretion. McLaren et al. proposed that an age adjustment factor be incorporated into the hydroxyproline index (39). Crowne et al. suggested that this index was useful as a measure of growth rate only in young children (17). Wenlock, in 1977, showed that infestation with malaria was a major factor responsible for decreased hydroxyproline excretion in children from Zambia (90).

Thus, many factors influence urinary hydroxyproline excretion and must be considered when interpreting results. The reliability of urinary hydroxyproline excretion as a component of nutritional assessment remains to be proven.

## BODY COMPONENTS

### Body Composition Studies

Direct analysis of body composition in malnourished patients was initially performed by autopsy study. Garrow et al. found that total body fat and protein were reduced to 18% and 62% of normal, respectively, in severe malnutrition (21). Total body potassium was severely depleted to 40% of normal. Although the absolute value of total body water showed great variation, all malnourished patients were relatively overhydrated with increased total body water. Similar results of fat, protein, and potassium depletion in a state of relative overhydration were reported by others.

Protein depletion is a generalized response by all tissues during developing malnutrition. Picou et al., in 1966, demonstrated that this protein loss occurs predominantly in the noncollagen protein fraction (54). In this study of severely malnourished infants from Jamaica, it was shown that the noncollagen protein level fell to 50% of normal despite no significant change in the collagen fraction. Skeletal muscle catabolism to provide substrates for gluconeogenesis during periods of inadequate intake accounts for a large proportion of this protein loss.

Muscle biopsies from patients who recovered from malnutrition confirmed these autopsy findings (51). Decreases in potassium and noncollagen nitrogen were accompanied by an increase in water content. These changes were shown to be reversible with successful treatment of malnutrition.

Tissue analyses by autopsy or biopsy techniques have been performed on relatively few malnourished human subjects but have revealed extreme changes in body composition. These findings led to the development of indirect tests for evaluating body composition. Creatinine–height index, total body potassium, and total body water measurements are three such techniques which are important in assessing nutritional status.

### Urinary Creatinine–Height Index

The creatinine–height index is a ratio of the milligrams of creatinine excreted by a subject over a 24-hour period to the expected amount excreted by a normal individual of the same height (86). Height has been chosen as a standard of comparison in preference to body weight, since the latter is subject to variations with adipose tissue content. The creatinine–height index is principally dependent upon muscle mass and is markedly lower in patients with protein calorie malnutrition (6,8,11). This index has been a useful indicator of muscle mass during protein depletion and during repletion. The creatinine–height index and potassium–height index correlate well in the estimation of muscle mass in malnourished children. Various other studies have revealed a relationship between urinary creatinine excretion and total body weight, fat-free mass, red blood cell mass, and total body potassium (87).

Several limitations, however, jeopardize the reliability of the creatinine–height index. The most serious problems inherent in monitoring the creatinine–height index are sampling errors and the tremendous variability of urinary creatinine excretion in a given individual from day to day. Viteri et al. demonstrated the standard deviation of 24-hour urinary creatinine excretion to be 25% of the mean amount (16). This degree of variability has been confirmed by several investigators. In addition, the dietary intake of creatine may significantly influence creatinine excretion. Consumption of a creatine-free diet may decrease the urinary creatinine excretion by as much as 30% despite adequate noncreatine protein intake (12). Single determinations of the creatinine–height index are subject to large errors. Serial measurements, however, may be important in assessing muscle mass, both during depletion and during recovery from the malnourished state.

## Total Body Potassium

The lean body mass is composed of the body cell mass and the extracellular mass. The body cell mass is the living, energy-exchanging, oxygen-consuming component of the body. The supporting, nonliving structures in the body comprise the extracellular mass. Total body potassium (TBK), total exchangeable potassium ($K_e$), and intracellular water are indirect measures of the body cell mass. Extracellular water and total exchangeable sodium ($Na_e$) represent measures of the extracellular mass (43).

Of the TBK, 98% is present within the body cell mass. The remainder exists within the extracellular fluid compartment and body fat. Gamma ray emission by the naturally occurring isotope $^{40}K$ and radioisotopic dilution techniques utilizing $^{42}K$ or $^{43}K$ provide two measures of body potassium content.

$^{40}K$ accounts for 0.012% of the potassium distributed throughout nature. This radioisotope decays either by beta particle emission or by emission of gamma rays with an energy of 1.46 MeV. Whole-body gamma counters have been developed to assay total body content of $^{40}K$. Total body potassium is subsequently derived from the simple linear relationship between $^{40}K$ and TBK mentioned above. The normal range of TBK depends on several factors including sex, age, weight, and height. Various equations relating these factors to TBK have been proposed.

Total exchangeable potassium ($K_e$) is a measurement based upon radioisotopic dilutions of $^{42}K$ or $^{43}K$. The difference between the $K_e$ and TBK, as determined by gamma counters, is small. Numerous studies have indicated that the ratio of $K_e$ to TBK in both normal and malnourished populations approximates 90% (56,81). Moore et al. described the following linear relationship between body cell mass and $K_e$ (43):

$$BCM = K_e \times 0.00833$$

This relationship has formed the basis for analysis of TBK and $K_e$ in the field of malnutrition.

Total body potassium and total exchangeable potassium are consistently below normal in patients with protein–calorie malnutrition. Smith et al., in 1960, found $K_e$ values reduced by 25% to 30% during malnutrition (76). Garrow et al., in 1965, discovered TBK deficits as great as 42% of normal in severely malnourished children (20). Alleyne et al. noted similar results in malnourished patients on admission, with significant increases following therapy (3).

Total body weight is poorly correlated with TBK or $K_e$. A much more significant correlation exists between changes in TBK or $K_e$ and total body water (81). Low TBK or $K_e$ values are associated with an increase in total body water during states of malnutrition. Subclinical degrees of total body water expansion may be present with significant TBK depletion (3). The resultant effects on total body weight cancel each other out.

Total body potassium and total exchangeable potassium have recently been used to monitor the efficacy of nutritional therapy in patients with a variety of catabolic disease states. Bernard et al., in 1973, reported changes in TBK before significant increases in body weight in patients receiving intravenous hyperalimentation (10). Spanier et al., in 1977, studied a group of 35 critically ill patients with a variety of diseases (78). This study demonstrated a positive correlation between the number of calories consumed and a change in $K_e$ per day. A linear regression was established, indicating that the average patient in a catabolic disease state required 46 Kcal/kg/day in order to effectively increase $K_e$.

In summary, TBK and $K_e$ represent indirect measurements of body cell mass. It is predominantly this component of lean body mass that suffers during malnutrition and is treated with nutritional therapy. Changes in TBK and $K_e$ may be valuable in detecting early stages of malnutrition and in monitoring the efficacy of therapy of many catabolic states. Further investigation is required to compare the results of these techniques with other indices of nutritional assessment.

## Total Body Water

Changes in total body water and extracellular fluid occur in a variety of disease states. Various methods are available for measuring the total body water and extracellular fluid compartments. Intracellular fluid volume represents the difference between these two values. Total body water is measured by dilution techniques employing tritiated water, a radioisotope, or deuterium oxide, a heavy, stable isotope of water. Extracellular fluid volume measurements are performed by dilution of radioisotopes of sodium, bromine, or sulfate. Electrical impedance techniques have recently been applied to determine total body water and extracellular fluid volume in clinical situations.

Protein–calorie malnutrition is associated with significant increases in both total body water and extracellular fluid volume. Smith, in 1960, discovered that total body water represented 84.5% of total body weight in 28 malnourished Jamaican infants (75). After recovery, total body water decreased to 62.6% of body weight in these same patients. Alleyne et al., in 1968, found an increase in total body water with malnutrition and determined that this increase occurred in the extracellular fluid compartment (3). The extracellular volume before and after therapy was 37.4% and 23.0%, respectively, of body weight. Extracellular fluid volume expansion was detected even in children without edema, suggesting that clinical assessment is an unreliable index of changes in extracellular fluid. Brinkman et al. found comparable changes in the extracellular fluid compartments, but noted a decrease in the intracellular fluid volume with malnutrition (13). Numerous studies of malnourished patients have subsequently demonstrated similar results.

Electrical impedance techniques have recently been introduced to determine fluid compartments within the human body (82). It has been demonstrated that electrical impedance measurements at low frequency ($Z_{LF}$) correlate linearly with extracellular fluid volume and that electrical impedance at high frequency ($Z_{HF}$) is a linear function of total body water. Jenin et al. found that the ratio of $Z_{LF}/Z_{HF}$ is normally 1.50 (32). This ratio is decreased in almost all pathological states, with values as low as 1.10 in malnutrition associated with cancer.

The changes in total body water and extracellular fluid volume in severe malnutrition are well documented. Subclinical levels of extracellular volume expansion are detectable by radioisotopic and electrical impedance techniques. Further analyses of these volume changes are required at early stages of malnutrition and other pathological states. The electrical impedance method requires further refinement and validation.

## CONCLUSIONS

Many different biochemical tests have been used for nutritional assessment; however, no single marker can identify the malnourished state in all instances. More difficult is the detection of preclinical or subclinical malnutrition.

There are several problems associated with the identification of an ideal nutritional marker. First, "protein–calorie malnutrition" represents a spectrum of undernutrition ranging from kwashiorkor to marasmus. The organism's response is different in each case, and different nutritional parameters may be needed to characterize these states. Second, dietary deficiencies vary in different parts of the world. Deficiencies other than those involving protein and calories may prove significant, so that a universally applicable nutritional parameter may not exist. Third, the majority of studies have been performed on severely malnourished patients or during their recovery phase. The most important aspect of nutritional assessment is predicting changes that occur during the early stages of dietary deficiency. Fourth, a dilemma confounds the attempts to discover a parameter that changes with nutritional status without simply reflecting recent dietary history. Fifth, all of the biochemical parameters thus far studied lack absolute specificity. The ideal biochemical marker would be one that responds exclusively to changes in nutritional status.

A single, ideal marker for detecting early malnutrition does not exist at the present time. Mullen et al. developed and validated a Prognostic Nutritional Index (PNI) which is able to predict accurately nutritionally based morbidity and mortality in surgical patients (47). The PNI was derived from a linear regression model, with serum albumin, serum transferrin, triceps skinfold, and delayed hypersensitivity included as follows:

$$PNI\ (\%) = 158 - 16.6\ (ALB) - 0.78\ (TSF) - 0.20\ (TFN) - 5.8\ (DH)$$

In a high-risk group of patients undergoing major cancer surgery, Smale et al. were able to demonstrate the reduction of operative morbidity and mortality with preoperative nutritional therapy (71). This predictive model may allow the rational use of nutritional therapy to reduce morbidity in other clinical situations as well.

## REFERENCES

1. Adams, E. B., and Scragg, J. N. (1965): Iron in the anaemia of kwashiorkor. *Br. J. Haematol.,* 11:676–681.
2. Albanese, A. A., Lorenze, E. J., Orto, L. A., et al. (1972): Nutritional and metabolic effects of some newer steroids. VI. Serum ribonuclease. *N.Y. State J. Med.,* 72:1595–1600.
3. Alleyne, G. A. O. (1968): Studies on total body potassium in infantile malnutrition: The relation to body fluid spaces and urinary creatinine. *Clin. Sci.,* 34:199–209.
4. Anasuya, A., and Rao, B. S. N. (1968): Plasma amino acid pattern in kwashiorkor and marasmus. *Am. J. Clin. Nutr.,* 21:723–732.
5. Antia, A. V., McFarlane, H., and Soothill, J. F. (1968): Serum siderophilin in kwashiorkor. *Arch. Dis. Child.,* 43:459–462.
6. Arroyave, G. (1962): The estimation of relative nutrient intake and nutritional status by biochemical methods: Proteins. *Am. J. Clin. Nutr.,* 11:447–461.
7. Arroyave, G. (1970): Comparative sensitivity of specific amino acid ratios versus "essential to nonessential" amino acid ratio. *Am. J. Clin. Nutr.,* 23:703–706.
8. Arroyave, G., Wilson, D., DeFunes, C., and Behar, M. (1962): The free amino acids in blood plasma of children with kwashiorkor and marasmus. *Am. J. Clin. Nutr.,* 11:517–524.
9. Balmer, S. E., and Ruishauser, I. H. E. (1968): Serum creatine kinase in malnutrition. *J. Pediatr.,* 73:783–787.
10. Bernard, R. W., and Stahl, W. M. (1973): Total body potassium as a guide to IV alimentation. *Ann. Surg.,* 178:559–562.
11. Bistrian, B. R., Blackburn, G. L., Sherman, M., and Scrimshaw, N. S. (1975): Therapeutic index of nutritional depletion in hospitalized patients. *Surg. Gynecol. Obstet.,* 141:512–516.

12. Bleiler, R. E., and Schedl, H. P. (1962): Creatinine excretion: Variability and relationships to diet and body size. *J. Lab. Clin. Med.,* 59:945–955.
13. Brinkman, G. L., Bowie, M. D., Hansen, B. F., and Hansen, J. D. L. (1965): Body water composition in kwashiorkor before and after loss of edema. *Pediatrics,* 36:94–103.
14. Chandra, R. K. (1975): Serum complement and immunoconglutinin in malnutrition. *Arch. Dis. Child.,* 50:225–229.
15. Cohen, S., and Hansen, J. D. L. (1962): Metabolism of albumin and γ-globulin in kwashiorkor. *Clin. Sci. Mol. Med.,* 23:351–359.
16. Creatinine–height index in malnourished children (1971): *Nutr. Rev.,* 29:134–137.
17. Crowne, R. S., Wharton, B. A., and McCance, R. A. (1969): Hydroxyproline indices and hydroxyproline/creatinine ratios in older children. *Lancet,* 1:395–396.
18. El-Shobaki, F. A., El-Hawary, M. F. S., Morcos, S. R., et al. (1972): Iron metabolism in Egyptian infants with protein–calorie deficiency. *Br. J. Nutr.,* 28:81–89.
19. Gabr, M., El-Hawary, M. F., and El-Dali, M. (1971): Serum transferrin in kwashiorkor. *J. Trop. Med. Hyg.,* 74:216–221.
20. Garrow, J. S. (1965): The use and calibration of a small whole body counter for the measurement of total body potassium in malnourished infants. *W. Indian Med. J.,* 14:73–81.
21. Garrow, J. S., Fletcher, K., and Halliday, D. (1965): Body composition in severe infantile malnutrition. *J. Clin. Invest.,* 44:417–425.
22. Gitlin, D., Cravioto, J., Frenk, S., et al. (1958): Albumin metabolism in children with protein malnutrition. *J. Clin. Invest.,* 37:682–686.
23. Goodman, D. S. (1974): Vitamin A transport and retinol-binding protein metabolism. *Vitam. Horm.,* 32:167–180.
24. Holt, L. E., Jr., Snyderman, S. E., Norton, P. M., et al. (1963): The plasma aminogram in kwashiorkor. *Lancet,* 2:1342–1348.
25. Houck, J. C., and Berman, L. B. (1958): Serum ribonuclease activity. *J. Appl. Physiol.,* 12:473–476.
26. Hydroxyproline creatinine ratio as an index of nutritional status. (1966): *Nutr. Rev.,* 24:324–326.
27. Ingenbleek, Y., Van Den Schrieck, H. G., De Nayer, P., and De Visscher, M. (1975): The role of retinol-binding protein in protein–calorie malnutrition. *Metabolism,* 24:633–641.
28. Ittyerah, T. R., Dumn, M. E., and Buchhawat, B. K. (1967): Urinary excretion of lysosomal arylsulfatases in kwashiorkor. *Clin. Chim. Acta,* 17:405–414.
29. Kelman, L., Saunders, S. J., Frith, L., et al. (1972): Effects of dietary protein restriction on albumin synthesis, albumin catabolism, and the plasma aminogram. *Am. J. Clin. Nutr.,* 25:1174–1178.
30. Kirsch, R., Frith, L., Black, E., and Hoffenberg, R. (1968): Regulation of albumin synthesis and catabolism by alteration of dietary protein. *Nature,* 217:578–579.
31. Kirsch, R. E., Saunders, S. J., Frith, L., et al. (1969): Plasma amino acid concentration and the regulation of albumin synthesis. *Am. J. Clin. Nutr.,* 22:1559–1562.
32. Jenin, P., Lenoir, J., Roullet, C., et al. (1975): Determination of body fluid compartments by electrical impedance measurements. *Aviat. Space Environ. Med.,* 46:152–155.
33. Lahey, M. E., Behar, M., Viteri, F., and Scrimshaw, N. S. (1958): Values for copper, iron, and iron-binding capacity in the serum in kwashiorkor. *Pediatrics,* 22:72–79.
34. Long, C. L., Schiller, W. R., Blakemore, W. S., et al. (1977): Muscle protein catabolism in the septic patient as measured by 3-methylhistidine excretion. *Am. J. Clin. Nutr.,* 30:1349–1352.
35. Mancini, G., Carbonara, A. O., and Heremans, J. F. (1965): Immunochemical quantitation of antigens by single radial immunodiffusion. *Immunochemistry,* 2:235–254.
36. Marliss, E. B., Murray, F. T., and Nakhooda, A. F. (1978): The metabolic response to hypocaloric protein diets in obese man. *J. Clin. Invest.,* 62:468–479.
37. McFarlane, A. S. (1963): Measurement of synthesis rates of liver produced plasma proteins. *Biochem. J.,* 89:277–290.
38. McFarlane, H., Reddy, S., Adcock, K. J., et al. (1970): Immunity, transferrin, and survival in kwashiorkor. *Br. Med. J.,* 4:268–270.
39. McLaren, D. S., Loshkajian, H., and Kanawati, A. A. (1970): Urinary creatinine and hydroxyproline in relation to childhood malnutrition. *Br. J. Nutr.,* 24:641–651.

40. McLaren, D. S., Kamel, W. W., and Ayyoub, N. (1965): Plasma amino acids and the detection of protein–calorie malnutrition. *Am. J. Clin. Nutr.,* 17:152–157.
41. McLean, A. E. M. (1966): Enzyme activity in the liver and serum of malnourished children in Jamaica. *Clin. Sci. Mol. Med.,* 30:129–137.
42. McLean, A. E. (1962): Serum enzymes during recovery from malnutrition. *Lancet,* 2:1294–1295.
43. Moore, F. D., Olesen, K. H., McMurray, J. D., et al. (1963): The body cell mass and its supporting environment. In: *Body Composition in Health and Disease.* Saunders, Philadelphia.
44. Morgan, E. H. (1974): Transferrin and transferrin iron in iron. In: *Biochemistry and Medicine,* edited by A. Jacobs and M. Worwood, pp. 29–71. Academic Press, London.
45. Morgan, E. H., and Peters, T., Jr. (1971): The biosynthesis of rat serum albumin. V. Effect of protein depletion and refeeding on albumin and transferrin synthesis. *J. Biol. Chem.,* 246:3500–3501.
46. Muhilal, H., and Glover, J. (1974): Effects of dietary deficiencies of protein and retinol on the plasma level of retinol-binding protein in the rat. *Br. J. Nutr.,* 32:549–558.
47. Mullen, J. L., Buzby, G. P., Waldman, M. T., et al. (1979): Prediction of operative morbidity and mortality by preoperative nutritional assessment. *Surg. Forum,* 30:80–82.
48. Mullen, J. L., Gertner, M. H., Buzby, G. P., et al. (1979): Implications of malnutrition in the surgical patient. *Arch. Surg.,* 114:121–125.
49. Munro, H. N., and Young, V. R. (1978): Urinary excretion of N-methylhistidine (3-methylhistidine): A tool to study metabolic responses in relation to nutrient and hormonal status in health and disease of man. *Am. J. Clin. Nutr.,* 31:1608–1614.
50. Muto, Y., Smith, J. E., Milch, P. O., and Goodman, D. S. (1972): Regulation of retinol-binding protein metabolism by vitamin A status in the rat. *J. Biol. Chem.,* 247:2542–2550.
51. Nichols, B. L., Alleyne, G. A. O., Barnes, D. J., and Hazlewood, C. F. (1969): Relationship between muscle potassium and total body potassium in infants with malnutrition. *J. Pediatr.,* 74:49–57.
52. Peterson, P. A., Nilsson, S. F., Ostberg, L., et al. (1974): Aspects of the metabolism of retinol-binding protein and retinol. *Vitam. Horm.,* 32:181–214.
53. Picou, D., Alleyne, G. A. O., and Seakins, A. (1965): Hydroxyproline and creatinine excretion in infantile protein malnutrition. *Clin. Sci. Mol. Med.,* 29:517–523.
54. Picou, D., Halliday, D., and Garroro, J. S. (1966): Total body protein, collagen, and non-collagen protein in infantile protein malnutrition. *Clin. Sci.,* 30:345–351.
55. Picou, D., and Waterlow, J. C. (1962): The effect of malnutrition on the metabolism of plasma albumin. *Clin. Sci. Mol. Med.,* 22:459–468.
56. Johnson, I. D. A., editor (1978): *Advances in Parenteral Nutrition.* Proceedings of an international symposium held in Bermuda, May 16–19, 1977, pp. 557–572. MTP Press Limited, Lancaster, England.
57. Rao, B. S. N., and Nagabhushan, V. S. (1973): Urinary excretion of 3-methylhistidine in children suffering from protein–calorie malnutrition. *Life Sci.,* 12:205–210.
58. Razaban, S. Z., Olusi, S. O., Ade-Serrano, M. A., et al. (1975): Acute phase proteins in children with protein–calorie malnutrition. *J. Trop. Med. Hyg.,* 78:264–266.
59. Reeve, E. B., Pearson, J. R., and Martz, D. C. (1963): Plasma protein synthesis in the liver: Method for measurement of albumin formation in vivo. *Science,* 139:914–916.
60. Reindorp, W., and Whitehead, R. G. (1971): Changes in serum creatine kinase and other biological measurements associated with musculature in children recovering from kwashiorkor. *Br. J. Nutr.,* 25:273–283.
61. Rothschild, M. A., Oratz, M., Mongelli, J., et al. (1969): Amino acid regulation of albumin synthesis. *J. Nutr.,* 98:395–403.
62. Rothschild, M. A., Oratz, M., and Schreiber, S. S. (1972): Albumin synthesis. *N. Engl. J. Med.,* 286:748–757.
63. Ruddy, S., Gigli, I., and Austen, K. F. (1972): The complement system of man. *N. Engl. J. Med.,* 287:489–495.
64. Saunders, S. J., Truswell, A. S., and Hansen, J. D. L. (1967): Plasma free amino acid pattern in protein–calorie malnutrition. *Lancet,* 2:795–797.
65. Schelp, F. P., Mugasina, P., Pongpaew, P., and Schreurs, W. H. P. (1978): Are proteinase inhibitors a factor for the derangement of homeostasis in protein–energy malnutrition? *Am. J. Clin. Nutr.,* 31:451–456.

66. Schelp, F. P., Thanangkul, O., Supawan, V., et al. (1979): Serum proteinase inhibitors and acute-phase reactants from protein–energy malnutrition children during treatment. *Am. J. Clin. Nutr.*, 32:1415–1422.

67. Scriver, C. R., Chow, C. L., and Lamm, P. (1971): Plasma amino acids: Screening, quantitation, and interpretation. *Am. J. Clin. Nutr.*, 24:876–890.

68. Shenkin, A., Citrin, D. L., and Rowan, R. M. (1976): An assessment of the clinical usefulness of plasma ribonuclease assays. *Clin. Chim. Acta*, 72:223–231.

69. Sigulem, D. M., Brasel, J. A., Velasio, E. G., et al. (1973): Plasma and urine ribonuclease as a measure of nutritional status in children. *Am. J. Clin. Nutr.*, 26:793–797.

70. Sirisinha, S., Suskind, R., Edelman, R., et al. (1973): Complement and C3-proactivator levels in children with protein–calorie malnutrition and effect of dietary treatment. *Lancet*, 1:1016–1020.

71. Smale, B. F., Mullen, J. L., Buzby, G. P., and Rosato, E. F. (1981): The efficacy of nutritional assessment and support in cancer surgery. *Cancer, (in press)*.

72. Smith, F. R., Goodman, D. S., Arroyave, G., and Viteri, F. (1973): Serum vitamin A, retinol-binding protein, and prealbumin concentrations in protein–calorie malnutrition. II. Treatment including supplemental vitamin A. *Am. J. Clin. Nutr.*, 26:982–987.

73. Smith, F. R., Goodman, D. S., Zaklama, M. S., et al. (1973): Serum vitamin A, retinol-binding protein, and prealbumin concentration in protein–calorie malnutrition. I. A functional defect in hepatic retinol release. *Am. J. Clin. Nutr.*, 26:973–981.

74. Smith, F. R., Suskind, R., Thanangkul, O., et al. (1975): Plasma vitamin A, retinol-binding protein, and prealbumin concentrations in protein–calorie malnutrition. III. Response to varying dietary treatments. *Am. J. Clin. Nutr.*, 28:732–738.

75. Smith, R. (1960): Total body water in malnourished infants. *Clin. Sci.*, 19:275–285.

76. Smith, R., and Waterlow, J. C. (1960): Total exchangeable potassium in infantile malnutrition. *Lancet*, 1:147–149.

77. Smith, S. R., Pozefsky, T., and Chhetri, M. K. (1974): Nitrogen and amino acid metabolism in adults with protein–calorie malnutrition. *Metabolism*, 23:603–618.

78. Spanier, A. H., and Shizgal, H. M. (1977): Caloric requirements of the critically ill patient receiving intravenous hyperalimentation. *Am. J. Surg.*, 133:99–104.

79. Stecher, V. J., and Thorbecke, G. J. (1967): Sites of synthesis of serum proteins. I. Serum proteins produced by macrophages in vitro. *J. Immunol.*, 99:643–652.

80. Stephen, J. M. L., and Waterlow, J. C. (1968): Effect of malnutrition on activity of two enzymes concerned with amino acid metabolism in human liver. *Lancet*, 1:118–119.

81. Talso, P. J., Miller, C. E., Carballo, A. J., and Vasquez, I. (1960): Exchangeable potassium as a parameter of body composition. *Metabolism*, 9:456–471.

82. Thomasset, A. (1962): Bio-electrical properties of tissue impedance measurements. *Lyon Med.*, 207:107–118.

83. Truswell, A. S., Wannenburg, P., Wittmann, W., and Hansen, J. (1966): Plasma-amino acids in kwashiorkor. *Lancet*, 1:1162–1163.

84. Venkataswamy, G., Glover, J., Cobby, M., and Pirie, A. (1977): Retinol-binding protein in serum of xerophthalmic malnourished children before and after treatment at a nutrition center. *Am. J. Clin. Nutr.*, 30:1968–1973.

85. Verhaegen, H., De Cock, W., De Cree, J., and Verbruggen, F. (1976): Increase of serum complement levels in cancer patients with progressing tumors. *Cancer*, 38:1608–1613.

86. Viteri, F. E., and Alvarado, J. (1970): The creatinine–height index: Its use in the estimation of the degree of protein depletion and repletion in protein–calorie malnourished children. *Pediatrics*, 46:696–706.

87. Waterlow, J. C., Neale, R. J., Rowe, L., and Palin, I. (1972): Effects of diet and infection on creatine turnover in the rat. *Am. J. Clin. Nutr.*, 25:371–375.

88. Waterlow, J. C., and Patrick, S. J. (1954): Enzyme activity in fatty livers in human infants. *Ann. N.Y. Acad. Sci.*, 57:750–763.

89. Waterlow, J. C., and Stephen, J. M. L. (1969): Enzymes and the assessment of protein nutrition. *Proc. Nutr. Soc.*, 28:234–242.

90. Wenlock, R. W. (1977): Hydroxyproline index as a tool for nutrition status surveys in malarial regions. *Br. J. Nutr.*, 38:239–243.

91. Whitehead, R. G. (1964): Rapid determination of some plasma amino acids in subclinical kwashiorkor. *Lancet*, 1:250–252.

92. Whitehead, R. (1965): Hydroxyproline creatinine ratio as an index of nutritional status and growth rate. *Lancet,* 2:567–570.
93. Whitehead, R. G., and Alleyne, G. A. O. (1972): Pathophysiological factors of importance in protein–calorie malnutrition. *Br. Med. Bull.,* 28:72–79.
94. Whitehead, R. G., and Dean, R. F. A. (1964): Serum amino acids in kwashiorkor. II. An abbreviated method of estimation and its application. *Am. J. Clin. Nutr.,* 14:320–330.
95. Whitehead, R. G., Frood, J. D. L., and Poskitt, E. M. E. (1971): Value of serum-albumin measurements in nutritional surveys: A reappraisal. *Lancet,* 2:287–289.
96. Young, G. A., Chem, C., and Hill, G. L. (1978): Assessment of protein–calorie malnutrition in surgical patients from plasma proteins and anthropometric measurements. *Am. J. Clin. Nutr.,* 31:429–435.

*Nutrition and Cancer: Etiology and Treatment,*
edited by G. R. Newell and N. M. Ellison.
Raven Press, New York © 1981.

# Radiographic Analysis of Body Composition by Computerized Axial Tomography

Steven B. Heymsfield and Robert A. Noel

*Emory University Hospital, Clinical Research Facility, Atlanta, Georgia 30322*

The energy required to fuel basal metabolic reactions in the adult human is about 1600 calories/day. Six organs, together making up less than one-half of total body weight (Table 1), account for over 90% of this basal energy expenditure. Classic studies relating metabolic activity to body composition have pooled these organs and the remaining oxygen-consuming tissues into the "lean body mass" (LBM) (15). Over the last four decades, a wide variety of techniques has been perfected to measure the total mass of these lean tissues (5,19). Until recently, it was impractical in living subjects to further compartmentalize LBM into the mass of individual organs. Since 1978, however, accurate noninvasive techniques have enabled investigators to measure the size of all of the organs presented in Table 1 (9,10) in living man. Thus, the interrelationship between nutritional status, metabolic activity, and organ weight can now be investigated in patients with cancer and noncancer cachexia.

The specific focus of this chapter is the measurement, by computerized axial tomography (CT), of the mass of liver, kidney, and spleen. Together, these visceral organs represent only 3% to 4% of total body mass, but they account for more than one-third of whole-body basal energy expenditure (Table 1). In the following section, we will review early X-ray studies investigating soft-tissue body composition. A simplified view of CT theory and technique will follow, and we will conclude by reviewing recent CT studies of organ mass and composition in living subjects.

## EARLY RADIOGRAPHIC TECHNIQUES

The functional unit of X-ray, the photon, comes into existence when energetic electrons interact with matter at the atomic level. Following emission from the X-ray tube, the beam of photons is "attenuated" as it passes through air and tissue before final impact on the radiographic receptor. In general, the degree of photon attenuation will be proportional to the density[1] of the tissues

---

[1] The total rate of attentuation is actually related to the so-called Compton and photoelectric interactions (18).

TABLE 1. *Organ–tissue composition and oxygen consumption of the standard 20–30-year-old, 70 kg man[a]*

| Organ | Total weight (kg) | Organ oxygen consumption (cc/min) | Percent of body weight | Percent of basal oxygen consumption |
|---|---|---|---|---|
| Skeletal muscle | 30.00 | 64 | 42.90 | 25.6 |
| Liver | 1.70 | 66 | 2.40 | 26.4 |
| Brain | 1.40 | 46 | 2.00 | 18.3 |
| Heart | 0.35 | 23 | 0.50 | 9.2 |
| Kidney | 0.30 | 18 | 0.43 | 7.2 |
| Spleen | 0.15 | 9 | 0.21 | 3.6 |

[a]From Behnke (2) and Diem (4), with permission.

through which the X-ray beam has passed (18). Soft tissues near the density of water (1 g/cc) are therefore easily discriminated from bone (1.8 to 2.0 g/cc). However, conventional radiographic methods are only able to detect differences in attenuation of ±2% to 4%, and this low contrast does not always enable the various soft tissues to be distinguished from one another (16,17). This applies to muscle (D = 1.06 g/cc) and visceral organs (D = 1.05 to 1.08 g/cc), which cannot be clearly defined radiographically as separate structures.

Despite these limitations, as early as 1920 X-ray methods were successfully applied to the study of body composition in humans. Garn (6), Behnke (1), Tanner (20), and other early workers were able to measure fat, muscle, and bone widths in the upper or lower limbs and then to extrapolate these dimensions by use of various formulas to estimate total body fat and LBM.

In addition to low image contrast, these early methods had three shortcomings. First, the recorded view represented a two-dimensional "shadow" of fat, muscle, and bone within the limb; X-ray was thus unable to provide an accurate three-dimensional fat, muscle, or bone "volume." The second problem involved transfer of the data from the X-ray film. Measurements were made by hand directly from the radiograph, and the data were then corrected by application of a predetermined magnification factor. The third problem was that quantitative information describing the X-rayed soft tissues was lacking. Specifically, what was the X-ray attentuation value of fat, muscle, bone, or visceral organs?

## COMPUTERIZED AXIAL TOMOGRAPHY

The problems presented above have been largely overcome by the development, in the last decade, of the quantitative radiographic method of computerized tomography (CT). The CT scanner can be envisioned as consisting of two components, (a) the X-ray tube and detector (Fig. 1) and (b) a computer which processes the scan data and produces an X-ray image on a cathode-ray tube. The data from each CT scan can be stored in computer memory, magnetic tape, or disc, and the radiologist can perform a wide array of measurements and calculations by use of a variety of scanner computer programs.

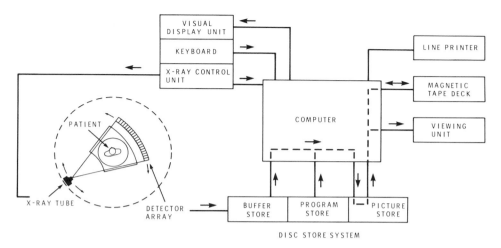

**FIG. 1.** Schematic illustration of CT scanner components.

## The CT Scan

The scanning sequence is as follows. The patient lies recumbent on a platform within the scanner gantry. Housed within the gantry, at right angles to the patient, is a large bearing. At one pole of the bearing is the X-ray tube (Fig. 1), and at the opposite pole is fastened a photon detector.[2] The desired scanning location on the patient is moved into the gantry, and the bearing rotated through one or several complete revolutions, usually requiring 2 to 30 seconds. The X-ray beam, 5–10 mm in width, exposes a cross-sectional "slice" through the patient; attenuated photons are captured by the detector, which generates an electrical impulse throughout the entire scan. These data are then relayed to the computer for reconstruction of the final image. The patient is moved a predetermined distance into the gantry, usually 1–2 cm, and the scanning sequence repeated for the next "slice." An axial slice image is reconstructed from each set of tomographic projections with the computer. The axial image can be reconstructed from the projection data by a number of methods (see footnote). The image is a two-dimensional representation of the axial slice of the patient. This matrix is normally displayed on a cathode-ray tube, with each numerical value converted to a shade of gray.

## Physical Properties of the CT Radiograph

Differences in X-ray attenuation of less than ±0.5% can be discriminated by CT (16), and this high image contrast allows a clear demarcation of different

---

[2] The scanner construction described is that of the General Electric CT/T 8800; other instruments may differ with respect to detector placement.

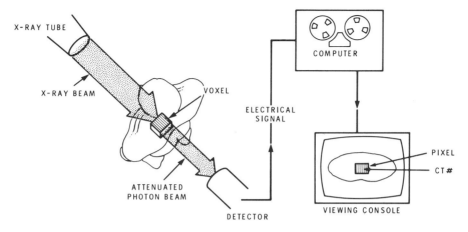

**FIG. 2.** Penetration of the voxel matrix by X-ray beam and reconstruction of the image pixel on the cathode-ray tube.

soft tissues. The reconstructed image has two important properties with respect to the study of body composition: (a) the image is composed of *pixels,* and (b) each pixel is assigned an attenuation value or CT number (CT#). The pixels (picture elements) are approximately 1 mm x 1 mm squares which are ultimately combined to form the cross-sectional image. Another term, *voxel* (volume element), includes slice thickness, and may, for example, represent a 1 mm x 1 mm x 10 mm block. The X-rayed cross-sectional body slice is divided by the CT scanner into a matrix of voxels. During the scanning sequence described above, the voxel matrix (Fig. 2) is penetrated by the X-ray beam. Following tissue interactions, the attenuated photon beam activates the detector, and the resulting signal is then computer-processed by either Fourier analysis or filtered-back projection (13). The result is the calculation of an attenuation value for each voxel. The actual attenuation values in all CT systems are processed to a simpler term, referred to as CT number (CT#).[3]

The total number of pixels collected during the scan represents slice volume. The CT# of each voxel provides the shading or contrast for each pixel. For example, a cross-sectional 60 cm² CT slice through the chest is composed of about 50,000 pixels, ranging in CT# from very low (air in lung) to high (bone). The absolute value of the CT# depends on the manufacturer; for example, on the General Electric System which uses the "Hounsfield scale", a CT# of −500 represents air, 0 water, and +500 bone; typical values are fat −70, muscle +20, and liver +25 to +30.

---

[3] $CT\# = \dfrac{K\ \mu p - \mu w}{\mu w}$, where K = contrast constant and $\mu p$ and $\mu w$ are the linear attentuation coefficients of the pixel in question and water, respectively (3).

## CT IN THE STUDY OF BODY COMPOSITION

Two types of CT soft-tissue studies have been reported. The first type measures cross-sectional area and/or volume of visceral organs, adipose tissue, or muscle. The second group of studies provides quantitative information on the composition of these respective tissues.

## MEASUREMENT OF AREA AND VOLUME BY CT

### Accurate Prediction of Liver, Kidney, and Spleen Volume by CT

As noted above, the effects of nutritional status and cancer on visceral organ size are difficult to assess using low-contrast radiography. However, the CT image of the abdomen readily allows measurement of liver, kidney, and spleen cross-sectional area at the viewing console (5). If contiguous, evenly spaced slices proceeding from cephalad to caudad are made through these respective organs, then organ volume can be calculated from the following equations:

(A) Volume of each slice$_i$ = area $\times$ slice width

(B) Volume of organ $= \sum\limits_{i=1}^{n}$ (volume of liver slice)$_i$

The reassembly of eight successive human CT liver slices, each separated by 2 cm, into a three-dimensional organ is demonstrated by the styrofoam model in Fig. 3. The accuracy of CT radiography in predicting organ volume by this method is ±5% (Fig. 4).

### Radiographic Quantification of Protein–Calorie Undernutrition

In a study similar to the early radiographic body composition studies presented above, Heymsfield and coworkers used CT to obtain the cross-sectional area of midarm adipose, muscle, and bone tissue (Fig. 5). The study had a twofold purpose. The first was to develop a simple radiographic method of quantifying the three aforementioned midarm tissues as indices of nutritional status. The second purpose was to validate empirically derived anthropometric formulas used in the calculation of midarm muscle and fat areas from skinfold measurements.

### Adipose and Lean Body Mass

The CT scanner has the capability of plotting a histogram of the image CT numbers. Since fat and lean tissues differ in density and attenuation, we can expect the CT# of each pixel representing these two tissues to differ markedly. A histogram of the pixels from a cross sectional X-ray of the abdomen is plotted

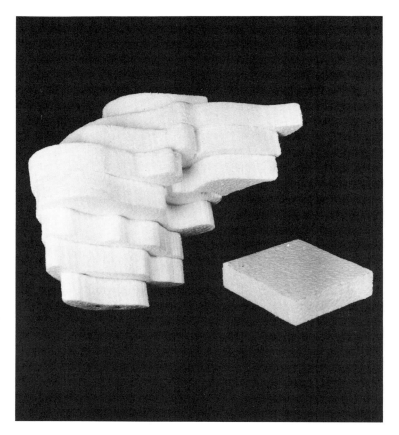

**FIG. 3.** Reconstructed "liver" from CT radiograph. Calibration block is 10 cm x 10 cm x 2 cm or 200 cm³. (From Heymsfield et al., ref. 10, with permission.)

in Fig. 6. This graph shows how low density–low attenuation adipose tissue pixels (D = 0.91 g/cc, CT# = −70) are clearly separated from lean tissue pixels, which are higher in density and attenuation (D = 1.05 to 1.1 g/cc, CT# = 15 to 30). Bone pixels appear mostly at the extreme end of the CT# scale, which currently ends at the arbitrarily chosen value of 512. By calculating the area (i.e., the number of pixels) under the fat, visceral lean tissue, and bone curves, the area and volume of each of these respective tissues can be calculated (Fig. 7). Another feature of CT abdominal radiography is that a separate histogram can be prepared from each slice that separates peritoneal from subcutaneous fat (Fig. 7). This is accomplished by selecting at the viewing console the appropriate pixels to be plotted. Finally, by preselecting regions of the body to be scanned, the nutritionist can quantitatively assess fat and lean tissue distribution (e.g., abdomen versus thigh).

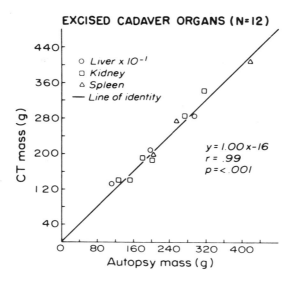

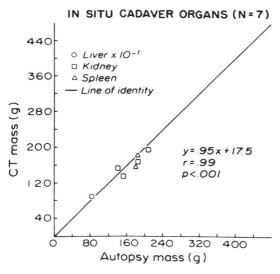

**FIG. 4.** Plot of CT mass on the ordinate and autopsy mass on the abscissa. CT mass calculated by multiplying CT volume times organ density, the latter determined in a density balance. **(Top)** Twelve observations of excised liver (N = 3), kidney (N = 6), and spleen (N = 3). CT mass agreed with actual mass ±5%. **(Bottom)** Seven observations of *in situ* cadaver liver (N = 1), kidney (N = 4), and spleen (N = 2). CT mass agreed with actual mass ±5%. (Adapted from Heymsfield et al., ref. 10.)

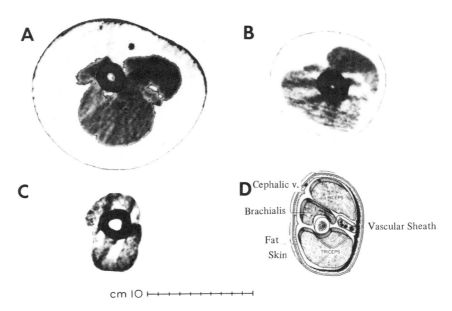

**FIG. 5.** CT radiograph of the midarm in an obese **(A)**, normal **(B)**, and undernourished **(C)** subject. The major mid-arm structures are diagrammed in panel **D.** (From Heymsfield et al., ref. 11, with permission.)

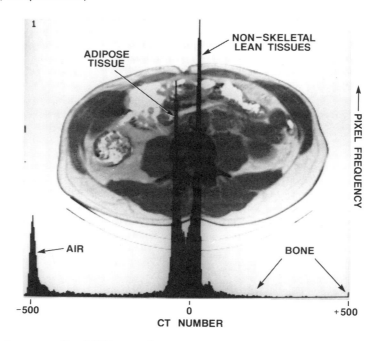

**FIG. 6.** A cross-sectional CT image of the abdomen in a healthy subject and a histogram of all of the image pixels.

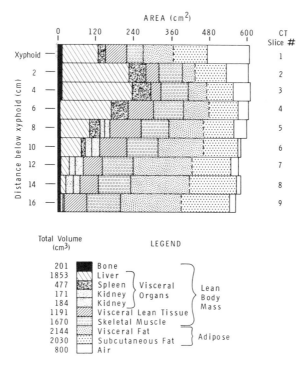

**FIG. 7.** Organ–tissue composition of a cancer patient, from the xyphoid process to the lower pole of the right kidney. Each slice was prepared in three steps. The liver, kidney and spleen pixels were first measured by tracing the outline of each respective organ. Next, the outline of the whole body slice was traced, and a pixel CT# histogram (Fig. 6) plotted; adipose, nonskeletal lean tissue, and bone pixels were then measured from the histogram. The third step was to trace an outline of the abdominal compartment, and repeat Step 2 to obtain total visceral lean tissue and mesenteric adipose pixels. The following equations were used to derive the data presented: subcutaneous adipose pixels = (total slice adipose pixels)–(visceral fat pixels), and skeletal muscle pixels = (total nonskeletal lean tissue pixels)–(visceral lean tissue pixels).

## CT in the Study of Tissue Composition

Pathological changes that alter tissue density in a tissue or cell will be recorded as a change in CT#. In addition, attenuation is also influenced by pathological tissue accumulation of elements with high atomic number. CT therefore may be used to quantitate liver and muscle triglyceride, liver iron stores, and bone density.

### Liver Triglyceride Content in Cases of Hepatic Steatosis

In fatty metamorphosis of the liver, the progressive increase in hepatocyte lipid content lowers cellular density, and therefore decreases CT# in a linear fashion. This method has proved highly accurate in the prediction of liver fat content in experimentally induced fatty liver in animals (22), and early results in man appear to be encouraging (8).

### Muscle Lipid Content in Muscular Dystrophy Cases

Some forms of muscular dystrophy (e.g., Duchenne's) are characterized by fatty replacement of the atrophic muscle group. Using the same principles as presented above for fatty liver, the severity of muscle atrophy and the rate of muscle disease progression can be quantitatively monitored by CT (7).

### Liver Iron Stores

In iron storage diseases, pathological accumulation of hepatocyte iron (atomic number 26) is registered as an increase in liver CT#. Preliminary studies indicate that hepatic iron can be estimated noninvasively by CT (14).

### Bone Density and Calcium Content

A number of investigators are now examining CT as a noninvasive method of studying bone composition, with special attention to the various demineralization diseases. The details of these studies are presented elsewhere (21).

## TECHNICAL LIMITATIONS OF CT

No discussion of a new quantitative method, such as CT radiography, would be complete without briefly mentioning some limitations of the technique. The first problem is that the CT# has a large coefficient of variation. Several factors influence the final CT# of a given tissue, including instrument calibration and noise, scanning parameters (e.g., KVP, reconstruction format, etc.) (12), patient positioning, and X-ray beam hardening. The latter problem occurs because the X-ray beam is polychromatic, and X-rays of low energy are preferentially absorbed as they pass through tissue; the result is a somewhat unpredictable attenuation value. For example, the CT# of subcutaneous adipose tissue (D = 0.91 g/cc) may differ slightly from that of visceral adipose tissue (D = 0.91 g/cc), because a different spectrum of X-rays passes through each respective tissue. Methods of improving these problems are being developed, and we can expect less CT# variability in future generation CT scanners.

A second problem, termed the partial volume effect (3), occurs when a voxel encloses two substances that differ in attenuation; the voxel CT# then has a value intermediate between the CT# of each respective substance. The investigator studying body composition is therefore unable to separate precisely the adipose and lean body mass curves presented in Fig. 6, because voxels at the interface between fat and lean tissue will have a CT# intermediate between the values for each of these two respective tissues. In general, the partial volume error will be proportional to voxel size and to the surface area-to-volume ratio (SA/V) of the structure under study. Voxel size can be minimized by closely spacing CT slices, but currently available scanners cannot reduce the voxel much below 1 mm x 1 mm x 2 mm. The volume or mass of structures with a low SA/V ratio, such as liver, are accurately predicted by CT. Prediction of organ or tissue mass by CT is less accurate in high SA/V structures, such as mesentery or intestinal tract.

In conclusion, CT radiography, although in only a relatively early phase of development and application, is proving to be a valuable instrument in the study of body composition. The technical limitations are not serious, and engineering advances should partially resolve these problems over the next several years. The wide availability of CT scanners should make the above-mentioned applications practical, but cost and radiation dosage must be considered before each study. A unique advantage of CT in the study of body composition in cancer cachexia, however, is that CT studies are often part of the clinical oncologic evaluation, and thus, the "data" are already being collected for clinical purposes. Harvesting this "free" information will be of great value in providing an understanding of the interrelationships between metabolic activity and body composition.

## REFERENCES

1. Behnke, A. R., and Siri, W. E. (1957): The estimation of lean body weight from anthropometric and X-ray measurements. Research and Development Technical Report USNRDL-TR-203, *Biology and Medicine*, 1–38.
2. Behnke, A. R., and Wilmore, J. H. (1974): Application of The Various Field Methods. In: *Evaluation and Regulation of Body Build and Composition*, pp. 58–59. Prentice-Hall, Inc., Englewood Cliffs, New Jersey.
3. Christensen, E. E., Curry, T. S., and Dowdey, J. E. (1978): Computed Tomography. In: *Introduction to the Physics of Diagnostic Radiology*, 2nd edition, pp. 329–360. Lea and Febiger, Philadelphia.
4. Diem, K., and Lentner, C. (1970): *Documenta Geigy Scientific Tables*, p. 539. J. R. Geigg, S. A. Baale, Switzerland.
5. Forbes, G. B., and Lewis, D. M. (1956): Total sodium, potassium and chloride in adult man. *J. Clin. Invest.*, 35:596–600.
6. Garn, S. (1961): Radiographic analysis of body composition. In: *Techniques for Measuring Body Composition*, edited by J. Brozek and A. Henschel. National Academy of Sciences National Research Council, Washington, D.C.
7. Galloway, J., Noel, R., Heymsfield, S., and Sones, P. (1980): Computerized axial tomography in the evaluation and management of Duchenne muscular dystrophy. *Clin. Res.*, (in press).
8. Goldberg, H. I., Thaler, M., Royal, S., and Ohto, M. (1979): Evaluation of fat and iron in the liver using computed tomography (CT) quantitative and qualitative study in dogs. *Gastroenterology*, (Abstract), 76:1139.
9. Heymsfield, S. B., Bethel, R. A., Ansley, J. D., Gibbs, D. M., Felner, J. M., and Nutter, D. O. (1978): Cardiac abnormalities in cachectic patients before and during nutritional repletion. *Am. Heart J.*, 95:584–594.
10. Heymsfield, S. B., Fulenwider, T., Nordlinger, B., Barlow, R., Sones, P., and Kutner, M. (1979): Accurate measurement of liver, kidney, and spleen volume and mass computerized axial tomography. *Ann. Intern. Med.*, 90:185–187.
11. Heymsfield, S. B., Olafson, R. P., Kutner, M. H., and Nixon, D. W. (1979): A radiographic method of quantifying protein–calorie undernutrition. *Am. J. Clin. Nutr.*, 32:693–702.

12. Heymsfield, S. B., Noel, R., Lynn, M., and Kutner, M. (1979): Accuracy of soft tissue density predicted by CT. *J. Comput. Assist. Tomogr.,* 3:859–60.
13. Kuhl, D. E., and Edwards, R. Q. (1968): Reorganizing data from transverse section scans of the brain using digital processing. *Radiology,* 91:975–980.
14. Mills, S. R., Doppman, J. L., and Niehuis, A. W. (1977): Computed tomography in the diagnosis of disorders of excessive iron storage of the liver. *J. Comput. Assist. Tomogr.,* 1:101–104.
15. Moore, F. D. (1963): The body cell mass and its supporting environment. W. B. Saunders, Philadelphia.
16. Phelps, M. E., Hoffman, E. J., and Ter-Pogossian, M. M. (1975): Attenuation coefficients of various body tissues, fluids and lesions at photon energies of 18 to 136 KeV. *Radiology,* 117:573–583.
17. Phelps, M. E., Gads, M. H., and Hoffman, E. J. (1975): Correlation of effective atomic number and electron density with attenuation coefficients measured with polychromatic X-rays. *Radiology,* 117:585–588.
18. Sprawls, P. (1977): Interaction of X-rays with matter. In: *The Physical Principles of Diagnostic Radiology,* pp. 101–117. University Park Press, Baltimore. 365 pp.
19. Rathburn, E. N., and Pace, N. (1945): Studies on body composition. *J. Biol. Chem.,* 158:667–676.
20. Tanner, J. M. (1964): *The Physique of the Olympic Athlete.* George Allen and Irwin, Ltd., London.
21. Ullrich, C. G., Binet, E. F., Sanecki, M. G., and Kieffer, S. A. (1980): Quantitative assessment of the lumbar spinal canal by computed tomography. *Radiology,* 134:137–143.
22. Vigil, V., and Heymsfield, S. B. (1979): Accurate prediction of liver fat content by computerized axial tomography (CT). *Clin. Res.,* 27:743A.

*Nutrition and Cancer: Etiology and Treatment,*
edited by G. R. Newell and N. M. Ellison.
Raven Press, New York © 1981.

# Fat and Cancer

## David Kritchevsky and David M. Klurfeld

*The Wistar Institute of Anatomy and Biology, Philadelphia, Pennsylvania 19104*

The association of nutritional state with development or promotion of cancer has been a topic of interest for many years and the subject of numerous reviews. A recent review by Carroll and Khor (12) provides references to the earlier works.

A role for dietary components in human cancer has been suggested by various epidemiological studies. Burkitt (6,7) has suggested that insufficient dietary fiber may contribute to the development of colon cancer. Drasar and Irving (17), on the other hand, find little correlation between low levels of fiber and colon cancer, but report a strong positive correlation between the latter and high levels of animal protein intake. Carroll and Khor (12) find a high positive correlation between per capita fat consumption and age-adjusted mortality from cancers of certain sites, such as the breast, intestine, and prostate. Negative correlations have been seen between fat consumption and cancers of the esophagus, stomach, and liver.

These dietary data reflect the availability of fat, rather than actual consumption. Furthermore, although a plot of age-adjusted death rates from intestinal cancer and dietary fat intake shows a definite correlation, in countries with the same death rates apparent fat intake may vary by as much as 100%. Thus, South African males have a death rate from intestinal cancer similar to that for Dutch males (11/100,000), but apparent fat intake of South African males is 68 g/day, whereas that of the Dutch is about 155 g/day. Portuguese and Norwegian males have the same death rate (6/100,000) from intestinal cancer, although their apparent fat intakes are about 75 and 135 g/day, respectively. Nevertheless, a general correlation between incidence of certain types of tumor and diet does exist and demands careful investigation.

Although it is hard to conceive of any normal dietary component as carcinogenic, certain nutrients may modify the neoplastic process by affecting transport of a procarcinogen or cocarcinogen, altering intestinal flora that may be involved in activation or detoxification of carcinogens, influencing hormone levels, affecting the host immune system, and affecting cell membrane permeability or enzymatic function. All of the above can be influenced by diet, but no definite connection between one of these actions and the effect of a carcinogen has been demonstrated experimentally.

In discussing fat, it is necessary to differentiate among neutral fats (triglycerides and fatty acid esters), steroids (cholesterol and bile acids), and phospholipids. In work on lipids and cancer, most attention has been paid to dietary cholesterol, fecal steroids, and total fat intake. Animal experiments provide more definitive answers, since tumors can be produced at specific sites and their presence and proliferation verified at autopsy. Work with human data is limited to epidemiological observations and certain biochemical measurements. In this brief review, we shall attempt to cover both the animal and human data, with the knowledge that interspecies extrapolation is of questionable value.

## ANIMAL STUDIES

The first study to demonstrate clearly that dietary fat could influence tumorigenesis was that of Watson and Mellanby (56). They found that addition of 12.5% to 25.0% butter to the basal diet (3% fat) of coal tar-treated mice increased the incidence of skin tumors from 34% to 57%. Carroll and Khor (12) summarized a number of other experiments in which the incidence of tumors was increased in mice whose diets contained between 15% and 30% partially hydrogenated vegetable oils.

Lavik and Baumann (33,34) tested the effect of topically administered methylcholanthrene on mice and found a relationship between tumorigenesis and diet. Addition of 15% fat (shortening) to the diet increased the yield of tumors from 12% to 83%. The authors found that the fat was especially effective when ingested 6 to 12 weeks after institution of treatment with the carcinogen. They also compared diets containing 10% corn oil, coconut oil, or lard for ability to promote tumors and found a minor effect for unsaturation, the incidences of tumors at 5 months being 33% (control), 61% (lard), 66% (coconut oil), and 76% (corn oil).

The level of dietary fat is obviously important, as is the amount of carcinogen used. Table 1 shows the effects of high and low doses of carcinogen and corn oil. At the low dose of carcinogen, the 20% corn oil diet leads to more tumors and a shorter latent period, but no difference in the number of tumors per

TABLE 1. *Effect of fat and carcinogen on induction of mammary tumors in rats* [a]

|  | 1 mg DMBA [b] | | 2.5 mg DMBA [b] | |
| --- | --- | --- | --- | --- |
|  | 0.5% corn oil | 20% corn oil | 0.5% corn oil | 20% corn oil |
| Percent rats with tumors | 3.6 | 6.6 | 33.3 | 56.6 |
| Tumors per rat | $0.17 \pm 0.02$ | $0.33 \pm 0.11$ | $0.6 \pm 0.17$ | $1.5 \pm 0.28$ |
| Tumors per tumor-bearing rat | $1.25 \pm 0.25$ | $1.25 \pm 0.78$ | $1.4 \pm 0.15$ | $1.9 \pm 0.26$ |
| Latent period (days) | 111 | 97 | 84 | 79 |

[a] After Carroll and Khor, ref. 10.
[b] 7,12-dimethylbenz(a)anthracene.

TABLE 2. *Effect of dietary fats on induction of mammary tumors in rats given DMBA[a]*

| Fat (20%) | Iodine value[b] | Rats with tumors (%) | No. tumors per tumor-bearing rat | Tumors per 30 rats |
|---|---|---|---|---|
| Sunflower seed oil | 148 | 96.6 | 4.8 ± 0.31 | 130 |
| Corn oil | 130 | 90.0 | 4.0 ± 0.62 | 110 |
| Cottonseed oil | 123 | 93.3 | 4.5 ± 0.75 | 127 |
| Soybean oil | 139 | 100.0 | 3.4 ± 0.46 | 103 |
| Olive oil | 84 | 86.6 | 4.5 ± 0.42 | 117 |
| Lard | 59 | 93.3 | 3.4 ± 0.47 | 97 |
| Tallow | 39 | 80.0 | 3.0 ± 0.49 | 72 |
| Butter | 34 | 86.6 | 3.3 ± 0.41 | 88 |
| Coconut oil | 6 | 96.6 | 2.5 ± 0.38 | 73 |

[a] After Carroll and Khor, ref. 11.
[b] Calculated from published data on fatty acid spectra.

tumor-bearing rat. When 2.5 mg 7,12-dimethylbenz(a)anthracene (DMBA) is used, the effect of the high-fat diet on the number of tumors is accentuated, but not in the latent period.

Several studies show that fewer tumors are produced in animals fed saturated fat than in those fed unsaturated fat. Carroll and Khor (11) fed female Sprague–Dawley rats fats (20%) of differing degrees of unsaturation and treated them with DMBA. A definite effect of saturation was observed (Table 2). The effect might be lost if the amount of fat fed is high enough. Reddy (50) treated rats with 1,2-dimethylhydrazine and fed them diets containing 5% or 20% lard or corn oil. Fewer colonic tumors were observed in rats fed 5% lard, but when the level of fat was 20%, the tumor incidence was the same in both diets (Table 3). Broitman et al. (5) fed rats 5% or 20% coconut oil or 20% safflower oil and treated them with 1,2-dimethylhydrazine. The percentages of rats with tumors and average numbers of tumors per rat were as follows: 5% coconut oil, 50% and 0.8 ± 0.3; 20% coconut oil, 85% and 2.2 ± 0.3; and 20% safflower oil, 100% and 3.8 ± 0.7. Burns et al. (8) found that the average survival time

TABLE 3. *Influence of dietary fat on tumor incidence in rats treated with DMH[a]*

| Dietary fat | Percent | No. rats | Rats with colon tumors | Rats with multiple colon tumors | Colon tumors per rat |
|---|---|---|---|---|---|
| Corn oil | 5 | 22 | 8 | 3 | 0.77 |
| Lard | 5 | 23 | 4 | 1 | 0.22 |
| Corn oil | 20 | 22 | 14 | 7 | 1.55 |
| Lard | 20 | 24 | 16 | 7 | 1.50 |
| Control | — | 20 | 5 | 0 | 0.25 |

[a] 1,2-dimethylhydrazine. After Reddy, ref. 50.

of leukemic mice fed 16% safflower oil was 188 hours, and that for mice fed 16% coconut oil was 202 hours.

What is the mechanism by which unsaturated fat enhances tumor growth? Carroll and Hopkins (9) found that 20% coconut oil added to a commercial ration resulted in a 28% incidence of DMBA-induced tumors in rats. When the rats were fed 17% coconut oil and 3% safflower oil the tumor incidence was 85%, and when 20% safflower oil was fed the tumor incidence was 66%. When the study was carried out using a semipurified diet (28), similar results were obtained. Newberne et al. (44) studied the effect of diet on aflatoxin B-induced liver tumors in rats. When the source of fat was beef, the number of tumors induced in two groups of rats was the same, regardless of whether the beef was fed only after induction (51%) or before and after induction (53%). Feeding corn oil before and after induction resulted in a 100% tumor yield, and when the oil was fed only after tumor induction, the yield was 66%. The studies of Carroll and his co-workers (9–12) suggest that unsaturated fat may promote carcinogenesis. Hillyard and Abraham (27) have shown that the growth of transplantable tumors is affected as much by 0.1% pure linoleic acid as by 15% corn oil. They suggest that unsaturated fat affects the immune system, possibly via prostaglandin synthesis. As evidence, they cite the inhibition of the tumor growth-promoting effect of polyunsaturated fat by inhibitors of prostaglandin synthesis, such as 5,8,11,14-eicosatetraynoic acid and indomethacin.

The data summarized above suggest that high-fat diets stimulate tumor growth to a greater extent than low-fat diets, and that polyunsaturated fats are more effective in this regard than saturated fats.

The role of cholesterol and bile acids in enhancing tumor growth has also been investigated. The fact that cholic or deoxycholic acid can be chemically converted to methylcholanthrene has stimulated interest in the premise that the chemical reaction that occurs on pyrolysis may take place *in vivo* at 37°C if proper enzymes are present.

Nigro et al. (45) found that addition of a bile acid-binding resin (cholestyramine) to the diet of rats treated with any of three carcinogens significantly increased the number of large bowel tumors (Table 4). Chomchai et al. (14) showed that diverting bile to the distal half of the small intestine significantly increased the number of tumors at that site. Thus, the presence of additional bile salt, either bound to a resin or introduced by surgical manipulation, enhanced tumorigenesis. Whether the mechanism of action is metabolic or physical is still a moot question.

The presence of bile salts bound to resins or to certain types of dietary fiber has been shown to disrupt the integrity of the intestinal mucosa (13). There are data suggesting a cocarcinogenic effect of bile acids, possibly owing to their action on the gut mucosa. Narisawa et al (42) have reported that intrarectal instillation of N-methyl-N'-nitro-N-nitrosoguanidine (MNNG) causes a 25% incidence of tumors in rats. When MNNG is given with lithocholic or taurodeoxycholic acid, the tumor incidence rises to 52% and 62%, respectively. The two

TABLE 4. *Influence of cholestyramine on incidence of chemically induced large bowel tumors in rats* [a]

|  | Number of tumors | |
| --- | --- | --- |
| Regimen | Proximal | Distal |
| 1,2-dimethylhydrazine | | |
|   ND [b] | 15 | 1 |
|   ND + 2% cholestyramine | 31 | 29 |
| Azoxymethane | | |
|   ND | 19 | 8 |
|   ND + 2% cholestyramine | 33 | 36 |
| Methylazoxymethanol | | |
|   ND | 4 | 2 |
|   ND + 2% cholestyramine | 18 | 15 |

[a] After Nigro et al., ref. 45.
[b] Normal diet.

bile acids exert no tumorigenic effect when given alone. The presence of high levels of beef fat in the diet increases the fecal excretion of deoxycholic acid, as noted by Nigro et al. (46), suggesting increased bacterial degradation of cholic acid. This diet also increases the incidence of tumor formation by 78%. Reddy et al. (52) reported increased fecal excretion of primary bile acid metabolites in rats treated with 1,2-dimethylhydrazine, but since their data were given in mg/kg body weight and neither body nor fecal weight was reported, the true level of excretion is hard to judge. The high beef-fat diet had no significant effect upon excretion of cholesterol degradation products.

## HUMAN STUDIES

The data linking human cancer with dietary fat are epidemiological in nature. Lea (35) found a correlation between geographic latitude and mortality from breast cancer, and attributed this to consumption of fats and oils. He also found a negative correlation between fat consumption and carcinoma of the stomach or corpus uterus. Wynder and his associates (57,58,59) have found increased mortality from colon cancer in those countries in which per capita intake of animal fats has risen. They also discovered a correlation between breast cancer and colon cancer, and suggested that both might be affected by dietary factors, such as fat intake, or by related socioeconomic variables. The link between these and other cancers and diet appears to be overnutrition. Berg (2) has suggested that hormone-dependent cancers are cancers of affluence.

Devesa (16) has summarized current trends in the incidence of the ten tumors most common in the United States. Between 1940 and 1970, there were dramatic changes in the incidence (rate per 100,000) of stomach cancer (down from 32 to 9), uterine cancer (down from 33 to 21), and lung cancer (up from 8.5 to 38); there was also an increase in lymphoma from 9 in 1950 to 15 in 1970.

The incidence of intestinal cancer has risen from 20 to 27 and of breast cancer from 32 to 39, whereas that of cancer of the rectum has fallen from 15 to 13. Newberne (43) has summarized data on the age-adjusted death rates for stomach, intestinal, and breast cancer from six countries (Table 5). It is evident that the U.S. has the lowest burden of deaths from all causes, and that the two countries with very low death rates from intestinal and breast cancer have very high death rates for stomach cancer. Higginson (24) has shown that when Japanese from Japan migrate to the U. S., their incidence of stomach cancer decreases but that of colon cancer increases. He has warned that dietary treatment aimed at reducing the incidence of colon cancer may increase the incidence of stomach cancer. Those who study diet and cancer would do well to examine the effects at all sites. Obviously, our aim is to reduce the incidence of all cancer, but when it is possible that a dietary regimen may decrease the development of one type of cancer while increasing the incidence of another, the overall impact of dietary changes should be addressed.

A large portion of the current research effort is directed towards identification of a metabolic connection between dietary fat and colon cancer. One aspect of this search has been the examination of patterns of fecal steroid excretion. Persons subsisting on diets high in animal fat excrete more fecal steroids than do vegetarians. The fecal steroids represent products of cholesterol metabolism, as well as sterols from sloughed intestinal mucosa and bacterial matter. It is not surprising, then, that subjects who ingest more of the steroid precursor cholesterol, excrete more steroids. Antonis and Bersohn (1) showed that the levels of both fat and fiber influenced the ratio of neutral to acidic steroid. Hill (25) showed that mean fecal bile acid concentration was a function of dietary fat (Table 6). Thus, the amount of excreted steroid may not be as important a clue as the ratios of metabolites. Cholesterol is stereospecifically hydrogenated by the intestinal microflora to yield coprostanol, which, in turn, is oxidized to coprostanone. Cholesterol is also converted to the primary bile acids, cholic and chenodeoxycholic, by liver enzymes. These bile acids are dehydroxylated

TABLE 5. *Age-adjusted death rate per 100,000 (1968–1969)*[a]

| Country | Primary cancer site | | | |
|---|---|---|---|---|
| | Stomach[b] | Colon and rectum[b] | Breast[c] | Total |
| U.S.A. | 13 | 35 | 22 | 70 |
| Netherlands | 39 | 35 | 26 | 100 |
| Scotland | 35 | 46 | 26 | 107 |
| W. Germany | 51 | 38 | 19 | 108 |
| Chile | 95 | 14 | 11 | 120 |
| Japan | 100 | 16 | 4 | 120 |

[a] After Newberne, ref. 43.
[b] Male and female.
[c] Female.

TABLE 6. *Relationship between dietary fat and fecal bile acids* [a]

| Subjects | No. | Mean fat intake (g/day) | Fecal bile acids (mg/g dry wt) |
|---|---|---|---|
| Volunteers | | | |
| Low fat | 5 | <30 | 1.5–2.0 |
| Controls | 5 | 100–120 | 6.0–6.8 |
| Volunteers | | | |
| Liquid diet | 4 | <5 | 1.5–2.0 |
| Controls | 4 | 100 | 5.5–6.5 |
| Vegetarians | 20 | 60–80 | 3–4 |

[a] After Hill, ref. 25.

at the 7 position by intestinal bacteria to yield the secondary bile acids, deoxy-cholic and lithocholic. Many other bile acids appear in the feces, practically all of which are derived from bacterial action.

Reddy (51) has reviewed various aspects of nutrition and colon cancer. The levels of neutral and acidic steroids found in the feces of subjects with colon cancer or adenomatous polyps and in controls are given in Table 7. The controls excreted considerably less of these steroids than did the patients. Proportionately, the control subjects excreted much less cholesterol than coprostanol, which suggested that the increased levels of cholesterol in the patients' feces included sloughed cells as well as ingested or synthesized sterol. The ratio of cholesterol to its neutral degradation products was high in patients with colon cancer, which suggested reduced metabolic (hydrogenating) activity. The levels of primary bile acids in the feces of the three groups were similar, but levels of secondary bile acids were much lower in the feces of controls. These data suggest accelerated synthesis of primary bile acids, enhanced turnover of the secondary

TABLE 7. *Fecal steroids (mg/g dry feces) in colon cancer patients, patients with adenomatous polyps, and controls* [a]

| | Colon cancer (35) | Adenomatous polyps (15) | Control (40) |
|---|---|---|---|
| Neutral steroids | | | |
| Cholesterol (CH) | 12.6 ± 1.50 | 6.4 ± 0.80 | 3.2 ± 0.41 |
| Coprostanol (CO) | 18.7 ± 1.78 | 19.6 ± 3.20 | 12.9 ± 0.82 |
| Coprostanone (CN) | 3.9 ± 0.42 | 4.0 ± 1.01 | 1.9 ± 0.19 |
| CH/CO | 0.67 | 0.33 | 0.25 |
| CH/CO + CN | 0.56 | 0.27 | 0.22 |
| Acidic steroids | | | |
| Cholic acid | 0.5 ± 0.12 | 0.4 ± 0.10 | 0.4 ± 0.08 |
| Chenodeoxycholic acid | 0.5 ± 0.18 | 0.3 ± 0.06 | 0.2 ± 0.08 |
| Deoxycholic acid | 7.0 ± 0.44 | 6.1 ± 0.70 | 3.7 ± 0.40 |
| Lithocholic acid | 6.5 ± 0.40 | 5.4 ± 0.50 | 3.1 ± 0.22 |
| Other bile acids | 5.1 ± 0.44 | 4.2 ± 0.50 | 3.5 ± 0.32 |
| Primary/secondary | 0.007 | 0.006 | 0.088 |

[a] After Reddy, ref. 51.

bile acids, or decreased conversion of primary to secondary bile acids. The ratios of primary to secondary bile acids reflect these differences.

Problems with interpretation of these data lie in the differences between the diets of healthy subjects and those of colon cancer patients and the relationship between excretion patterns and disease, i.e., do the patterns reflect susceptibility or are they after-the-fact manifestations of disease? One of these problems has been addressed by Moskovitz et al. (40), who used three groups of subjects (normal, N; colon cancer, CC; and nongastric or intestinal cancer, NGC) whose diets were similar in caloric content and composition. Fecal steroid excretion was lowest in group CC. The ratios of primary to secondary bile acids were 0.23, 0.32, and 0.22 in groups N, CC, and NGC, respectively. The ratios of cholesterol to coprostanol plus coprostanone were as follows: N, 0.44; CC, 0.73; and NGC, 0.55. The observed differences reflect impaired degradation of cholesterol and primary bile acids in the patients with colon cancer. The authors conclude that excretion of neutral and acidic steroid was similar in the three groups, since no significant differences were observed.

Reddy (51) presents data on bile acid composition of feces from healthy males in New York City (which has a high incidence of colon cancer) and Kuopio, Finland (where the incidence of colon cancer is low). New Yorkers excrete twice as much bile acid as Finns, based on mg/g feces, but equal amounts based on mg/day, since the Finns produce a greater bulk of feces. Based on the mg/g data, ratios of primary to secondary bile acids for New Yorkers and Finns are 0.67 and 0.106, respectively; the ratios based on mg/day data are the same. On a daily basis, the Finns excrete almost twice as much primary bile acid as New Yorkers, but only 10% more secondary bile acid. Clearly, excretion data must be presented in both mg/g feces and mg/day. Fecal excretion data for five different populations (Table 8) show that total steroid excretion can be related to dietary fat; the ratio of sterols to bile acids is the same for Japanese and for Americans eating a high-fat diet. The ratio of primary to secondary bile acids is lower in American Seventh-Day Adventists (who have

TABLE 8. *Daily fecal steroid excretion in five populations*[a]

| Group | Steroids[b] | | | | |
|---|---|---|---|---|---|
| | Total steroids (mg/day) | Total bile acids (mg/day) | S/BA | CO/CH | P/S |
| U.S. high fat diet (17) | 818 | 256 | 3.20 | 26.3 | 0.043 |
| U.S. vegetarian (12) | 318 | 133 | 2.39 | 3.7 | 0.127 |
| U.S. SDA[c] (11) | 266 | 54 | 4.92 | 2.6 | 0.025 |
| Japanese (17) | 266 | 83 | 3.20 | 7.7 | 0.079 |
| Chinese (11) | 195 | 54 | 3.61 | 1.6 | 0.071 |

[a] After Reddy, (ref. 51.).
[b] S/BA = Sterols/bile acids; CO/CH = coprostanol + coprostanone/cholesterol; P/S = primary/secondary bile acids.
[c] Seventh-Day Adventists.

a relatively low incidence of colon cancer) than in Americans on either high-fat or vegetarian diets. Mower et al. (41) assessed the fecal bile acids of Japanese populations with low (Akita) and high (Hawaii) cancer incidences. Amounts of total bile acid excretion (mg/g dry weight) were similar, 8.61 in Hawaii and 7.45 in Akita. Mower and co-workers found 16 bile acids, nine of which could not be identified. Ratios of primary to secondary bile acids were 0.61 in Hawaii and 0.65 in Akita; ratios of primary bile acids to all other bile acids were 0.53 in Hawaii and 0.41 in Akita. The authors concluded that the data "were suggestive, but not strongly supportive, of a relationship between fecal bile acid patterns and colon cancer risk."

It has been suggested that consumption of animal fat is highly correlated with mortality from colon cancer (12). Leveille (36) analyzed colon cancer incidence in Connecticut and found a strong positive correlation with meat intake. However, Blot et al. (4) have shown great geographical variations in colon cancer incidence within the United States that cannot be readily correlated with patterns of diet. Over 95% of all counties in the Northeast exhibit colon cancer rates above the U.S. median, but only 27% of the counties in the Southeast do. Seventh-Day Adventists, many of whom are vegetarians, exhibit a low incidence of colon cancer (49), but so do Latter-Day Saints, who are not vegetarians (38). Enstrom (19) has shown that beef consumption has almost doubled in the U.S. since 1940, whereas colon cancer mortality has remained the same (Table 9). Graham and Mettlin (21) have shown that the frequency of meat eating in a large number of colon cancer patients is similar to that of the general population (Table 10).

Berg (2) suggested that the cancers seen in the Western world might be due to overnutrition rather than to any specific nutrient. In other words, the culprit may be total calories. Despite the changing picture of fat availability in the U.S. (Table 11), caloric availability has been relatively constant (20). Gregor et al. (22) analyzed data relating to calorie intake and gastric and intestinal cancers concluding that with higher food intake, the gastric cancer mortality rate falls but rises for intestinal cancer. This observation may explain the frequently quoted differences among Japanese in Japan, Hawaii,

TABLE 9. *Colorectal cancer and beef consumption in the U.S.*[a]

| Year | Beef consumption (weekly lb. per capita) | Colon cancer[b] | |
|------|------------------------------------------|-----------------|-----------|
| | | Incidence | Mortality |
| 1940 | 1.1 | – | 20 |
| 1950 | 1.3 | 44 | 20 |
| 1960 | 1.6 | – | 19 |
| 1965 | 1.9 | – | 19 |
| 1970 | 2.1 | 33 | 19 |

[a] After Enstrom, ref. 19.
[b] Annual rate/100,000 standardized to 1950.

TABLE 10. *Association between monthly frequency of meat ingestion and colon cancer*[a]

| Frequency | Colon cancer patients (192) % | Controls (620) % |
|---|---|---|
| 0–20 | 14.1 | 9.2 |
| 21–30 | 33.3 | 33.4 |
| 31–40 | 30.7 | 33.9 |
| 41–50 | 19.3 | 17.9 |
| 51+ | 2.6 | 5.6 |

[a] After Graham and Mettlin, ref. 21.

TABLE 11. *Food lipids available in the U.S. per capita per day*[a]

| Years | Total fat (g) | Fatty acids | | | Cholesterol (mg) | Total calories |
|---|---|---|---|---|---|---|
| | | Saturated (g) | Oleic (g) | Linoleic (g) | | |
| 1909–1913 | 125 | 50.3 | 51.5 | 10.7 | 509 | 3,480 |
| 1925–1929 | 135 | 53.3 | 55.2 | 12.5 | 524 | 3,470 |
| 1935–1939 | 133 | 52.9 | 54.5 | 12.7 | 493 | 3,270 |
| 1947–1949 | 141 | 54.4 | 58.0 | 14.8 | 577 | 3,230 |
| 1957–1959 | 143 | 54.7 | 58.2 | 16.6 | 578 | 3,130 |
| 1965 | 145 | 53.9 | 58.8 | 19.1 | 540 | 3,140 |
| 1970 | 157 | 53.9 | 63.1 | 23.3 | 556 | 3,300 |
| 1974 | 158 | 56.0 | 62.9 | 24.2 | — | 3,350 |

[a] After Gortner, ref. 20.

and California. Some of Gregor's findings are shown in Table 12. Hill et al. (26) presented data on colorectal cancer mortality in three socioeconomic groups in Hong Kong. Colorectal cancer mortality rose with income, as did fecal bile acids and every component of the diet, including fat, protein, carbohydrates, and fiber. The mortality observed in the richest group (26.7/100,000) was more than twice that in the poorest (11.7/100,000); fat intake was 61% higher, carbohydrate intake 40% higher, meat intake 47% higher, and intake of fiber-rich foods 29% higher. A crude estimate of daily calorie intake (based on data in Hill's paper) for the three groups is 2,700, 3,000, and 3,900, respectively.

In animal studies, Tannenbaum (55) showed that the mean time for appearance of tumors in mice varied inversely with daily calorie intake. Lavik and Baumann (34) showed that incidence of methylcholanthrene-induced skin tumors in mice was related more to calorie intake than to fat intake (Table 13). Many of the observed differences in fecal steroids may be related to calorie intake rather than to fat intake.

Since diets high in fat and calories are related to higher incidences of both atherosclerosis and colon cancer, and given the statistical relationship between elevated serum cholesterol levels and atherosclerosis, there has been interest

TABLE 12. *Mortality rates for stomach and intestinal cancer and intake of animal protein* [a]

| Country [b] | Animal protein (1962–63) g/day | Standardized mortality rate | |
| | | Stomach cancer | Intestinal cancer |
|---|---|---|---|
| Japan | 16.9 | 67.96 | 2.97 |
| Columbia | 20.0 | 21.20 | 2.24 |
| Spain | 23.4 | 30.37 | 6.15 |
| Venezuela | 25.3 | 33.00 | 4.10 |
| Italy | 29.8 | 34.22 | 7.97 |
| Hungary | 37.0 | 46.40 | 6.26 |
| France | 43.0 | 23.03 | 11.34 |
| Netherlands | 46.1 | 29.50 | 10.53 |
| W. Germany | 49.2 | 38.41 | 9.15 |
| Switzerland | 51.3 | 27.81 | 10.53 |
| Finland | 54.7 | 44.80 | 5.20 |
| Australia | 59.6 | 17.06 | 12.68 |
| Canada | 63.8 | 18.69 | 13.88 |
| United States | 64.2 | 14.87 | 12.25 |
| New Zealand | 74.8 | 17.90 | 12.45 |

[a] After Gregor et al., ref. 22.
[b] Selected from 28 countries.

in relating serum cholesterol levels to the incidence of colon cancer. Pearce and Dayton (48) carried out an eight-year clinical trial in which groups of 422 and 424 men were fed a conventional diet and one containing high levels of polyunsaturated fat, respectively. Fatal atherosclerotic events were significantly more frequent in the control group, but the total mortality rates in the two groups were similar because of the greater incidence of cancer deaths in the group on the experimental diet. Miettinen et al. (39) conducted a similar experiment in Finland and also found more carcinomas in the test group. A study group was convened to examine cancer incidences in men on cholesterol-lowering diets, and although the group found little difference in relative risks, it concluded, in part: "Much more data are needed to determine whether serum-cholesterol-lowering diets increase, decrease, or leave unaltered the cancer risk"

TABLE 13. *Influence of fat and calories on methylcholanthrene-induced skin tumors in mice* [a]

| Diet | Tumor incidence (%) |
|---|---|
| Low fat, low calorie | 0 |
| Low fat, high calorie | 54 |
| High fat, low calorie | 28 |
| High fat, high calorie | 66 |

[a] After Lavik and Baumann, ref. 34.

(18). The recently published findings of a long-term study on the use of clofibrate (ethyl *p*-chlorophenoxyisobutyrate) for lowering serum lipids and treating ischemic heart disease show a reduction in the number of myocardial infarctions, but more deaths caused by gastrointestinal malignancies in men taking the hypolipidemic agent (15). These findings raise the question of the relationship between low serum lipid levels and cancer. Wynder and Shigematsu (60) studied total serum cholesterol levels in patients with large bowel cancer (Table 14). They found that 46% of the men and 29% of the women had serum cholesterol levels below 200 mg/dl, and 84% of the men and 75% of the women had cholesterol levels below 249 mg/dl. Cholesterol levels between 200 and 249 mg/dl are considered to be in the normal range. Rose et al. (53) also examined the relationship between colon cancer and blood cholesterol. They examined data from six large studies and found 90 colon cancer patients in a population of several thousand. They reported, "The initial levels of blood-cholesterol in these men were found surprisingly to be lower than the expected values." The mean deviation in persons without colon cancer was relatively high. Bjelke (3) reported a similar correlation between colon cancer and low levels of blood cholesterol. Nydegger and Butler (47) examined total serum cholesterol levels and $\alpha_1$ and $\beta$ lipoprotein levels in 186 control subjects and 122 patients with malignant tumors. The data (Table 15) show generally lower cholesterol levels and lower $\alpha/\beta$ ratios in the cancer patients. Thus, the cancer patients exhibited relatively higher $\beta$ lipoprotein levels, despite their lower cholesterol levels. If the data for all the patients are averaged, the serum cholesterol levels of the normal and cancer subjects were 221 and 197 mg/dl, respectively. The cancer patients were generally older than the controls. Average cholesterol levels in the subjects below 50 years of age were similar (210 mg/dl in controls and 201 mg/dl in cancer patients), but in the 50+-year-old group the normal subjects exhibited an average serum cholesterol level of 246 mg/dl and the cancer patients had an average of 195 mg/dl. Average levels for total serum lipids, esterified fatty acids, triglycerides, and phospholipids (all in mg/100 ml) for controls

TABLE 14. *Total serum cholesterol levels in patients with cancer of large bowel*[a]

| Total serum cholesterol (mg/dl) | No. of men | No. of women |
|---|---|---|
| 100–149 | 9 | 2 |
| 150–199 | 14 | 12 |
| 200–249 | 19 | 22 |
| 250–299 | 2 | 10 |
| 300+ | 6 | 2 |

[a]Excluded were patients with 10 lb or more recent weight loss; after Wynder and Shigematsu, ref. 60.

TABLE 15. *Serum lipid levels in cancer patients* [a]

| Age group (yrs) | Control | | Cancer | |
|---|---|---|---|---|
| | $\alpha_1/\beta$ [b] | Cholesterol (mg/dl) | $\alpha_1/\beta$ | Cholesterol (mg/dl) |
| <30 | 1.14 | 198 | 0.88 | 193 |
| 30–39 | 1.04 | 212 | 0.78 | 204 |
| 40–49 | 1.31 | 227 | 0.67 | 212 |
| 50–59 | 1.07 | 256 | 0.80 | 196 |
| 60–69 | 1.16 | 234 | 0.76 | 205 |
| 70–79 | 0.90 | 258 | 0.71 | 185 |
| 80–89 | 1.07 | 221 | 0.81 | 176 |
| 90–99 | 1.21 | — | — | — |

[a] After Nydegger and Butler, ref. 47.
[b] Ratio of $\alpha_1$ to $\beta$ lipoproteins.

and cancer patients were 823 and 771, 337 and 338, 121 and 142, and 175 and 140, respectively.

Liu et al. (37) report a high correlation between intake of cholesterol and colon cancer mortality in a study of data from 20 countries. The data reflect high fat, and hence high calorie, intake. This suggests that high fat intake is correlated with elevations in serum lipid levels, but that all components of the diet affect hypercholesterolemia (32). We have already discussed data (22) relating to total caloric intake and the inverse relationship between gastric and intestinal cancer.

Serum and leukocyte membrane cholesterol levels are low in leukemia patients (30). When Inbar and Shinitzky (29) enriched lymphoma cells with cholesterol *in vitro*, they observed inhibition of tumor growth and increased host survival time after those cells were transplanted into mice. Dietary cholesterol has been found to enhance lymphocyte function (31), and inhibition of cholesterol synthesis to decrease T-lymphocyte cytotoxicity (23). In addition to theories that attribute the observed high colon cancer–low serum cholesterol relationship to flux through the intestine and enhanced bile acid synthesis, investigators must consider the influence of cholesterol and lipoproteins on the immune system.

To summarize, the available data relate diets high in fat to a high incidence of colon cancer. Polyunsaturated fat is more effective than saturated fat in this regard. A role for bile acids (possibly as procarcinogens) has been suggested, but bile acid production is a function of the level of fat in the diet. Ultimately, the entire effect may revolve around the caloric content of the diet. A role for fat as a mediator in the immune system cannot be ruled out.

There are extensive data, epidemiological and experimental, related to diet, fat, and cancer. These are what Stavraky (54) has called "hypothesis-generating data." The hypotheses have been generated; their confirmation remains to be established.

## ACKNOWLEDGMENTS

This investigation has been supported in part by Research Career Award HL-00734 from the National Institutes of Health and grants in aid from the National Dairy Council, the National Livestock and Meat Board, and the W. W. Smith Charitable Trust.

## REFERENCES

1. Antonis, A., and Bersohn, I. (1962): The influence of diet on fecal lipids in South African white and Bantu prisoners. *Am. J. Clin. Nutr.,* 11:142–155.
2. Berg, J. W. (1975): Can nutrition explain the pattern of international epidemiology of hormone-dependent cancers? *Cancer Res.,* 35:3345–3350.
3. Bjelke, E. (1974): Colon cancer and blood-cholesterol. *Lancet,* 1:1116–1117.
4. Blot, W. J., Fraumeni, F. J., Jr., Stone, B. J., and McKay, F. W. (1976): Geographic patterns of large bowel cancer in the United States. *J. Natl. Cancer Inst.,* 57:1225–1231.
5. Broitman, S. A., Vitale, J. J., Vavrousek-Jakuba, E., and Gottlieb, L. S. (1977): Polyunsaturated fat, cholesterol and large bowel tumorigenesis. *Cancer,* 40:2453–2463.
6. Burkitt, D. P. (1971): Epidemiology of cancer of the colon and rectum. *Cancer,* 28:3–13.
7. Burkitt, D. P. (1975): Benign and malignant tumors of the large bowel. In: *Refined Carbohydrate Foods and Disease,* edited by D. P. Burkitt and H. C. Trowell, pp. 117–133. Academic Press, London.
8. Burns, C. P., Luttenegger, D. G., and Spector, A. A. (1978): Effect of dietary fat saturation on survival of mice with L1210 leukemia. *J. Natl. Cancer Inst.,* 61:513–515.
9. Carroll, K. K., and Hopkins, G. J. (1978): Dietary polyunsaturated fat versus saturated fat in relation to mammary carcinogenesis. *Lipids,* 14:155–158.
10. Carroll, K. K., and Khor, H. T. (1970): Effects of dietary fat and dose level of 7,12-dimethylbenz(a)anthracene on mammary tumor incidence in rats. *Cancer Res.,* 30:2260–2264.
11. Carroll, K. K., and Khor, H. T. (1971): Effect of level and type of dietary fat on incidence of mammary tumors induced in female Sprague–Dawley rats by 7,12-dimethylbenz(a)anthracene. *Lipids,* 6:415–420.
12. Carroll, K. K., and Khor, H. T. (1975): Dietary fat in relation to tumorigenesis. *Prog. Biochem. Pharmacol.,* 10:308–353.
13. Cassidy, M. M., Grund, B., Lightfoot, F., Vahouny, G., Gallo, L., Kritchevsky, D., Story, J., and Treadwell, C. (1978): Alterations in topographical ultrastructure of rat jejunum and colon induced by feeding with alfalfa and cholestyramine. *Fed. Proc.,* 37:543.
14. Chomchai, C., Bhadrachari, N., and Nigro, N. D. (1974): The effect of bile on the induction of experimental intestinal tumors in rats. *Dis. Colon Rectum,* 17:310–312.
15. Committee of Principal Investigators (1978): A cooperative trial in the primary prevention of ischemic heart disease using clofibrate. *Br. Heart J.,* 40:1069–1118.
16. Devesa, S. (1980): Trends in the incidence and mortality in the United States. *J. Environ. Pathol. Toxicol. (In press).*
17. Drasar, B. S., and Irving, D. (1973): Environmental factors and cancer of the colon and breast. *Br. J. Cancer,* 27:167–172.
18. Ederer, F., Leren, P., Turpeinen, O., and Frantz, I. D., Jr. (1971): Cancer among men on cholesterol-lowering diets: Experience from five clinical trials. *Lancet,* 2:203–206.
19. Enstrom, J. E. (1975): Colorectal cancer and consumption of beef and fat. *Br. J. Cancer,* 32:432–439.
20. Gortner, W. A. (1975): Nutrition in the United States, 1900 to 1974. *Cancer Res.,* 35:3246–3253.
21. Graham, S., and Mettlin, C. (1979): Diet and colon cancer. *Am. J. Epidemiol.,* 109:1–20.
22. Gregor, O., Toman, P., and Prušová, F. (1969): Gastrointestinal cancer and nutrition. *Gut,* 10:1031–1034.
23. Heiniger, H. J., Brunner, K. T., and Cerottini, J. C. (1978): Cholesterol is a critical cellular component for T-lymphocyte cytotoxicity. *Proc. Natl. Acad. Sci. USA,* 75:5683–5687.

24. Higginson, J. (1980): Multiplicity of factors involved in cancer patterns and trends. *J. Environ. Pathol. Toxicol. (In press).*
25. Hill, M. J. (1974): Colon cancer: A disease of fibre depletion or of dietary excess? *Digestion,* 11:289–306.
26. Hill, M. J., MacLennon, R., and Newcombe, K. (1979): Diet and large-bowel cancer in three socioeconomic groups in Hong Kong. *Lancet,* 1:436.
27. Hillyard, L. A., and Abraham, S. (1979): Effect of dietary polyunsaturated fatty acids on growth of mammary adenocarcinomas in mice and rats. *Cancer Res.,* 39:4430–4437.
28. Hopkins, G. J., and Carroll, K. K. (1979): Relationship between amount and type of dietary fat in promotion of mammary carcinogenesis induced by 7,12-dimethylbenz(a)anthracene. *J. Natl. Cancer Inst.,* 62:1009–1012.
29. Inbar, M., and Shinitzky, M. (1974): Increase of cholesterol level in the surface membrane of lymphoma cells and its inhibitory effect on ascites tumor development. *Proc. Natl. Acad. Sci. USA,* 71:2128–2130.
30. Inbar, M., and Shinitzky, M. (1974): Cholesterol as a bioregulator in the development and inhibition of leukemia. *Proc. Natl. Acad. Sci. USA,* 71:4229–4231.
31. Klurfeld, D. M., Allison, M. J., Gerszten, E., and Dalton, H. P. (1979): Alteration of host defenses paralleling cholesterol-induced atherogenesis. II. Immunologic studies of rabbits. *J. Med.,* 10:49–64.
32. Kritchevsky, D. (1976): Diet and atherosclerosis. *Am. J. Pathol.,* 84:615–632.
33. Lavik, P. S., and Baumann, C. A. (1941): Dietary fat and tumor formation. *Cancer Res.,* 1:181–187.
34. Lavik, P. S., and Baumann, C. A. (1943): Further studies on the tumor-promoting action of fat. *Cancer Res.,* 3:749–756.
35. Lea, A. J. (1966): Dietary factors associated with death-rates from certain neoplasms in man. *Lancet,* 2:332–333.
36. Leveille, G. A. (1975): Issues in human nutrition and their probable impact on foods of animal origin. *J. Anim. Sci.,* 41:723–727.
37. Liu, K., Stamler, J., Moss, D., Gorside, D., Persky, V., and Soltero, I. (1979): Dietary cholesterol, fat, and fibre, and colon cancer mortality. *Lancet,* 2:782–785.
38. Lyon, J. L., Klauber, M. R., Gardner, J. W., and Smart, C. R. (1976): Cancer incidence in Mormons and non-Mormons in Utah 1966–1970. *N. Engl. J. Med.,* 294:129–133.
39. Miettinen, M., Turpeinin, O., Karvonen, M. J., Elosus, R., and Paavilainin, E. (1972): Effect of cholesterol-lowering diet on mortality from coronary heart-disease and other causes. *Lancet,* 2:835–838.
40. Moskovitz, M., White, C., Barnett, R. N., Stevens, S., Russell, E., Vargo, D., and Floch, M. H. (1979): Diet, fecal bile acids, and neutral sterols in carcinoma of the colon. *Dig. Dis. Sci.,* 24:746–751.
41. Mower, H. F., Ray, R. M., Shoff, R., Stemmermann, G. N., Nomura, A., Glober, G. A., Kamiyama, S., Shimada, A., and Yamakawa, H. (1979): Fecal bile acids in two Japanese populations with different colon cancer risks. *Cancer Res.,* 39:328–331.
42. Narisawa, T., Magadia, N. E., Weisburger, J. H., and Wynder, E. (1974): Promoting effect of bile acids on colon carcinogenesis after intrarectal instillation of MNNG in rats. *J. Natl. Cancer Inst.,* 55:1093–1097.
43. Newberne, P. M. (1978): Diet and nutrition. *Bull. N.Y. Acad. Med.,* 54:385–396.
44. Newberne, P. M., Weigert, J., and Kula, N. (1979): Effects of dietary fat or hepatic mixed-function oxidases and hepatocellular carcinoma induced by aflatoxin $\beta_1$ in rats. *Cancer Res.,* 39:3986–3991.
45. Nigro, N. D., Bhadrachari, N., and Chomchai, C. (1973): A rat model for studying colonic cancer: Effect of cholestyramine on induced tumors. *Dis. Colon Rectum,* 16:438–443.
46. Nigro, N. D., Campbell, R. L., Singh, D. V., and Lin, Y. N. (1976): Effect of diet high in beef fat on the composition of fecal bile acids during intestinal carcinogenesis in the rat. *J. Natl. Cancer Inst.,* 57:883–888.
47. Nydegger, U. E., and Butler, R. E. (1972): Serum lipoprotein levels in patients with cancer. *Cancer Res.,* 32:1756–1760.
48. Pearce, M. L., and Dayton, S. (1971): Incidence of cancer in men on a diet high in polyunsaturated fat. *Lancet,* 1:464–467.

49. Phillips, R. L. (1975): Role of life-style and dietary habits in risk of cancer among Seventh-Day Adventists. *Cancer Res.,* 35:3513–3522.
50. Reddy, B. S. (1975): Role of bile metabolites in colon carcinogenesis. *Cancer,* 36:2401–2406.
51. Reddy, B. S. (1979): Nutrition and colon cancer. In: *Adv. Nutritional Res.,* 2:199–218, edited by H. H. Draper. Plenum Press, New York.
52. Reddy, B. S., Weisburger, J. H., and Wynder, E. L. (1974): Effects of dietary fat level and dimethylhydrazine on fecal acid and neutral sterol excretion and colon carcinogenesis in rats. *J. Natl. Cancer Inst.,* 52:507–511.
53. Rose, G., Blackburn, H., Keys, A., Taylor, H. L., Kannel, W. B., Paul, O., Reid, D. D., and Stamler, J. (1974): Colon cancer and blood-cholesterol. *Lancet,* 1:181–183.
54. Stavraky, K. M. (1976): The role of ecological analysis in the etiology of disease: A discussion with reference to large bowel cancer. *J. Chronic Dis.,* 29:435–444.
55. Tannenbaum, A. (1945): The dependence of tumor formation on the degree of caloric restriction. *Cancer Res.,* 5:609–615.
56. Watson, A. F., and Mellanby, E. (1930): Tar cancer in mice. II. The condition of the skin when modified by external treatment or diet, as a factor in influencing the cancerous reaction. *Br. J. Exp. Pathol.,* 11:311–322.
57. Wynder, E. L. (1976): Nutrition and cancer. *Fed. Proc.,* 35:1309–1315.
58. Wynder, E., Graham, S., and Eisenberg, H. (1966): Conference on the etiology of cancer in the gastro-intestinal tract: Report of the Research Committee, World Health Organization, on Gastroenterology, New York, N.Y., June 10–11, 1965. *Cancer,* 19:1561–1566.
59. Wynder, E. L., Hyams, L., and Shigematsu, T. (1967): Correlations of international cancer death rates: An epidemiological exercise. *Cancer,* 20:113–126.
60. Wynder, E. L., and Shigematsu, T. (1967): Environmental factors of cancer of the colon and rectum. *Cancer,* 20:1520–1561.

*Nutrition and Cancer: Etiology and Treatment,*
edited by G. R. Newell and N. M. Ellison.
Raven Press, New York © 1981.

# Fiber and Other Constituents of Vegetables in Cancer Epidemiology

## *Saxon Graham and **Curtis Mettlin

*Department of Social and Preventive Medicine, State University of New York at Buffalo,
Buffalo, New York 14261;
**Department of Cancer Control and Epidemiology, Roswell Park Memorial Institute,
Buffalo, New York 14263

It is likely that agents exogenous to an organism may either enhance or reduce the likelihood that it will develop disease. Such agents may gain access to the organism via the emotions, skin, or respiratory system, or alimentary tract. Thus, diet should figure importantly in studies of epidemiology, especially epidemiology of cancer at various sites. Many hypotheses link diet and cancer. Those that link the ingestion of meats or fats to increased risk of a variety of cancers, notably those of the colon and breast, are important. In this chapter, however, we shall concentrate on the relationships between vegetable substances and risk of cancer.

One hypothesis dealing with vegetables holds that ingestion of fiber reduces the risk of cancer of the colon. This may be the best known of the various hypotheses linking vegetable consumption to an alteration in cancer risk. A number of other hypotheses, mainly arising from studies of cell cultures and carcinogenesis in animals, link the various antioxidants, particularly vitamin C, to a reduced risk of cancer. Another class of nutrients that has been found in animal studies to reduce the risk of colon cancer includes compounds found in the cruciferous vegetables, such as cabbage, brussels sprouts, broccoli, and cauliflower. A few epidemiological studies of cancer patients and controls seem to corroborate this finding. Finally, researchers using both cell cultures and laboratory animals have noted a substantial inhibition of tumor growth in tissue challenged with known carcinogens and treated by vitamin A or synthetic retinols. Here again, a few epidemiological studies of diet in cancer patients and controls appear to corroborate the experimental findings.

Although there appears to be a growing mass of data linking various food substances to a reduced risk of a variety of cancers, and almost none linking vegetable substances to an enhanced risk, there are enough difficulties with the methods used in all the studies to make the findings less than fully convincing. Although corroborative findings have been reported, the methodology of the studies has enough potential for bias to make further substantial research necessary, not only on the hypotheses but, in some cases, on the methodology.

## METHODS OF STUDYING DIET

Researchers have used a number of methods to study diet. Chief among these methods have been international comparisons of disease rates and food consumption patterns, applications of information from animal studies, and comparisons of biological and interview materials from patients and controls. In the typical international comparison, the rates of consumption of various foods in different countries are related to death rates for relevant diseases. The authors of one such attempt (66) found that the greater the fat consumption in a country, the higher is the mortality from colon cancer (Fig. 1). The dangers in concluding from this that dietary fats cause colon cancer are many, and because the approach has been widely used, we need to evaluate it in some detail. In the case of fats and mortality from colon cancer, considerable error may be inherent in the diagnosis of the cause of mortality; indeed, for many of the countries studied, this error may completely account for the differences observed. For example, the low mortality from colon cancer in Chile, Portugal, and Italy may be related to the fact that this difficult-to-diagnose cancer tends to be underreported as a cause of death.

In addition, inferring rates of fat consumption by cancer patients from a national average may be faulty. There is good evidence that in the more industrialized nations, diet varies widely from individual to individual. It is obviously impossible to extrapolate from the millions of people who make up a national

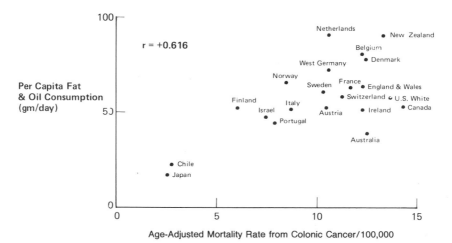

**FIG. 1.** From Graham, S., and Mettlin, C. (1979): Diet and colon cancer. *Am. J. Epidemiol.*, 109:1–20, with permission.

average to the comparative few who develop colon cancer. There are no data on the rate of fat consumption by colon cancer patients themselves. They may be very different from the average.

A variety of other factors could be correlated with mortality from colon cancer in an international comparison. Higginson (21) has shown that as industrialization increases, so do colon cancer rates. We could hypothesize with some confidence that high per capita consumption of starchy foods, refined carbohydrates, expensive garden vegetables, and aspirin, not to mention more telephones, cars, and refrigerators per capita, might also characterize nations with high colon cancer rates.

There are other anomalies in this approach. Although a rather high correlation may be indicated, exceptions are important. For example, although U.S. whites and Canadians have the same per capita fat and oil consumption as Finns, Israelis, Portuguese, and Italians, they have twice as high a rate of colon cancer. Enstrom (12) has illustrated the difficulty of using ecological data by showing the substantial increase in consumption of meats and fats over 40 years in the United States, during which time colon cancer incidence changed little. Similarly, he showed that the upper classes ingested more meats and fats without experiencing a concomitant higher risk of colon cancer.

We are interested in the traits of colon cancer patients specifically, not of the populations they come from. It appears that a much safer way of drawing inferences about the diets of persons with and without a given disease would be to study those individuals directly.

One way of doing this is to determine levels of ingestion of various nutrients from studies of blood, urine, feces, or other materials from patients and controls. On the basis of such findings, inferences might be drawn as to the kinds of diet that might produce the disease. Studies have shown a correlation between amounts of thiamine, riboflavin, and vitamin C ingested and their appearance in the urine and plasma, and leukocyte studies have been done on ingestion of vitamins E and A. However, as with all approaches in this difficult area, there are certain drawbacks. A patient's disease may substantially alter the way dietary factors are transformed in the alimentary system. Moreover, certain dietary components involved in current hypotheses of cancer etiology may be influenced by variations in individual metabolism and in other factors. For example, the microbial contents of and activity in the gut have been observed to vary with changes in psychological or physical stress, as well as with changes in diet (24,56). Similarly, although the level of serum cholesterol may be lowered by manipulating diet, the levels of serum cholesterol observed in a cross-sectional study may also be affected by such factors as psychological and physical stress, and may not faithfully reflect diet. Thus, although much more research is needed and may be quite useful, attempts to draw generalizations from findings in patients and controls may involve some error. Other drawbacks are the high cost of this approach and the difficulty in getting materials from enough subjects to perform adequate statistical, especially multivariate, analyses. On the other hand, as Reddy and Wynder showed (47), the method can supply useful data, and in spite of cost, it should be applied to large numbers of patients and controls.

Attempts to generalize from animal to human diseases are also fraught with difficulty. Studies of animals have been useful, but in many instances conclusions drawn on the basis of such studies do not hold up when applied to humans. Although DDT may be carcinogenic in animals, it has not been shown to be so in humans. Numerous animal studies have indicated that saccharine is associated with cancer, but a number of epidemiological studies of human bladder cancer patients and controls indicate no risk associated with the use of nonnutritive sweeteners (27,39,52). Two studies do find a risk, but strangely only for males (25). No one has been able to produce cancer in animals with alcohol, but five large epidemiologic interview studies have linked alcohol to oral cancer in humans (15,26,32,51,65). Although animal and vegetable fats have been shown to produce colon cancer in rodents, only three epidemiologic interview studies have shown this effect in humans (3,8,17). Many others have not, and the negative epidemiologic results suggest that further study is needed. Although we can determine the potential pathogenicity of various factors from studies of animals, it would seem prudent, before drawing conclusions regarding human disease causation, to determine whether evidence on human epidemiology corroborates findings from animal studies.

When we are dealing with something as complex as diet, particularly in the developed nations, it appears that one logical and inexpensive method would be to ask people what they eat. The prime difficulty is the possibility of misrecollection of amounts and frequencies of eating various foods. However, social intercourse, indeed, the whole structure of society, is based on verbal communication. The interview method is relatively cheap and fast, can be used to study many parameters at once, and can be applied to the large numbers of people necessary for statistical testing of hypotheses. No other method has these properties, and if we are to test the many dietary hypotheses now before us, we must consider this method along with the others. It appears that an assessment of the nature, sources, and seriousness of error in the diet interview or questionnaire should be undertaken before the method is discarded out of hand. A small body of research on this subject has accumulated, but a great deal more needs to be done.

Approaches to ascertaining individuals' diets are many; they include asking individuals what their usual diet is (for example, what they usually eat for dinner). In a developed society, however, diet is so varied from meal to meal that this method is relatively ineffective. Another approach is to ask respondents to keep a diary. The lack of enthusiasm for this task exhibited by most laymen selects in unknown ways those who will respond. Moreover, there is evidence that diet diaries underestimate intake, and the act of keeping the record may itself affect the amounts and types of food eaten.

A variation on the "usual diet" method is to obtain the subject's estimate of his usual frequency, per day, week, or month, of ingesting specific foods. This may be used in combination with asking about all foods eaten in the previous 24 hours.

A number of studies of the reliability of the food frequency method have been conducted on small numbers of subjects. Those by Dawber and co-workers (10) and Reshef and Epstein (49) compared the quantities of calories, carbohydrates, protein, and the like, estimated from diet interviews carried out on two occasions. Nutrients were determined by multiplying the frequency of eating by the amount of nutrients in an average serving. In a much larger study, Nomura and co-workers (43) determined the frequency with which specific items of food were eaten by subjects reinterviewed after six months and two years. In this study, the percentage of subjects agreeing with their original estimates ranged from 78% to 97% for the six-month group and from 63% to 95% for the two-year group.

Some years ago, we (17) compared frequencies reported by 99 patients interviewed 18 months apart and found an average of 89% in agreement on the two interviews. In the largest and most definitive study published to date, Morgan and colleagues (40) asked 400 persons to report the amounts of and frequencies with which a series of food items were usually consumed during the preceding two months and for the two months six months before that. In addition, the subjects were asked to list everything they had eaten during the 24 hours immediately prior to the interview. Finally, each was asked to maintain a diary over the four days following the interview. The investigators found a low correlation between the 24-hour recall, the diet diary, and the food-frequency history. For frequency of eating fat, they found a Pearsonian correlation of 0.92 between the histories recorded six months apart. High correlations were also found for other nutrients.

In our western New York interview study of diet and cancer, we are comparing all colon cancer patients with neighborhood controls in the three most populous counties. We have used a variety of quality-control procedures, including the diet diary, the 24-hour recall, the reinterview of subjects, and the comparison of spouses' reports of subjects' frequencies of ingesting various foods. Our findings, reported by Marshall (31), like those of Kolonel and co-workers in a similar study (28), indicate levels of spouse agreement on frequency of food ingestion consistent with those found in the studies described above. It is interesting that we and Kolonel and co-workers found similar degrees of agreement on the possibly sensitive subject of alcohol ingestion, as well as on cigarettes smoked. Although error in reports of cigarette smoking has, to our knowledge, not been much studied, there very likely is some; our study and that of Kolonel et al. suggest that cigarette data are no more accurate than food-frequency data. However, such interview and questionnaire data on smoking frequency were in large part responsible for establishing the relationship between cigarette smoking and lung cancer.

Of course, a comparison of spouses' estimates of the frequency with which a given item is eaten, like a reinterview with an individual, does not reveal the accuracy of the report. Nevertheless, the studies of Jain and co-workers suggest that the truth lies near the two estimates provided. In the study by Hankin et al. (19), subjects were visited in their homes and instructed how to weigh foods and use forms on which each item ingested at each meal for one week was to be recorded. Later, subjects were interviewed about their frequency of ingesting various foods during the period they had kept the records. A comparison of the records with the frequencies obtained on the interviews indicated substantial agreement, ranging from 80% to 100%. Jain and Miller conducted a study of similar design with comparable results (Jain, *personal communication*).

In an English study (2), entries on a seven-day diet diary kept by individuals in the British National Food Survey were compared with estimates derived from 63 Cambridgeshire housewives who were instructed by a nutritionist how to weigh and record everything ingested and who were later visited several times to check on the accuracy of their weighing. Total dietary fiber per person was 19.9 grams per day for the group of housewives, as compared with 19.7 grams per day in the National Food Survey. Jensen and MacLennan (Jensen, *personal communication*) attempted to assess the reliability and validity of interview estimates of nutrients ingested in Finland and Denmark for a study of colon cancer patients. A nutritionist instructed participants in weighing foods eaten in a four-day period. Duplicate portions of foods eaten by subjects were collected for chemical analysis, and nitrogen analysis of 24-hour urine samples was used to estimate protein intake. They have yet to report their results.

James Marshall (31) has assessed the degree to which various levels of error in interview reports could mask an actual relative risk or find a relative risk when in fact there is none. It is well known that the existence of error randomly distributed between patients and controls provides an estimate of relative risk smaller than that which actually exists. This has been known for some time for four-fold tables and, as Marshall's study indicates, it holds also in the $2 \times 3$ or $2 \times 4$ tables needed for assessing whether risk increases with exposure. Given the amount of error that the reliability and validity studies cited above suggest may exist (about 10% to 20%), it is possible that actual relative risks of around 1.5 might be masked. Larger ones, however, would still be identified. To produce the appearance of a risk when there is none, the error would have to be much larger than we suspect exists, and distributed differently in patients and controls. Errors of 30% or more involving overreporting among patients or underreporting among controls would be required. These studies suggest that the kinds of error we encounter in interview investigations of frequency of ingestion of foods may not seriously limit their use in epidemiology investigations.

Although these few studies give us some confidence in inquiries about the current diets of patients and controls, many methodological problems in diet interview studies remain. In investigating diseases with a long latency, we must know the extent to which recall of diet prior to the onset of symptoms may reflect diet 15 to 20 years earlier. We also need to know such basic things as the extent to which diet changes throughout life, not only with fluctuations in price or availability, but also with changes in the life-cycle, such as marriage, divorce, widowhood, and lessening of physical exercise. One study of those issues is under way. Michel Ibrahim of the University of North Carolina has conducted diet interviews of subjects first interviewed 15 years earlier *(personal communication)*. This is enabling him to determine changes that occur over time and the extent to which estimates obtained in a recent interview correlate with diet reported some years earlier.

In the absence of opportunities such as Ibrahim's, respondents are being asked to recall changes in diet throughout life in current studies. The error in this type of recall may be large. Essentially, all of the findings in studies of diet and diseases of long latency are predicated on stability of diet throughout life, and we now have little evidence that such stability exists. It is possible, however, that lifetime diet patterns are set at a young age, that there is enough consistency in individuals' dietary patterns throughout life, and that diets recalled for periods before onset of symptoms are similar enough to those 20 years earlier to distinguish large groups of patients from controls.

Thus, although there are a number of drawbacks to the various methods of study, numerous findings in tests of the various hypotheses of etiology have accumulated, some replicated and some not, some congruent with findings in other fields and some not. These are reviewed and evaluated below.

## THE FIBER HYPOTHESIS

Dietary fiber derives from cell walls of all parts of the plant, including the leaves, stem, root, and seeds. It is that part of plant material that resists digestion by the human gastrointestinal system. Although studies have frequently concentrated on crude fiber, this represents only a small proportion of the total fiber ingested. Crude fiber is the residue of plant material left after treatment with boiling sulfuric acid, sodium hydroxide, water, alcohol, and ether, and it consists mainly of cellulose and lignin. Dietary fiber, on the other hand, consists not only of the above-mentioned compounds, but also of hemicellulosic and noncellulosic polysaccharides, various starches, waxes, and a small amount of protein. Bingham and co-workers (2) feel that estimates of crude fiber provide totally inadequate estimates of relevant fiber, and that dietary fiber is not fully appreciated as a factor in the etiology of disease.

The fiber hypothesis for the etiology of colon cancer is based on a simple and logical-sounding theory, which maintains that high-fiber foods take less time to pass through the gut. This reduced time presumably reduces the opportunity for bacteria in the bowel to produce carcinogens and for carcinogens to work on the gut wall. In addition, a high-fiber diet increases total bulk, so any carcinogenic materials passing through do so in a more dilute form. Eastwood et al. (11) and Burkitt et al. (6) furnished some evidence for a dilution effect.

However, there is disagreement in the literature on many of these points. No one has come up with unequivocal evidence that high fiber content in the diet always shortens transit time. Some researchers have found that fiber speeds transit time, others that it has no effect, and still others, such as Harvey et al. (20), that transit time is shortened in those with originally long transit times, extended in those with short times, and affected not at all in those with moderate times.

A few studies on the effects of dietary fiber on experimentally induced colon cancer in animals have produced equivocal results. Some show a reduction in tumor incidence upon administration of fiber, some no effect, and some an enhanced incidence. Fleiszer et al. (13) found that a diet containing 28% by weight of bran reduced the incidence of colonic tumors induced by dimethylhydrazine (DMH). Ward et al. (57) studied the effect of cellulose in the diet of rats exposed to the colon carcinogen azomethane. Contrary to the hypothesis, more colon tumors were observed in rats receiving the fiber supplementation. However, some reduction in the incidence of tumors of the small intestine was observed. Similarly, Asp et al. (1) supplemented the diets of rats challenged with DMH with wheat bran, carrot fiber, or citrus pectin. The incidence of colon tumors observed in the citrus pectin-supplemented group was higher than in controls. No protective effects were observed with wheat bran or carrot fiber. Wilson et al. (63) studied DMH-induced colon tumors in rats fed diets with or without wheat bran. They found no significant difference in the percentage of rats with malignant tumors of the colon, but the incidence of nonmalignant lesions was higher in the low-fiber group. Cruse et al. (8) compared groups of DMH-treated rats given diets containing 4.8% fiber, 20% bran, or no fiber. At the conclusion of the experiment, no differences in the incidence of colon carcinoma were observed among the experimental and control groups.

Although animal studies to date lend little support to the fiber hypothesis, it may be that chemically induced cancer in rats does not resemble the natural history of the disease in humans. Virtually all animals in the experiments evidenced some form of neoplasia within a short time. Because of lower levels of challenge from the carcinogenic stimuli usually present in human carcinogenesis, fiber may have effects that could not be detected in these experiments.

On the epidemiologic level, there have been few studies. Burkitt and Trowell (5) studied the relationship between fiber and transit times in English and African boarding-school boys. They found the Africans ate more fiber and had shorter transit times and less colon cancer. In later studies of occupational groups in England and Africa, their findings were similar. Note that the authors did not study cancer patients and controls, but merely generalized from entire societies to the few who develop colon cancer. In a similar study, Glober et al. (14) studied transit time using the Hinton method, by which 23 Caucasian and 63 Japanese males swallowed barium-impregnated plastic pellets and the time until the appearance of the pellets in the stool was measured. Although Japanese living in Hawaii have rates of colon cancer similar to those of Caucasian Hawaiians, their average transit time was found to be significantly less than that of the Caucasians.

One epidemiologic study that suggests a low risk of colon cancer for individuals who frequently eat fibrous foods is that by Modan et al. (38) on populations in Israel. The authors compared 198 colon cancer patients with age- and sex-matched hospitalized patients with other diseases and healthy neighbors. The researchers found that the only foods of which the cancer patients ate less than both sets of controls were those containing at least 0.5% fiber. In San Francisco, Dales et al. (9) studied the reported dietary habits of 99 black colorectal cancer patients and 280 matched controls. Colon cancer patients were found to report less frequent consumption of meats and foods with at least 0.5% crude fiber content than controls, but the difference was not statistically significant. It is interesting, however, that individuals with a high-fat, low-fiber diet had a risk 2.68 times that of those with a low-fat, high-fiber diet (P < .05). Bjelke (3), in studies of 259 cancer patients and 1,659 controls in Minnesota and 162 patients and 1,394 controls in Norway, found that colon cancer patients reported less frequent consumption of both vegetables and fibrous foods.

MacLennan and Jensen (30) furnish indirect evidence that consumption of fiber may reduce the risk of colon cancer. They examined the diets of individuals from Copenhagen, Denmark, and Finland. These two groups were of interest because Danes have a high incidence of colon cancer and Finns a low incidence. The authors found that the two populations ingest similar amounts of fats, but Finns eat substantially more fiber. Reddy et al. (46) found something similar in their comparison of residents of Kuopio, Finland, and New York City. The New Yorkers had a substantially higher incidence of colon cancer than the Finns and ate similar amounts of fat and substantially less fiber.

Some other studies fail to support the link between vegetables or fibrous foods and colon cancer. Higginson (21), in 1966, reported no difference between the dietary habits of U.S. colon cancer patients and controls, and Haenszel et al. (18) found no risk reduction for vegetables or crude fiber consumption in their study of 179 Japanese-Hawaiian patients and 357 controls. In fact, in that study one fibrous food, string beans, was found to be associated with an increased risk of colon cancer, even when possibly related food habits were controlled for.

In short, some findings support the fiber hypothesis on the etiology of colon cancer, but few of those are uncontradicted. There seems little doubt that fiber increases fecal bulk, possibly diluting carcinogens carried in the stool. Evidence on the effect of dietary fiber on stool transit time is equivocal. Data from studies of the effect of fiber on chemically induced colon cancer in rodents are inconsistent. It is evident from previous research, as well, that fiber obtained from different sources has different effects. This may account for some of the inconsistencies in research findings in animal studies and in studies of stool transit time in humans. Even when findings do suggest a protective effect for dietary fiber, additional research is needed to clarify the role of fiber vis-à-vis other nutritional qualities of foods rich in fiber. Fruits and vegetables not only contribute fiber to the diet, but account for nearly all the typical person's intake of vitamin C, two-thirds of the vitamin A, and substantial amounts of vitamin E, and contain numerous chemicals having antioxidant or other potential cancer-inhibiting properties.

## VITAMIN C

The attribution of a protective effect from fruit and vegetable consumption to the vitamin C that these foods may contain stems mainly from evidence that formation of carcinogenic nitrosamines can be inhibited by vitamin C (37). Such evidence comes from both *in vitro* and *in vivo* studies, and Weisburger (62) reasons that, since gastric cancer is less common in populations consuming large amounts of lettuce, green vegetables, and other sources of vitamin C, a simple way to inhibit carcinogenesis is year-round consumption of foods containing vitamin C.

Other hypotheses involving vitamin C as an inhibitor of carcinogenesis have been studied. Pipkin et al. (45) reported inhibition of 3-hydroxyanthranilic acid-induced bladder tumors in mice by ascorbic acid supplementation of drinking water. Wattenberg (59) found no evidence of tumor suppression in benz(a)pyrene-induced tumors of the mouse forestomach, whereas Migliozzi (36) found that tumor growth was dependent on the presence of vitamin C in the diet of guinea pigs and that a low vitamin C diet favored tumor growth.

Few actual epidemiological data identify vitamin C as the specific factor in fruit and vegetable consumption that accounts for risk reduction. Bjelke (3), in the aforementioned studies in Norway and the United States, found that gastric cancer patients reported lower intake of vitamin C, as measured by an index multiplying the vitamin C content of various foods by the frequency of their consumption. Sorenson and Lyon (54), in an unpublished report based on extensive dietary interviews with 300 colon cancer patients and 600 age-matched controls, found that the controls reported significantly higher usual intake of vitamin C than the cancer patients.

Since vitamin C is found in a great many vegetables, as are fiber and vitamin A, inquiries into a relationship of cancer with vitamin C may not have discriminated vitamin C sufficiently from other constituents of these vegetables, such as fiber or vitamin A or E. Further in-depth studies of diet are necessary to provide the large amounts of data necessary to develop indices distinguishing among vitamins A, C, and E, fiber, and other constituents of possible value.

In this chapter, we are primarily concerned with fiber and vitamins A, C, and E; the most important sources of these are shown in Table 1. This table sets forth the amounts of the nutrients in specific foods, but there is also interest in identifying those foods that contribute the largest amounts of the vitamins we are concerned with to the diet of average individuals. The amount of a given vitamin that a particular food contributes to the diet is a function of

TABLE 1. Foods containing largest amounts of indicated nutrients, in order of amount per 100-gram helping

| Vitamin A[a] (International units) | Vitamin C[a] (mg) | Vitamin E[b] (mg) | Dietary fiber[c] (g) | Fats[a] (g) |
|---|---|---|---|---|
| Liver (lamb, beef, calf, turkey, hog, chicken) (34,220) | Hot red chili pepper, raw (369) | Cottonseed oil (43.6) | All-Bran cereal (Kellogg's) (26.7) | Butter (81.0) |
| Hot red chili pepper, raw (21,600) | Hot green chili pepper, raw (235) | Walnuts (22.0) | Dried fruits (apricots, figs, prunes, peaches, dates), raw (16.3), cooked (8.2) | Mayonnaise (79.9) |
| Dandelion greens, raw (14,000), cooked (11,700) | Sweet red pepper, raw (204) | Almonds (15.0) | Puffed Wheat cereal (Quaker) (15.4) | Nuts (macadamia, pecans, Brazil, hazel, walnuts, almonds, cashews) (61.6) |
| Carrots, raw (11,000), cooked (10,500) | Currants, raw (200) | Olive oil (14.4) | Almonds (14.3) | Salad dressing (French, Italian, Blue Cheese, Russian, Thousand Island, Mayonnaise-type) (52.1) |
| Dried apricots, uncooked (10,900) | Kale, leaves only, raw (186), cooked (93) | Wheat germ, crude, commercially milled (13.5) | Coconuts (13.6) | Bacon (52.0) |
| Hot chili sauce, canned (9,590) | Parsley, raw (172) | Margarine (12.5) | Shredded Wheat cereal (Nabisco) (12.3) | Peanuts, peanut butter (49.1) |
| Kale, leaves only, raw (10,000), cooked (8,300) | Collards, leaves only, raw (152), cooked (76) | Soy bean oil (12.1) | Potato chips (11.9) | Capicola (cold cuts) (45.8) |
| Parsley, raw (8,500) | Turnip greens, raw (139), cooked (69) | Mayonnaise (11.9) | Crispbread, rye (Ryvita) (11.7) | Pork sausage, cooked (39.9) |
| Spinach, raw (8,100), cooked (8,100) | Sweet green pepper, raw (128), cooked (96) | Italian salad dressing (9.1) | Cornflake cereal (Kellogg's) (11.0) | Potato chips (39.8) |
| Sweet potato, cooked (7,900) | Broccoli, raw (113), cooked (90) | Cabbage, raw (7.8), cooked (7.6) | Parsley, raw (9.1) | Dried salami (38.1) |
| Liverwurst (6,530) | Puffed corn breakfast cereal, fruit flavored, added nutrients (106) | Peanuts, peanut butter (6.6) | Brazil nuts (9.0) | Cream cheese (37.7) |
| Pumpkin, canned (6,400) | Brussels sprouts, raw (102), cooked (87) | Collards, leaves only, cooked (5.9) | Wholemeal bread (8.5) | Heavy cream (37.6) |
| Greens (collards, turnip, beet, mustard, watercress), raw (6,980), cooked (6,250) | Mustard greens, raw (97) | Salad dressing, mayonnaise-type (5.3) | Currants, black and red, raw (8.5), cooked (7.2) | Goose, cooked (36.0) |
| | Pimiento, canned, solids and liquid (95) | Cashews (5.1) | Peanuts, peanut butter (7.9) | Greek-style olives, salt-cured, oil-coated (35.8) |
| | Cauliflower, raw (78) | Cream (4.9) | Raspberries, raw (7.4), cooked (7.8) | Chocolate (35.7) |
| | | Popcorn (4.4) | Blackberries, raw (7.3), cooked (6.3) | Deviled ham, canned (32.3) |
| | | Potato chips (4.3) | | Cheddar cheese (32.2) |
| | | Spinach, raw (2.9) | | |
| | | Summer squash, cooked (2.4) | | |
| | | Vegetable fat (2.3) | | |

TABLE 1. (Continued)

| Vitamin A[a] (International units) | Vitamin C[a] (mg) | Vitamin E[b] (mg) | Dietary fiber[c] (g) | Fats[a] (g) |
|---|---|---|---|---|
| Chicken giblets (5,760) | Persimmon, raw (66) | | Baked beans, canned in to- mato sause (7.3) | Beef, cooked (31.6) |
| Sweet red pepper, raw (4,450) | Red cabbage, raw (61) | | Grapenuts cereal (General Foods) (7.0) | Light cream (31.3) |
| Winter squash, cooked (3,500) | Strawberries, raw (59) | | Raisins (6.8) | Egg yolks (30.6) |
| Cantaloupe (3,400) | Papaya, raw (56) | | Spinach, cooked (6.3) | |
| Egg yolk (3,400) | Chives, raw (56) | | | |
| Endive (3,300) | | | | |
| Butter, margarine (3,300) | | | | |

[a] B. K. Watt and A. L. Merrill, Composition of Foods, Raw, Processed, Prepared. Agricultural Handbook No. 8. United States Department of Agriculture, Washington, D.C., 1963.
[b] J. Pennington, Dietary Nutrient Guide. AVI Publishing Company, Westport, Conn., 1976.
[c] A. A. Paul and D. A. T. Southgate, McCance and Widdowson's Composition of Foods. Her Majesty's Stationery Office, London, England, 1978.

the amount of the vitamin that is contained in the food times the frequency with which the food is eaten (Table 2). This table lists those foods most highly correlated in multiple correlation analyses with various levels of an index of total nutrients for each of 282 individuals in western New York State. For each individual in the survey, the total intake from all foods of the nutrients in question was calculated. Listed in Table 2, in order of their importance, are the individual foods that were most highly correlated, in terms of frequency of ingestion times amount of the vitamin contained per serving of food.

## VITAMIN A

Several laboratory investigations, both animal and *in vitro* studies, have shown tumor inhibition by vitamin A in its various forms. Saffiotti et al. (50) treated Syrian golden hamsters with a series of intratracheal instillations of the carcinogen benzo(a)pyrene. Half of the animals were then fed 5 mg of vitamin A palmitate in corn oil by stomach tube twice weekly. The vitamin A group developed markedly fewer respiratory tumors, particularly squamous tumors, and a reduction in squamous metaplasia (Table 3). A lower incidence of tumors at nonrespiratory sites were also observed. Chu and Malmgren (5) inhibited the induction of squamous cell carcinomas of the hamster uterine cervix by dimethylbenz(a)anthracene (DMBA) with vitamin A palmitate supplementation of the diet. In a related study, Nettesheim and Williams (41) demonstrated inhibition of metaplastic lung nodules by all-transretinyl acetate in rats with no symptoms of vitamin deficiency and adequate liver stores of vitamin A challenged by 3-methylcholanthrane.

Sporn and co-workers (55) have observed that the toxicity inherent in naturally occurring vitamin A may limit its potential as an antineoplastic agent. They and others have investigated the effectiveness of various synthetic retinoids that may effectively inhibit carcinogenesis without tending to concentrate in tissue at toxic levels. Newberne and Suphakarn (42), for example, report enhanced inhibition of DMH-induced colon tumors by one of the synthetic retinoids, 13-*cis* retinoic acid, even when diets of control animals are amply supplemented by retinyl acetate (Table 4). Merriman and Bertram (33) observed similar inhibitory properties of 13-*cis* retinoic acid *in vitro*. In their study of 3-methylcholanthrane-induced neoplastic transformations in cultured mouse fibroblasts, they were able to inhibit cell transformation dramatically by administering retinyl acetate up to three weeks after the initial treatment with the carcinogen.

Several epidemiologic case-control interview studies corroborate these experimental findings. In Japan, green and yellow vegetable consumption accounts for an average 44% and 23% of the typical dietary intake of vitamins A and C, respectively. Hirayama (23), in a 10-year prospective study of 256,118 Japanese adults, found associations between frequency of green and yellow vegetable consumption and rates of mortality from cancer of different sites. Figure 2 shows that lung cancer death rates for male and female smokers and nonsmokers

TABLE 2. Association of frequency of eating various foods with indices of total consumption of different nutrients [a]

| Vitamin A | Vitamin C | Vitamin E | Dietary fiber | Fats |
|---|---|---|---|---|
| Liver (.327) | Grapefruit (.175) | Peanuts (.244) | Peaches (.186) | Pork chops (.244) |
| Greens (.531) | Greens (.310) | Greens (.412) | Peas (.333) | Doughnuts, pastry (.359) |
| Carrots (.597) | Orange, grapefruit juice (.427) | Other nuts (.498) | Baked beans (.408) | Hot dogs (.427) |
| Brussels sprouts (.637) | Tomatoes (.507) | Pineapples (.548) | Greens (.468) | Ham other than canned (.472) |
| Peas (.667) | Rice (.562) | Macaroni (.593) | Cookies (.520) | Peanuts (.515) |
| Tomatoes (.691) | Tangerines, oranges (.601) | Tomatoes (.630) | Apricots (.559) | Salami (.547) |
| Apricots (.699) | Brussels sprouts (.636) | Pies (.665) | Tomatoes (.592) | Milk (.583) |
| Spinach (.720) | Peas (.668) | Spinach (.693) | Potatoes (.624) | Canned ham (.612) |
| Hot dogs (.730) | Sausage (.690) | Potatoes (.714) | Pork chops (.652) | Candy (.635) |
| Hot peppers (.739) | Potatoes (.705) | Apples (.732) | Apples (.671) | Pineapples (.656) |
| Eggplant (.747) | Spaghetti (.715) | Baked beans (.745) | Corn (.682) | Potatoes (.677) |
| Pies (.752) | Tomato juice (.725) | Red cabbage (.757) | Pies (.692) | Baked beans (.693) |
| Smoked, dried meats (.758) | Hot peppers (.734) | Salami (.766) | Macaroni (.700) | Sausage (.706) |
| Bacon (.764) | Apricots (.743) | Summer squash (.774) | Milk (.709) | Meat spreads (.716) |
| Salami (.770) | Green peppers (.752) | Doughnuts, pastry (.781) | Pineapples (.717) | Cookies (.726) |
| Cucumbers (.775) | Kale (.758) | Apricots (.786) | Orange, grapefruit juice (.724) | Spaghetti (.734) |
| Green beans (.779) | Pineapples (.768) | Cucumbers (.791) | lemons, limes (.731) | Rice (.741) |
| Tangerines, oranges (.783) | Cucumbers (.775) | Canned ham (.796) | Berries (.737) | Liverwurst, other cold cuts (.748) |
| Onions (.786) | Eggplant (.781) | Cookies (.801) | Nonwhite bread (.741) | Hamburger (.754) |
| | Salami (.786) | Hot peppers (.806) | White bread (.750) | Lima beans (7.60) |

[a] Cumulative percents of variation explained in order of contribution (multiple $R^2$).

TABLE 3. *Effects of vitamin A on benzo(a)pyrene-induced tumors*[a]

| | | Animals with | | | | | |
|---|---|---|---|---|---|---|---|
| | Effective no. of animals at risk[b] | Respiratory tumors (all types) | | Squamous changes | | Squamous tumors | |
| Treatment | | No. | (%) | No. | (%) | No. | (%) |
| BP only | 53 | 17 | (32) | 18 | (34) | 11 | (21) |
| BP + vitamin A | 46 | 5 | (11) | 2 | (4) | 1 | (2) |

[a] From Saffiotti et al., ref. 50, with permission.
[b] Survivors at time of first respiratory tumor (33 weeks), less animals lost through cannibalism.

TABLE 4. *Effects of 13-cis retinoic acid on DMH-induced tumors in the rat*[a]

| Treatment | No. of animals at risk | No. with colon tumors | Percent with tumors | Average no. tumors/animal |
|---|---|---|---|---|
| 3 $\mu$g retinyl acetate/g | 20 | 20 | 100 | 3.1 |
| 3 $\mu$g retinyl acetate + 67 $\mu$g/g 13-*cis* retinoic acid | 20 | 8 | 40 | 2.3 |

[a] From Newberne and Suphakarn, ref. 42, with permission.

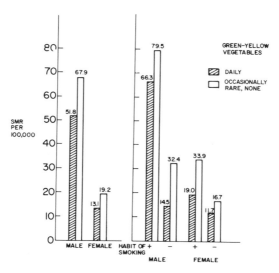

**FIG. 2.** Standardized mortality rate for lung cancer by sex, by smoking habit, and by habit of green-yellow vegetables intake. From Hirayama, T. (1979): Epidemiological evaluation of the role of naturally occurring carcinogens and modulators of carcinogenesis, edited by E. C. Miller et al., p. 359, University Park Press, Baltimore.

were elevated for those who, in 1965, reported infrequent green and yellow vegetable consumption. Age- and smoking-adjusted prostatic cancer mortality rates were also found to be higher among those who had previously reported infrequent eating of green and yellow vegetables.

Bjelke (4) surveyed the dietary habits of more than 8,000 Norwegian men and observed the incidence of lung cancer among them five years later. He found consumption of vitamin A to be negatively associated with lung cancer incidence at all levels of cigarette smoking. The lung cancer incidence among persons having high levels of vitamin A intake was 38% that of persons who reported low levels of intake. Comparable reductions in risk have been observed in retrospective studies in Singapore, where a lower risk of lung cancer was observed for Chinese women who reported frequent consumption of green leafy vegetables, which are typically rich in vitamins A and C (29).

In our study of 292 male lung cancer and 801 control patients at Roswell Park Memorial Institute (35), we found significant risk reduction associated with increased amounts of dietary vitamin A. In Table 5, the inverse dose–response relationship between vitamin A intake and risk of disease is evident. Risk reduction was also specifically associated with frequent consumption of carrots and milk. The effect of vitamin A on the risk of lung cancer was found to be similar in persons from different social classes and geographic areas (urban versus rural) and, most importantly, with degrees of smoking. The effect was particularly marked in heavy smokers, but was also observed in light smokers. A similar risk reduction with carrot and milk consumption and overall vitamin A intake was found in a study of 569 patients with bladder cancer and 1,025 age- and sex-matched controls (34). Bladder cancer risk has been found to be enhanced by increased ingestion of coffee, as well as by cigarette smoking. Because milk is an important component on the vitamin A index, and because individuals who drink coffee drink less milk, we felt it necessary to examine

TABLE 5. *Estimated vitamin A intake and risk of lung cancer*[a]

| Level of vitamin A intake[b] (1000 IU) | Relative risk by number of cigarettes smoked | | |
|---|---|---|---|
| | ≤ Pack/day (176 patients, 600 controls) | > Pack/day (98 patients, 122 controls) | Smoking-adjusted (274 patients, 722 controls) |
| < 25 | 1.9[c] | 3.8[c] | 2.4[c] |
| 25–49 | 2.3[c] | 2.5[c] | 2.4[c] |
| 50–74 | 1.8 | 1.8 | 1.8 |
| 75–99 | 2.1[c] | 1.0 | 1.7 |
| 100–124 | 1.9 | 1.5 | 1.7 |
| 125–150 | 2.1[c] | .8 | 1.5 |
| > 150 | 1.0 | 1.0 | 1.0 |

[a] From Mettlin et al., ref. 35, with permission.
[b] Weighted index of monthly consumption of 23 vitamin A-containing edibles.
[c] Differs from 1.0, $P < .05$.

the vitamin A relationship for individuals who drink large and small amounts of coffee. The risk reduction associated with vitamin A was observed in both groups. Similarly, bladder cancer risk has long been recognized to be raised by increasing cigarette smoking. Here again, when we examined the effects of increased ingestion of vitamin A, we found the risk of bladder cancer to be reduced for heavy and light smokers, as well as for nonsmokers.

The effect of vitamin A obtained from regular use of preparations such as multivitamin tablets was studied by Smith and Jick (53) in 800 patients with cancer at various sites and 3,333 controls. Among males, a two-fold reduction in risk was found to be associated with taking such tablets. This finding is comparable to those in the other investigations we have described. Curiously, the authors found no effect among women, perhaps because most of the cancers in men involved the squamous epithelium (lung cancer) and those in women were glandular (breast cancer).

We conclude that, although a few *in vitro, in vivo,* and human case-control studies have produced congruent findings, much work must be done to corroborate those findings.

## CRUCIFEROUS VEGETABLES

We have noted already that Bjelke (4), in a prospective study, found cancer risk inversely related to ingestion of foods containing vitamin A. This was also true in the case-control studies (3) conducted in Minnesota and Norway. As shown in Table 6, Bjelke found less frequent consumption by colorectal cancer patients of vegetables in general and, in Minnesota, of cabbage in particular. At about the same time Bjelke was doing this epidemiologic work, Wattenberg (58) was studying aryl hydrocarbon hydroxylase (AHH) activity in various organs of rodents. Evidence had accumulated that such activity occurs in tissues of all the major portals, including the gastrointestinal tract, lung, and skin. This activity could represent an initial metabolic barrier to noxious chemicals

TABLE 6. *Relative risk of colorectal cancer by intake of vegetables in Norway and U.S.A.*[a]

| | Value of vegetables index | Retrospective | | Prospective | |
|---|---|---|---|---|---|
| | | No. of patients | Relative risk[b] | No. of patients[c] | Relative risk[d] |
| Norway | < 30 | 101 | 1.00 | 29 | 1.00 |
| | ≥ 30 | 177 | 0.72 | 14 | 1.18 |
| U.S.A. | < 30 | 98 | 1.00 | 21 | 1.00 |
| | ≥ 30 | 275 | 0.74 | 28 | 0.67 |

[a] From Bjelke, ref. 3, with permission.
[b] Adjusted for sex.
[c] For U.S.A., number of deaths.
[d] Adjusted for age, based on males only.

in the external environment. Mice and rats that are starved or fed purified diets show weak AHH activity in the intestines and lungs. However, as shown in Table 7, a number of cruciferous plants, including brussels sprouts, cabbage, turnips, cauliflower, and broccoli, increase this activity. Benzopyrene (BP) hydroxylase activity in the small intestine of rats was considerably enhanced among those whose diets contained 25% ground brussels sprouts, cabbage, turnips, and broccoli (58).

Wattenberg and Loub (60) determined that the inducers in these vegetables are indoles. They wished to determine whether those compounds inhibit carcinogenesis by polycyclic hydrocarbons. Table 8 shows the results of their experiments on the effects of indoles on DMBA-induced mammary tumor formation. When no indoles were added to the diet, 91% of the rats developed tumors, with an average of 1.45 tumors per rat. When indole 3-carbinol and diindolylmethane were added to the diet, the proportion of animals with tumors dropped 21% to 27% and the mean numbers of tumors dropped to 0.4. Table 9 shows the results of two experiments in which benzpyrene-induced gastric tumors were substantially reduced in mice receiving a diet containing indole 3-acetonitrile. In the second experiment, the BP dose was only one-third as large and was given over eight weeks, instead of four. All the animals so challenged developed tumors, but when the indole was added, only 44% developed tumors. The mean number of tumors per animal dropped from 7 to 1. It would appear that Wattenberg and Loub have identified chemicals in cabbage, cauliflower, turnips, broccoli, and brussels sprouts that can reduce the number of tumors that ordinarily appear when animals are challenged by DMBA and BP. They have also inhibited tumor formation in animals simply by feeding them these vegetables, raw or cooked.

TABLE 7. *Effect of vegetables on the benzo(a)pyrene hydroxylase activity of the small intestine* [a]

| Additions to purified diet [b] | Diet intake (g/day) | Benzo(a)pyrene hydroxylase activity (units/mg wet weight) [c] |
|---|---|---|
| Brussels sprouts | 11 | 23.8 ± 2.0 |
| Cabbage | 12 | 11.6 ± 0.7 |
| Turnips (greens) | 12 | 5.4 ± 0.2 |
| Broccoli | 10 | 3.5 ± 1.4 |
| Cauliflower | 11 | 1.0 ± 0.0 |
| Alfalfa | 13 | 2.6 ± 0.3 |
| Spinach | 9 | 0.6 ± 0.1 |
| Lettuce | 12 | 0 |
| Artichokes | 11 | 0 |
| None | 13 | 0.1 ± 0.1 |

[a] From Wattenberg, ref. 58, with permission.
[b] Rats were fed the diets for 7 days, 4 rats per group except for last group, which contained 20.
[c] Mean ± S.D.

TABLE 8. *Effects of indoles on DMBA-induced mammary tumor formation* [a]

| Experiment | Material administered [b] | Dose (mmole) | Route of indole administration | No. of rats at risk | Weight gain (g) [c] | Percentage of rats with tumors at 21 weeks | Tumors per rat, mean ± S.D. |
|---|---|---|---|---|---|---|---|
| 1 | DMSO-solvent control | — | By oral intubation | 11 | 138 | 91 | 1.45 ± 0.28 |
|   | Indole-3-carbinol | 0.10 | | 14 | 146 | 21 [e] | 0.29 ± 0.16 [e] |
|   | 3,3'-Diindolylmethane | 0.05 | | 11 | 139 | 27 [e] | 0.36 ± 0.20 [e] |
|   | Indole-3-acetonitrile | 0.10 | | 11 | 145 | 73 | 1.55 ± 0.46 |
| 2 | DMSO-solvent control | — | By oral intubation | 10 | 149 | 60 | 0.90 ± 0.28 |
|   | Indole-3-carbinol | 0.10 | | 14 | 142 | 14 [d] | 0.21 ± 0.16 [d] |
|   | 3,3'-Diindolylmethane | 0.05 | | 14 | 175 | 36 | 0.57 ± 0.25 |
|   | Indole-3-acetonitrile | 0.10 | | 14 | 175 | 50 | 0.86 ± 0.29 |
| 3 | DMSO-solvent control | — | By oral intubation | 14 | 149 | 64 | 1.00 ± 0.28 |
|   | Indole-3-carbinol | 0.10 | | 14 | 147 | 21 [d] | 0.21 ± 0.11 [d] |
|   | Indole-3-acetaldehyde | 0.10 | | 14 | 125 | 36 | 0.43 ± 0.17 |
|   | Indole-3-acetaldehyde oxime | 0.10 | | 16 | 107 | 19 [d] | 0.19 ± 0.10 [d] |
| 4 | None | — | Addition to diet | 15 | 169 | 73 | 1.20 ± 0.30 |
|   | Indole-3-carbinol | 0.014/g of diet | | 15 | 178 | 20 [e] | 0.33 ± 0.19 [d] |
|   | Indole-3-acetonitrile | 0.030/g of diet | | 16 | 173 | 54 | 1.00 ± 0.39 |

[a] From Wattenberg and Loub, ref. 60, with permission.
[b] Female Sprague–Dawley rats 7 weeks of age were given, by oral intubation, a single dose of the indicated indole in 1 ml DMSO or 1 ml DMSO only 20 hours prior to administration of 12 mg of DMBA in 1 ml olive oil, also by oral intubation. In experiment 4 the indoles were added to the diet, which was administered for 8 days prior to administration of 12 mg DMBA by oral intubation.
[c] From 7 to 28 weeks of age for experiments 1–3 and from 6 to 28 weeks of age for experiment 4.
[d] P < 0.05.
[e] P < 0.01.

TABLE 9. Effects of indoles on BP-induced gastric tumor formation[a]

| Experiment | Additions to the diet[b] | Carcinogen and dose schedule[c] | No. of mice at risk | Diet intake (g/day) | Age at death (wks) | Wt. gain (g)[d] | Percentage of mice with tumors | Tumors per mouse (mean ± S.D.) |
|---|---|---|---|---|---|---|---|---|
| 1 | None | BP 1 mg by oral intubation 2×/week × 4 weeks | 39 | 4.2 | 31 | 5.9 | 93 | 5.0 ± 0.54 |
| | Indole-3-carbinol 0.03 mmole/g | | 20 | 4.2 | 31 | 6.6 | 80 | 1.9 ± 0.35[e] |
| | 3,3'-Diindolylmethane 0.02 mmole/g | | 18 | 4.2 | 31 | 7.8 | 94 | 3.2 ± 0.51[f] |
| | Indole-3-acetonitrile 0.03 mmole/g | | 19 | 4.1 | 31 | 6.4 | 68 | 1.6[c] ± 0.43[e] |
| 2 | None | BP 0.3 mg by oral intubation 3×/week × 8 weeks | 33 | 3.1 | 41 | 20.2 | 100 | 7.1 ± 0.64 |
| | Indole-3-acetonitrile 0.03 mmole/g | | 18 | 2.8 | 41 | 15.8 | 44[e] | 1.1 ± 0.33[e] |
| 3 | None | None | 19 | 3.5 | 41 | 19.4 | 0 | 0 |
| | 3,3'-Diindolylmethane 0.02 mmole/g | | 17 | 3.3 | 41 | 20.2 | 0 | 0 |
| | Indole-3-carbinol 0.03 mmole/g | | 20 | 2.8 | 41 | 18.2 | 0 | 0 |
| | Indole-3-acetonitrile 0.03 mmole/g | | 18 | 3.5 | 41 | 21.9 | 0 | 0 |

[a] From Wattenberg and Loub, ref. 60, with permission.
[b] Female ICR/Ha mice were fed a semipurified diet, Normal Protein Test Diet (ICN Pharmaceuticals, Cleveland), containing the indicated indole, starting at 63 days of age and continuing until 98 days of age in experiment 1 or 126 days of age in experiments 2 and 3.
[c] The initial dose of carcinogen was given 8 days after the start of the experimental diets.
[d] Weight gain from 8 weeks of age to 31 weeks of age in experiment 1 and 41 weeks of age in experiments 2 and 3.
[e] P < 0.01.
[f] P < 0.05.

In an epidemiologic study carried out with a rather primitive instrument on a series of 257 patients and 783 controls from Roswell Park Memorial Institute (16), we produced results quite similar to those of Wattenberg. We found a lower risk of colon cancer for individuals ingesting cabbage, broccoli, and brussels sprouts in particular, and vegetables in general. Table 10 lists the monthly frequency with which colon cancer patients and controls reported they ate vegetables that they usually consumed raw. The possibilities included cole slaw, tomatoes, red cabbage, lettuce, cucumbers, and carrots. Note that, although there is only a low probability that most of the differences occurred by chance, the relative risks and the differences in frequencies are small. On the other hand, risk does increase with decreases in the frequency of eating vegetables. When we looked at monthly frequencies of ingesting any of the 19 vegetables included in our study, we again found an increased risk with decreases in amounts ingested (Table 11).

An item-by-item analysis of each vegetable produced some interesting results. As Table 12 indicates, a decreasing frequency of eating cabbage is associated with an increased risk for cancer of the colon. There is a suggestion of a dose-response relationship and larger case-control differences than observed before. A similar dose–response relationship was encountered in analyses of ingestion of two other forms of cabbage, sauerkraut and cole slaw, as well as the related vegetables brussels sprouts and broccoli.

Our finding of a decreased risk of colon cancer for humans eating vegetables seems to parallel Wattenberg's finding in animals. Some results of the few previ-

TABLE 10. *Reported monthly frequencies of eating vegetables, usually raw, by colon cancer patients and controls[a]*

| Monthly frequency | Patients (N = 193) | Controls (N = 627) | Relative risk | P |
|---|---|---|---|---|
| 21+ | 23.8% | 34.0% | 1.00 | – |
| 11–20 | 23.3% | 23.1% | 1.44 | .06 |
| 0–10 | 52.9% | 42.9% | 1.75 | .002 |

[a]From Graham et al., ref. 16, with permission.

TABLE 11. *Reported monthly frequencies of eating 19 vegetables by colon cancer patients and controls[a]*

| Monthly frequency | Patients (N = 183) | Controls (N = 627) | Relative risk | P |
|---|---|---|---|---|
| 61+ | 25.7% | 31.4% | 1.00 | – |
| 41–60 | 39.3% | 40.1% | 1.20 | .19 |
| 21–40 | 27.9% | 24.4% | 1.40 | .07 |
| 0–20 | 7.1% | 4.1% | 2.12 | .02 |

[a]From Graham et al., ref. 16, with permission.

TABLE 12. *Reported frequencies of ingesting cabbage by colon cancer patients and controls* [a]

| Frequency | Patients (N = 195) | Controls (N = 625) | Relative risk | P |
|---|---|---|---|---|
| At least once a week | 8.7% | 19.7% | 1.00 | – |
| Once every 2–3 weeks | 14.9% | 18.9% | 1.78 | .04 |
| Once a month | 27.1% | 20.2% | 3.04 | .0001 |
| Less than once a month | 26.7% | 24.1% | 2.49 | .001 |
| Never | 22.6% | 17.1% | 2.98 | .0003 |

[a] From Graham et al., ref. 16, with permission.

ous epidemiologic studies on the role of vegetables in colon cancer also seem consistent with this finding. The discovery by Modan et al. (38) of a lower risk with a higher ingestion of fiber may implicate not only fiber, but other constituents of vegetables as well. Indeed, those authors found that cancer patients consumed cabbage significantly less frequently than did controls, and a similar directional difference was found for other cruciferous vegetables, such as kohlrabi, sauerkraut, turnips, and cauliflower. Bjelke's findings for vegetables in general and cabbage in particular are also congruent (3). The evidence that Seventh-Day Adventists, who abstain from meat, are at a low risk of colon cancer (44) may as reasonably suggest that vegetables are associated with low risk as that meat promotes high risk.

On the other hand, Haenszel et al. (18) and Higginson (21) specifically examined risk associated with various vegetables and found no interesting relationships with colon cancer. Furthermore, the relative risks of colon cancer associated with rarely eating vegetables observed in our research reach only to the level of 2 for vegetables in general and to the level of 3 for cabbage. This finding of higher risk was borne out for several cruciferous vegetables and supported Wattenberg's findings. Nevertheless, systematic error may have entered into the study. For example, because of abdominal distress, patients may have stopped eating vegetables to avoid symptoms. However, our interviewers continually emphasized our interest in eating habits during the year prior to the appearance of discomfort. Moreover, such discomfort occurs infrequently prior to the diagnosis of colon cancer, so it is likely that few recent changes in eating habits were made. We are reluctant to extrapolate findings from animal studies, such as Wattenberg's, to humans, without confirmation in human epidemiologic research, but it may be that more sophisticated inquiries will furnish that confirmation. The congruence of Wattenberg's results with epidemiologic results suggests the need for further interview and animal studies on the relation between colon cancer and vegetables, especially the cruciferae.

The logic of the approaches of Wynder (64), Hill (22), Weisburger (61), and Reddy and Wynder (48), as well as many of their findings, suggests the importance of continuing investigations into the relationship between meat and colon cancer. That a carefully controlled study by Haenszel et al. (18) revealed a dose–response relationship between beef ingestion and risk of colon cancer in a low-risk population suggests that similar studies are necessary. As Wynder suggests, other epidemiologic studies may have discovered no relationship because everyone in the societies studied had at least moderate exposure to meat and because above a certain threshold no dose–response is visible. Studying a low-risk population, with less exposure to meat, may provide detailed information about dose response associated with low levels of meat ingestion, such as those encountered by Haenszel and co-workers. However, a still unpublished study by Haenszel *(personal communication)* found no relationship between colon cancer and meat among Japanese, although reduction in risk was found with an increase in the amount of cabbage eaten.

The findings regarding meat and vegetables are not necessarily contradictory. Indeed, they may be complementary. In the future, a positive relationship between meat and colon cancer may be confirmed, together with a negative relationship between cruciferous vegetables and colon cancer. Meat ingestion could promote a high risk, with the vegetables inducing activity in the gut that protects against carcinogenesis. The same model might be proposed for meat and fiber, as Reddy et al. suggest in their study on Finns (46). Those authors found that Finns (with a low incidence of colon cancer) and New Yorkers (with a high incidence) eat about the same amounts of meat, but the Finns eat more vegetables. MacLennan and co-workers (29) reported similar findings when they compared Finns (low risk) with Danes (high risk). Most recently, Dales et al. (9) found no significant relation between either animal fats or fiber and colon cancer in a small study of blacks in San Francisco. However, they did find that blacks with a high-fat, low-fiber diet had a substantially higher risk than blacks with a low-fat, high-fiber diet.

## SUMMARY

Fiber and other constituents of vegetables have been hypothesized to be related to risk of cancer at a number of sites. It is unique in studies of etiology that these constituents almost always reduce risk. It is not unique that, in spite of their potential value, they have been studied relatively little. Almost no definitive research has been done on the theory that is best known and most widely accepted, that ingestion of fiber is related to reduced risk of cancer of the large bowel. Animal studies of fiber are equivocal, with some showing that fiber increases risk, others showing that it reduces risk, and still others that it affects risk not at all. The evidence for the theory that fiber shortens transit time in humans is equally equivocal. However, there is little doubt that fiber increases fecal bulk and therefore may dilute potential carcinogens.

Case-control interview studies have been conducted to examine the effects of fiber, vitamins, and individual vegetables without reference to nutrient content. One case-control interview study showed that fiber significantly reduced risk for cancer of the large intestine; two others have furnished evidence that is congruent but others have not. Several studies have shown a reduced risk for colon, stomach, bladder, and lung cancer associated with diets containing large amounts of green and yellow vegetables. In the case of gastric cancer, this could be related to the vitamin C content of these vegetables, but there is a paucity of good epidemiologic evidence on this matter. Animal studies show tumor inhibition with ingestion of cruciferous vegetables and the indoles found in them, and two or three interview studies provide corroborative data for colon cancer, but not cancer of other sites. Finally, *in vivo, in vitro,* and interview studies show the risk of human lung, larynx, and bladder cancer is reduced with vitamin A and synthetic retinols. More experimental research has probably been done on the retinols and cancer than on any other constituent of vegetables, and the results are uniformly consistent, but the body of case-control epidemiologic work is primarily distinguished by its unimpressive size.

More *in vivo, in vitro,* and interview studies are obviously called for. Many more studies on the effect of the cruciferous vegetables, the retinols, other vitamins, and fiber on humans are needed to confirm their association with the tumors studied to date (colon, lung, bladder, and stomach) and to discover any relationships they may have with cancer at other sites. Inquiries to date suggest that these approaches may help uncover relations with factors that may reduce the risk of human cancer.

## ACKNOWLEDGMENT

This study was supported by Public Health Service Grant CA-11535 from the National Cancer Institute.

## REFERENCES

1. Asp, N., Bauer, H., Dahlquist, A., Fredhind, P., and Oste, R. (1979): Dietary fibre and experimental colon cancer in the rat. *Nutr. Cancer,* 1:70–73.
2. Bingham, S., Cummings, J. H., and McNeil, N. I. (1979): Intakes and sources of dietary fibre in the British population *(unpublished manuscript).*
3. Bjelke, E. (1973): Epidemiologic studies of cancer of the stomach, colon and rectum, with special emphasis on the role of diet. *Thesis,* University of Minnesota. University Microfilms, Ann Arbor.
4. Bjelke, E. (1975): Dietary vitamin A and human lung cancer. *Int. J. Cancer,* 15:561–565.
5. Burkitt, D. P., and Trowell, H. C. (1975): *Refined Carbohydrate Foods and Disease.* Academic Press, London.
6. Burkitt, D. P., Walker, A. R., and Painter, N. S. (1972): Effect of dietary fibre on stools and transit-times, and its role in the causation of diseases. *Lancet,* 2:1408–1412.
7. Chu, S. W., and Malmgren, R. A. (1965): An inhibitory effect of vitamin A on the induction of tumors of the forestomach and cervix in the Syrian hamster by carcinogenic polycyclic hydrocarbons. *Cancer Res.,* 25:884–895.
8. Cruse, J. P., Lewin, M. R., and Clark, C. G. (1978): Failure of bran to protect against experimental colon cancer in rats. *Lancet,* 2:1278–1279.
9. Dales, L. G., Friedman, G. D., Ury, H. K., Grossman, S., and Williams, S. R. (1978): A case-control study of relationships of diet and other traits to colorectal cancer in blacks. *Am. J. Epidemiol.,* 109:132–144.

10. Dawber, T. R., Pearson, G., Anderson, P., Mann, G. V., Kannel, W. B., Shurtleff, D., and McNamara, P. (1962): Dietary assessment in the epidemiologic study of coronary heart disease: The Framingham Study. II. Reliability of measurement. *Am. J. Clin. Nutr.,* 11:226–233.
11. Eastwood, M. A., Kirkpatrick, J. R., Mitchell, W. D., Bone, A., and Hamilton, T. (1973): Effects of dietary supplements of wheat bran and cellulose on faeces and bowel function. *Br. Med. J.,* 4:392–394.
12. Enstrom, J. E. (1975): Colorectal cancer and consumption of beef and fat. *Br. J. Cancer,* 32:432–439.
13. Fleiszer, D., Murray, D., MacFarlane, J., and Brown, R. A. (1978): Protective effect of dietary fibre against chemically induced bowel tumors in rats. *Lancet,* 1:552–553.
14. Glober, G. A., Klein, K. L., Moore, J. O., and Abba, B. C. (1974): Bowel transit-times in two populations experiencing similar colon-cancer risks. *Lancet,* 2:80–81.
15. Graham, S., Dayal, H., Rohrer, T., Swanson, M., Sultz, H., Shedd, D., and Fischman, S. (1977): Dentition, diet, tobacco, and alcohol in the epidemiology of oral cancer. *J. Natl. Cancer Inst.,* 59:1611–1618.
16. Graham, S., Dayal, H., Swanson, M., Mittelman, A., and Wilkinson, G. (1978): Diet in the epidemiology of cancer of the colon and rectum. *J. Natl. Cancer Inst.,* 61:709–714.
17. Graham, S., Lilienfeld, A. M., and Tidings, J. E. (1967): Dietary and purgation factors in the epidemiology of gastric cancer. *Cancer,* 20:2224–2234.
18. Haenszel, W., Berg, J. W., Segi, M., Kurihara, M., and Locke, F. B. (1973): Large-bowel cancer in Hawaiian Japanese. *J. Natl. Cancer Inst.,* 51:1765–1779.
19. Hankin, J. H., Rhoads, G. G., and Globe, G. (1975): A dietary method for an epidemiologic study of gastrointestinal cancer. *Am. J. Clin. Nutr.,* 28:1055–1061.
20. Harvey, R. F., Pomare, E. W., and Heaton, K. W. (1973): Effects of increased dietary fibre on intestinal transit. *Lancet,* 1:1278–1280.
21. Higginson, J. (1966): Etiological factors in gastrointestinal cancer in man. *J. Natl. Cancer Inst.,* 37:527–545.
22. Hill, M. J. (1975): Metabolic epidemiology of dietary factors in large bowel cancer. *Cancer Res.,* 35:3398–3402.
23. Hirayama, T. (1979): Diet and cancer. *Nutr. Cancer,* 1:67–81.
24. Holdeman, L. V., Good, I. J., and Moore, W. E. (1976): Human fecal flora: Variation in bacterial composition within individuals and possible effect of emotional stress. *Appl. Environ. Microbiol.,* 31:359–375.
25. Howe, G. R., Burch, J. D., Miller, A. B., Morrison, B., Gordon, P., Weldon, L., Chambers, L. W., Fodor, G., and Winsor, G. M. (1977): Artificial sweeteners and human bladder cancer. *Lancet,* 2:578–581.
26. Keller, A. (1967): Cirrhosis of the liver, alcoholism, and heavy smoking associated with cancer of the mouth and pharynx. *Cancer,* 20:1015–1022.
27. Kessler, I., and Clark, J. P. (1978): Saccharin, cyclamate and human bladder cancer. *J.A.M.A.,* 240:349–355.
28. Kolonel, N., Hirohata, T., and Nomura, A. (1977): Adequacy of survey data collection from substitute respondents. *Am. J. Epidemiol.,* 106:476–484.
29. MacLennan, R., DaCosta, J., Day, N. E., Law, C. H., Ng, Y. K., and Shanmugaratnam, K. (1977): Risk factors for lung cancer in Singapore Chinese, a population with high female incidence rates. *Int. J. Cancer,* 20:854–860.
30. MacLennan, R., and Jensen, O. M. (1977): Dietary fibre, transit-time, faecal bacteria, steroids, and colon cancer in two Scandinavian populations. *Lancet,* 2:207–211.
31. Marshall, J. (1979): *Verification by spouses of reported dietary behavior.* Paper presented at the Twelfth Annual Meeting of the Society for Epidemiologic Research, New Haven, Conn., June 13, 1979.
32. Martinez, I. (1969): Factors associated with cancer of the esophagus, mouth, and pharynx, in Puerto Rico. *J. Natl. Cancer Inst.,* 42:1069–1094.
33. Merriman, R., and Bertram, J. (1979): Reversible inhibition by retinoids of 3-methylcholan-threne-induced neoplastic transformation in c3L/10T½/2/8 cells. *Cancer Res.,* 39:1661–1666.
34. Mettlin, C., and Graham, S. (1979): Dietary risk factors in human bladder cancer. *Am. J. Epidemiol.,* 110:255–263.
35. Mettlin, C., Graham, S., and Swanson, M. (1979): Vitamin A and lung cancer. *J. Natl. Cancer Inst.,* 62:1435–1438.

36. Migliozzi, J. A. (1977): Effect of ascorbic acid on tumor growth. *Br. J. Cancer,* 35:448–453.
37. Mirvish, S. S. (1975): Blocking the formation of N-nitroso compounds with ascorbic acid in vitro and in vivo. *Ann. N.Y. Acad. Sci.,* 258:175–180.
38. Modan, B., Barell, V., Lubin, F., Modan, M., Greenberg, R. A., and Graham, S. (1975): Low-fiber intake as an etiologic factor in cancer of the colon. *J. Natl. Cancer Inst.,* 55:15–18.
39. Morgan, R. W., and Jain, M. G. (1974): Bladder cancer: Smoking beverages and artificial sweeteners. *Can. Med. Assoc. J.,* 111:1067–1070.
40. Morgan, R. W., Jain, M., Miller, A. B., Choi, N. W., Matthews, V., Munan, L., Burch, J. D., Feather, J., Howe, G. R., and Kelley, A. (1978): A comparison of dietary methods in epidemiologic studies. *Am. J. Epidemiol.,* 107:488–498.
41. Nettesheim, P., and Williams, M. L. (1976): The influence of vitamin A on the susceptibility of the rat lung to 3-methylcholanthrene. *Int. J. Cancer,* 17:351–357.
42. Newberne, P. M., and Suphakarn, V. (1977): Preventive role of vitamin A in colon carcinogenesis in rats. *Cancer,* 40:2553–2556.
43. Nomura, A., Hankin, J. H., and Rhoads, G. G. (1976): The reproducibility of dietary intake data in a prospective study of gastrointestinal cancer. *Am. J. Clin. Nutr.,* 29:1432–1436.
44. Phillips, R. L. (1975): Role of life-style and dietary habits in risk of cancer among Seventh-Day Adventists. *Cancer Res.,* 35:3513–3522.
45. Pipkin, G. F., Schlegel, J. U., Nishimura, R., and Schultz, G. N. (1969): Inhibitory effect of L-ascorbate on tumor formation on urinary bladders implanted with 3-hydroxyanthranilic acid. *Proc. Soc. Exp. Biol. Med.,* 131:522–524.
46. Reddy, B. S., Hedges, A., Laakso, K., and Wynder, E. L. (1978): Fecal constituents of a high-risk North American and a low-risk Finnish population for the development of large bowel cancer. *Cancer Lett.,* 4:217–222.
47. Reddy, B. S., and Wynder, E. L. (1973): Large bowel carcinogenesis: Fecal constituents of population with diverse incidence rates of colon cancer. *J. Natl. Cancer Inst.,* 50:1437–1442.
48. Reddy, B. S., and Wynder, E. L. (1977): Metabolic epidemiology of colon cancer: Fecal bile acids and neutral sterols in colon cancer patients and patients with adenomatous polyps. *Cancer,* 39:2533–2539.
49. Reshef, A., and Epstein, L. M. (1972): Reliability of a dietary questionnaire. *Am. J. Clin. Nutr.,* 25:91–95.
50. Saffiotti, U., Montesano, R., Sellakumar, A. R., and Boorg, S. A. (1964): Experimental cancer of the lung. *Cancer,* 20:857–864.
51. Schwartz, D., Lellouch, J., Flamant, R., and Denoix, P. F. (1962): Alcool et cancer: Resultats d'une enquete retrospective. *Rev. Franc. Etudes Clin. Biol.,* 7:590–604.
52. Simon, D., Yen, S., and Cole, P. (1975): Coffee drinking and cancer of the lower urinary tract. *J. Natl. Cancer Inst.,* 54:587–591.
53. Smith, P. G., and Jick, H. (1978): Cancers among users of preparations containing vitamin A. *Cancer,* 42:808–811.
54. Sorenson, A., and Lyon, L. (1979): *A case-control study of diet and cancer.* Paper presented at the Twelfth Annual Meeting of the Society for Epidemiologic Research, New Haven, Conn., June 13, 1979.
55. Sporn, M. B., Dunlop, N. M., Newton, D. L., and Smith, J. M. (1979): Prevention of chemical carcinogenesis by vitamin A and its synthetic analogs (retinoids). *Fed. Proc.,* 35:1332–1338.
56. Tannock, G. W., and Savage, C. (1974): Influences of diet and environmental stress on microbial populations in the murine gastrointestinal tract. *Infect. Immun.,* 9:591–598.
57. Ward, J. M., Yamanoto, R. S., and Weisburger, J. H. (1973): Cellulose dietary bulk and azoxy-methane-induced intestinal cancer. *J. Natl. Cancer Inst.,* 51:713–715.
58. Wattenberg, L. W. (1971): Studies of polycyclic hydrocarbon hydroxylases of the intestine possibly related to cancer. *Cancer,* 28:99–102.
59. Wattenberg, L. W. (1979): Inhibitors of carcinogenesis. In: *Carcinogens: Identification and Mechanisms of Action,* edited by A. C. Griffin and C. R. Shaw, pp. 299–316. Raven Press, New York.
60. Wattenberg, L. W., and Loub, W. D. (1978): Inhibition of polycyclic aromatic hydrocarbon induced neoplasia by naturally occurring indoles. *Cancer Res.,* 38:1410–1413.
61. Weisburger, J. H. (1975): Large bowel cancer: Metabolic epidemiology and carcinogenesis. *Cancer,* 36:2385–2386.
62. Weisburger, J. H. (1977): Vitamin C and prevention of nitrosamine formation. *Lancet,* 2:607.

63. Wilson, R. B., Hutcheson, D. P., and Wideman, L. (1977): Dimethylhydrazine-induced colon tumors in rats fed diets containing beef fat or corn oil with and without wheat bran. *Am. J. Clin. Nutr.,* 30:176–181.
64. Wynder, E. L. (1975): The epidemiology of large bowel cancer. *Cancer Res.,* 35:3388–3394.
65. Wynder, E. L., and Bross, I. R. (1957): Aetiological factors in mouth cancer: An approach to its prevention. *Br. Med. J.,* 1:1137–1143.
66. Wynder, E. L., Graham, S., and Eisenberg, H. (1966): Conference on the etiology of cancer in the gastro-intestinal tract: Report of the Research Committee, World Health Organization, on Gastroenterology, New York, New York, June 10–11, 1965. *Cancer,* 19:1561–1566.

*Nutrition and Cancer: Etiology and Treatment,*
edited by G. R. Newell and N. M. Ellison.
Raven Press, New York © 1981.

# Vitamin A, Retinoids, and Cancer

## Paul M. Newberne and Adrianne E. Rogers

*Department of Nutrition and Food Science, Massachusetts Institute of Technology,
Cambridge, Massachusetts 02139*

Vitamin A and related compounds can retard or inhibit tumor development and cause tumor regression under certain conditions (59). This discovery, based on studies in many laboratories, represents one of the most exciting areas in cancer research because it holds the promise of developing effective methods for tumor prevention and of increasing our understanding of mechanisms of carcinogenesis. Vitamin A alcohol (retinol), acid (retinoic acid) (Fig. 1), esters and ethers of the alcohol, and numerous synthetic analogues of the acid, a class of compounds referred to as retinoids, have prophylactic or therapeutic activity against spontaneous and chemically induced cancers of some target organs (37,61). The naturally occurring forms of vitamin A are not sufficiently effective or are too toxic to be useful, but synthetic compounds closely related to them are proving effective and less toxic in experimental animals. One exception to the generalization about toxicity of naturally occurring forms of vitamin A is a recently isolated, naturally occurring metabolite of vitamin A, 5,6-epoxy-retinoic acid, which may prove to be effective in nontoxic doses (41).

Vitamin A is essential to the differentiation and maintenance of several epithelial and other tissues, an observation first made more than 50 years ago (72,73). Wolbach and Howe observed replacement of the normal columnar and transitional epithelium by squamous, frequently keratinizing, epithelial cells in several tissues in vitamin A-deficient rats. They noted that in the epithelium of the urinary bladder, ureter, and renal pelvis, the original epithelium was replaced by keratinizing epithelium that developed from underlying nests of cells. The authors described the rapid growth of the epithelium, with increased mitotic figures in all epithelial layers. In the bladder, ureter, and renal pelvis, downgrowth and vascularization of the epithelium was observed. The authors concluded that "The behavior indicates growth power suggestive of neoplastic potentiality." The early studies of Wolbach and Howe have been confirmed many times, but it has been unequivocally shown that, in contrast to true neoplasia, the changes associated with vitamin A deficiency are fully reversible by ingestion of a diet containing enough vitamin A (75). In support of the suggestion of neoplastic change in epithelia of deficient animals, evidence has been presented

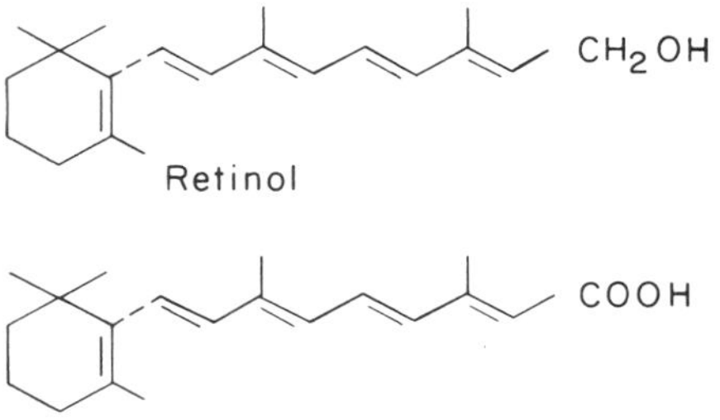

Retinol

Retinoic Acid (all trans)

**FIG. 1.** Structural formulas for retinol and retinoic acid.

that mucous membranes of vitamin A-deficient rats may have heightened suscep-tibility to chemical carcinogenesis (6,61).

The past several years have seen a significant increase in research related to vitamin A, its analogues, and how these may relate to the prevention of some forms of cancer. These studies have followed lines of investigation involving *in vivo* and *in vitro* experimental systems and epidemiologic approaches. Each line will be discussed separately, with specific examples provided where appropri-ate. Before describing these investigations, a brief note on vitamin A metabolism is necessary.

## METABOLISM OF VITAMIN A

Ingested vitamin A is absorbed through the intestinal epithelium, transported to the liver, and stored as esters of retinol. It is released into the blood bound to a specific transport protein, retinol-binding protein (RBP), which complexes with prealbumin (48). The complex of retinol–RBP–prealbumin delivers retinol to target cells, where uptake appears to depend on specific membrane receptors for the complex (30). Only retinol, not the transport protein, is taken into the cell. A small part of a physiological dose of retinol is oxidized to retinoic acid (21). Recent work has suggested that both retinol and retinoic acid are active forms of the vitamin but are not interchangeable in function, and that each has a specific intracellular binding protein that mediates its activity (15).

Vitamin A activity of natural or synthetic compounds can be assayed *in vivo* by measurement of growth, reproduction, and organ weight, evaluation of vision, and histologic assessment of epithelial differentiation. *In vitro* assays have been developed that are more convenient, highly sensitive, and do not require binding to serum RBP. Trachea and prostate organ cultures have been the most useful for *in vitro* assay methods (61).

The demonstration of specific cellular receptors has suggested to some that there are similarities in activity between vitamin A and steroid hormones (50). A small protein that binds retinol specifically is found in most tissues and, in particular, in all vitamin A-responsive tissues examined (2,3). The binding pro-tein, termed cellular retinol binding protein (CRBP), has been shown to bind all-trans retinol, the natural isomer, and to be distinctly different from the transport protein in the serum (15). Evidence has been compiled that substantiates the assumption that CRBP mediates the action of retinol in normal tissues (44,47). CRBP is depleted of vitamin A in the deficiency state, but the level of the binding protein does not change. In normal animal tissues, such as lung and testis, the protein is 50% to 70% saturated with retinol. CRBP permits specific binding of retinol to nuclei; the number of binding sites is greater in nuclei from vitamin A-deficient animals than from control animals. When depleted animals are resupplemented, nuclei show a decrease in binding sites in as little as two hours (63). CRBP has been purified to homogeneity from rat liver and testis and from bovine retina (45,46,52,55).

Tissues also contain a small protein that specifically binds retinoic acid and certain synthetic derivatives of it (44). This cellular retinoic acid binding protein (CRABP) has been reported in a number of animal tissues, including chick embryo skin, bovine eye epithelium, and transformed mammalian cells (16, 54,70). The identification of a separate binding protein for retinoic acid supports the view that retinoic acid acts as a physiological compound separate from retinol. The protein has now been purified to homogeneity (46,55,57). The distribution of CRABP in rat tissue is different from the distribution of CRBP (44).

CRBP and CRABP are present in all fetal tissues that have been examined. CRBP is maintained in all tissues except muscle as animals mature, but CRABP falls to undetectable levels in most tissues, including lung, liver, and kidney. It is maintained, however, in testis, uterus, ovary, eye, and brain. The perinatal development of the two vitamin A-binding proteins appears to be different for each protein and organ, suggesting that requirements for retinol and retinoic acid change during the development of each organ and on into advanced age (45). The binding specificity of CRABP for several analogues of retinoic acid correlates well with the activity of the analogues in maintaining differentiation of epithelial cells in culture, as evaluated in either of two systems (Table 1) (14,59). This supports the view that CRABP mediates the ability of retinoic acid and its analogues to reverse metaplasia and promote normal growth.

TABLE 1. *CRABP binding capacity and physiological effects of retinoic acid and its analogues*

| Chemical | Growth promotion (percent increase in DNA) | Percent binding inhibition | Metaplasia reversal |
|---|---|---|---|
| Furyl analogue | 1 | 34 | ± |
| Pyridyl analogue | 9 | 22 | ± |
| Phenyl analogue | 23 | 42 | ± |
| DACP analogue | 54 | 100 | +++ |
| TMMP analogue | 65 | 100 | +++ |
| All-transretinoic acid | 46 | 100 | +++ |

Adapted from Chytil and Ong, ref. 6, and Sporn, ref. 60.

## VITAMIN A BINDING IN TUMORS

The finding of the two binding proteins for retinol and retinoic acid and the indications that the action of these chemicals on normal tissues and neoplasms may be mediated through their binding proteins have led to some interesting results and suggestions. Several human tumors (breast, lung, skin, and stomach) contain considerable amounts of CRABP, whereas the adjacent histologically normal tissues have no detectable CRABP (Table 2) (15,47). This may have a bearing on differences in susceptibility of epithelial and other tissues to carcinogenesis, and on the effect of retinoids on carcinogenesis in those tissues or in tumors derived from them.

Skin papillomas induced in mice by DMBA and croton oil can be prevented by systemic treatment with retinoic acid and some of the retinoic acid analogues, which will be discussed later (7,10). The degree of binding of retinoic acid and its various analogues by CRABP of mouse papillomas and human breast tumor, reversal of metaplasia *in vitro,* and growth promotion are all closely correlated (Table 1) (14). If the binding protein is mediating the activity of retinoids in epithelial or other cells, its presence may be necessary but not sufficient for the compounds to have an effect on carcinogenesis (45).

Ong et al. studied cellular binding proteins for vitamin A in colorectal adenocarcinoma in rats (46). CRBP and CRABP were measured in rat colon mucosa during 1,2-dimethylhydrazine (DMH) carcinogenesis. The adenocarcinomas contained low levels of CRABP, similar to those found in adjacent mucosa, but levels of CRBP that were dramatically higher than CRBP levels in adjacent mucosa. These CRBP levels were only slightly higher than levels in normal or DMH-treated rats before tumors developed. This indicated that the increase in CRBP occurred only with tumor appearance and not with the earlier general hyperplasia of the crypts that accompanies DMH carcinogenesis. CRBP of the tumor was saturated with endogenous retinol to about 77% to 100%, and its fluorescence spectra were similar to those of the CRBP of normal tissues.

The study of Ong et al. contains the first report of a tumor that shows elevated CRBP but not CRABP. If CRBP is required to mediate the effect of retinol,

TABLE 2. *Vitamin A-binding proteins in human tumors*

| Tumor site | Binding Protein | |
|---|---|---|
| | CRBP | CRABP |
| Skin | ± | + |
| Thyroid | ± | + |
| Breast | − | + |
| Lung | − | + |
| Uterus | + | + |
| Kidney | + | + |

From Chytil and Ong, ref. 15, with permission.

then pharmocological doses of retinol or its esters would not be expected to affect the tumor because the binding sites would already be virtually saturated. We found that toxic doses of retinyl palmitate provided no significant protection against DMH carcinogenesis, although prolonged elevation of serum vitamin A was produced (51). Another factor that may reduce the effect of natural retinoids is that, in hypervitaminotic A rats, serum vitamin A is composed of two fractions, one bound normally to RBP and the other to lipoproteins. The lipoprotein-bound fraction may not be as readily available to tissues as the RBP fraction (36).

Other questions concerning the significance of mediators and tissue retinoid content are raised by observations in different tumor model systems. Cohen et al. (17) reported that retinyl palmitate, given in pharmacological amounts, had no effect on bladder carcinogenesis by N-[4-(5-nitro-2-furyl)-2-thiazolyl] (FANFT), despite the fact that the level of vitamin A in the bladder was two to three times normal. The vitamin A-binding proteins or complexes were not measured. Two studies have been reported in which the synthetic retinoic acid analogue 13-*cis* retinoic acid was given to rats treated with a colon carcinogen, DMH in one case and N-nitrosomethylurea (NMU) in the second. The analogue delayed or prevented tumor induction by DMH in one study (42) but had no effect on NMU activity in the other study (68). The 13-*cis* analogue binds to CRABP, which is present at low levels in colon mucosa and tumor, and this may influence its effect on tumor induction. The acid analogue's ability to block DMH carcinogenesis, although the natural retinyl ester did not, may have been related to its greater therapeutic index, differences in affinity of the two binding proteins, differences in activity of the retinoid-binding protein complex, or differences in experimental conditions. Because 13-*cis* retinoic acid retarded NMU carcinogenesis in the bladder of rats, apparently it can interact with NMU under some experimental conditions (62). The generally greater antitumor activity of retinoic acid and its analogues than of retinol or retinyl esters suggests that CRABP complexes may be more potent anticarcinogens than CRBP complexes. The significant relationships between retinoids, their binding proteins, and their physiological and pharmacological effects require definition in further studies.

## RETINOIDS AND PREVENTION OR TREATMENT OF TUMORS

The areas of interest in retinoids today and the lines of research that are uncovering promising areas are the prophylactic effects of retinoids on development of neoplasms and the therapeutic uses of the retinoids in treatment of neoplasms. Natural and synthetic retinoids in pharmacological amounts are effective in reducing the incidence or delaying the appearance of carcinogen-induced epithelial metaplasia and tumors. Organ sites that have exhibited such responses include the forestomach and cervix (13), the respiratory tract in some experiments (18,56), skin, bladder, and mammary gland (4,7,26,39). Species in

TABLE 3. *Retinoid intake and bladder carcinogenesis in rats*

| Rats | | | | | % Incidence bladder tumor | | |
| --- | --- | --- | --- | --- | --- | --- | --- |
| Strain | Sex | Carcinogen[a] | | Retinoid | + Retinoid | − Retinoid | Reference |
| W/L | F | NMU | | 13-*cis* retinoic acid | 40 | 57 | Sporn et al. 1977 |
| F344 | M | OH-BBN | 1,200 mg | 13-*cis* retinoic acid | 17 | 36 | Becci et al. 1978 |
| | | | 1,800 mg | | 52 | 72 | |
| | | | 2,400 mg | | 57 | 87 | |
| SD | F | FANFT | | Retinyl palmitate | 84 | 80 | Cohen et al. 1976 |

[a] NMU, 1-methyl-1-nitrosourea; OH-BBN, N-butyl-N-(4-hydroxybutyl) nitrosamine; FANFT, N-[4-(5-nitro-2-furyl)-2-thiazolyl] formamide.

which the effects of retinoids on these organs sites have been demonstrated include rats, mice, and hamsters, as well as rabbits in the case of the Shope papilloma (38,66). It may be through this mechanism that the retinoids prevent or modify carcinogenesis. This subject will be examined below in the discussion of studies by Boutwell and colleagues.

Squamous carcinoma in the skin and forestomach of experimental animals may be prevented by topical application of high concentrations of retinoids. Another site in which positive results have been obtained is the urinary bladder, although there is also a negative study (Table 3). The positive results were obtained with 13-*cis* retinoic acid against two nitrosocarcinogens, and the negative result with the natural retinoid, retinyl palmitate, against a chemically different carcinogen.

A number of transplanted tumors are not affected by retinoid treatment (8), but some are inhibited, such as murine melanoma (23) and rat chondrosarcoma (29).

## In Vitro Tests

Retinoids block phenotypic cell transformation by carcinoma growth factor (64), inhibit carcinogen-induced metaplasia of hamster trachea (19) and mouse prostate (12,33), growth of malignant murine melanoma and other tumors (34,35), radiation-induced oncogenic transformation of transformed mouse fibroblasts, and restore anchorage-dependent growth to them (20,28). In humans, retinoids have induced regression of basal cell carcinoma and actinic keratoses (11), leukoplakia of the mouth and larynx (53), and recurrent papillomas of the urinary bladder (22).

In an evaluation of this area in 1976, Sporn et al. (61) concluded that problems of interpretation and inconsistency of data arose because of systemic and local toxicity of natural retinoids and failure to achieve continuously high tissue levels

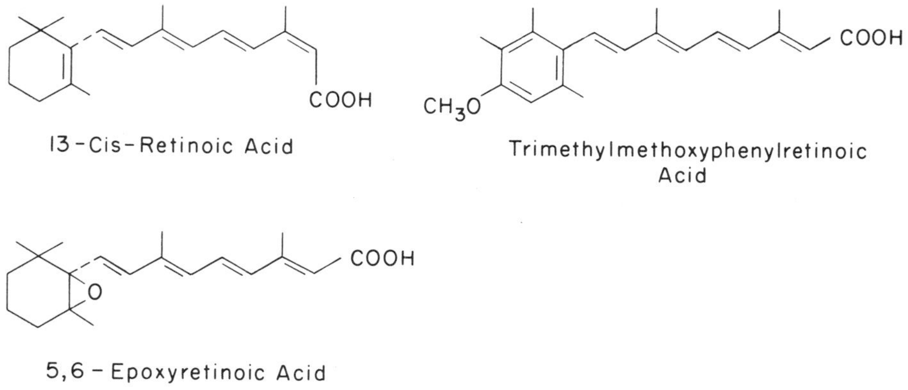

13-Cis-Retinoic Acid

Trimethylmethoxyphenylretinoic Acid

5,6-Epoxyretinoic Acid

**FIG. 2.** Analogues of retinoic acid active in modifying epithelial carcinogenesis.

outside the liver, which takes up and stores retinol and its esters. Variations in experimental methods were also cited, but the authors concluded that problems of toxicity and distribution precluded the obtaining of meaningful results in experimental animals, and urged that research with synthetic compounds be pursued. They delineated some of the new directions that appeared most promising in studies of synthetic retinoids. Arguing by analogy to synthetic adrenal steroids, they pointed out that compounds with greater activity in direct *in vitro* tests (organ cultures, cell cultures, or cell-free systems) and greater affinity for cell receptors than the natural compounds might have greater anticarcinogenic potency, and they urged further studies of synthetic compounds.

The retinoid molecule can be modified in the hydrocarbon ring, the hydrocarbon side chain, and the polar terminal group (Fig. 2). The first successful efforts to show that synthetic retinoids are less toxic and more potent in cancer prevention than the natural retinoids were reported by Bollag (8,9). The synthetic compounds he used have a tenfold greater therapeutic index than retinoic acid when tested for induction of regression of skin papillomas in mice. In these compounds, the cyclohexenyl ring of retinoic acid has been replaced with an aromatic trimethylmethoxyphenol ring (TMMP), and the terminal carboxyl group has been replaced with an ester or an ethyl amide (Fig. 2). Both of these analogues are considerably more effective than retinoic acid in inducing regression of papillomas, and the ethyl amide derivative is considerably less toxic. This demonstrates that tumor regression is not necessarily accompanied by toxicity. The aromatic (TMMP) analogues of retinoic acid and its esters are active in controlling tracheal epithelial cell differentiation. Both compounds reverse keratinizing squamous metaplasia in the trachea in organ culture (59). They maintain weight gain in and permit survival of hamsters fed vitamin A-deficient diets (61).

Early demonstration of inhibition by natural retinoids of polycyclic aromatic hydrocarbon respiratory tract carcinogenesis in hamsters has not been convincingly repeated in hamsters or shown consistently in rats in several large experiments (58). One study in hamsters, discussed briefly in a review article, gave results suggesting inhibition by 13-*cis* retinoic acid, a compound altered in the side chain and less toxic than all-trans retinoic acid. In that study, 134 control animals were treated with a low dose of benzo(*a*)pyrene and ferric oxide, which induced respiratory tract carcinoma in about 10%. Following completion of carcinogen treatment, other groups of animals were given lifetime treatment with 13-*cis* retinoic acid and the incidence of cancer was markedly decreased. Two of 152 hamsters (1.3%) given 3 mg of 13-*cis* retinoic acid weekly developed respiratory tract carcinoma. A higher dose of 13-*cis* retinoic acid, 9 mg, prevented respiratory carcinoma in all 158 animals treated and elicited no toxic response. Thus, again, inhibition of carcinogenesis was not accompanied by the toxicity associated with the natural retinoids.

Modification of the ring with retention of activity was shown using alpha-retinylacetate and alpha-retinoic acid, in which the ring double bond was shifted to the 4–5 position. Both compounds were essentially equivalent to the natural beta analogues in controlling differentiation of tracheal epithelium in culture (24,60). The compounds also supported growth in hamsters and rats, although less effectively than beta analogues (24). Other modifications of the hydrocarbon ring have been studied, and at least four have biological activity. Further research is expected to produce other modifications of the ring that may be useful in preventing or inhibiting tumor induction or in treating tumors.

A difficult task in synthetic organic chemistry is alteration of the terminal side chain, an area in which little progress has been made. The 13-*cis* retinoic acid is one compound found to be active. Morton pointed out in 1960 that the side chain was an important part of the molecule that might yield hydroxylated derivatives with biological activity (40). The presence of the individual double bonds in the side chain is important for activity, particularly the 9–10, 11–12, and 13–14 double bonds. Saturation of the 7–8 double bond does not appear to cause significant loss of activity (61).

A final site that can be modified with varying degrees of effectiveness is the polar terminal group. The presence of the carboxyl group in retinoic acid confers properties on the molecule different from those of retinol, e.g., it is not stored in the liver, and it is transported in the blood by serum albumin rather by RBP, which transports retinol. However, there are undesirable side effects associated with the terminal carboxyl group on the side chain (8,9,24). These compounds have varying antitumor activity and are toxic, presumably because they can be converted back to the carboxylic acid. Less polar terminal groups, such as ethers, have been examined. Retinyl methyl ether is as potent as retinol or retinyl acetate in supporting growth of rats and is less toxic than the natural compounds (27,31,74). Organ culture and other studies have indicated that the ether analogues should be further examined.

There is little understanding of the normal physiologic functions of vitamin

A and how they relate to its antitumor effect, if indeed they do. Several vitamin A analogues that have potent antitumor activity have little, if any, vitamin A effect when fed to vitamin A-deficient animals, although they are active *in vitro* in reversing squamous metaplasia (61). Since these compounds do not combine with RBP, and therefore are not carried by it to the vitamin A target tissues, one would not necessarily expect them to have vitamin A activity *in vivo* (61).

An exception is a metabolite of retinoic acid which Napoli et al. isolated from the small intestine of vitamin A-deficient rats by high-pressure liquid chromatography and identified by mass spectrometry as 5, 6-epoxyretinoic acid (41). This compound, described some time ago, has vitamin A activity *in vivo* (32). It reverses keratinization of hamster trachea epithelium cultured in vitamin A-deficient medium, and is as effective as retinoic acid itself. It inhibits promoter-mediated induction or ornithine decarboxylase (ODC) in lymphocyte cell cultures (see below) (69). One interesting difference from retinoic acid is that this compound appears to inhibit ODC induction only when it is applied simultaneously with the promoter, whereas retinoic acid must be applied an hour before the promoter to be effective. This suggests that retinoic acid must be activated to the 5,6-epoxy form before it can inhibit induction of ODC.

In summary, the following observations can be made about *in vitro* studies of vitamin A and its various synthetic analogues: the growth of some, but not all, normal or transformed cells can be inhibited; the expression of some phenotypic markers characteristic of transformed cells is inhibited; the transformation of fibroblast cultures by chemical and physical agents can be inhibited; and natural and synthetic retinoids can inhibit carcinogen-induced hyperplasia and metaplasia in organ cultures of the prostate. These effects can be readily achieved with some of the less toxic synthetic retinoids.

*In vivo* studies indicate that some synthetic retinoids are much more effective therapeutically in the prevention or treatment of cancer than are naturally occurring vitamin A compounds. Some established primary or transplanted tumors regress partially or totally under intensive retinoid therapy. Tumor induction by chemical carcinogens can be effectively inhibited by retinoids under some conditions in certain organs, but results using natural retinoids are not consistent. At this time, it is not possible to determine why some studies of vitamin A interactions with carcinogenesis are contradictory. Undoubtedly there are effects involving the dose of the carcinogen, the type of retinoid, the mode of administration of retinoid or carcinogen, the vitamin A status of the animal, and the tumor studied. It is clear that some tissues and tumors are refractory and that others are sensitive to the effects of retinoids.

A note of caution must be inserted into this discussion of use of retinoids for tumor prevention. In at least three experiments, treatment of experimental animals with high doses of a natural or synthetic retinoid has increased tumor incidence. All three experiments were performed in hamsters. Increased tumor incidence and severity were induced in the cheek pouch by exposure to topical DMBA and retinyl palmitate (49), and increased incidence of respiratory tract tumors was induced in hamsters given benzo(*a*)pyrene intratracheally and fed retinyl acetate (58) or given NMU intratracheally and fed 13-*cis* retinoic acid. Enhancement of tumor growth by retinoids is rare within the large number of studies that have been reported and, considering all the studies as a group, not significant statistically.

### Activity of Retinoids in the Two-Stage Model of Skin Carcinogenesis

The effects of retinoids on tumor induction can be explained most clearly using the model of skin carcinogenesis. Two well-defined stages of carcinogenesis are observed in the process of skin tumor induction. The two steps, initiation and promotion, can be studied separately. Initiation is induced by application of a carcinogen to the skin. If a carcinogenic dose is given, initiation is followed by tumor development. If a subcarcinogenic dose is applied, it produces the initiation stage, but tumor does not develop unless the application is followed by repeated applications of a promoter, such as croton oil or phorbol esters. The combined treatment leads to skin papillomas and finally carcinomas. There is a correlation between the tumor-promoting activity of chemicals and their ability to produce ODC (65), which converts ornithine to putrescine, the precursor of the polyamines spermine and spermidine. The induction can result in a 200-fold increase in ODC activity. Since ODC is the rate-limiting enzyme in polyamine biosynthesis, and since the polyamines play a role in cell proliferation and malignant transformation, it may be significant that agents without tumor-promoting activity do not induce ODC.

In studies significant for retinoid research (1,66), Boutwell's group applied the promoter phorbol ester, 12-0-tetradecanoyl-phorbol-13-acetate (TPA) to the skin of mice and measured ODC activity in the supernatant fractions of epidermal homogenates. Maximum activity appeared about four hours after TPA application. Following TPA treatment, there was a three- to four-fold increase in putrescine in as little as 6 h; the spermine level was unaffected by TPA, and spermidine increased.

The researchers then tested retinoic acid to determine whether it counteracted ODC induction by a promoter, and found a significant and dose-dependent inhibition when 0.5 $\mu$g of retinoic acid was applied to the skin in a single dose one hour before TPA application. Retinoic acid was less effective the longer the interval before TPA application. Retinoic acid blocked the increase in putrescine but not in spermidine. Studies were performed to determine whether, under the same conditions, retinoic acid inhibited the induction of skin tumors. The carcinogenic initiator dimethylbenzanthracene (DMBA) was applied to mouse skin in acetone. TPA was administered twice weekly, beginning 10 days later, for 14 weeks, and the experimental group was given retinoic acid by application to the skin one hour before each TPA treatment. Retinoic acid decreased papilloma incidence by 55% and inhibited epidermal ODC induction by the promoter. A number of naturally occurring retinoids, including retinoic acid, retinol, retinal, and retinyl esters, were studied, and the degree of inhibition of ODC induction correlated with the inhibition of skin tumors. This clearly indicated a relationship between induction of ODC and promotion of skin carcinogenesis.

The same group of investigators tested synthetic vitamin A analogues for inhibition of ODC induction by a promoter (66). Retinoic acid and a more active cyclopentenyl analogue were the most effective compounds tested. 13-*cis* retinoic acid, 13-*cis* retinal, and alpha-retinoic acid also were effective, as were a number of other derivatives. Some analogues were inactive. The active compounds were shown by Sporn et al. to be effective in hamster trachea or chick embryo skin *in vitro* (60,71). The retinoids were about equally active, even if given *per os* rather than by skin application one hour before TPA application. Again, inhibition of ODC induction and of tumor formation were correlated.

In studies in mice treated with DMBA, retinoic acid applications to the skin one hour before each promoter treatment reduced skin tumor incidence by about 75%. If retinoic acid was applied before, during, or immediately after carcinogen treatment and was followed by standard promoter treatment, there was no reduction in tumor incidence.

If the retinoid was applied 24 hours after TPA, when ODC activity had returned to normal, skin tumor development was not inhibited. Therefore, it appears that retinoic acid exerts its antitumor activity during promotion and not during initiation, possibly by inhibition of ODC induction (67).

## VITAMIN A DEFICIENCY AND ENHANCED SUSCEPTIBILITY TO CARCINOGENESIS

Retrospective and prospective epidemiologic studies indicate that the risk of developing lung cancer is inversely proportional to vitamin A intake (5,25,30a). Such studies are necessarily less specific than experimental studies because so many variables are present, but the similarity of results of studies in different parts of the world, using somewhat different methods, lends weight to the observation. The conclusion to be drawn is that segments of the population may be marginally deficient in vitamin A, since clinical deficiencies were not reported, and that their susceptibility to environmental carcinogens, such as tobacco smoke, is increased. This hypothesis is supported by experimental results demonstrating that deficiency of vitamin A enhances the susceptibility of the epithelium of the respiratory tract, colon, and urinary bladder to chemical carcinogenesis (17,42).

In the study of Cohen et al. (17) (Table 3), rats fed vitamin A-deficient diets and given FANFT had marked acceleration of bladder tumor development compared to normal or hypervitaminotic A rats, and developed tumors at other sites in the urinary tract as well.

Vitamin A-deficient rats have increased susceptibility to the induction of colon carcinoma by aflatoxin $B_1$ ($AFB_1$) (42). This hepatocarcinogen rarely induces

TABLE 4. *Enhancement of AFB₁ colon carcinogenesis by vitamin A deficiency*[a]

| Vitamin A intake | Sex | Percent tumor incidence | |
|---|---|---|---|
| | | Colon | Liver |
| Adequate | M | 0 | 48 |
| Deficient | M | 12 | 22 |
| Excessive | M | 0 | 38 |
| Adequate | M | 4 | 88 |
| | F | 8 | 79 |
| Deficient | M | 29 | 89 |
| | F | 28 | 76 |
| Excessive | M | 8 | 92 |
| | F | 10 | 84 |

[a] From ref. 51, with permission.

colon tumors in normal rats (Table 4). Using another colon carcinogen, DMH, we obtained evidence suggesting that tumor induction was accelerated by vitamin A deficiency, but found no significant effect on tumor incidence or number (51).

In unpublished studies in our own laboratories, we found that hepatic and colon mucosal microsomal oxidases and microsomal protein were not significantly affected by vitamin A deficiency, but levels were reduced in both normal and vitamin A-deficient animals by $AFB_1$ treatment. An exception was p-nitroanisole demethylase, production of which was increased in liver but decreased in colon mucosa by $AFB_1$ treatment. The response of the enzyme was not influenced by vitamin A. Vitamin A-deficient rats had decreased hepatic glutathione levels but increased levels of $AFB_1$-glutathione conjugates compared to normal rats; results in the colon were not affected by diet. Finally, and probably most significantly, vitamin A-deficient rats had greater binding of $AFB_1$ to colon mucosal DNA than normal rats; if deficient rats were given vitamin A, the binding decreased to normal levels within 48 hours.

The entire area of retinoids and synthetic analogues is one of intense activity today. The demonstrated capacity of both natural and synthetic molecules to modify or control cellular differentiation of normal and preneoplastic epithelial cells, as well as some fully formed tumors, offers a great deal of promise for preventing or treating cancers of some sites. It appears that the natural retinoids at normal tissue concentrations are useful in the prevention of cancer, and that increasing this level has no further obvious effects, aside from toxicity. Alteration of the molecule to decrease or prevent toxicity and increase tissue exposure holds promise of producing more effective compounds. Evidence that retinoids play a critical role in controlling DNA synthesis, mitotic activity, and differentiation in target epithelia, and the exciting work of Boutwell and his group showing that retinoids act during the promotion stage of cancer induction, indicate mechanisms by which this class of compounds can prevent or retard tumor development. Populations at high risk for tumors of vitamin A-responsive target organs, such as smokers or people exposed to different forms of radiation, may expect to benefit from preventive treatment. Second, the observations on inhibition or promoter-mediated induction of ODC may be of enormous importance in basic studies to increase understanding of carcinogenesis. Finally, the demonstration that a naturally occurring vitamin A metabolite, 5,6-epoxyretinoic acid, is active in the skin tumor model has added considerable thrust to research in this area of carcinogenesis and tumor prevention.

## ACKNOWLEDGMENTS

Part of the work by Newberne and Rogers referred to in this paper was supported by NIH National Cancer Institute Contract 69–2083 and by Hoffmann-La Roche, Nutley, New Jersey.

## REFERENCES

1. Boutwell, R. K., and Verma, A. K. (1978): Inhibition of 12-0-tetradecanoylphorbol-13-acetate (tpa)-induced epidermal ornithine decarboxylase activity (ODC) by vitamin A analogues (retinoids) a screen for their anti-promoting properties. *Fed. Proc.*, 37:1429.
2. Bashor, M. N., and Chytil, F. (1975): Cellular retinol binding protein. *Biochim. Biophys. Acta.*, 411:87–96.
3. Bashor, M. N., Toft, D. O., and Chytil, F. (1972): Binding of retinol to rat tissue components. *Proc. Nat. Acad. Sci., USA.*, 70:3483–3487.
4. Becci, P. J., Thompson, H. J., Grubbs, C. J., Squire, R. A., Brown, C. C., Sporn, M. B., and Moon, R. C. (1978): Inhibitory effect of 13-cis-retinoic acid on urinary bladder carcinogenesis induced in C57BL/6 mice by N-butyl-N-(4-hydroxybutyl)-nitrosamine. *Cancer Res.*, 38:4463–4466.
5. Bjelke, E. (1975): Dietary vitamin A and human lung cancer. *Int. J. Cancer*, 15:561.
6. Bollag, W. (1970): Vitamin A and vitamin A acid in the prophylaxis and therapy of epithelial tumors. *Int. J. Vitam. Nutr. Res.*, 40:299–314.
7. Bollag, W. (1972): Prophylaxis of chemically induced benign and malignant epithelial tumors by vitamin A acid (retinoic acid). *Eur. J. Cancer*, 8:689–693.
8. Bollag, W. (1974): Therapeutic effects of an aromatic retinoic acid analogue on chemically induced skin papillomas and carcinomas of mice. *Eur. J. Cancer*, 10:731–737.
9. Bollag, W. (1975): Therapy of epithelial tumors with an aromatic retinoic acid analogue. *Chemotherapy*, 21:236–247.
10. Bollag, W. (1975): Prophylaxis of chemically induced epithelial tumors with an aromatic retinoic acid analog (RO10-9359). *Eur. J. Cancer*, 11:721–724.
11. Bollag, W., and Ott, F. (1971): Therapy of actinic keratoses and basal cell carcinomas with local application of vitamin A acid (NSC-122758). *Cancer Chemother. Rep.*, 55:59–6.
12. Chopra, D. P., and Wilkoff, L. J. (1977): Reversal by vitamin A analogues (retinoids) of hyperplasia induced by N-methyl-N-nitro-N-nitrosoguanidine in mouse prostate organ cultures. *J. Natl. Cancer Inst.*, 58:923–930.
13. Chu, E. W., and Malmgren, R. A. (1965): An inhibitory effect of vitamin A on the induction of tumors of forestomach and cervix in the Syrian hamster by carcinogenic polycyclic hydrocarbons. *Cancer Res.*, 25:884–895.
14. Chytil, G., and Ong, D. E. (1976): Mediation of retinoic acid-induced growth and anti-tumour activity. *Nature* (London), 260:48–51.
15. Chytil, F., and Ong, D. E. (1978): Cellular vitamin A binding proteins. *Vitam. Horm.*, 36:1–17.
16. Chytil, F., Page, D., and Ong, D. E. (1975): Presence of cellular retinol and retinoic acid binding protein in human uterus. *Int. J. Vitam. Nutr. Res.*, 45:293–298.

17. Cohen, S. M., Wittenberg, J. F., and Bryan, G. T. (1976): Effect of avitaminosis A and hypervitaminosis A on urinary bladder carcinogenicity of N-[4-(5-Nitro-2-furyl)-2-thiazolyl] formamide. *Cancer Res.,* 36:2334–2339.
18. Cone, M. V., and Nettesheim, P. (1973): Effects of vitamin A on 3-methylcholanthrene-induced squamous metaplasias and early tumors in the respiratory tract of rats. *J. Nat. Cancer Inst.,* 50:1599–1606.
19. Crocker, T. T., and Sanders, L. L. (1970): Influence of vitamin A and 3, 7-dimethyl-2,6-octadienal (citral) on the effect of benzo(a)pyrene on hamster trachea in organ culture. *Cancer Res.,* 30:1312–1318.
20. Dion, L. D., Blalok, J. E., and Gifford, G. E. (1978): Retinoic acid and the restoration of anchorage dependent growth to transformed cells. *Exp. Cell Res.,* 117:15–22.
21. Emerick, R. J., Zile, M., and DeLuca, H. F. (1967): Formation of retinoic acid from retinol in the rat. *Biochem. J.,* 102:606–611.
22. Evard, J. P., and Bollag, W. (1972): Konservative behandling der rezidinierenden harnblasen-papillomatose mit vitamin A saure. *Schweiz. Med. Wochenschrift,* 102:1880–1883.
23. Felix, E. L., Loyd, B., and Cohen, M. H. (1975): Inhibition of the growth and development of a transplantable murine melanoma by vitamin A. *Science,* 189:886–888.
24. Goodman, D. S., Smith, J. E., Hembrz, R. M., and Dingle, J. T. (1974): Comparison of vitamin A and its analogs in culture and in rats. *J. Lipid Res.,* 15:406–414.
25. Gregor, A., Lee, P. N., Frances, J. C. R., Wilson, M. J., and Melton, A. (1979): Comparison of dietary histories in lung cancer cases and controls with special reference to vitamin A. *Nutr. and Cancer (in press).*
26. Grubbs, C. J., Moon, R. C., Sporn, M. B., and Newton, D. L. (1977): Inhibition of mammary cancer by retinyl methyl ether. *Cancer Res.,* 37:599–602.
27. Hanze, A. E., Conger, T. W., Wise, E. C., and Weisblat, V. I. (1948): Crystalline vitamin A methyl ether. *J. Am. Chem. Soc.,* 70:1253–1256.
28. Harisiadis, L., Miller, R. C., Hall, E. J., and Borek, C. (1978): A vitamin A analogue inhibits radiation-induced oncogenic transformation. *Nature,* 274:486–487.
29. Heilman, C., and Swarm, R. L. (1975): Effects of 13-cis vitamin A acid on chondrosarcoma (abstract #3406). *Fed. Proc.,* 34:822.
30. Heller, J. (1975): Characterization of bovine plasma retinol-binding protein and lack of binding other plasma proteins. *J. Biol. Chem.,* 250:6549–6554.
30a. Hirayama, T. (1979): Diet and cancer. *Nutr. Cancer,* 1:67–81.
31. Isler, O., Ronco, R., Geux, W., Hindley, N. C., Huber, W., Dialer, K., and Kofler, M. (1949): Uber die ester und ather des synthelischen vitamins A. *Helv. Chim. Acta.,* 32:489–505.
32. John, K. V., Lakshmanan, M. R., and Cama, H. R. (1967): Preparation, properties and metabolism of 5,6-monoepoxyretinoic acid. *Biochem. J.,* 103:539–543.
33. Lasnitzki, H., and Goodman, D. S. (1974): Inhibition of the effects of methylcholanthrene on mouse prostate in organ culture by vitamin A and its analogs. *Cancer Res.,* 34:1564–1571.
34. Lotan, R., Giotta, G., Nork, E., and Nicolson, G. L. (1978): Characterization of the inhibitory effects of retinoids on the in vitro growth of two malignant murine melanomas. *J. Natl. Cancer Inst.,* 60:1035–1041.
35. Lotan, R., and Nicolson, G. L. (1977): Inhibitory effects of retinoic acid or retinyl acetate on the growth of untransformed, transformed, and tumor cells in vitro. *J. Natl. Cancer Inst.,* 59:1717–1722.
36. Mallia, A. K., Smith, J. E., and Goodman, D. S. (1975): Metabolism of retinol-binding protein and vitamin A during hypervitaminosis A in the rat. *J. Lipid Res.,* 16:180–188.
37. McMichael, H. (1965): Inhibition of growth of Shope rabbit papilloma by hypervitaminosis A. *Cancer Res.,* 25:947–955.
38. Moon, R. C., Grubbs, C. J., Sporn, M. B., and Goodman, D. J. (1977): Retinyl acetate inhibits mammary carcinogenesis induced by N-methyl-N-nitrosourea. *Nature,* 267:620–621.
39. Morton, R. A. (1960): Summary discussion on vitamin A symposium. *Vitam. Horm.,* 18:543–569.
40. Napoli, J. L., McCormick, A. M., Schnoes, H. K., and DeLuca, H. F. (1978): Identification of 5,8-oxyretinoic acid isolated from small intestine of A-deficient rats dosed with retinoic acid. *Proc. Natl. Acad. Sci.,* 75:2603–2605.
41. Newberne, P. M., Rogers, A. E., and Gross, R. L. (1976): Nutritional modulation of carcinogenesis. Proceedings, International Congress, Cancer Detection and Prevention. Marcel Dekker Inc., New York, pp. 665–691.

42. Newberne, P. M., and Suphakarn, V. (1977): Preventive role of vitamin A in colon carcinogenesis in rats. *Cancer,* 40:2553.
43. Ong, D. E., and Chytil, F. (1975): Retinoic acid binding protein in rat tissue. *J. Biol. Chem.,* 250:6113–6117.
44. Ong, D. E., and Chytil, F. (1978): Cellular retinoic acid binding protein from rat testes. *J. Biol. Chem.,* 253:4551–4555.
45. Ong, D. E., and Chytil, F. (1978): Cellular retinol binding protein from rat liver. *J. Biol. Chem.,* 253:828–832.
46. Ong, D. E., Marker, C., and Chiu, J. F. (1978): Cellular binding proteins for vitamin A and colorectal adenocarcinoma of the rat. *Cancer Res.,* 38:4422–4426.
47. Ong, D. E., Tasi, H., and Chytil, F. (1976): Cellular retinol binding protein and retinoic acid binding protein in rat testes: Effect of retinol depletion. *J. Nutr.,* 106:204–211.
48. Peterson, P. A., Nilsson, S. F., Ostberg, L., and Vahlquist, A. (1974): Aspects of the metabolism of retinol binding protein and retinol. *Vitam. Horm.,* 32:181–214.
49. Polliack, A., and Levij, I. S. (1969): The effect of topical vitamin A on papillomas and intraepithelial carcinomas induced in hamster cheek pouches with 9,10-dimethyl-1,2-benzanthracene. *Cancer Res.,* 29:327–332.
50. Prutkin, L., and Bogart, B. (1970): The uptake of labeled vitamin A acid in keratocanthoma. *J. Invest. Dermatol.,* 55:249–255.
51. Rogers, A. E., Herndon, B. J., and Newberne, P. M. (1973): Induction by dimethylhydrazine of intestinal carcinoma in normal rats and rats fed high or low levels of vitamin A. *Cancer Res.,* 33:1003–1009.
52. Ross, A. C., Takahashyi, Y. I., and Goodman, D. S. (1978): The binding protein for retinol from rat testes cytosol. *J. Biol. Chem.,* 253:6591–6598.
53. Ryssel, H. J., Bruner, K. W., and Bollag, W. (1971): Die perorale anwendungvon vitamin A-Saure bei Leukepalkien, hyperkeratosin und plattenepithelkarzinonmen Ergbnisse und Bertraglichkeit. *Schweiz. Med. Wochenschr.,* 101:1027–1030.
54. Saari, J. C., Futterman, S., Stubbs, D. W., Heffernan, J. T., Bredberg, L., Chan, A. Y., and Albert, D. M. (1978): Cellular retinol and retinoic acid binding protein in transformed mammalian cells. *Invest. Ophth. Vis. Sci.,* 17:988–992.
55. Saari, J. C., Futterman, S., and Bredberg, L. (1978): Cellular retinol and retinoic acid binding proteins of bovine retina. *J. Biol. Chem.,* 253:6432–6436.
56. Saffiotti, U., Montesano, R., Sellakumar, A. R., and Borg, S. A. (1967): Experimental cancer of the lung. Inhibition by vitamin A of the induction of tracheobronchial squamous metaplasia and squamous cell tumors. *Cancer,* 20:857–864.
57. Banerjee, C. K., and Sani, B. P. (1978): Purification and properties of retinoic acid binding protein (abstract). *Fed. Proc.,* 37:485.
58. Smith, D. M., Rogers, A. E., Herndon, B. J., and Newberne, P. M. (1975): Vitamin A (retinyl acetate) and benzo(a)pyrene-induced respiratory tract carcinogenesis in hamsters fed a commercial diet. *Cancer Res.,* 35:11–16.
59. Sporn, M. B. (1977): Retinoids and carcinogenesis. *Nutr. Rev.,* 35:65–69.
60. Sporn, M. B., Clamon, G. H., Dunlop, N. M., Newton, D. L., Smith, J. M., and Saffiotti, U. (1975): Activity of vitamin A analogues in cell cultures of mouse epidermis and organ cultures of hamster trachea. *Nature,* 253:47–50.
61. Sporn, M. B., Dunlop, N. M., Newton, D. L., and Smith, J. M. (1976): Prevention of chemical carcinogenesis by vitamin A and its synthetic analogs (retinoids). *Fed. Proc.,* 35:1332–1338.
62. Squire, R. A., Sporn, M. B., Brown, C. C., Smith, J. M., Wenk, M. L., and Springer, S. (1977): Histopathological evaluation of the inhibition of rat bladder carcinogenesis by 13-cis-retinoic acid. *Cancer Res.,* 37:2930–2936.
63. Takase, S., Ong, D. E., and Chytil, F. (1979): Cellular retinol-binding protein allows specific interaction of retinol with the nucleus in vitro. *Proc. Natl. Acad. Sci. USA,* 76:2204–2208.
64. Todaro, O. J., DeLarco, J. E., and Sporn, M. B. (1978): Retinoids block phenotypic cell transformation produced by sarcoma growth factor. *Nature,* 276:272–274.
65. Verma, A. K., and Boutwell, R. K. (1977): Vitamin A acid (retinoic acid), a potent inhibitor of 12-0-tetradecanoyl-phorbol-13-acetate-induced ornithine decarboxylase activity in mouse epidermis. *Cancer Res.,* 37:2196–2201.
66. Verma, A. K., Rice, H. M., Shapas, B. G., and Boutwell, R. K. (1978): Inhibition of 12-0-tetradecanoylphorbol-13-acetate-induced ornithine decarboxylase activity in mouse epidermis by vitamin A analogs (retinoids). *Cancer Res.,* 38:793–801.

67. Verma, A. K., Shopas, B. G., Rice, H. M., and Boutwell, R. K. (1979): Correlation of the inhibition by retinoids of tumor promoter-induced mouse epidermal ornithine decarboxylase activity and of skin tumor promotion. *Cancer Res.,* 39:419–425.
68. Ward, J. M., Sporn, M. B., Wenk, M. L., Smith, J. M., Feeser, D., and Dean, R. J. (1978): Dose response to intrarectal administration of N-methyl-N-nitrosourea and histopathologic evaluation of the effect of two retinoids on colon lesions induced in rats. *J. Natl. Cancer Inst.,* 60:1489–1493.
69. Wertz, P. W., Kensler, T. W., Mueller, G. C., Verma, A. K., and Boutwell, R. K. (1979): 5,6-epoxyretinoic acid opposed the effects of TPA in bovine lymphocytes. *Nature,* 277:227–229.
70. Wiggert, P. N., and Charder, G. J. (1975): A receptor for retinol in the developing retina and pigment epithelium. *Exp. Eye Res.,* 21:143–151.
71. Wilkoff, L. J., Peckham, J. C., Dulmadge, E. A., Mowry, R. W., and Chopra, D. P. (1976): Evaluation of vitamin A analogs in modulating epithelial differentiation of 13-day chick embyro metatarsal skin explants. *Cancer Res.,* 36:964–972.
72. Wolbach, S. B., and Howe, P. R. (1925): Tissue changes following deprivation of fat soluble A vitamin. *J. Exp. Med.,* 43:753–777.
73. Wolbach, S. B., and Howe, P. R. (1933): Epithelial repair in recovery from vitamin A deficiency. *J. Exp. Med.,* 57:511–526.
74. Wolbach, S. B., and Maddock, C. L. (1951): Hypervitaminosis A an adjunct to present methods of vitamin A identification. *Proc. Soc. Exp. Biol. Med.,* 77:825–829.

*Nutrition and Cancer: Etiology and Treatment,*
edited by G. R. Newell and N. M. Ellison.
Raven Press, New York © 1981.

# Vitamins E and C and Their Relationship to Cancer

*Neil M. Ellison and **Harold Londer

*Department of Hematology/Oncology, Geisinger Medical Center, Danville, Pennsylvania 17821; **Minnesota Medical Specialists, Minneapolis, Minnesota 55440*

Vitamins E and C have received increased publicity in the lay press as effective agents in the prevention or treatment of numerous maladies, including cancer. The substantial scientific data on the relationship between these vitamins and cancer are the subject of this review.

## VITAMIN E

Vitamin E was first described by Evans and Bishop (9) in 1922 as a substance essential for rat spermatogenesis. The primary form of vitamin E is alpha-tocopherol, a methyl-substituted 6-hydroxychroman derivative with a 16-carbon side chain. It is most often found in vegetable oils, and its concentration is usually proportional to the amount of linoleic acid present, with safflower oil having the highest concentration. The minimum daily requirement is estimated to be approximately 30 International Units (15 mg), an amount that is present in virtually all diets (16). It is apparently fairly nontoxic in moderate doses, because 800 IU ingested daily for three years has been observed to have no ill effects in man (10). The major physiologic role of vitamin E is generally considered to be its ability to function as an antioxidant and as a "free radical scavenger." The vitamin's lipid solubility and antioxidant role make it especially active in inhibiting lipid peroxidation (31).

The biological effects of vitamin E deficiency in animals have been well described, and vary greatly from species to species. Included are disorders of the reproductive, musculoskeletal, central nervous, and vascular systems (16). The effects of vitamin E deficiency in humans are much less certain. No notable clinical disorders were observed when human volunteers were maintained on vitamin E-deficient diets for six years; however, the volunteers' red blood cells became more sensitive to *in vitro* oxidative hemolysis (17). A hemolytic anemia correctable with vitamin E has been described in premature infants; this condition is felt to be caused by insufficient development of free radical defense mechanisms

(31). Many other clinical phenomena have been attributed to vitamin E deficiency, but no substantial scientific evidence supports these claims.

### Vitamin E and Carcinogenesis

Several investigators have studied the influence of vitamin E on experimental tumors. Shamberger and Rudolph (39) studied the effects of several antioxidants, including vitamin E, on croton oil-induced skin neoplasms in mice. When applied topically for several days after the carcinogen, vitamin E was able to significantly decrease the number of tumors induced. Similar anticarcinogenic effects were noted by Bonmassar et al. (3), who observed that mice with benzo(*a*)pyrene-induced sarcomas had an increased median survival if given alpha-tocopherol treatment. Haber and Wissler (13) also observed a marked decrease in carcinogenicity of methylcholanthrene in mice fed diets containing supplemental vitamin E. In an interesting paper, Sadaat-Noori and Afnan (36) demonstrated depression of plasma vitamin E levels in chicks with leukemia. No follow-up of this study has been presented, and its significance remains obscure.

Thus, with several carcinogen-induced tumors, dietary, topical, or parenteral vitamin E has been shown to decrease the rate of tumor induction or growth. In none of these studies was an attempt made to identify the mechanism of action of vitamin E. To date, no studies have examined any potential relationship of vitamin E to human carcinogenesis.

### Vitamin E and Radiation

Radiation energy is a potent source of free radical generation in biologic systems. Depending on the number of free radicals formed, radiation effects may be directly toxic, carcinogenic, or of little consequence. Several investigators have studied the ability of parenteral and enteral vitamin E to alter the mortality rates associated with total body irradiation in mice. These studies have yielded conflicting results, with some observers noting a protective effect (37) and others reporting no effect or increased mortality in a group of animals pretreated with high doses of vitamin E (15). In a study by Londer and Myers (22), treatment with parenteral vitamin E before total body irradiation of $CDF_1$ weanling mice significantly decreased the lethality of the radiation (Fig. 1). It should be noted that these animals were treated at a very steep portion of the radiation dose–response curve, and that minimal changes in the radiation administered could dramatically affect the results. Therefore, many other variables, such as diet, age and breed of mouse, and timing of vitamin E administration, must be examined in future studies to explain previously reported conflicting results. Finally, it has also been observed that whole-body irradiation of mice induces a mild *in vivo* hemolysis that is not so marked if vitamin E treatment is given prior to irradiation (18,33).

Studies investigating the interaction of vitamin E with irradiated animal tu-

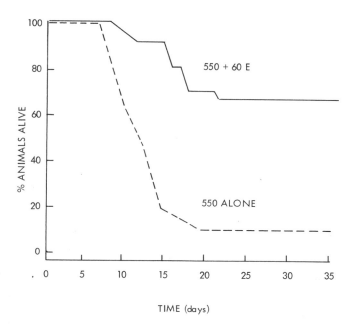

TIME (days)

**FIG. 1.** Effect of vitamin E pretreatment on mortality of 550 rads tbi. Influence of pretreatment with 60 units of intraperitoneal α-tocopherol (E) 30 minutes before 550 rads total body irradiation of CDF$_1$ male weanling mice. (Londer and Myers, 1978)

mors and tumor cell lines have yielded conflicting results. Prasad et al. (32) showed that vitamin E treatment enhanced the morphologic differentiation of neuroblastoma cells in culture and increased the effect of radiation on these cells. Other antioxidants, such as ascorbate and glutathione, did not share this property. Other researchers have also reported enhancement by vitamin E of irradiation's antitumor effects (19). At the same time, vitamin E-depleted lymphosarcoma cells have been observed to be more sensitive to radiation damage than normal lymphosarcoma cells in culture (11,20). This effect has been postulated to be caused by stabilization of cell membranes by vitamin E.

No studies on vitamin E interaction with human tumors and radiation have been published to date. It has been suggested that vitamin E treatment can improve radiation cystitis, but this observation is based on a small number of cases and has not been further tested (47). Obviously, studies of long-term radiation effects (such as carcinogenesis) and the interrelationships of radiation with vitamin E are necessary to resolve this controversy.

### Vitamin E and Adriamycin

Perhaps the most interesting and clinically relevant observations regarding vitamin E and cancer are the recent studies regarding the interaction of vitamin

E and adriamycin (Doxorubicin). Adriamycin is an antitumor antibiotic of the anthracyclene type that has proved effective in the treatment of human neoplasms (2). Its usefulness has been limited by its cardiotoxic effects. Since vitamin E deficiency in certain animals can also produce cardiomyopathy (43), parenteral vitamin E was used as a pretreatment in an experimental attempt to alleviate adriamycin's cardiac toxicity (30). A significant improvement was observed in survival of animals pretreated with vitamin E (Fig. 2). In a later report (29), the same investigators used the appearance of malondialdehyde, a naturally occurring product of lipid peroxidation, as a marker of adriamycin cardiac toxicity. A wave of malondialdehyde formation in cardiac tissues was noted after adriamycin treatment, confirming that lipid peroxidation had occurred.

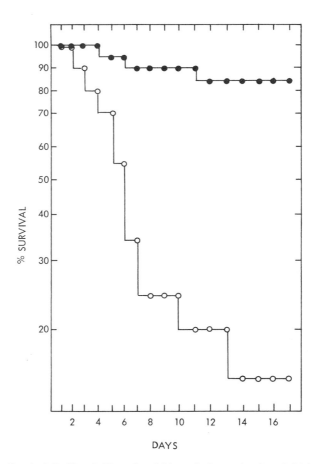

**FIG. 2.** Reduction in lethality of 15 mg/kg Adriamycin by pretreatment 24 hours prior with 85 units intraperitoneal α-tocopherol. (Reprinted with permission of author, Myers et al, 1976.) Adriamycin, open circles; Adriamycin + pretreatment α-tocopherol; closed circles

This wave was essentially abolished by pretreatment with vitamin E. Electron microscopic examination of cardiac tissues also demonstrated this protective effect. Of particular interest, this paper also reported that there was no vitamin E effect on the responsiveness of an experimental tumor (P388 ascites) to adriamycin.

Several additional investigators have confirmed these observations. Sonneveld (41) demonstrated that vitamin E pretreatment in a rat model of adriamycin-induced cardiac disease was able to decrease toxicity, as measured by heart weight and light microscopic and electrocardiographic changes. The neoplastic response to adriamycin was not affected by this pretreatment. Lubawy et al. (23) were able to show inhibition of adriamycin-induced cardiac toxicity in mice by pretreatment with vitamin E. Van Vleet et al. (42) studied the effects of a selenium–vitamin E combination in weanling rabbits treated with adriamycin and demonstrated a significant decrease in cardiac pathology in pretreated animals. Minnaugh et al. (26) found that there were no effects on adriamycin metabolism and, interestingly, plasma levels of adriamycin were higher in vitamin E-pretreated mice.

The relationship of these observations to human clinical cardiac toxicity remains unclear. Doroshow et al. (8) have reviewed the various experimental models of adriamycin cardiotoxicity and stress the difficulties in extrapolating from these models to humans. Several clinical studies are currently under way to evaluate the effects of vitamin E on adriamycin toxicity and antineoplastic activity.

## VITAMIN C

Few nutrients have received such wide publicity for possible anticancer activity as has vitamin C (ascorbic acid). It has been claimed to act as both a cancer preventative and a specific treatment for diagnosed cancers. Both claims are controversial.

### Vitamin C and Carcinogenesis

One of the best-substantiated claims for vitamin C's anticancer effect is the role it plays in preventing the formation of carcinogens from ingested food stuffs. Many fresh vegetables and preserved foods contain nitrates and nitrites, which can undergo *in vitro* and *in vivo* conversion to nitrosamines (24). The latter compounds are potent mutagens and animal carcinogens. Ascorbic acid has been shown to effectively block this spontaneous conversion *in vitro* when it is added to a mixture of nitrates and food homogenates, and *in vivo* when it is ingested with foods containing nitrates (28,34). This protective action by vitamin C has been postulated to account for the decreased incidence of gastric carcinoma that has been observed in populations that frequently consume fruits and vegetables with high vitamin C content (45).

Since a relatively high incidence of gastric carcinoma in Japan has been attributed, at least in part, to the Japanese custom of ingesting nitrate-preserved smoked Sanma fish, Weisburger et al. (44) studied the mutagenesis and carcinogenesis induced by this particular foodstuff. They demonstrated that fish homogenates incubated with nitrates at an acid pH were mutagenic in the *Salmonella typhimurium* TA-1535 bioassay. If vitamin C was added to these nitrated homogenates, the formation of mutagens was blocked. Furthermore, they showed that the nitrite-preserved fish were carcinogenic in a rat gastric tumor model. Carcinogenesis was observed to occur even in rats fed the mutagenic extract early in life and then given a nonmutagenic diet.

Other animal tumor carcinogenic systems have been studied and vitamin C has been shown to protect against (38), have no effect on (40), or even possibly enhance (27) the carcinogens used. However, when all the data are weighed, it is most probable that, in experimental systems, moderate doses of ascorbic acid are protective against some food carcinogens or procarcinogens. This is also supported by human epidemiologic data which indicate that vitamin C intake is negatively associated with the development of gastric cancer (12,14,46). Of course, because of the enormous number of variables in any human subpopulation, a direct one-to-one correlation between vitamin C intake and gastric cancer is impossible. However, enough data are present to support the recommendation that vitamin C-containing foods or supplements be eaten throughout the year, and especially with foods containing nitrates or nitrites.

### Vitamin C as a Cancer Treatment

Besides its activity as a carcinogen inhibitor, vitamin C has also been heralded as a treatment for existing cancer. This has received broad coverage by the lay press, and it is probably not unusual for cancer patients to self-medicate with large quantities of this vitamin.

Lowered leukocyte ascorbic acid levels have been reported in patients with malignant disease (1,21), but the studies fail to describe a number of factors concerning their patient groups and are also lacking in adequate controls. At best, the reports can be described as interesting observations that require much further documentation. However, one of the papers states that patients with malignant disease should receive vitamin C replacement (21). This conclusion is completely unsupported by the data presented. In fact, Miglozzi's data on the effects of ascorbic acid on tumor growth in guinea pigs could be cited as contraindicating vitamin C treatment of cancer (25). The guinea pig, like man but unlike mice and rats, cannot synthesize vitamin C and is dependent upon ingested ascorbate to meet its requirements for this vitamin. When sarcoma-bearing animals were fed diets without vitamin C, tumor regression was noted in the majority of animals. Animals fed diets containing small amounts of vitamin C showed tumor growth inhibition without regression, whereas animals ingesting high doses of vitamin C had tumor growth without any signs of retardation.

When vitamin C was added to the diet of the ascorbate-depleted group, enhanced tumor growth was observed.

Others have reported possible benefits of ascorbic acid therapy in human premalignant conditions. DeCosse et al. (7) described disappearance or regression of rectal polyps in five of eight patients with familial polyposis who ingested 3 g of vitamin C daily. These investigators hypothesized that ascorbic acid's protective effects were the result of alterations in intestinal bacteria, with subsequent changes in fecal steroid metabolism. An association has been observed between microbially modified bile acids, cholesterol metabolites, and colon cancer risk in different populations (35).

Cameron and Pauling (4) reported that 100 "terminal" cancer patients treated with 10 g of vitamin C daily survived 4.16 times longer than 1,000 untreated controls and also had an "improved quality of life." The controls were retrospective and were not shown to be well matched for known prognostic features of the tumors involved. The evidence of objective benefits in the treated group was anecdotal. The paper was of interest to those treating cancer patients, but its conclusions required substantiation in a controlled setting. This was performed at the Mayo Clinic, where 150 advanced cancer patients were treated in a double-blind controlled study of high-dose vitamin C therapy (5). The vitamin C- and placebo-treated patients were well matched for age, sex, site of primary tumor, performance score, tumor grade, and previous chemotherapy. No difference was noted in median survival between the groups. Similarly, no differences between the vitamin C- and placebo-treated groups were observed in terms of subjective improvement in symptoms, performance status, appetite, or weight gain. Although this paper has been criticized by vitamin C advocates because of the possible negative effects that prior chemotherapy could have had on vitamin C antitumor effect (6), it remains the best study of ascorbic acid in the treatment of human cancer, and its results are convincingly negative.

## SUMMARY

Vitamin E functions as an antioxidant and has the ability to inhibit free radical-induced lipid peroxidation. It has been shown to protect against certain carcinogens in animal systems, and, in some test situations, to protect against radiation-induced damage. Vitamin E eases the cardiac toxicity of adriamycin in several animal systems, apparently without interfering with the antineoplastic activity of the drug. Although many of these observations are quite provocative, virtually all have dealt with specific experimental animal systems, and any potential relevance to human carcinogenesis or cancer therapy remains conjectural.

Vitamin C probably possesses significant activity as a carcinogen inhibitor in some animal models. By extrapolating these data to man, one can conclude that it would be advisable to ingest vitamin C in its natural or supplemental form daily throughout the year, especially when eating nitrate- or nitrite-containing foods. There are no convincing data that vitamin C is effective in the treatment of already diagnosed cancer.

## REFERENCES

1. Basu, T. K., Raven, R. W., Dickerson, J. W. T., and Williams, D. C. (1974): Leukocyte ascorbic acid and urinary hydroxyproline levels in patients bearing breast cancer with skeletal metastases. *Eur. J. Cancer,* 10:507–511.
2. Blum, R., and Carter, S. (1974): Adriamycin. *Ann. Intern. Med.,* 80:249–254.
3. Bonmassar, E., Dallavalle, R., and Giuliani, G. (1968): Influence of vitamin E and propylgallate on carcinogenesis with benzopyrene in mice. *Arch. Ital. Pathol. Clin. Tumor,* 11:245–250.
4. Cameron, E., and Pauling, L. (1976): Supplemental ascorbate in the supportive treatment of cancer: Prolongation of survival times in terminal human cancer. *Proc. Nat. Acad. Sci. USA,* 73:3685–3689.
5. Creagan, E. T., Moertel, C. G., O'Fallon, J. R., Schutt, A. J., O'Connell, M. J., Rubin, J. and Frytak, S. (1979): Failure of high-dose vitamin C (ascorbic acid) therapy to benefit patients with advanced cancer. *N. Engl. J. Med.,* 301:687–690.
6. Creagan, E. T., and Moertel, C. G. (1979): Vitamin C therapy of advanced cancer. *N. Engl. J. Med.,* 301:1300.
7. DeCosse, J. J., Adams, M. B., Kuzma, J. F., Logerfo, P., and London, R. E. (1975): Effect of ascorbic acid on rectal polyps of patients with familial polyposis. *Surgery,* 78:608–612.
8. Doroshow, J., Locker, G., and Myers, C. E. (1979): Experimental animal models of adriamycin cardiotoxicity. *Cancer Treat. Rep.,* 63:855–860.
9. Evans, H., and Bishop, K. (1922): On the existence of hitherto unrecognized factor essential for reproduction. *Science,* 56:650–651.
10. Farrell, P., and Biere, J. (1975): Megavitamin E supplementation in man. *Am. J. Clin. Nutr.,* 28:1381–1385.
11. Fonck, K., and Konings, A. (1978): The effect of vitamin E on cellular survival after X-irradiation of lymphoma cells. *Br. J. Radiol.,* 51:832–833.
12. Graham, S., Schotz, W., and Martino, P. (1968): Alimentary factors in the epidemiology of gastric cancer. *Cancer,* 20:163–172.
13. Haber, S., and Wissler, R. (1962): Effect of vitamin E on carcinogenicity of methylcholanthrene. *Proc. Soc. Exp. Biol.,* 111:774–775.
14. Haenszel, W., and Correa, P. (1975): Developments in the epidemiology of stomach cancer over the past decade. *Cancer Res.,* 35:3452–3459.
15. Haley, T., McCulloh, E., and McCormick, W. (1954): Influence of water soluble vitamin E on survival time in irradiated mice. *Science,* 131:126–127.
16. Howritt, M. (1980): Vitamin E. In: *Modern Nutrition in Health and Disease,* edited by R. Goodhart and M. Shils, pp. 181–191. Lea & Febiger, Philadelphia.
17. Howritt, M., Harvey, C., Duncan, G., and Wilson, W. (1956): Effect of limited tocopherol intake in man with relationship to erythrocyte hemolysis and lipid oxidation. *Am. J. Clin. Nutr.,* 4:408–419.
18. Hoffer, A., and Roy, R. (1975): Vitamin E decreased erythrocyte fragility after whole body irradiation. *Radiat. Res.,* 61:439–443.
19. Kagerud, A., Holm, G., Larsos, H., and Peterson, H. (1978): Tocopherol and local X-ray irradiation of two transplantable rat tumors. *Cancer Lett.,* 5:123–129.
20. Konings, A., and Trieling, W. (1977): The inhibition of DNA synthesis in vitamin E depleted lymphosarcoma cells by X ray and cystostatics. *Int. J. Radiat. Biol.,* 31:397–400.
21. Krasner, N., and Dymock, I. W. (1974): Ascorbic acid deficiency in malignant diseases: A clinical and biochemical study. *Br. J. Cancer,* 30:142–145.
22. Londer, H., and Myers, C. (1978): Radioprotective effects of vitamin E (abstract). Presented at American Society of Clinical Nutrition, p. 284A.
23. Lubawy, W., Whaley, J., and Hurley, L. (1979): Coenzyme $Q_{10}$ or alpha-tocopherol reduce the acute toxicity of anthracyclenes in mice. *Res. Commun. Clin. Pathol. Pharmacol.,* 24:401–404.
24. Marquardt, H., Rufino, R., and Weisburger, J. H. (1977): On the etiology of gastric cancer: Mutagenicity of food extracts after incubation with nitrite. *Food Cosmet. Toxicol.,* 15:97–100.

25. Miglozzi, J. A. (1977): Effect of ascorbic acid on tumor growth. *Br. J. Cancer,* 35:448–453.
26. Minnaugh, E., Siddik, Z., Drew, R., Sikic, B., and Gram, T. (1979): The effects of alpha-tocopherol on the toxicity, disposition and metabolism of adriamycin in mice. *Toxicol. Appl. Pharmacol.,* 49:119–126.
27. Mirvish, S. S., Pelfrene, A. F., Garcia, H., and Shubik, P. (1976): Effect of sodium ascorbate on tumor induction in rats treated with morpholine and sodium nitrate and with nitrosomorpholine. *Cancer Lett.,* 2:101–108.
28. Mirvish, S. S. (1975): Blocking the formation of N-nitroso compounds with ascorbic acid in vitro and in vivo. *Ann. NY Acad. Sci.,* 258:175–180.
29. Myers, C., McGuire, W., Liss, H., Ifrim, I., Grotzinger, K., and Young, R. (1977): Adriamycin: The role of lipid peroxidation in cardiac toxicity and tumor response. *Science,* 197:165–167.
30. Myers, C., McGuire, W., and Young, R. (1976): Adriamycin amelioration of toxicity by alpha-tocopherol. *Cancer Treat. Rep.,* 60:961–962.
31. Oski, F. (1977): Metabolism and physiologic role of vitamin E. *Hosp. Pract.,* 12:79–85.
32. Prasad, K., Ramanujam, S., and Gaudreau, P. (1979): Vitamin E induces morphologic differentiation and increases the effect of ionizing radiation on neuroblastoma cells in culture. *Proc. Soc. Exp. Biol. Med.,* 161:570–573.
33. Prince, E., and Little, J. (1973): The effect of dietary fatty acids and tocopherol on the radiosensitivity of mammalian erythrocytes. *Radiat. Res.,* 53:49–64.
34. Raineri, R., and Weisburger, J. H. (1975): Reduction of gastric carcinogens with ascorbic acid. *Ann. NY Acad. Sci.,* 258:181–189.
35. Reddy, B. S., Mastromarino, A., and Wynder, E. L. (1975): Further leads on metabolic epidemiology of large bowel cancer. *Cancer Res.,* 35:3403–3406.
36. Saadat-Noori, M., and Afnan, M. (1970): Depression of plasma tocopherol level in chicks infected with avian leukosis. *Poult. Sci. Rep.,* 49:358–359.
37. Sakamoto, K., and Sakka, M. (1973): Reduced effect of irradiation on normal and malignant cells irradiated in vivo in mice pretreated with vitamin E. *Br. J. Radiol.,* 56:538–540.
38. Schlegel, J. V., Pipkin, G. E., Nishimuro, R., and Shultz, G. N. (1970): The role of ascorbic acid in the prevention of bladder tumor formation. *J. Urol.,* 103:155.
39. Shamberger, R., and Rudolph, G. (1966): Protection against co-carcinogens by antioxidants. *Experientia,* 22:116.
40. Soloway, M. S., Cohen, S. M., Dekernion, J. B., and Persky, L. (1975): Failure of ascorbic acid to inhibit FANFT-induced bladder cancer. *J. Urol.,* 113:483–486.
41. Sonneveld, P. (1978): Effect of alpha tocopherol on the cardiotoxicity of adriamycin in the rat. *Cancer Treat. Rep.,* 62:1033–1036.
42. Van Vleet, J., Greenwood, L., Ferrans, V., and Rebar, A. (1978): Effects of selenium–vitamin E on adriamycin induced cardiomyopathy in rabbits. *Am. J. Vet. Res.,* 39:997–1010.
43. Van Vleet, J., Hall, B., and Simon, J. (1968): Vitamin E deficiency. *Am. J. Pathol.,* 52:1067–1079.
44. Weisburger, J. H., Marquardt, H., Hirota, N., Mori, H., and Williams, G. (1980): Induction of cancer of the glandular stomach in rats with an extract of nitrate treated fish. *J. Nat. Cancer Inst.,* 64:163–167.
45. Weisburger, J. H. (1977): Vitamin C and prevention of nitrosamine formation. *Lancet,* 17:607.
46. Weisburger, J. H., and Raineri, R. (1975): Dietary factors and the etiology of gastric cancer. *Cancer Res.,* 35:3469–3474.
47. Wojewski, A., and Roessler, R. (1965): Treatment of post-irradiation lesions of the urinary bladder. *Pol. Med. Sci. Hist. Bull.,* 8:110–113.

*Nutrition and Cancer: Etiology and Treatment,*
edited by G. R. Newell and N. M. Ellison.
Raven Press, New York © 1981.

# Minerals, Trace Elements, and Cancer

*Mason G. Stout and **Rulon W. Rawson

*LDS Hospital, Salt Lake City, Utah 84143 **Bonneville Center for Research on Cancer Cause and Prevention, University of Utah Research Institute, Salt Lake City, Utah 84108

In the past two decades there has been increasing awareness that environmental exposure to selected inorganic elements or their salts may be causally related to certain neoplastic diseases. In addition, there is evidence that some trace elements may inhibit the action of certain carcinogens. The interest stimulated by these observations has led to a great deal of basic research, not only into the mechanisms of the carcinogenic and mutagenic actions of these inorganic compounds but into the mechanisms by which inhibiting agents protect an organism. Epidemiological evidence for human carcinogenic effects has been presented for arsenic, cadmium, chromium, and nickel compounds. Of these, chromium and nickel salts are probably the most active carcinogens. Other compounds found to be carcinogenic in animal models include cobalt, iron, manganese, lead, titanium, and zinc compounds. In this review, we will consider inorganic compounds implicated in human carcinogenesis, compounds shown to initiate tumor formation in animals, and compounds that have shown a potential for carcinogenesis or mutagenesis in biochemical, chemical, microbiological, or *in vitro* systems. We will review a number of *in vitro* tests that correlate well for mutagenesis and carcinogenesis. The future looks promising for establishment of a battery of *in vitro* tests for screening potentially carcinogenic and mutagenic compounds.

To keep the number of references to a minimum, this review will be organized mainly by citing other reviews (34,35,41,42,44,45,61,136,161,162) and more recent pertinent references, with an emphasis on those reports detailing possible mechanisms of action and proposed approaches that elucidate the molecular activities of various metal ions. We will begin with a description of the most interesting studies on the proposed mechanisms and then, in the sections on each metal, briefly mention the metal's activity in that test. In their review, Furst and Radding (44) included several metals for which only one or two references exist in the literature. We did not include many of these metals in our review because of limited space.

## MECHANISTIC STUDIES OF METAL IONS AS CARCINOGENS

The mechanism of carcinogenesis by the known inorganic carcinogens is not understood, but a few studies implicate an interaction of metal ions with DNA or RNA, causing a change in conformation with subsequent misreading of the template, thus giving rise to changes in the DNA or RNA daughter strands. Some tests involve using a mutagenic strain of bacteria or a mutated natural DNA strand as a template, and results are measured by following mutagenic reversion to the natural form. Other tests evaluate the observed chromosomal breaks of leukocyte or fibroblast chromosomes following *in vivo* or *in vitro* exposure to various inorganic salts.

Eichhorn and co-workers (30,151) have used optical rotatory dispersion (ORD) and ultraviolet (uv) measurements of polyadenylic acid [poly(A)] at pH 6 and 7 with various metal ions to determine the stability and conformation of the complexes formed with those metal ions. Poly(A) is a compound with known, reproducible physical measurements. Because these measurements are subject to many factors, including pH, temperature, and ionic strength of the medium, careful technique is critical to achieving meaningful results. Poly(A) possesses a partially stacked, single-stranded helical structure at neutral and alkaline pHs, and in acidic solution it has a double-stranded helical form. The stability of the single-stranded helical form in alkaline and neutral media is caused by the stacking tendency of the nucleoside bases. Any factor that interferes with base stacking will cause a reduction in the helical form and thus a decrease in the ORD and uv spectra maximums. The random-coil form is produced at elevated temperatures and is indicative of denaturation. These studies were based on the observation that metal ions can bind to the phosphate groups of the backbone of a DNA or RNA strand, to the bases appended thereto, or to both. Most divalent metal ions bind to the phosphate, and many of the transition metal ions bind to both sites. Those that bind only to the phosphate tend to stabilize the double helix (increased Tm) and those that bind to the base destabilize the DNA double helix (decreased Tm), causing a rewinding of the two strands of denatured DNA with resulting displacement or change in absolute absorptivity of the uv and ORD absorption spectra.

With no added electrolyte in the media, the ORD and uv spectra are exquisitely sensitive to ions that change the configuration of poly(A) in solution. $Ca^{2+}$ and $Mg^{2+}$ produce minimal changes (and in the direction of increased stability), whereas $Cu^{2+}$, $Cd^{2+}$, $Ni^{2+}$, $Co^{2+}$, and $Zn^{2+}$ all shift the spectra, indicating instability of the poly(A). The stabilizing effects of $Ca^{2+}$ and $Mg^{2+}$ indicate that the ions are bound to the phosphate only, thus shielding the neighboring groups from the mutual repulsion of their negative charges. The effects of the other ions indicate some binding to the bases. These shifts are consistent with the formation of the random-coil structure for poly(A). The degree of denaturation caused by 2 moles of a given metal ion per mole of poly(A) corresponds to the same degree of denaturation that would be caused by the temperature in centigrade indicated for each ion: $Cu^{2+}$, 89°C; $Cd^{2+}$, 85°C; $Ni^{2+}$, 83°C; $Co^{2+}$, 82°C; $Zn^{2+}$, 60°C; and $Mn^{2+}$, 58°C.

The transition from a single to a double helix occurs near pH 6, when protonation is sufficient to stabilize the double helix. At this transition point, any change in ionic strength or pH is readily seen. Measurements at pH 6 with $5 \times 10^{-3}$ $M$ $Na^+$ showed that $Ni^{2+}$ and $Co^{2+}$ stabilize the single helix, $Mg^{2+}$, $Ca^{2+}$, $Mn^{2+}$, and $Zn^{2+}$ give a mixture of double and single helices, and $Cu^{2+}$ and $Cd^{2+}$ tend to produce the random-coil structure. These measurements indicate the strength of the metal-to-phosphate bond at pH 6, which, in turn, draws the electrons of the phosphate group toward the metal ion and thereby destabilizes the third hydrogen bond in the poly(A), which exists between the phosphate oxygen and the second hydrogen of the 6-amino group of adenine.

Sirover and Loeb (152,153) used poly(A)·oligo (dT) {poly[d(A-T)]} as a known template and avian myeloblastosis virus (AMV) DNA polymerase to determine the effect of various metal ions on the fidelity and accuracy of the AMV DNA polymerase in copying the poly[d(A-T)]. This method appears to be reliable in determining the potential for mutagenesis or carcinogenesis of metal ions. AMV DNA polymerase was chosen because it is well characterized, incorporates noncomplementary deoxynucleotides as single base substitutions, and lacks any associated exodeoxynuclease activity that might excise noncomplementary bases after incorporation, thus masking the errors of polymerization. Sirover and Loeb demonstrated that all the known metal mutagens or carcinogens were positive and all the noncarcinogenic metals were negative, and that of three potential mutagens one was positive ($Cu^{2+}$) and two were negative ($Fe^{2+}$ and $Zn^{2+}$). The degree of fidelity was determined using an $\alpha$-$^{32}$P-labeled complementary deoxynucleotide of low specific activity and a noncomplementary deoxynucleotide labeled with $^3$H of high specific activity in the reaction mixture. The differential measurement gave the degree of incorporation of the noncomplementary nucleotide, which was compared to the known degree of fidelity for the polymerase. Compounds that increased the error frequency by greater than 30% at two or more concentrations were scored as positive. The results for each metal tested are presented in the section for that metal, below.

Weymouth and Loeb (182) copied a natural $\phi$X174 DNA template using *Escherichia coli* DNA polymerase. They demonstrated that the substitution of $Mn^{2+}$ for $Mg^{2+}$ when an excess of deoxycytidine triphosphate was present significantly increased the error frequency at the *am 3* locus. This extension of Sirover and Loeb's earlier work with a natural DNA template makes that work even more exciting.

Another test for possible carcinogenicity or mutagenicity was performed by Hoffman and Niyogi (63). The authors used *E. coli* RNA polymerase with calf thymus DNA, which is not sigma factor-dependent, or phage $T_4$ DNA, which is sigma factor-dependent, as a template. They used the incorporation of [$^{14}$C]AMP to measure total RNA synthesis and [$\alpha$-$^{32}$P]ATP and [$\alpha$-$^{32}$P]GTP to measure RNA chain initiation. The authors suggest that new initiation sites on the DNA template are made available by the carcinogenic or mutagenic metals, which bind to the nucleic acid bases, altering the DNA configuration and potentially providing an increase in RNA chain initiating sites. Because these RNA chains start at abnormal sites, they are shorter and there is an overall decrease in absolute RNA quantity. The authors tested five known carcinogens or mutagens (Pb, Cd, Co, Cu, Mn) and five metals that are not carcinogens (Zn, Mg, Li, Na, K), according to the assay of Sirover and Loeb (152), and found complete agreement with the DNA fidelity assay.

In another screening procedure, using Syrian hamster embryo cells (HEC) and assessing the transformation of these cells by simian adenovirus SA7 and various metallic salts, Casto et al. (22) obtained results that correlate well with those of the mutagenesis/carcinogenesis assays of Sirover and Loeb (152), as well as with the combined data extracted from several animal studies of metal ion carcinogens and mutagens. This assay had previously shown good correlative data with organic carcinogens and has more recently been used with inorganic compounds.

Paton and Allison (124) examined chromosomal damage in human lymphocytes and fibroblasts caused by metals and metal ions. They showed that, of the ten metal salts tested, only arsenic, antimony, and tellurium salts cause chromosomal breaks. These chromatid breaks were frequent with the active salts and were often located near the ends of chromosomes. The authors noted that chromatid exchanges were more common in leukocytes than in fibroblasts. No biochemical explanation was offered for this observation.

Several researchers have used microbial systems in attempts to determine the mutagenic or carcinogenic potential of various metal salts. For an excellent review, see Sunderman (161). In this type of biological test, a strain of bacteria is used that has an easily evaluated mutation because of its single locus. The strain's rate of spontaneous reversion to the native state has been determined by observation. The mutated strain is exposed to the compound being evaluated and any increase in reversion is noted by observing the colonies grown after exposure. The increase in reversion is a measure of the mutation caused by that compound.

*Bacillus subtilis* strains H17 and M45 were used by Nishioka (114), following the assay of Kada et al. (74) for initial screening. The positive metal ions tested were $As^{3+}$, $As^{5+}$, $Cd^{2+}$, $Cr^{6+}$, $Hg^{2+}$, $Mn^{2+}$, and $Mo^{6+}$. It is interesting that strongly suspected carcinogenic salts, such as $Be^{2+}$, $Co^{2+}$, $Cr^{3+}$, $Ni^{2+}$, and $Pb^{2+}$, yielded negative results. Nishioka then tested those compounds that were active in the *B. subtilis* test in three strains of *E. coli* that have different DNA repair capacities but have a common tryptophan deficiency that is suppressible by ochre suppressor mutations. The two strains in which the rec-A postreplication repair pathway is intact showed induced tryptophan reversion mutations when treated with $As^{3+}$, $Cr^{6+}$, or $Mo^{6+}$. This list was expanded by Yagi and Nishioka (186) to include $As^{3+}$, $Cd^{2+}$, $Cr^{6+}$, $Hg^{2+}$, $Mo^{6+}$, $Se^{6+}$, $Te^{6+}$, and $V^{4+}$.

Kanematsu and Kada (76) have reported on several newly demonstrated active mutagens in the "rec-assay" using *B. subtilis* (M45) and the wild strain (H17). The mutagens include cesium chloride, germanium tetrachloride, osmic acid, chloroplatinic acid, rhodium trichloride, antimony compounds ($Sb_2O_3$, $SbCl_5$, $SbCl_3$), tellurium compounds ($Na_2H_4TeO_6$, $Na_2TeO_3$), and vanadium compounds ($VOCl_2$, $V_2O_5$, and $NH_4VO_3$). Some of these mutagenic compounds were tested in the *E. coli* B/r WP2 *try* and WP2 *try hcr* reverse mutation assay. $VOCl_2$ and $RhCl_3 \cdot 3H_2O$ were shown to cause base change mutations.

The properties of the various metals are described in this chapter in alphabetical order in three groupings: first, those metals closely associated with human carcinogenesis; second, those associated with carcinogenesis in animal studies; and third, those associated with positive biochemical tests or possibly useful in the prevention or treatment of carcinogenesis.

## METALS ASSOCIATED WITH HUMAN CARCINOGENESIS

### Arsenic

Inorganic arsenic is one of the few simple chemical agents implicated epidemiologically in human cancer. Exposure to arsenic has been implicated as a cause of cancer among employees of a copper smelter (87,113), among gold miners (120), in agricultural operations (46), in the manufacture of pesticides (122), and by accidental inclusion in food substances (175). Arsenic occurring naturally in drinking water has been causally associated with skin cancer in Taiwan, Argentina, Chile, and Poland (3,48,134,173,174,187,188). Fowler's solution, which contains arsenic and has been used to treat asthma and psoriasis, has been causally related to skin cancer (39).

Diseases associated with the above exposures include lung, skin, lymphatic, and visceral cancers. The estimates by various researchers of the latent period for human tumors associated with arsenic are quite long. Lee and Fraumeni (87) estimated average latent periods of 34 years for heavy exposure, 39 years for medium exposure, and 41 years for light exposure, and Tokudome and Kuratsune's (170) estimates of 34 years for medium exposure and 45 years for light exposure correlate quite well. Newman et al. (113) have demonstrated the interesting relationship between poorly differentiated epidermoid bronchogenic carcinomas and arsenic exposure.

Although circumstantial epidemiological evidence implicates arsenic as a carcinogen, to date no good animal models for arsenic carcinogenesis have been reported. The lymphocytes of smelter workers exposed to arsenic show a 6.7-fold increase in chromosomal aberrations. The effects of other exposures, including tobacco smoke, have not been investigated (11,116). Petres et al. (127) earlier demonstrated chromosomal aberrations in wine growers exposed to arsenic and in psoriasis patients who used Fowler's solution. Paton and Allison (124) have demonstrated chromosomal breaks in leukocytes and fibroblasts *in vitro* using arsenic. In workers whose last exposure to arsenic occurred up to 30 years prior to examination, chromosomes still showed increased numbers of aberrations (126). The finding of chromosomal changes in leukocytes, as well as in other cells, suggests that arsenic alters stem cells permanently without having a marked effect on mitosis. There is increased endoreduction, as demonstrated by an increase in tetraploid cells. The mechanism for damage offered by Petres and co-workers (126) is that arsenic inhibits cell metabolism and has a particularly strong affinity for sulfhydryl-containing enzymes. The authors also speculated on the possible substitution of $AsO_4^{3-}$ for $PO_4^{3-}$ in DNA and RNA on the basis of the observed blockage of the incorporation of $^{32}P$ nucleotides into DNA by large concentrations of arsenate. These studies indicate that DNA polymerase is more strongly inhibited by $AsO_4^{3-}$ than is RNA polymerase. The possibility that arsenate might replace phosphate in the backbone of DNA or RNA was originally proposed by Petres et al. (127) and later by Rosen (139). Rosen speculated that if such incorporation did indeed take place, it could increase the instability of the DNA or RNA chain.

Both lymphocytic tumors and leukemias have been reported in mice given sodium arsenate intravenously or subcutaneously (121), and in a study by Baroni et al. (7), skin papillomas developed in a small proportion of mice whose skins were painted with sodium arsenate in solution with Tween 60 or Tween 80.

Schiller et al. (144) and Fowler et al. (37) have recently shown that arsenic tends to accumulate in the mitochondria of liver cells, where it decreases the activity of pyruvate dehydrogenase, which, in turn, decreases the carbon flow through the TCA cycle, with an overall decrease in the storage of triglycerides. Furthermore, arsenic depresses hepatic δ-amino-levulinic acid (ALA) synthetase and heme synthetase activities in male rats. Concomitantly, urinary uroporphyrin levels increase up to 12-fold and coproporphyrins as much as ninefold. There is a uniquely greater increase in urinary uroporphyrin than in copropophyrin, and Woods and Fowler (185) suggest that the unusual ratio of uroporphyrin to coproporphyrin may be used in the future in a specific test for arsenic poisoning. In all other abnormally increased urinary uroporphyrin and coproporphyrin states, the ratio is reversed.

Studies with arsenic in bacterial systems have shown that $As^{3+}$ and $As^{5+}$ are positive in the postreplication repair assay of Nishioka (114) and negative in the frame-shift Salmonella typhimurium test of Lofroth and Ames (97), whereas only $As^{3+}$ is positive in the dark repair assay systems of Jung et al. (73).

Sunderman (161) speculates that arsenic may be a cocarcinogen rather than a direct carcinogen as are other carcinogenic metal ions. Indeed, when one combines all these facts with the reports that no animal models for reproducible carcinogenesis exist for arsenic, that prolonged chromosomal aberrations are found in workers exposed to arsenic, that there is a 25- to 40-year latency for cancer formation, that cigarette smoking is synergistic with arsenic exposure, and that arsenic appears to have one of its major effects on DNA repair enzymes, then Sunderman's hypothesis certainly has merit. Rossman and colleagues (142) have also pointed out the likelihood that arsenic is a cocarcinogen.

The actual role of arsenic in metabolism remains to be determined. There is a great deal of evidence that arsenic may be an essential element in nutrition. In a chapter entitled "The Arsenic Problems," D. V. Frost (40) details many of the misconceptions that have been perpetuated about arsenic and points out the fact that various animals have dietary requirements for arsenic. A recent report by Mertz (105) notes that lack of dietary arsenic leads to cardiomyopathy in lactating goats. It appears that there is a great need to establish definite limits for safe levels of arsenic in our diets and environment. If arsenic is indeed an essential element, a level too low might be more devastating than one too high. Pories et al. (131) reviewed several metals that appear to inhibit neoplastic growth. They noted that Kanisawa and Schroeder (77) found that mice whose diets were supplemented with arsenic had a decreased incidence of all tumors, especially lung adenomata and carcinomata. Furthermore, the arsenic-fed animals were smaller than controls.

The oxidation state of the carcinogenic species of arsenic remains to be determined, although both $As^{3+}$ and $As^{5+}$ inhibit bacterial strains deficient in DNA repair enzymes (114). Cell transformations have been reported only for $As^{3+}$ (124).

### Cadmium

Although cadmium is a relatively rare metal, it is used in many manufacturing industries. In the United States alone, an estimated 100,000 workers are exposed to cadmium-related products (1974 NIOSH Priority List for Development of Criteria for Toxic Substances and Physical Agents). Kipling and Waterhouse (78) have reported the occurrence of four prostatic cancers in 248 workers exposed to cadmium for more than one year. This was more than three times the expected number of prostatic carcinomas. A report by Lemen et al. (90) supports the thesis that cadmium exposure increases the risk of prostatic cancer.

Evidence for cadmium-associated renal cancers in man has been reported by Kolonel (80). He found an increased incidence of renal cancer among cigarette smokers, which he attributed to trace amounts of cadmium in cigarettes. Further studies are needed to support or refute this hypothesis. Ellis et al. (31) have demonstrated that smokers have a body burden of cadmium twice that of non-smokers.

In animal studies, a number of researchers have demonstrated the formation of interstitial cell testicular tumors in mice and rats 14 to 20 months after the administration of cadmium salts (56,79,98,137). Cadmium metal injected into the thigh muscle of hooded strain rats produced a high incidence of rhabdomyosarcomas (60). A later paper from the same laboratory (179) showed that, after physiologic dissolution of the metals from the injection sites, between 70% and 90% of each of the active metals is found within the cell nuclei. More than half of this amount is found in the nucleoli, with the remainder in the nuclear sap and chromatin.

Zasukhina and co-workers (189) claimed that, although they found cadmium salts to have no direct mutagenic effects, when rat embryo cell cultures were first infected with Kilham parvovirus (KRV) and then treated with $3.5 \times 10^{-6}$ $M$ CdCl$_2$, there was a fivefold increase in the natural mutation frequency. This result was nearly twice the additive effect of both parameters individually. Most of the chromosomal changes were breaks and chromatid exchanges. The authors pointed out that about 30% of the population carries parvovirus antibodies.

In another culture, using live Chinese hamster fibroblasts, (CHC), Rohr and Bauchinger (138) demonstrated that 16 hours after the cells were treated with Cd$^{2+}$ the mitotic index was reduced and the stickiness and pycnosis of the chromosomes increased. The assay of Casto et al. (22,23), using Syrian HEC with transformation by simian adenovirus SA7, showed Cd$^{2+}$ to be one of the most active of all metal salts tested in enhancing the transformation. Casto et al. (22) compared their results found with 38 metallic salts to those of Sirover and Loeb (152); the DNA polymerase fidelity was in excellent agreement as to which ions were mutagenic or carcinogenic as well as noncarcinogenic.

As implied in the preceding paragraph, Cd$^{2+}$ was positive in the fidelity-inhibition assay of Sirover and Loeb (152). Paton and Allison (124) demonstrated no increase in chromosomal breaks in leukocytes or fibroblasts incubated with Cd$^{2+}$ salt solution. Eichhorn and co-workers (30) reported physical measurements with mixtures of poly(A) and Cd$^{2+}$ indicative of random-coil structure, which indicates a strong bond by Cd$^{2+}$ to both the phosphate and the nucleoside bases. In an extension of Eichhorn's work, Murray and Flessel (109) have demonstrated that $10^{-3}$ $M$ Cd$^{2+}$ induces changes in the uv spectra of a solution of poly(I) and poly(C,U), indicating that Cd$^{2+}$ causes base mispairing. The assay of Hoffman and Niyogi (63), described in the introduction, was positive for Cd$^{2+}$ as a carcinogen. This test system used the initiation of RNA synthesis by $E.$ $coli$ RNA polymerase with calf thymus or phage T4 DNA templates.

## Chromium

Many reports associating chromium with cancer of the respiratory tract have been published since Lehmann's (88) initial paper. One of the earliest works reporting data on a large series was that of Baetjer (4,5). Baetjer found a 21.8% incidence of respiratory tract cancer in a group of men employed in the chromate-producing and chrome pigment industries, compared to an expected incidence of 1.4%. Mancuso and Hueper (102) published a study showing a 15-fold greater incidence of lung cancer deaths among chromate workers than in the general population in the same geographical area. They estimated the period from onset of exposure to diagnosis of lung cancer to be 10.6 years. They causally implicated insoluble chromium compounds, such as chromite dust and chromic oxides, in these tumors. Hueper (65) cited 123 cases of lung cancer among chromate workers and showed the histological types to be squamous-cell in 37% and adenocarcinoma in 9%, with the other 52% a mixture of anaplastic, undifferentiated, and round-cell cancers. All nasal cavity carcinomas were squamous-cell. A report from the USSR by Pokrovskaia and Shabynina (129) linked chromium ferroalloy industrial exposure with increased incidences of cancers of the esophagus, stomach, and lung. Okubo (118) described an apparent increase in cancer of the pancreas and liver among chromate workers in Japan. We have recently observed a 35-year-old man, who never used tobacco or alcohol, who had a squamous carcinoma of the tongue. He reported that for 10 years he had worked as a decorator hanging drapes, and while hanging them he had held zinc chromate screws in his mouth.

In animal studies, pulmonary adenomas were produced in mice exposed to calcium chromate dust (112) and also in guinea pigs exposed to potassium dichromate–sodium chromate dust. Calcium chromate suspended in cholesterol was used by Laskin et al. (85) to produce squamous-cell cancers of the bronchus in rats by the intrabronchial pellet technique. Exposure by other workers (156) of rats, mice, guinea pigs, and rabbits to an atmosphere simulating a chromate foundry failed to produce any malignancies.

In biochemical studies and studies of human carcinogenesis, hexavalent chromium is the species generally felt to be carcinogenic. In the Syrian HEC transformation assay with simian adenovirus SA7 (22), three chromate salts ($Pb^{2+}$, $K^+$, and $Zn^{2+}$) were positive. In a battery of microbiological tests, Nestmann et al. (111) demonstrated the mutagenic activity of $PbCrO_4$ in the *S. typhimurium* $His^+$ reversion (mutation), *S. cerevisiae* D5 reversion (recombination), and *E. coli* Trp reversion fluctuation test (mutation). Since one *Salmonella* test detects frame-shift mutations and the *E. coli* and another *Salmonella* test detect base substitutions, the authors concluded that $PbCrO_4$ can induce both types of mutation. Petrilli and DeFlora (128) had previously demonstrated similar findings in other systems. Green et al. (54) showed $Cr^{6+}$ to be mutagenic in *E. coli* in a fluctuation test. Lofroth and Ames (97) reported that both chromate and dichromate are frame-shift mutagens in *S. typhimurium his*D3052, *his*C3076, and *his*G46 strains. In Nishioka's (114) assay with *B. subtilis*, both potassium chromate and potassium dichromate were positive, with $K_2Cr_2O_4$ being the most potent of all salts tested. When $Cr^{6+}$ was reduced with $Na_2SO_3$, the mutagenic activity was lost. Gene mutation reversion induced by potassium dichromate has also been demonstrated in the eukaryote yeast *Schizosaccharomyces pombe* by Bonatti et al. (18).

Chromium has shown marked ability to participate in or initiate mutagenic or carcinogenic activity in many cell line systems. Casto et al. (22) have shown $Cr^{6+}$ to be one of the most active metal ions in enhancing the activity of simian adenovirus SA7 in transforming Syrian HEC, which enhancement is indicative of mutation or carcinogenesis.

In a series of papers, Levis et al. (91–93) demonstrated that $Cr_2O_7^{2-}$ stimulates the uptake of nucleosides, especially thymidine, into BHK cultured fibroblast cells and human epithelial-like cells (HEp). DNA synthesis is, however, inhibited by $Cr^{6+}$ and $Cr^{3+}$. Cells treated with $Cr^{3+}$ show about 1/20th the uptake of chromium compared to those cells treated with $Cr^{6+}$, but the cells do show accumulations of chromium in both ionic states. Even when $Cr^{6+}$ is the species with which cells are treated, only $Cr^{3+}$ is detectable within the cells. The mechanism for cell penetration by $CrO_4^{2-}$ is thought to be the sulfate transportation pathway according to Jennette (71); once inside the cell the $Cr^{6+}$ is reduced to $Cr^{3+}$ via the microsomal cytochrome P450 enzyme system, with NADH or NADPH as cofactors (71). The mode of action of chromium seems to be dependent not only on the oxidation state but also on the integrity of the system. Intact cell systems appear to require $Cr^{6+}$ for cell-wall penetration, but in disrupted cell component systems $Cr^{3+}$ is more active (55,152). Inside cells, $Cr^{3+}$ is bound to the anionic DNA and this binding may be the mode of mutagenicity (71). Langard (83) showed that $Cr^{3+}$ is the only state in which chromium binds to nucleic acids, and he indicated that $Cr^{3+}$ appears to bind to the phosphate groups of DNA and RNA. He also indicated that the endoplasmic reticulum in the mitrochondria is the site of reduction of $Cr^{6+}$. Adenine and guanine are the principle electron donors.

Venitt and Levy (177) used B/r $Wp_2$: $WP_2uvrA$: $WP_2exrA$ strains of *E. coli,* which differ in their sensitivity to and mutability by uv light, ionizing radiation, and alkylating and arylalkylating agents. The authors obtained negative results using salts of W, Mo, $Cr^{3+}$, Zn, Cd, and Hg. The only active ion in this series was $Cr^{6+}$. The interesting aspect of this research is the conclusion that $Cr^{6+}$ exerts its action by a direct effect on GC base pairs in the DNA, thus causing GC to AT transitions in subsequent DNA replications.

BHK 21 cells grown in the presence of $Cr^{6+}$ grew as shortened fibroblasts and in a random orientation. These changes appeared to be irreversible and the cells, even after removal of $Cr^{6+}$, remained shortened with apparent loss of contact inhibition. The authors felt that this represented a heritable change (38).

The questions still unanswered in chromium carcinogenesis appear to be how the metal ion interferes with cell replication and why the alterations require 10 to 20 years for the tumors to arise. Does the $Cr^{3+}$ cause a misreading of the DNA template, or does it bind tightly enough that separation of the strands cannot take place during mitosis? Is it the very slow reverse cell-wall penetration of $Cr^{3+}$ that makes this one of the most mutagenic of metals once it is in the cells after penetration of the $Cr^{6+}$ and subsequent reduction to $Cr^{3+}$? Is there a point, after human exposure to $Cr^{6+}$, at which the DNA repair enzymes no longer function fully, resulting in tumor formation secondary to the abnormality induced by $Cr^{3+}$ inside the cell?

## Nickel

The original report on cancer among nickel workers was made by Granfell and colleagues in 1932 (52,53). They reported 10 cases of nasal and paranasal sinus cancer. Subsequent reports by Doll (28), Morgan (108), and Doll and co-workers (29) have demonstrated that workers who were exposed to various forms of nickel and its compounds, such as nickel dust, nickel sulfides, nickel oxides, and nickel carbonyl, had a fivefold increase in the incidence of lung cancer and a 100- to 900-fold increase in the incidence of nasal cancer. Workers exposed to the above nickel compounds who later worked in cleaner atmospheres had a slightly reduced chance of getting lung cancer, but no change in the rate of nasal cancer. Workers who were exposed after 1924, when more stringent controls on dust, etc., were instituted, had only a slightly increased risk of lung cancer and no increased risk of nasal cancer. Other types of cancer associated with nickel exposure included soft-tissue sarcomas, gastric cancer, and laryngeal cancer.

A recent update on active and retired nickel workers by Torjussen and Andersen (171) showed that nickel concentrations in body fluids depended on the specific nickel compound to which the individual was exposed. If the inhaled compound was $Ni_3S_2$ or NiO, the highest nickel concentrations were in saliva, whereas with more soluble salts (chloride or sulfate), urine and plasma had the highest concentrations. From biopsies of nasal mucosa, the authors estimated the $T_{1/2}$ for inhaled or ingested nickel to be 3.5 years. They also noted prior work showing nickel to be an essential element for growth, enzymatic actions, and iron absorption from the gastrointestinal tract. A comprehensive update of nickel carcinogenesis was published by Sunderman (159).

In an analysis of particulate waste in the flue dust from a Canadian nickel refinery, Gilman (49) isolated 11 products (FeS, FeO, $Fe_2O_3$, $Ni_3S_2$, NiO, $NiSO_4 \cdot 6H_2O$, CuS, $Cu_2S$, CuO, CoS, and CoO) and determined that $Ni_3S_2$ was the most carcinogenic when injected intramuscularly into rats or mice. The test subsequently developed by Gilman (50) showed that rhabdomyosarcomas and fibrosarcomas induced by injection of $Ni_3S_2$ offer very good experimental models for the study of chemotherapeutic agents.

Sunderman's review (159) contains several references to the quantity of nickel found in tobacco and to the form in which nickel enters the body during tobacco smoking or inhaling snuff. Cigarettes expose smokers not only to nickel but also to several other trace metals, including cadmium. McEwan (104) suggests that nickel exposure is carcinogenic primarily in cigarette smokers.

Sunderman (159) has also speculated on the potential risks of nickel in the alloys in surgical and dental prosthetic devices and wires. Although there is a paucity of evidence for carcinogenesis by these devices, increased nickel concentrations in the tissues adjacent to the devices have been demonstrated. Sunderman cites two case reports of tumors, one a sarcoma and the other a hemangioendothelioma, that developed some 30 years after implantation of nickel-containing steel plates during orthopedic surgery. The screws in each case were of a dissimilar alloy to that in the prosthesis, and may have contributed as unnecessary additional risk secondary to electrolysis.

Animal studies (49,157,163) have shown an increased incidence of sarcomas in 28% of rats subjected to intrafemoral or subcutaneous injection of powdered nickel (64), as well as increases in undifferentiated sarcomas of lung, pleura, liver, pancreas, uterus, and abdominal wall, fibrosarcomas of neck, pinna, and orbit, carcinomas of liver, kidney, and breast, leukemia, and lymphomas (86).

Attempts to produce mutagenic transformations with nickel salts in *E. coli, B. subtilis,* and *S. typhimurium* have consistently proved unsuccessful (54,114). Specific effects in cellular and enzymatic systems include the following:

(A)  A decrease in the fidelity of DNA replication was found with the AMV DNA polymerase system of Sirover and Loeb (152).

(B)  In the Syrian HEC assay using simian adenovirus SA7 for the transformation, $Ni^{2+}$ showed intermediate enhancement (22).

(C)  $Ni(CO)_4$ inhibited DNA-dependent RNA polymerase in hepatic nuclei (9,164).

(D)  Syrian HEC exposed to $Ni_3S_2$ showed neoplastic transformation consisting of tightly packed, crisscrossed, and piled-up colonies that, when injected via the subcutaneous route into nude mice, produced fibrosarcomas (25).

(E)  $Ni^{2+}$ inhibited interferon synthesis in mouse L929 cells when challenged by Newcastle disease virus (132,172).

(F)  In three lines of human lymphoblastoid cells (one normal and two leukemic), the presence of $Ni^{2+}$ in the medium made a marked difference in susceptibility to the effects of X-irradiation of normal and leukemic cells, especially when the $Ni^{2+}$ was added after X-irradiation (12–16).

(G)  Eichhorn et al. (30) and Shin et al. (151) demonstrated that $Ni^{2+}$ in solution with poly(A) at neutral and alkaline pH binds to the phosphate group and to the nucleoside bases, thus causing instability of the helix, as shown by the ORD and uv spectra, whereas at acid pH the $Ni^{2+}$ appears to bind only to the phosphate and produces a single helix.

(H)  Nickel suppresses cell division and increases abnormal mitoses, as indicated by distorted bipolar and multipolar spindles, C-metaphase-like shapes, lagging chromosomes, and unequal cytoplasmic divisions in rat embryo muscle cells. Dissolution of the spindle mechanism is indicated by arrest of cell division in telophase and post-telophase. This type of chromosomal aberration is consistent with increased somatic mutation (carcinogen or mutagen) (167).

(I)  Webb and co-workers (60,179,180) have shown that when powdered nickel is injected into the thighs of rats, a high incidence of rhabdomyosarcomas results. This tumor-forming capability is shared by cobalt and cadmium, whereas iron, copper, zinc, manganese, beryllium, and tungsten are not carcinogenic under these conditions.

(J)  Nickel carbonyl ($Ni(CO)_4$), when given by IV injection to rats, shows marked inhibition of RNA synthesis by liver hepatocytes. This effect has also been demonstrated *in vitro* and is thought to be related to the effect of $Ni^{2+}$ on RNA polymerase activity. A 75% inhibition of [$^{14}C$]orotic acid incorporation into RNA and an 18% inhibition of [$^{14}C$]leucine incorporation into hepatic microsomal proteins was noted (9,10,158,164).

## METALS ASSOCIATED WITH ANIMAL CARCINOGENESIS

### Beryllium

Evidence for beryllium carcinogenesis is questionable at best. The only study that has implicated beryllium as a carcinogen in man was that of Mancuso (101), which showed an inverse relationship between degree of carcinogenesis and time of employment. A report by Bayliss not yet public (150) has recently implicated beryllium as a carcinogen. There is still much controversy over this report. In earlier reports by Bayliss (8), no association between beryllium and cancer was noted.

Animal testing has shown that pulmonary tumors are formed in rats and monkeys that inhale aerosols of beryllium salts (66,178). Gardner and Heslington (47) and Barnes et al. (6) reported that suspensions of beryllium oxide or zinc beryllium silicate injected intravenously into rabbits resulted in the development of malignant osteogenic sarcomas.

In the DNA replicative-fidelity assay using AMV DNA polymerase (152,153), beryllium did cause a decrease in fidelity. The results with beryllium using *Micrococcus luteus* DNA polymerase also showed a decrease in fidelity (99). In the transformation of Syrian HEC by simian adenovirus SA7, beryllium was found to be one of the intermediate enhancers of transformation (22). In Nishioka's (114) rec-assay, beryllium was negative in the *B. subtilis* strains tested. Witschi and co-workers (103,183,184) demonstrated marked inhibition in DNA synthesis if the beryllium was given shortly after partial hepatectomy. Neither RNA synthesis nor protein synthesis was affected. The apparent block was in the production of new enzymes for DNA synthesis, not in enzymes already present. Beryllium was taken up preferentially by lysozymes and nuclei in rat liver.

### Cobalt

Cobalt has not been implicated in human carcinogenesis, but there have been reports of the induction of rhabdomyosarcomas and fibrosarcomas in animals injected with cobalt and its salts (49,58,160). Studies by Heath and co-workers (60,179) on the distribution pattern of cobalt in rat tissues following injection of cobalt metal powder into the thigh muscle showed high concentrations of cobalt in liver, kidney, and spleen. Heath (59) showed that $Co^{2+}$ causes an extensive reversal of the normal process by which embryonic myoblasts associate to form a malignant variant from the breakdown of mature fibers to promote tumorigenesis. On fractionation of the cells in which cobalt accumulated, Heath found 97% of the incorporated metal accounted for and 52% of the cobalt in the nucleus or nucleolus. He suggested that the effect of $Co^{2+}$ might be on "the processing of the ribosomal precursor RNA."

Hoffman and Niyogi (63) listed cobalt as one of the metals that enhance the initiation of new RNA chain formation at concentrations that decrease the overall synthesis of RNA. Their findings are in good agreement with those of Sirover and Loeb (152), who used AMV DNA polymerase with a synthetic poly[d(A-T)] template and found that $Co^{2+}$ enhanced infidelity in new DNA synthesis. When Murray and Flessel (109) tried to extend Sirover and Loeb's work with $Co^{2+}$ to other synthetic polymers, no data were obtainable because of precipitation with $Co^{2+}$. In a paper by Casto et al. (22), $Co^{2+}$ was found to be one of the intermediate but positive metals that enhanced the transformation of Syrian HEC by simian adenovirus SA7. Komczynski et al. (81) and Glass (51) showed that $Co^{2+}$ causes aberrations in nuclear chromatin and nucleoli in broad beans *(Vicia faba)*.

Shin et al. (151) found that only $Co^{2+}$ and $Ni^{2+}$ stabilize the configuration of poly(A) in the single helix at pH 6, which indicates interference with one of the hydrogen bonds. At neutral and alkaline pH, $Co^{2+}$ binds to both the phosphate and the heterocyclic base.

The *B. subtilis* assay of Nishioka (114) and a test for the production of lung adenomas in strain A mice by Stoner et al. (157) were negative for mutagenesis with cobalt.

## Iron

In humans, three cases of sarcoma arising at the site of Fe–dextran injections have been reported (100,160). One of these tumors was similar in histologic type to tumors induced in animals by Fe–dextran injection (84). In addition, there have been reports from England and Sweden of increased incidences of respiratory cancer in iron miners, but because of several uncontrolled parameters in both studies, no positive correlation could be drawn (19,72). MacKinnon (100) reported studies with hamsters, rats, mice, and rabbits that also suggested Fe–dextran is carcinogenic.

The cellular systems showed $Fe^{2+}$ to be weakly positive in the Syrian HEC assay of Casto et al. (22). It was mutagenic in *S. typhimurium*, causing reverse mutations in TA-1537 and TA-1538 but not in TA-1535 (21). Iron salts gave negative results in the AMV DNA polymerase assay of Sirover and Loeb (152), the *B. subtilis* mutation test of Nishioka (114), and the chromosomal damage assay of Paton and Allison (124). It failed to produce lung adenomas in strain A mice (157).

## Lead

Notwithstanding the ubiquitousness of lead in the environment and the frequency of lead poisoning, especially in children, the only report that implicates lead as a possible human carcinogen is that of Cooper (24). His data covered 7,032 men with a minimum of one year of employment at six lead smelters and ten battery plants. There were simultaneous exposures to arsenic, cadmium, and sulfur dioxide that could not be quantified. The study showed "deaths from malignant neoplasms were somewhat elevated in both groups." The incidence of respiratory and gastrointestinal cancers was greater in the smelter workers. No increase in neoplasms of kidney or brain was found, as had been noted in laboratory animals.

In laboratory animals, the main site of neoplasia has been the kidney (20, 32,190). Lead plus 2-acetylaminofluorene produced gliomas in the CNS system of rats (123).

Severe chromosomal aberrations were noted in cultures of lymphocytes from zinc workers who had also been exposed to lead and cadmium (26). In follow-up studies with cultures of human lymphocytes, lead did not induce chromosomal aberrations *in vitro,* but in calcium-deficient mice both lead and zinc caused chromosomal aberrations in marrow leukocytes.

In the AMV DNA polymerase fidelity assay of Sirover and Loeb (152), lead was classified as a possible mutagen, whereas in the Syrian HEC transformation assay (22,23) it caused enhanced transformation. In Hoffman and Niyogi's (63) assay of RNA chain initiation and total RNA synthesis, lead was shown to fulfill the criteria for mutagenesis. Lead was the most active metal ion tested (as the subacetate) for the induction of lung adenomas in strain A mice in the assay of Stoner et al. (157). Lead, as the chromate salt, was a mutagen in several strains of *E. coli, S. typhimurium,* and *S. ceravisiae* (111).

## Manganese

There have been no reports of human carcinogenesis with manganese, but Furst (43) reported the formation of fibrosarcomas at the site of manganous acetylacetate injection. Neither manganese powder nor manganese dioxide in trioctanoin suspension was active, however. Manganous sulfate was shown by Stoner et al. (157) to produce a significant increase in the average number of lung adenomas in strain A mice. The authors concluded that it was weakly carcinogenic.

Sunderman et al. (165), in studying the effects of various metal dusts on the formation of sarcomas in rats injected with $Ni_3S_2$, noted that 96% to 100% of rats injected with $Ni_3S_2$ plus aluminum, copper or chromium dust developed sarcomas at the injection site within 24 months, whereas only 67% of those receiving manganese dust with $Ni_3S_2$ developed sarcomas; control animals developed no sarcomas. The role of manganese dust in this study remains to be determined, but the authors speculated that a direct displacement of nickel by manganese, macrophage stimulation by manganese, or antigonization of nickel-induced RNA polymerase inhibition by manganese might be the mechanism.

Casto et al. (22) noted that $Mn^{2+}$ enhances the transformation of Syrian HEC by simian adenovirus SA7. In the assay of RNA chain initiation with concomitant reduction of overall RNA synthesis for potential mutagenic compounds (63), $MnCl_2$ was one of the active compounds. Rao et al. (135) have shown that $Mn^{2+}$ significantly alters the ability of *E. coli* RNA polymerase to distinguish between ribo- and deoxyribonucleotides for incorporation into RNA. The manganous ion is also one of the ions that increases the infidelity of AMV DNA polymerase in copying poly[d(A-T)] (152). In an extension of Sirover and Loeb's work by Weymouth and Loeb (182), the manganous ion was found to increase the error frequency of *E. coli* DNA polymerase in copying a natural DNA strand from $\phi$X174 DNA containing amber mutant by about 10-fold over $Mg^{2+}$, as determined by the reversion frequency of the progeny DNA. In the rec-assay with *B. subtilis* of Nishioka (114), $Mn^{2+}$ was mildly positive for mutations. Putrament et al. (133) demonstrated that $Mn^{2+}$ is mutagenic in the eukaryote *Saccharomyces cerevisiae*.

Eichhorn et al. (30) and Shin et al. (151) noted that $Mn^{2+}$ is one of the metal ions that causes a mixture of single and double helices at acid pH. At neutral or alkaline pH, it causes a decrease in the ORD or uv spectra, indicative of a decrease in base stacking of poly(A). When Murray and Flessel (109) studied the effects of metal ions on base mispairing between poly(I) and poly(C,U) or poly(C,A), $Mn^{2+}$ and $Cd^{2+}$ showed increases in base mispairing. In his review, Sunderman (162) noted that Blagoi et al. (17) ascribed the altered thermal denaturation of bovine spleen DNA by $Mn^{2+}$ to the interaction of $Mn^{2+}$ with the GC base pairs. In a review of manganese mutagenesis (33), Flessel noted that manganese is a relatively nontoxic compound but "a potent mutagen whose genetic effects are strongly influenced by the condition of the organism." The mutagenesis of $Mn^{2+}$ is completely antagonized by equimolar $Mg^{2+}$, suggesting that the ions compete for the same enzyme sites. Flessel noted that the mutagenicity is primarily via base-pair substitution-type interactions.

## Zinc

Although there are no reports of carcinogenesis by zinc, Pories (130) has suggested that serum zinc levels may prove helpful in the diagnosis of certain types of cancer. In prostatic hyperplasia, zinc and magnesium levels are high, whereas they are low in cancer of the prostate, liver, or lung. In leukemia, zinc levels are low and rise with patient response to treatment. Petering (125) has noted that zinc is required for the proliferation of both normal and tumor cells, but in tumor growth there is a difference between serum zinc levels during initial carcinogenesis and later tumor growth. He theorizes that, since zinc is required for the mobilization of vitamin A from liver cells, low serum zinc levels during exposure to carcinogens might facilitate tumor initiation; on the other hand, zinc-deficient animals show a marked slowing of tumor growth, which may be the result of the fact that both DNA and RNA polymerases are zinc-requiring enzymes. DeWys and Pories (27) have demonstrated slowing of growth in Walker 256 carcinosarcoma, Lewis lung tumor, various leukemias, and ascites carcinomas in conditions of zinc deficiency.

In animal studies, zinc has produced testicular teratomas when injected intratesticularly (154). In the test of Stoner et al. (157), zinc failed to produce lung adenomas in strain A mice. Severe chromosomal aberrations were noted by Deknudt (26) in the lymphocytes of zinc workers. In follow-up work, zinc produced similar chromosomal aberrations in normal lymphocytes *in vitro* and in C57B1 mice. Deknudt noted that calcium deficiency was an important contributing factor for tumor growth.

Zinc was shown to be mutagenic in the indicator *Salmonella* strains of Ames, and the changes were due to frame-shift mutations (75). In the *B. subtilis* rec-assay, Nishioka (114) showed zinc to be negative. Casto et al. (22) showed zinc to be in the intermediate group in enhancing the transformation of Syrian HEC by simian adenovirus SA7. The AMV DNA polymerase fidelity assay of Sirover and Loeb (151) showed zinc to be negative, as did the RNA initiation–total synthesis test of Hoffman and Niyogi (63). Shin et al. (151) demonstrated that $Zn^{2+}$ at acid pH gave a mixture of single and double helices, and at neutral or alkaline pH appeared to bind to both phosphate and heterocyclic bases, indicating some instability induction. In Murray and Flessel's (109) assay with poly(I) and poly(C,U) or poly(C,A), zinc showed no tendency to enhance mispairing.

## METALS ASSOCIATED WITH POSITIVE TESTS

### Aluminum

Flessel stated, in his chapter "Metals as Mutagens" (34), that aluminum causes chromosomal aberrations or abnormal cell division, although no specific reference was cited. Aluminum foil implanted into rats produces local fibrosarcomas (117). This induction very likely occurs via the "Oppenheimer effect," in which fibrosarcomas are produced by nondegraded foreign-body implantation in animals (119).

Negative results with aluminum include its failure to enhance the simian adenovirus SA7 transformation of Syrian HEC (22), lack of mutagenicity in Nishioka's (114) assay in *B. subtilis,* and failure to increase AMV DNA polymerase infidelity in copying poly[d(AT)] (152).

### Antimony

Antimony was shown by Paton and Allison (124) to increase chromosomal breakage in human leukocytes. Recently, Casto et al. (22) found $Sb^{3+}$ to be one of the most active ions in their test for enhancement of Syrian HEC transformation by simian adenovirus SA7. Nishioka (114) found $Sb^{3+}$ to be negative in the *B. subtilis* mutation assay.

### Copper

Furst and Radding (44), at the 1979 IABS conference, stated that although copper is not generally carcinogenic, skin painting with copper compounds does enhance papilloma formation. This is the only reference known to the authors for any tumor enhancement by copper. Serum copper levels, like those of zinc, have been used to follow various hematologic cancers, particularly Hodgkin's disease and the leukemias. Flynn (36) noted that serum copper levels can be fairly well correlated with tumor growth and regression in breast, colorectal, and lung cancer.

In the carcinogenicity test in strain A mice of Stoner et al. (157), $Cu^{2+}$ was noted to be negative. The Syrian HEC transformation by simian adenovirus SA7 showed $Cu^{2+}$ to be intermediate in its ability to enhance transformation (22). In both the AMV DNA polymerase fidelity assay of Sirover and Loeb (152) and the RNA initiation–total synthesis assay of Hoffman and Niyogi (63), $Cu^{2+}$ was positive for mutagenesis; however, in the *B. subtilis* mutagen assay of Nishioka, $Cu^{2+}$ was negative. Weed (181) had previously demonstrated that the *B. subtilis* variant 16P (a tryptophan auxotroph) after exposure to $4 \times 10^{-4}$ $M$ $CuSO_4$ was transformed from auxotrophy to prototrophy and was stable after many transfers in the absence of $Cu^{2+}$. In the interaction determination of $Cu^{2+}$ with poly(A), the random-coil configuration was induced at acid pH, and at neutral or alkaline pH the spectra indicated that $Cu^{2+}$ induced the highest degree of denaturation of any metal tested.

## Gallium

Gallium nitrate is currently in Phase 2 trials as an agent against breast carcinoma.

## Germanium

Germanium tetrachloride was recently reported to be positive in the rec-assay using *B. subtilis* M45 (76).

## Magnesium

Seelig (146) noted that areas where the soil is low in $Mg^{2+}$ have increased incidences of human gastric, breast, and bladder cancer and of cattle leukemia. Jasmin (70) reported that when Sprague–Dawley rats were kept on a magnesium-deficient diet for more than 40 days, up to 40% developed thymic lymphosarcomas.

## Mercury

Ethylmercuric chloride, a component of pesticides, was recently shown to induce chromosomal aberrations in mice. It also induced recessive lethal sex-linked mutations in *Drosophila melanogaster,* (89). Two organomercury compounds ($CH_3HgCl$ and $C_6H_5HgOAc$) were positive in the rec-assay with *B.*

*subtilis* (114). This result was confirmed, using an unspecified mercury salt, by Kanematsu and Kada (76). Mercuric chloride was in the intermediate group of compounds capable of enhancing simian adenovirus SA7 transformation of Syrian HEC (22). It did not produce chromosomal breaks in the assay of Paton and Allison (124).

## Molybdenum

Molybdenum, in the form of $Mo_2O_3$, has been shown to be one of the metallic compounds capable of inducing a significant increase in the number of lung adenomas in strain A mice (157). In Nishioka's (114) rec-assay with *B. subtilis,* $K_2MoO_4$ and $(NH_4)_6Mo_7O_{24}$ were positive; however, $MoCl_5$ was negative. Nishioka noted that $(NH_4)_6Mo_7O_{24}$ was also mutagenic in an *E. coli* tester strain.

## Platinum

Rosenberg et al. (141) originally noted that platinum derivatives had marked antitumor activity. After many platinum derivatives were tested, *cis*-platinum diaminodichloride (PDD, NSC-119875) was selected for clinical trial. PDD is one of the newer anticancer agents, and is used particularly against testicular, ovarian, bladder, and head and neck neoplasms, with promise in breast and other cancers (140,166).

As with many cancer chemotherapeutic agents, questions arise concerning the mode of action and potential mutagenicity of platinum. Kanematsu and Kada (76) showed chloroplatinic acid to be mutagenic in the rec-assay with *B. subtilis,* and Casto et al. (22) showed $PtCl_4$ to be in the most active group of compounds capable of enhancing the transformation of Syrian HEC by simian adenovirus SA7. Further evidence for mutagenicity has been obtained for PDD itself by Turnbull et al. (176). To induce chromosomal aberrations and sister chromatid exchanges in Chinese hamster V79-4 cells and to cause Syrian HEC transformation, Meyne and Lockhart (106) noted a preferential binding of the PDD complex to guanine, followed by adenine and cytosine. They noted that chromosome No. 9 had a significant increase in breakpoints and that the breakpoints corresponded to light G-bands. The light G-bands seem to have a correlation with increased G–C content, and the authors speculated that the sites of interaction between PDD and chromosomal DNA may be specific.

## Rhodium

Rhodium was noted to be mutagenic in tester strains of *S. typhimurium* and *E. coli* SP2, as tested by Monti-Bragadin et al. (107). Kanematsu and Kada (76) showed $RhCl_3$ to be mutagenic in the *B. subtilis* (M45) rec-assay, and Nishioka (114) noted that $RhCl_2$ was negative in the same assay.

## Ruthenium

Ruthenium was reported to be mutagenic in the *S. typhimurium* assay of Monti-Bragadin et al. (107) and negative in the *B. subtilis* rec-assay of Nishioka (114).

## Selenium

There are no reports of human tumors induced by selenium. For years it was thought that selenium was a hepatocarcinogen, based on a study by Nelson et al. (110). More recent studies by Sprinker (155), Tinsley and associates (169), and Harr and associates (57) indicate that the tumors Nelson et al. reported were a manifestation of advanced cirrhosis, with resultant nonmalignant, regenerative, adenomatous hyperplasia. Jacobs (67) has demonstrated that the well-known carcinogenesis in rats by dimethylhydrazine (DMH), a procarcinogen, and methylazoxymethanol (MAM), an ultimate carcinogen, is reduced two- to threefold by the addition of 4ppm of $Na_2SeO_3$ to the rats' drinking water. Jacobs (68) also reported that selenium significantly inhibits the mutagenic effects of 2-acetylaminofluorene, N-hydroxyacetylaminofluorene, and N-hydroxyamino-fluorene. The addition of selenite to cultures of human leukocytes caused a threefold reduction in the number of sister chromatid exchanges (SCE) induced with methylmethane sulfonate. In similar studies, Shamberger (147) demonstrated that carcinogenesis by 7,12-dimethylbenz(*a*)anthracene (DMBA) was decreased by the addition of 1 ppm of $Na_2SeO_3$ to the drinking water, and that topical $Na_2SeO_3$ was effective against skin tumors induced by topical DMBA in croton oil, croton resin, or phenol. Schrauzer and Ishmael (145) have reported that only 10% of C3H mice that received 2 ppm of selenite in the drinking water developed spontaneous breast tumors, whereas 82% of those without selenite developed such tumors.

Yagi and Nishioka (186) showed that $Se^{6+}$ was a positive mutagen in a tester strain of *E. coli,* and Lofroth and Ames (97) showed that it caused base-pair substitution mutations, but not frame-shift mutations. Noda et al. (115) confirmed the mutagenicity of $SeO_3^{2-}$ and $SeO_4^{2-}$ in *S. typhimurium* and *B. subtilis.* Paton and Allison (124) were unable to demonstrate chromosomal breakage with $Se^{4+}$ or $Se^{6+}$ in human leukocytes, and neither $Se^{4+}$ nor $Se^{6+}$ was mutagenic in *B. subtilis* when tested by Nishioka (114). Lo et al. (96) demonstrated that sodium selenite causes fragmentation of DNA, can trigger DNA repair synthesis, and induces chromosomal aberrations, as well as inhibiting mitosis in cultured human fibroblasts. They also noted that sodium selenate is a weak inducer of DNA repair.

It appears that selenium has a narrow therapeutic index in animals. Although no selenium deficiency or toxicity diseases have been described for humans, veterinarians have described deficiency diseases in animals, including exudative diathesis associated with edema in chickens, a nutritional muscular dystrophy, liver necrosis in swine, and white-muscle disease in ruminants. In excess, selenium causes hepatic cirrhosis.

Selenium appears to protect animals and humans against various forms of cancer. Shamberger and Willis (149) coordinated the data of Kubota et al. (82) with regional death tables for various forms of cancer. They noted that incidences of cancers of the colon, rectum, and breast were markedly lower, in general, in areas where the soil was high in selenium, and were correspondingly higher in areas where the selenium content was lower. Jansson et al. (69) pointed out that the organs exposed to the environment (rectum, esophagus, tongue, larynx, lip, and colon) have a greater geographic dependence for tumor than those organs not exposed. Shamberger et al. (148) have reported the mean serum level of selenium in 48 normal persons to be $22.9 \pm 3.59$ $\mu$g/100 ml, whereas those for patients with gastrointestinal cancers were considerably lower (e.g., colon, $15.8 \pm 2.06$; stomach, $15.3 \pm 2.1$; liver metastases, 15.0; and pancreas, 13.2).

The exact role of selenium in cancer has yet to be defined. A close relationship between selenium and vitamin E has been suggested (168). Selenium does appear to protect red blood cells against the oxidative hemolysis characteristic of vitamin E deficiency (143). It is known that selenium is a component of glutathione peroxidase (62). The mechanism by which selenium inhibits carcinogenesis needs to be clarified. Most likely this essential element acts as an antioxidant and may be synergistic with other antioxidants, such as vitamin E.

Recent investigations by Andreesen and co-workers (1,2) and Ljungdahl and co-workers (94,95) indicate that selenium and molybdate are components of formate dehydrogenase, an enzyme found in *Clostridium thermoaceticum*. These investigators have demonstrated that these two trace elements are essential to the growth of the bacterial organism and to the function of the bacterial enzyme. Selenium and molybdenum act synergistically to promote the action of the enzyme. Of interest is their observation that molybdenum can be replaced by tungsten. It would be valuable to determine whether molybdenum or tungsten might act synergistically with selenium to inhibit the actions of certain carcinogens on mammalian cells.

### Silver

Reports of carcinogenesis by silver implanted or injected into animals are ambiguous. Casto et al. (22) showed that $Ag^+$ enhances the simian adenovirus SA7 transformation of Syrian HEC, and Sirover and Loeb (152) showed that it decreases the fidelity of AMV DNA polymerase; Nishioka (114) noted that it was negative in the rec-assay with *B. subtilis*.

### Tellurium

Tellurium has been reported by Paton and Allison (124) to increase chromosomal breaks in human leukocytes *in vitro* and to be mutagenic as $Na_2H_4TeO_6$

and $Na_2TeO_3$ in the *B. subtilis* rec-assay by Kanematsu and Kada (76), but negative in the same rec-assay as $TeCl_4$ by Nishioka (114).

## Thallium

Thallium was in the intermediate group of active compounds that enhanced the simian adenovirus SA7 transformation of Syrian HEC (22) and negative in the rec-assay with *B. subtilis* of Nishioka (114).

## Vanadium

Kanematsu and Kada (76) recently reported that $VOCl_2$, $V_2O_5$, and $NH_4VO_3$ are positive in the *B. subtilis* M45 rec-assay for mutagenesis. Sodium metavanadate did not produce chromosomal breakage in the assay of Paton and Allison (124), nor did vanadium$^{3+}$ 2,4-pentanedione cause an increased incidence of lung adenomas in strain A mice, as tested by Stoner et al. (157).

## CONCLUSIONS

The foregoing review of the carcinogenic and carcinogen-inhibiting actions of certain trace elements should open new and challenging research frontiers for cancer epidemiologists and cancer biologists, who should find it exciting to develop, with geochemists, cooperative programs to determine possible relationships of trace elements and metals in soil and water to the geographic distribution of certain human cancers. Cancer biologists should find exciting new frontiers collaborating with enzymologists and molecular biologists on research programs to determine the roles of trace elements in initiating, promoting, and preventing the carcinogenic process.

## REFERENCES

1. Andreesen, J. R., and Ljungdahl, L. G. (1973): Formate dehydrogenase of clostridium thermoaceticum: Incorporation of selenium-75, and the effects of selenite, molybdate, and tungstate on the enzyme. *J. Bacteriol.*, 116:867–873.
2. Andreesen, J. R., Schaupp, A., Neurauter, C., Brown, A., and Ljungdahl, L. G. (1973): Fermentation of glucose, fructose and xylose by clostridium thermoaceticum: Effect of metals on growth yield, enzymes, and the synthesis of acetate from $CO_2$. *J. Bacteriol.*, 114:743–751.
3. Arguello, R. A., Cenget, D. D., and Tello, E. E. (1939): Cancer and regional endemic chronic arsenicism. *Br. J. Dermatol.*, 51:548.
4. Baetjer, A. M. (1950): Pulmonary carcinoma in chromate workers. I. A review of the literature and report of cases. *AMA Arch. Indust. Hyg. Occupat. Med.*, 2:487–504.
5. Baetjer, A. M. (1950): Pulmonary carcinoma in chromate workers. II. Incidence on basis of hospital records. *AMA Arch. Indust. Hyg. Occupat. Med.*, 2:505–516.
6. Barnes, J. M., Denz, F. A., and Sissons, H. A. (1950): Beryllium bone sarcomata in rabbits. *Br. J. Cancer*, 4:212–222.
7. Baroni, C., Van Esch, G. J., and Saffiotti, U. (1963): Carcinogenesis tests of two inorganic arsenicals. *Arch. Environ. Health*, 7:668–674.
8. Bayliss, O. (1972): *National Institute for occupational Health and Safety: Criteria for a Recom-*

*mended Standard: Occupational Exposure to Beryllium.* U.S. Department of Health, Education and Welfare, Washington, D.C., pp. IV-22–IV-23, Tables VII–X.

9. Beach, D. J., and Sunderman, F. W., Jr. (1970): Nickel carbonyl inhibition of RNA synthesis by a chromatin–RNA polymerase complex from hepatic nuclei. *Cancer Res.,* 30:48–50.
10. Beach, D. J., and Sunderman, F. W., Jr. (1969). Nickel carbonyl inhibition of [14]C-orotic acid incorporation into rat liver RNA. *Proc. Soc. Exp. Biol. Med.,* 131:321–322.
11. Beckman, G., Beckman, L., and Nordenson, I. (1977): Chromosome aberrations in workers exposed to arsenic. *Environ. Health Perspect.,* 19:145–146.
12. Bensimon, J., and Rosenfeld, C. (1974): Influence du sulfate de nickel sur la croissance de deux lignees lymphoblastoides humaines d'origine normale et leucemique. *CR Acad. Sci. [D] (Paris),* 278:345–348.
13. Bensimon, J. (1977): Action combinee de sulfate de nickel et du rayonnement sur des cellules lymphoblastoides humaines d'origine leucemique. *CR Acad. Sci [D] (Paris),* 284:1959–1962.
14. Bensimon, J., and Rimbert, J. N. (1977): Sensibilite au rayonnement de cellules lymphoblas-toides humaines cultivees en milieu enrichis de sulfate de nickel. *CR Acad. Sci. [D] (Paris),* 284:867–869.
15. Bensimon, J., and Rosenfeld, C (1976): Etude de l'index de marquage de cellules lymphoblas-toides humaines cultivees en milieux enrichis de sulfate de nickel. *CR Acad. Sci. [D] (Paris),* 283:167–169.
16. Bensimon, J., and Rosenfeld, C. (1977): Dosages du nickel dans des cellules lymphoblastoides humaines cultivees en milieux enrichis en sulfate de nickel: Remarques sur les modes d'action du nickel. *CR Acad. Sci. [D] (Paris),* 285:123–126.
17. Blagoi, Y. P., Sorokin, V. A., Valeer, V. A., and Gladchenko, G. O. (1978): Ob osobennostiakh perekhoda spiral'-klubok v DNK v oblasti inversii otnositel'noi stabil'nosti GC i AT-par, obuslovlennoi ionami $Cu^{2+}$ i $Mn^{2+}$. *Dokl. Akad. Nauk. SSSR,* 240:459–462.
18. Bonatti, S., Meini, M., and Abbondandolo, A. (1976): Genetic effects of potassium dichromate in *Schizosaccharomyces pombe. Mutat. Res.,* 38:147–150.
19. Boyd, J. T., Doll, R., Faulds, J. S., and Leiper, J. (1970): Cancer of the lung in iron ore (haematite) miners. *Br. J. Ind. Med.,* 27:97–105.
20. Boyland, E., Dukes, C. E., Grover, P. L., and Mitchley, B. C. V. (1962): The induction of renal tumours by feeding lead acetate to rats. *Br. J. Cancer,* 16:283–288.
21. Brusick, D., Gletten, F., Jagannath, D. R., and Weekes, U. (1976): The mutagenic activity of ferrous sulfate for *Salmonella typhimurium. Mutat. Res.,* 38:386–387.
22. Casto, B. C., Meyers, J., and DiPaolo, J. A. (1979): Enhancement of viral transformation for evaluation of the carcinogenic or mutagenic potential of inorganic metal salts. *Cancer Res.,* 39:193–198.
23. Casto, B. C., Pieczynski, W. J., Nelson, R. L., and DiPaolo, J. A. (1976): *In vitro* transformation and enhancement of viral transformation with metals. *Proc. Am. Assoc. Cancer Res.,* 17:46.
24. Cooper, W. C. (1976): Cancer mortality patterns in the lead industry. *Ann. NY Acad. Sci.,* 271:250–259.
25. Costa, M., Nye, J., and Sunderman, F. W., Jr. (1980): Morphological transformation of Syrian hamster fetal cells induced by nickel compounds. *Ann. Clin. Lab. Sci. (in press).*
26. Deknudt, G. (1978): Mutagenicity of heavy metals. *Mutat. Res.,* 53:176.
27. DeWys, W., and Pories, W. (1972): Inhibition of a spectrum of animal tumors by dietary zinc deficiency. *J. Natl. Cancer Inst.,* 48:375–381.
28. Doll, R. (1958): Cancer of the lung and nose in nickel workers. *Br. J. Ind. Med.,* 15:217.
29. Doll, R., Morgan, L. G., and Speizer, F. E. (1970): Cancers of the lung and nasal sinuses in nickel workers. *Br. J. Cancer,* 24:623–632.
30. Eichhorn, G. L., Richardson, C., and Pitha, J. (1971): Mispairing of nucleotide bases induced by metal ions. In: *162nd National Meeting, Am. Chem. Soc.,* Abstr. 17, Biol. Chem. Div., Washington, D.C..
31. Ellis, K. J., Vartsky, D., Zanzi, I., Cohn, S. H., and Yasumura, S. (1979): Cadmium: In vivo measurement in smokers and nonsmokers. *Science,* 205:323–325.
32. Esch, G. J. Van, Genderen, H. Van, and Vink, H. H. (1962): The induction of renal tumors by feeding basic lead acetate to rats. *Br. J. Cancer,* 16:289–297.
33. Flessel, C. P. (1979): Manganese mutagenesis (abstract). In: *Second International Conference on Inorganic and Nutritional Aspects of Cancer,* La Jolla, Calif., p. 11.
34. Flessel, C. P. (1978): Metals as mutagens. In: *Inorganic and Nutritional Aspects of Cancer,* edited by G. N. Schrauzer. Plenum Press, New York, p. 117–128.

35. Flessel, C. P., Furst, A., and Radding, S. B. (1979): A comparison of carcinogenic metals. In: *Metal Ions in Biological Systems,* edited by H. Sigel. Marcel Dekker, New York *(in press).*
36. Flynn, A. (1979): Copper and zinc metabolism with solid tumor growth. In: *Second International Conference on Inorganic and Nutritional Aspects of Cancer,* La Jolla, Calif., p. 23.
37. Fowler, B. A., Woods, G. S., and Schiller, C. M. (1977): The ultrastructural and biochemical effects of prolonged oral arsenic exposure on liver mitochondria of rats. *Environ. Health Perspect.,* 19:197–204.
38. Fradkin, A., Janoff, A., Lane, B. P., and Kuschner, M. (1975): *In vitro* transformation of BHK21 cells grown in the presence of calcium chromate. *Cancer Res.,* 35:1058–1063.
39. Franseen, C. C. (1940): Occupational and industrial cancer. In: *Cancer: A Manual for Practitioners,* edited by C. C. Simmons. Committee on Publications, Massachusetts Medical Society, Boston, pp. 227–234.
40. Frost, D. V. (1978): The arsenic problems. In: *Inorganic and Nutritional Aspects of Cancer,* edited by G. N. Schrauzer. Plenum Press, New York, pp. 259–279.
41. Furst, A. (1977): Inorganic agents in carcinogens. In: *Advances in Modern Toxicology,* edited by H. F. Kraybill and M. A. Mehlman. John Wiley & Sons, New York, pp. 209–229.
42. Furst, A. (1978): An overview of metal carcinogenesis. In: *Inorganic and Nutritional Aspects of Cancer,* edited by G. N. Schrauzer. Plenum Press, New York, pp. 1–12.
43. Furst, A. (1978): Tumorigenic effect of an organomanganese compound on F344 rats and Swiss albino mice: Brief communication. *J. Natl. Cancer Inst.,* 60:1171–1173.
44. Furst, A., and Radding, S. B. (1979): Carcinogenicity of less common metals (abstract). In: *Second International Conference on Inorganic and Nutritional Aspects of Cancer,* La Jolla, Calif., p. 1.
45. Furst, A., and Radding, S. B. (1979): Unusual metals as carcinogens. *Biol. Trace Element Res.,* 1:169–181.
46. Galy, P., Touraine, R., Brune, J., Gallois, P., Roudier, P., Loire, R., Lheureux, P., and Wiesendanger, T. (1963): Les cancers bronchopulmonaires de l'intoxication arsenicale chronique chez les viticulteurs du Beaujolais. *Lyon Med.,* 210:735.
47. Gardner, L. U. and Heslington, H. F. (1946): Osteosarcoma from intravenous beryllium compounds in rabbits. *Fed. Proc.,* 5:221.
48. Geyer, L. (1898): Uber die chronischen hautveranderungen beim arsenicismus und betrattingen uber der massenerkrankunger in reichenstein in schlesien. *Arch. Dermatol. Syph.,* 43:221.
49. Gilman, J. P. W. (1962): Metal carcinogenesis. II. A study on the carcinogenic activity of cobalt, copper, iron and nickel compounds. *Cancer Res.,* 22:158–162.
50. Gilman, J. P. W. (1964): Muscle tumorigenesis. In: *Proceedings of the Sixth Canadian Cancer Research Conference, Honey Harbor, Ontario.* Pergamon Press, Oxford, pp. 209–233.
51. Glass, E. (1956): Untersuchungen uber die einwirkung von schwermetallsalzen auf die wurzelspitzenmitose von Vicia faba. *Z. Botanik.,* 44:1–58.
52. Granfell, D., and Gilmour, J. (1932): Cancer among nickel workers. *Lancet,* 2:1086–1087.
53. Granfell, D., and Samuel, H. (1932): Cancer among Welsh nickel workers. *Lancet,* 1:375.
54. Green, M. H. L., Muriel, W. J., and Bridges, B. A. (1976): Use of a simplified fluctuation test to detect low levels of mutagens. *Mutat. Res.,* 38:33–41.
55. Gruber, J. E., and Jennette, K. W. (1978): Metabolism of the carcinogen chromate by rat liver microsomes. *Biochem. Biophys. Res. Commun.,* 82:700–706.
56. Gunn, S. A., Gould, T. C., and Anderson, W. A. D. (1963): Cadmium-induced interstitial cell tumors in rats and mice and their prevention by zinc. *J. Natl. Cancer Inst.,* 31:745–753.
57. Harr, J. R., Exon, J. H., Weswig, P. H., and Whanger, P. D. (1973): Relationship of dietary selenium concentration, chemical cancer induction, and tissue concentration of selenium in rats. *Clin. Toxicol.,* 6:487–495.
58. Heath, J. C. (1956): The production of malignant tumors by cobalt in the rat. *Br. J. Cancer,* 10:668–673.
59. Heath, J. C. (1960): The histogenesis of malignant tumours induced by cobalt in the rat. *Br. J. Cancer,* 14:478–482.
60. Heath, J. C., and Webb, M. (1967): Content and intracellular distribution of the inducing metal in the primary rhabdomyosarcomata induced in the rat by cobalt, nickel and cadmium. *Br. J. Cancer,* 21:768–779.
61. Hernberg, S. (1977): Incidence of cancer in population with exceptional exposure to metals. In: *Origins of Human Cancer, Book A, Vol. 4,* edited by H. H. Hiatt, J. D. Watson, and

J. A. Winsten. Cold Spring Harbor Conferences on Cell Proliferation, Cold Spring Harbor, New York, pp. 147–157.

62. Hoekstra, W. G. (1975): Biochemical function of selenium and its relation to vitamin E. *Fed. Proc.,* 34:2083–2089.

63. Hoffman, D. J., and Niyogi, S. K. (1977): Metal mutagens and carcinogens affect RNA synthesis rates in a distinct manner. *Science,* 198:513–514.

64. Hueper, W. C. (1958): Experimental studies in metal cancerigenesis. IX. Pulmonary lesions in guinea pigs and rats exposed to prolonged inhalation of powdered metallic nickel. *Arch. Path.,* 65:600–607.

65. Hueper, W. C. (1966): *Occupational and Environmental Cancers of the Respiratory System.* Springer–Verlag, New York.

66. Infante, P. F., and Wagoner, J. K. (1975): *Proceedings of the International Conference on Heavy Metals in the Environment,* edited by T. C. Hutchinson. Institute for Environmental Studies, Toronto, pp. 329–338.

67. Jacobs, M. M. (1977): Inhibitory effects of selenium on 1,2-dimethylhydrazine and methylazoxy-methanol colon carcinogenesis. *Cancer,* 40:2557–2564.

68. Jacobs, M. M., Matney, T. S., and Griffin, A. C. (1977): Inhibitory effects of selenium on the mutagenicity of 2-acetylaminofluorene (AAF) and AAF derivatives. *Cancer Lett.,* 2:319–322.

69. Jansson, B., Seibert, G. B., and Speer, J. F. (1975): Gastrointestinal cancer. Its geographic distribution and correlation to breast cancer. *Cancer,* 36:2373–2384.

70. Jasmin, G. (1979): Thymic lymphosarcoma in magnesium-deficient rats (abstract). In: *Second International Conference on Inorganic and nutritional Aspects of Cancer,* La Jolla, Calif., p. 17.

71. Jennette, K. W. (1979): Chromate metabolism in liver microsomes (abstract). In: *Second International Conference on Inorganic and Nutritional Aspects of Cancer,* La Jolla, Calif., p. 4.

72. Jorgensen, H. S. (1973): A study of mortality from lung cancer among miners in Kiruna, 1950–1970. *Work Environ. Health,* 10:107.

73. Jung, E. G., Traschel, B. Y., and Immich, H. (1969): Arsenic as an inhibitor of the enzymes concerned in cellular recovery (dark repair). *Germ. Med. Monthly,* 14:614–616.

74. Kada, T., Sadaie, Y., and Tutikawa, K. (1972): *In vitro* and host-mediated "rec-assay" procedures for screening chemical mutagens, and phloxine, a mutagenic red dye detected. *Mutat. Res.,* 16:165–174.

75. Kalinina, L. M., Polukhina, G. N., and Lukasheva, L. I. (1977): Salmonella typhimurium—test-system for indication of mutagenic activity of environmental hazards. *Genetika,* 13:1089–1092.

76. Kanematsu, K., and Kada, T. (1978): Mutagenicity of metal compounds. *Mutat. Res.,* 53:207–208.

77. Kanisawa, M., and Schroeder, H. A. (1967): Life term studies on the effect of arsenic germanium, tin, and vanadium on spontaneous tumors in mice. *Cancer Res.,* 27:1192–1195.

78. Kipling, M. D., and Waterhouse, J. A. H. (1967): Cadmium and prostatic carcinoma. *Lancet,* 1:730–731.

79. Knorre, V. D. (1971): Zur induktion von hodenzwischenzelltumoren an der albinrate durch kadmiumchlorid. *Arch. Geschwulstforsch,* 38:257–263.

80. Kolonel, L. N. (1976): Association of cadmium with renal cancer. *Cancer,* 37:1782–1787.

81. Komczynski, L., Nowak, H., and Rejniak, L. (1963): Effect of cobalt, nickel and iron on mitosis in the roots of the broad bean (Vicia faba). *Nature,* 198:1016–1017.

82. Kubota, J., Allaway, W. H., Carter, D. L., Cary, E. E., and Lazar, V. A. (1967): Selenium in crops in the United States in relation to selenium responsive diseases in animals. *J. Agric. Food Chem.,* 15:448–453.

83. Langard, S. (1979): The distribution of chromium in the rat and in the rat liver cell after intravenous administration (abstract). In: *Second International Conference on Inorganic and Nutritional Aspects of Cancer,* La Jolla, Calif., p. 3.

84. Langvad, E. (1966): *Proceedings of the Third Quadrennial Conference on Cancer,* edited by L. Severi. University of Perugia, Perugia, Italy, p. 897.

85. Laskin, S., Kuschner, M., and Drew R. T. (1976): Studies in pulmonary carcinogenesis. In: *Inhalation Carcinogenesis,* edited by M. G. Hanna, Jr., P. Nettesheim, and J. R. Gilbert. U.S. Atomic Energy Commission, Symposium Series No. 18, pp. 321–351.

86. Lau, T. J., Hackett, R. L., and Sunderman, F. W., Jr. (1972): The carcinogenicity of intravenous nickel carboyl in rats. *Cancer Res., 32:2253–2258.*

87. Lee, A. M., and Fraumeni, J. F., Jr. (1969): Arsenic and respiratory cancers in man: An occupational study. *J. Natl. Cancer Inst., 42:1045–1052.*

88. Lehmann, K. B. (1932): 1st grund zu liner besonderen beunruhigung wegen des auftretens von lungenkrebs bei chromatarbeitern vorhanden? *Zentralb. Gewerbehyg., 19:168.*

89. Lekevichus, R., Vijanskaja, T., and Stukiene, R. (1978): Mutagenic activity of ethylmercurichloride and its disintegration product mercury. *Mutat. Res., 53:218–219.*

90. Lemen, R. A., Lee, J. S., Wagoner, J. K., and Blejer, H. P. (1976): Cancer mortality among cadmium production workers. *Ann. NY Acad. Sci., 271:273–279.*

91. Levis, A. G., Bianchi, V., Tamino, G., and Pegoraro, B. (1978): Cytotoxic effects of hexavalent and trivalent chromium on mammalian cells *in vitro. Br. J. Cancer, 37:386–396.*

92. Levis, A. G., and Buttignol, M. (1977): Effects of potassium dichromate on DNA synthesis in hamster fibroblasts. *Br. J. Cancer, 35:496–499.*

93. Levis, A. G., Buttignol, M., Bianchi, V., and Sponga, G. (1978): Effects of potassium dichromate on nucleic acid and protein synthesis and on precursor uptake in BHK fibroblasts. *Cancer Res., 38:110–116.*

94. Ljungdahl, L. G. (1976): Tungsten, a biologically active metal. *Trends Biochem. Sci., 1:63–65.*

95. Ljungdahl, L. G., and Andreesen, J. R. (1975): Tungsten, a component of active formate dehydrogenase from *Clostridium thermoaceticum. FEBS Lett., 54:279–282.*

96. Lo, L. W., Koropatnick, J., and Stich, H. F. (1978): The mutagenicity and cytotoxicity of selenite, "activated" selenite and selenate for normal and DNA repair-deficient human fibroblasts. *Mutat. Res., 49:305–312.*

97. Lofroth, G., and Ames, B. N. (1978): Mutagenicity of inorganic compounds in *Salmonella typhimurium:* Arsenic, chromium and selenium. *Mutat. Res., 53:65–66.*

98. Lucis, O. J., Lucis, R., and Aterman, K. (1972): Tumorigenesis by cadmium. *Oncology, 26:53–67.*

99. Luke, M. Z., Hamilton, L., and Hollocher, T. C. (1975): Beryllium-induced misincorporation by a DNA polymerase: A possible factor in beryllium toxicity. *Biochem. Biophys. Res. Commun., 62:497–501.*

100. MacKinnon, A. E., and Bancewicz, J. (1973): Sarcoma after injection of intramuscular iron. *Br. Med. J., 2:277–279.*

101. Mancuso, T. F. (1970): Relation of duration of employment and prior respiratory illness to respiratory cancer among beryllium workers. *Environ. Res., 3:251–275.*

102. Mancuso, T. F., and Hueper, W. C. (1951): Occupational cancer and other health hazards in a chromate plant: A medical appraisal. I. Lung cancers in chromate workers. *Ind. Med. Surg., 20:358–363.*

103. Marcotte, J., and Witschi, H. P. (1972): Synthesis of RNA and nuclear proteins in early regenerating rat livers exposed to beryllium. *Res. Commun. Chem. Pathol. Pharmacol., 3:97–104.*

104. McEwan, J. C. (1976): A study of sputum cytology in two industrial groups (abstract). In: *Proceedings of the 18th International Congress on Occupational Health.* Brighton, p. 308.

105. Mertz, W. (1979): The newer trace elements (abstract). In: *Second International Conference on Inorganic and Nutritional Aspects of Cancer,* La Jolla, Calif., p. 21.

106. Meyne, J., and Lockhart, L. H. (1978): Cytogenetic effects of cis-platinum (II) diaminedichloride on human lymphocyte cultures. *Mutat. Res., 58:87–97.*

107. Monti-Bragadin, C., Tamaro, M., Banfi, E., and Zassinovich, G. (1977): Mutagenic activity of metal compounds (abstract). *IUPAC International Symposium on Clinical Chemistry and Chemical Toxicology of Metals,* Monte Carlo, Monaco.

108. Morgan, J. G. (1958): Some observations on the incidence of respiratory cancer in nickel workers. *Br. J. Indust. Med., 15:224–234.*

109. Murray, M. J., and Flessel, C. P. (1976): Metal–polynucleotide interactions. A comparison of carcinogenic and non-carcinogenic metals *in vitro. Biochim. Biophys. Acta, 425:256–261.*

110. Nelson, A. A., Fitzhugh, O. G., and Calvery, H. O. (1943): Liver tumors following cirrhosis caused by selenium in rats. *Cancer Res., 3:230–236.*

111. Nestmann, E. R., Matula, T. I., Douglas, G. R., Bora K. C., and Kowbel, D. J. (1979): Detection of the mutagenic activity of lead chromate using a battery of microbial tests. *Mutat. Res. 66:357–365.*

112. Nettesheim, P., Hanna, M. G., Jr., Doherty, D. G., Newell, R. F., and Hellman, A. (1971): Effect of calcium chromate dust, influenza virus and 100 R whole body X-radiation on lung tumor incidence in mice. *J. Natl. Cancer Inst.*, 47:1129–1144.
113. Newman, J. A., Archer, V. E., Saccomanno, G., Kuschner, M., Auerbach, O., Grondahl, R. D., and Wilson, J. C. (1976): Histologic types of bronchogenic carcinoma among members of copper-mining and smelting communities. *Ann. NY Acad. Sci.*, 271:260–268.
114. Nishioka, H. (1975): Mutagenic activities of metal compounds in bacteria. *Mutat. Res.*, 31:185–189.
115. Noda, M., Takano, T., and Sakurai, H. (1979): Mutagenic activity of selenium compounds. *Mutat. Res.*, 66:175–179.
116. Nordenson, I., Beckman, G., Beckman, L., and Nordstrom, S. (1978): Occupational and environmental risks in and around a smelter in northern Sweden. II. Chromosomal aberrations in workers exposed to arsenic. *Hereditas*, 88:47–50.
117. O'Gara, R. W., and Brown, J. M. (1967): Comparison of the carcinogenic actions of subcutaneous implants of iron and aluminum in rodents. *J. Natl. Cancer Inst.*, 38:947–957.
118. Okubo, T. (1979): Epidemiological study among chromium platers in Japan (abstract). In: *Second International Conference on Inorganic and Nutritional Aspects of Cancer*, La Jolla, Calif., p. 3..
119. Oppenheimer, B. S., Oppenheimer, E. T., Danishefsky, I., and Stout, A. P. (1956): Carcinogenic effect of metals in rodents. *Cancer Res.*, 16:439–441.
120. Osburn, H. S. (1960): Lung cancer in a mining district in Rhodesia. *S. Afr. Med. J.*, 43:1307–1312.
121. Osswald, H., and Goerttler, K. (1971): Leukosen beider maus nach diaplazentare und post natale arsenic application. *Verh. Dtsch. Ges. Pathol.*, 55:289.
122. Ott, M. G., Holder, B. B., and Gordon H. L. (1974): Respiratory cancer and occupational exposure to arsenicals. *Arch. Environ. Health*, 29:250–255.
123. Oyasu, R., Battifora, H. A., Clasen, R. A., McDonald, J. H., and Hass, G. M. (1970): Induction of cerebral gliomas in rats with dietary lead subacetate and 2-acetylaminofluorene. *Cancer Res.*, 30:1248–1261.
124. Paton, G. R., and Allison, A. C. (1972): Chromosome damage in human cell cultures induced by metal salts. *Mutat. Res.*, 16:332–336.
125. Petering, D. H. (1979): Mechanism of control of Ehrlich cell division by zinc (abstract). In: *Second International Conference on Inorganic and Nutritional Aspects of Cancer*, La Jolla, Calif., p. 16.
126. Petres, J., Baron, D., and Hagedorn, M. (1977): Effects of arsenic cell metabolism and cell proliferation: Cytogenetic and biochemical studies. *Environ. Health Perspect.*, 19:223–227.
127. Petres, J., Schmid-Ullrich, K., and Wolf, U. (1970): Chromosomen-aberrationen an menschlichen lymphozyten bei chronischen arsenschaden. *Dtsch. Med. Wochenschr.*, 95:79–80.
128. Petrilli, F. L., and DeFlora, S. (1977): Toxicity and mutagenicity of hexavalent chromium on *Salmonella typhimurium*. *Appl. Environ. Microbiol.*, 33:805–809.
129. Pokrovskaia, L. V., and Shabynina, N. K. (1974): Carcinogenesis hazards in the production of chromium ferroalloys. *Gig. Tr. Prof. Zabol.*, 17:23–26.
130. Pories, W. J., Mansour, E. G., and Flynn, A. (1979): Trace element profiles in cancer patients (abstract). In: *Second International Conference on Inorganic and Nutritional Aspects of Cancers*, La Jolla, Calif., p. 22.
131. Pories, W. J., Mansour, E. G., and Strain, W. H. (1972): Trace elements that act to inhibit neoplastic growth. *Ann. NY Acad. Sci.*, 199:265–273.
132. Pribyl, D., and Treagan, L. (1977): A comparison of the effect of metal carcinogens chromium, cadmium and nickel on the interferon system. *Acta Virol.*, 21:507.
133. Putrament, A., Baranowska, H., Ejchart, A., and Prazmo, W. (1975): Manganese mutagenesis in yeast. A practical application of manganese for the induction of mitochondrial antibiotic-resistant mutations. *J. Gen. Microbiol.*, 62:265–270.
134. Quiroga Micheo, E. (1979): Epidemiology of blood neoplasms in the Argentine (abstract). In: *Second International Conference on Inorganic and Nutritional Aspects of Cancer*, La Jolla, Calif., p. 5.
135. Rao, K. G., Wu, F. Y. H., Sethi, S., and Eichhorn, G. L. (1977): Effects of divalent ions on the structure and sugar fidelity of *E. coli* RNA polymerase (abstract). In: *174th National Meeting Am. Chem. Soc. Biol. Chem. Div.*, Washington, D.C.
136. Rawson, R. W. (1976): Inorganic carcinogens. In: *Proceedings of the Third International Sympo-*

*sium on Detection and Prevention of Cancer,* edited by H. E. Nieburgs. M. Dekker, New York, pp. 1893–1906.

137. Roe, F. J. C., Dukes, C. E., Cameron, K. M., Pugh, R. C. B., and Mitchley, B. C. V. (1964): Cadmium neoplasia: Testicular atrophy and Leydig cell hyperplasia and neoplasia in rats and mice following the subcutaneous injection of cadmium salts. *Br. J. Cancer,* 18:674–681.

138. Rohr, G., and Bauchinger, M. (1976): Chromosome analyses in cell cultures of the Chinese hamster after application of cadmium sulphate. *Mutat. Res.,* 40:125–130.

139. Rosen, P. (1971): Theoretical significance of arsenic as a carcinogen. *J. Theor. Biol.,* 32:425–426.

140. Rosenberg, (1978): Noble metal complexes in cancer chemotherapy. In: *Inorganic and Nutritional Aspects of Cancer,* edited by G. N. Schrauzer. Plenum Press, New York, pp. 129–150.

141. Rosenberg, B., VanCamp, L., Trosko, J. E., and Mansour, V. H. (1969): Platinum compounds: A new class of potent antitumour agents. *Nature,* 222:385–386.

142. Rossman, T. G., Meyn, M. S., and Troll, W. (1977): Effects of arsenite on DNA repair in *Escherichia coli. Environ. Health Perspect.,* 19:229–233.

143. Rotruck, J. T., Pope, A. L., Ganther, H. E., Swanson, A. B., Hafeman, D. G., and Hoekstra, W. G. (1973): Selenium: Biochemical role as a component of clatathione. *Science,* 179:588–590.

144. Schiller, C. M., Fowler, B. A., and Woods, J. S. (1977): Effects of arsenic on pyruvate dehydrogenase activation. *Environ. Health Perspect.,* 19:205–207.

145. Schrauzer, G. N., and Ishmael, D. (1974): Effects of selenium and arsenic on the genesis of spontaneous mammary tumors in inbred C3H mice. *Ann. Clin. Lab. Sci.,* 4:441–447.

146. Seelig, M. S. (1979): Magnesium and trace mineral deficiences in the pathogenesis of cancer (abstract). In: *Second International Conference on Inorganic and Nutritional Aspects of Cancer,* La Jolla, Calif., p. 18.

147. Shamberger, R. J. (1970): Relationship of selenium to cancer. I. Inhibitory effect of selenium on carcinogenesis. *J. Natl. Cancer Inst.,* 44:931–936.

148. Shamberger, R. J., Rukovena, E., Longfield, A. K., Tytko, S. H., Deodhar, S., and Willis, C. E. (1973): Antioxidants and cancer. I. Selenium in the blood of normals and cancer patients. *J. Natl. Cancer Inst.,* 50:863–870.

149. Shamberger, R. J., and Willis, C. E. (1971): Selenium distribution and human cancer mortality. *Crit. Rev. Clin. Chem.,* 2:211–221.

150. Shapley, O. (1977): Occupational cancer: Government challenged in beryllium proceeding. *Science,* 198:898–901.

151. Shin, Y. A., Heim, J. M., and Eichhorn, G. L. (1972): Interaction of metal ions with polynucleotides and selected compounds. XX. Control of the conformation of polyriboadenylic acid by divalent metal ions. *Bioinorg. Chem.,* 1:149–163.

152. Sirover, M. A., and Loeb, L. A. (1976) Infidelity of DNA synthesis *in vitro:* Screening for potential metal mutagens on carcinogens. *Science,* 194:1434–1436.

153. Sirover, M. A., and Loeb, L. A. (1976): Metal-induced infidelity during DNA synthesis. *Proc. Natl. Acad. Sci. USA,* 73:2331–2335.

154. Smith, A. G., and Powell, L. (1957): Genesis of teratomas of the testes. A study of normal and zinc-injected testes of roosters. *Am. J. Pathol.,* 33:653–669.

155. Sprinker, L. H., Harr, J. R., Newberne, P. D., Whanger, P. D., and Weswig, P. H. (1971): Selenium deficiency lesions in rats fed vitamin E supplemented rations. *Nutr. Rep. Int.,* 4:335–340.

156. Steffee, C. H., and Baetjer, A. M. (1965): Histopathologic effects of chromate chemicals: Report on studies in rabbits, guinea pigs, rats and mice. *Arch. Environ. Health,* 11:66–75.

157. Stoner, G. D., Shimkin, M. B., Troxell, M. C., Thompson, T. L., and Terry, L. S. (1976): Test for carcinogenicity of metallic compounds by the pulmonary tumor response in strain A mice. *Cancer Res.,* 36:1744–1747.

158. Sunderman, F. W., Jr. (1970): Effect of nickel carbonyl upon incorporation of $^{14}$C-leucine into hepatic microsomal proteins. *Res. Commun. Chem. Pathol. Pharmacol.,* 1:161–168.

159. Sunderman, F. W., Jr. (1973): The current status of nickel carcinogenesis. *Ann. Clin. Lab. Sci.,* 3:156–180.

160. Sunderman, F. W., Jr. (1977): Metal carcinogenesis. In: *Advances in Modern Toxicology, Vol. 1,* edited by R. A. Goyer and M. A. Mehlman. Washington Hemisphere Corporation, Washington, D.C., pp. 257–295.

161. Sunderman, F. W., Jr. (1978): Carcinogenic effects of metals. *Fed. Proc.,* 37:40–46.

162. Sunderman, F. W., Jr. (1979): Mechanisms of metal carcinogenesis. In: *The Clinical Biochemistry of Cancer. Proceedings of the Second Arnold O. Beckman Conference in Clinical Chemistry.* American Association for Clinical Chemistry, San Antonio, Texas, pp. 265–297.
163. Sunderman, F. W., and Donnelly, A. J. (1965): Studies of nickel carcinogenesis. Metastasized pulmonary tumors in rats induced by the inhalation of nickel carboyl. *Am. J. Pathol.,* 46:1027–1041.
164. Sunderman, F. W., Jr., and Esfaheni, M. (1968): Nickel carbonyl inhibition of RNA polymerase activity in hepatic nuclei. *Cancer Res.,* 28:2565–2567.
165. Sunderman, F. W., Jr., Lau, T. J., and Cralley, L. J. (1974): Inhibitory effect of manganese upon muscle tumorigenesis by nickel subsulfide. *Cancer Res.,* 34:92–95.
166. Sutton, B. M. (1978): Metals in treatment of disease. *Ann. Rep. Med. Chem.,* 14:321–329.
167. Swierenga, S. H., and Basrur, P. K. (1968): Effect of nickel on cultured rat embryo muscle cells. *Lab. Invest.,* 19:663–674.
168. Tappel, A. L. (1965): Free lipid peroxidation damage and its inhibition by vitamin E and selenium. *Fed. Proc.,* 24:73–78.
169. Tinsley, I. J., Harr, J. R., and Bone, J. F. (1967): Selenium toxicity in rats. I. Growth and Longevity. In: *Selenium in Biomedicine.* International Symposium, Oregon State University, AVI Publishing Co., Westport, Conn., pp. 141–152.
170. Tokudome, S., and Kuratsune, M. (1976): A cohort study on mortality from cancer and other causes among workers at a metal refinery. *Int. J. Cancer,* 17:310–317.
171. Torjussen, W., and Andersen, I. (1979): Nickel concentration in nasal mucosa, plasma, and urine in active and retired nickel workers. *Ann. Clin. Lab. Sci.,* 9:289–298.
172. Treagan, L., and Furst, A. (1970): Inhibition of interferon synthesis in mammalian cell cultures after nickel treatment. *Res. Commun. Chem. Pathol. Pharmacol.,* 1:395–402.
173. Tseng, W. P. (1977): Effects and dose–response relationship of skin cancer and blackfoot disease with arsenic. *Environ. Health Perspect.,* 19:109–119.
174. Tseng, W. P., Chu, H. M., How, S. W., Fong, J. M., Lin, C. S., and Yeh, S. (1968): Prevalence of skin cancer in an endemic area of chronic arsenicism in Taiwan. *J. Natl. Cancer Inst.,* 40:453–463.
175. Tsuchiya, K. (1977): Various effects of arsenic in Japan depending on the type of exposure. *Environ. Health Perspect.,* 19:35–42.
176. Turnbull, D., Popescu, N. C., DiPaolo, J. A., and Myhr, B. C. (1979): *Cis*-Platinum (II) diamine dichloride causes mutation, transformation, and sister-chromatid exchanges in cultured mammalian cells. *Mutat. Res.,* 66:267–275.
177. Venitt, S., and Levy, L. S. (1974): Mutagenicity of chromates in bacteria and its relevance to chromate carcinogenesis. *Nature,* 250:493–495.
178. Vorwald, H. J., Reeves, A. L., and Urban, E. C. J. (1966): Experimental beryllium toxicology. In: *Beryllium: Its Industrial Hygiene Aspects,* edited by H. E. Stokinger. Academic Press, New York, p. 201 ff.
179. Webb, M., Heath, J. C., and Hopkins, T. (1972): Intranuclear distribution of the inducing metal in primary rhabdomyosarcomata induced in the rat by nickel, cobalt, and cadmium. *Br. J. Cancer,* 26:274–278.
180. Webb, M., and Weinzierl, S. M. (1972): Uptake of $^{63}Ni^{+2}$ from its complexes with proteins and other ligands by mouse dermal fibroblasts *in vitro. Br. J. Cancer,* 26:292–298.
181. Weed, L. L. (1963): Effects of copper on *Bacillus subtilis. J. Bacteriol.,* 85:1003–1010.
182. Weymouth, L. A., and Loeb, L. A. (1978): Mutagenesis during *in vitro* DNA synthesis. *Proc. Natl. Acad. Sci. USA,* 75:1924–1928.
183. Witschi, H. P. (1970): Effects of beryllium on deoxyribonucleic acid-synthesizing enzymes in regenerating rat liver. *Biochem. J.,* 120:623–634.
184. Witschi, H. P., and Aldridge, W. N. (1968): Uptake, distribution and binding of beryllium to organelles of the rat liver cell. *Biochem. J.,* 106:811–820.
185. Woods, J. S., and Fowler, B. A. (1977): Effects of chronic arsenic exposure on hematopoietic function in adult mammalian liver. *Environ. Health Perspect.,* 19:209–213.
186. Yagi, T., and Nishioka, H. (1977): DNA damage and its degradation by metal compounds. *Doshisha Daigaku Rikogaku Kenkyu Hokoku,* 18:63–70.
187. Yeh, S. (1973): Skin cancer in chronic arsenicism. *Hum. Pathol.,* 4:469–485.
188. Zaldivar, R. (1974): Arsenic contamination of drinking water and foodstuffs causing endemic chronic poisoning. *Beitr. Pathol.,* 151:384–400.
189. Zasukhina, G. D., Shalunova, N. V., Shvetsova, T. P., and Lomanova, G. A. (1975): Increase

of virus mutagenic potential in presence of cadmium salt. *Dokl. Akad. Nauk. SSSR*, 224:1189–1191 (Engl. trans. pp. 425–427).
190. Zollinger, H. U. (1953): Kidney adenomas and carcinomas in rats induced by chronic lead poisoning and their relationship to corresponding human neoplasms. *Virchows Arch. Pathol. Anat.*, 323:694–710.

*Nutrition and Cancer: Etiology and Treatment,*
edited by G. R. Newell and N. M. Ellison.
Raven Press, New York © 1981.

# Artificial Sweeteners and Cancer

## Guy R. Newell

*The University of Texas System Cancer Center, M. D. Anderson Hospital and Tumor
Institute, Houston, Texas 77030*

In 1879, saccharin was discovered by Constantine Fahlberg at Johns Hopkins
University. Since that time, its history has been stormy and controversial (Table
1). Saccharin, a white crystalline powder synthesized from toluene, has a sweetness several hundred times that of cane sugar. It became popular as a sugar
substitute for persons suffering from diabetes, obesity, and gout. When sugar
was rationed or unavailable during World Wars I and II, the use of saccharin
increased substantially. It is used as a flavoring agent in toothpaste, mouthwash,
dietetic foods, and cosmetics. Soft-drink manufacturers introduced saccharin-
containing diet sodas in response to America's weight consciousness.

## ANIMAL STUDIES

Three studies (3,4,10) have demonstrated that high-saccharin diets fed to
rats over a long period produced bladder tumors in second-generation rats.
Rats of the first generation were placed on diets containing saccharin at the
time of weaning. These animals were bred while on this diet, and the resulting
offspring were fed saccharin throughout their lives. Members of the second
generation were thus exposed to saccharin from the moment of conception.
The two earlier studies (3,10), although statistically significant, were not considered to be conclusive evidence of saccharin's carcinogenicity. The Canadian
study (4), which prompted a proposed ban on saccharin by the Food and Drug
Administration (FDA), exposed rats to a high dose of saccharin (5% of the
diet). Five percent of the diet is equal to about 2.5 g of saccharin/kg/body
weight/day. Under these conditions, only male rats developed significantly more
bladder tumors than did rats not exposed to saccharin. In contrast, several
studies conducted by feeding saccharin to a single generation of animals from
weaning until death reported negative or ambiguous results (1). These findings
are not considered absolute proof of saccharin's safety, but they do indicate
that, for a wide range of exposures in several species of animals, saccharin
did not cause cancer.

TABLE 1. *Historical highlights of saccharin*

| | |
|---|---|
| 1879 | Discovery by Constantine Fahlberg at Johns Hopkins. |
| 1885 | U.S. patent awarded by Fahlberg for the manufacture of saccharin. |
| 1911 | President Theodore Roosevelt authorized review of charges against safety of saccharin. Food Inspection Decision prohibited use of saccharin in foods. Decision overturned 12 days later, eventually allowing limited general use. |
| 1914 | Saccharin use increased during World War I because of short sugar supplies. |
| 1938 | Food, Drug and Cosmetic Act passed by Congress. |
| 1939 | Saccharin use increased during World War II, especially in Europe. |
| 1955 | [a]NAS reported saccharin and cyclamate safe for human consumption. |
| 1958 | Congress passed Delaney Clause, which prohibits food additives if found to be carcinogenic in animal or man. |
| 1960 | Approximate start of consumer demand for low-calorie products. |
| 1968 | [b]WHO reported saccharin safe for human use. [a]NAS/[c]NRC stated that up to 1 g of saccharin per day is safe. |
| 1969 | Cyclamate, only other artificial sweetener, banned from U.S. food supply. |
| 1970 | [a]NAS/[c]NRC reported saccharin safe for use in foods. |
| 1972 | Saccharin removed from [d]GRAS list by [e]FDA on basis of preliminary results of animal tests. |
| 1974 | [a]NAS/[c]NRC determined saccharin to be safe under previous conditions. |
| 1977 | |
| March | [e]FDA announced proposed ban on saccharin based on Canadian studies in male rats. |
| September | Canadian epidemiologic study suggested artificial sweetener related to bladder cancer in males only. |
| October | Congress voted an 18-month moratorium on proposed ban. |
| November | President Carter signed moratorium (P.L. 95-203). Congressional [f]OTA reported laboratory evidence that saccharin is carcinogenic. |
| 1978 | [a]NAS reported saccharin a weak carcinogen in male rats, therefore potential risk for humans. |
| 1979 | 100th anniversary of discovery of saccharin. |
| December | [g]NCI/[e]FDA study noted on increased cancer risk for general population but small increases in cancer risk among heavy artificial-sweetener users and heavy smokers. |
| 1980 | |
| March | [h]HSPH study reported no evidence of an association between artificial-sweetener use and bladder cancer. |
| March | [i]AHF study reported no association between artificial-sweetener use and bladder cancer. |

[a] NAS = National Academy of Science; [b] WHO = World Health Organization; [c] NRC = National Research Council; [d] GRAS = Generally Regarded as Safe; [e] FDA = Food and Drug Administration; [f] OTA = Office of Technology Assessment; [g] NCI = National Cancer Institute; [h] HSPH = Harvard School of Public Health; [i] AHF = American Health Foundation.
    Adapted from "Saccharin," a report by the American Council on Science and Health, New York.

## Extrapolation from Animals to Humans

Because carcinogenicity cannot be directly tested in humans, indirect methods are necessary, including animal bioassays. Standard procedure in animal experiments is to feed substances at the "maximum tolerated dose," which for saccharin is 5% of the rat's diet. If cancer is produced in animals at these high doses, it will probably also be produced at low-dose levels, but in fewer animals. To test low doses of saccharin in rats directly (doses closer to those ingested by humans) would require thousands of rats. Such studies are neither technically possible nor economically feasible. So that a smaller number of animals can be used, higher doses are tested. Most of the evidence suggests that this procedure is reasonable.

Saccharin was found to be among the weakest carcinogens ever detected in rats. Chemical carcinogens vary in their carcinogenic potency by more than a millionfold range of doses. Potency is measured by comparing the dose that will cause cancer in 50% of rats. For example, aflatoxin, a substance produced by certain fungi and found on moldy peanuts and grains, causes cancer in 50% of rats at a dose of more than one million times *less* than the dose of saccharin. Other known chemical carcinogens fall somewhere in between. There is evidence to suggest that the potency of carcinogens in rodents may be roughly comparable to their potency in humans. Thus, it is likely that saccharin is a relatively weak carcinogen in humans.

Although saccharin is likely to be a weak carcinogen in humans, based on animal extrapolation, it should still be a cause for public health concern. In addition to potency, one must consider the amount or dose to which people may be exposed and the number of people exposed. The degree of uncertainty in animal extrapolations may be wrong by a factor of 10 or even 100, thus possibly misinterpreting carcinogenic potency. Since saccharin is not the only carcinogen to which people are exposed, multiple exposures to other substances could act synergistically.

## HUMAN STUDIES

Although most epidemiologic evidence did not link saccharin use to human bladder cancer, one study from Canada (5) suggested that males with bladder cancer were more frequent users of artificial sweeteners than were persons without bladder cancer, inferring that saccharin was a potential cause of bladder cancer in humans. In the fall of 1977, the FDA used the results of this study to support their proposed ban on saccharin, which had been based on rat studies only. The limitations of this study in humans were enumerated by several individuals, including the editor of the journal in which it was published (2).

The Commissioner of the FDA assembled a group of scientists from the FDA and the National Cancer Institute (NCI) to review all available human epidemiologic studies pertaining to saccharin and cancer. The group came to the following conclusion: "The conclusion of the Saccharin Working Group is that at the present time, there is neither enough evidence to accept nor to reject the hypothesis that use of artificial sweeteners, specifically saccharin, increases the risk of bladder cancer in humans" (7).

This conclusion was based on a review of two time-trend studies, three studies of diabetic populations, and three case-control studies. The detailed review of these studies has been summarized (6). Likewise, the Congress of the United

States Office of Technology and Assessment (OTA) concluded: "Epidemiological studies of human experience have not been sensitive enough to determine whether or not saccharin is a carcinogen when ingested" (1).

Following the Saccharin Working Group's initial report (7), a large-scale investigation designed to meet the criticisms of earlier efforts and to resolve some of the conflicting results of former studies was launched. A case-control interview study (8) of bladder cancer involving almost 9,000 persons was conducted in five states and five metropolitan areas, in order to evaluate the possible risks associated with the use of artificial sweeteners. Overall, 3,010 persons with newly diagnosed cases of bladder cancer occurring during 1978 in the study areas were interviewed, along with 5,783 controls from a stratified random sample of the population. The 15-month study did not discover greater risks of bladder cancer among users of artificial sweeteners in the overall population, but did find higher risk rates in certain subgroups. The study cited these as evidence that, although saccharin and cyclamate are weak carcinogens, they should be regarded as potential risk factors in causing human bladder cancer.

## POTENTIAL BENEFITS

The benefits of a non-nutritive sweetner, such as saccharin, are unusually difficult to assess. This is because such sweeteners have become integral to the diet of many Americans and thus are perceived to be beneficial (and safe) because of the absence of controlled studies on their effectiveness in any situation. The Congressional OTA study found no scientific data to prove or disprove that use of a non-nutritive sweetener leads to any health benefits (1).

Perceived benefits from saccharin were identified for four groups:

A. Diabetics, in whom saccharin may help avoid consumption of sugar and maintenance of dietary control. Although saccharin is not essential to a diabetic's treatment, many physicians and patients believe that saccharin contributes to the quality of their lives.

B. Persons with obesity or who are overweight.

C. Persons susceptible to dental caries.

D. Persons using drugs or oral products in which saccharin is added to improve taste.

Thus, at issue is the presumed carcinogenicity of saccharin for humans based on animal studies and the perceived benefits of having an artificial sweetener available for use by the public.

## ALTERNATIVE SWEETENERS

Although saccharin is the only non-nutritive sweetener currently available to Americans, others have been used in the past. Cyclamate was introduced into the market in 1950, but the FDA banned its use in all foods and drugs in 1970. This action was taken because some tests resulted in bladder tumor in rats. Cyclohexylamine, a metabolite of cyclamate, caused chromosomal abnormalities and testicular atrophy in test animals, and dermatitis and convulsions in humans. An NCI review panel concluded that the present evidence does not establish the carcinogenicity of cyclamate or its principal metabolite, cyclohexylamine, in experimental animals (9). Because of unresolved questions about the other toxic effects, the FDA has not allowed cyclamate back on the market.

Aspartame was approved as a food additive for a number of foods in 1974; however, this was revoked in 1975. Objections to aspartame center on the potential risk of brain damage, primarily in infants and children. In addition, elevated levels of phenylalanine, an amino acid present in aspartame, are associated with development of mental retardation.

There has been recent interest in neohesperidian dihydrochalcone, a substance present in grapefruit rinds and sweet oranges. Two petitions are before the FDA for approval. Although the FDA may approve these petitions, the taste characteristics of neohesperidian dihydrochalcone may not be conducive to widespread acceptance. Its sweet sensation is slow in onset, usually long in duration, and it has a slight licorice aftertaste.

Miraculin is a substance found in the berries of the Nigerian fruit, *Synsepalum dulcificum,* commonly eaten by children in West Africa. It is a taste modifier that causes sour foods to taste sweet. The FDA has not permitted the marketing of "miracle fruit" because its safety for long-term use has not been demonstrated.

Monellin is a sweetener isolated from the fruit of a West African plant. Two proteins, thaumatin I and II, were extracted from a Nigerian fruit. Interest in these focuses on the reasons for their sweet taste. No petitions requesting their use as food additives have been filed with the FDA.

## ACKNOWLEDGMENT

This study was supported by Grant Number 2 R18 CA16413-04A1, awarded by the National Cancer Institute, DHEW.

## REFERENCES

1. Congress of the United States, Office of Technology Assessment (1977): *Cancer Testing Technology and Saccharin* (Library of Congress Catalog Card No. 77-600051). U.S. Government Printing Office, Washington, D.C.
2. Editorial (1977): Bladder cancer and saccharin. *Lancet,* 8038:592.
3. Food and Drug Administration (1973): *Histopathologic Evaluation of Tissues from Rats Following Continuous Dietary Intake of Sodium Saccharin and Calcium Cyclamate for a Maximum Period of Two Years: Final Report.* Project P-169-70.
4. Health Protection Branch, National Health and Welfare Department. *Toxicity and Carcinogenicity Study of Orthotoluenesulfonamide and Saccharin.* Project E405/405E. Canada.
5. Howe, G. R., Burch, J. D., Miller, A. B., Morrison, B., Gordon, P., Weldon, L., Chambers, L. W., Fodor, G., and Wisnor, G. M. (1977): Artificial sweeteners and human bladder cancer. *Lancet,* 8038:578–581.

6. Newell, G. R., Hoover, R. N., and Kolbye, A. C. (1978). Status report on saccharin in humans. *J. Natl. Cancer Inst.,* 61:275–276.

7. *Preliminary Findings and Recommendations of the Interagency Saccharin Working Group,* submitted to the Commissioner, Food and Drug Administration, December 21, 1977.

8. *Progress Report to the Food and Drug Administration from the National Cancer Institute Concerning the National Bladder Cancer Study.* December, 1979.

9. Public Health Service: *Report of the Temporary Committee for the Review of Data on Carcinogenicity of Cyclamate.* DHEW Publication No. (NIH) 77–1437.

10. WARF Institute: *Preliminary Report: Chronic Toxicity Study–Sodium Saccharin.* Presented at Harrison House, Glen Cove, N. Y., April 26–28, 1972.

*Nutrition and Cancer: Etiology and Treatment,*
edited by G. R. Newell and N. M. Ellison.
Raven Press, New York © 1981.

# Food Additives and Contaminants as Modifying Factors in Cancer Induction

## Thomas J. Slaga

*Biology Division, Oak Ridge National Laboratory, Oak Ridge, Tennessee 37830*

On the basis of knowledge derived from epidemiological studies, it is currently thought that the majority of cancers in humans are caused by environmental factors. Other than skin cancer, for which solar ultraviolet light is an important causative factor (7), emphasis has been placed on environmental chemicals as major factors in the etiology of cancers in man. Furthermore, studies with experimental animals have provided evidence that some chemicals in our environment are responsible for a significant proportion of human cancers. For example, polycyclic aromatic hydrocarbons (PAH) are widespread contaminants in our environment, occuring primarily as a result of combustion and pyrolysis of organic materials, e.g., cigarette smoke, automobile exhaust, industrial combustion products, etc. Concern over PAH has increased as evidence establishing that a significant number of these compounds are carcinogenic has accumulated. It has been estimated that approximately 2,000 tons of benzo($a$)pyrene [B($a$)P], a widely studied PAH carcinogen, find their way into the atmosphere in the United States annually (6). A wide variety of other environmentally occurring, structurally diverse chemicals, including aromatic amines, nitrosamines, nitrosamides, and aflatoxins, are also known to be carcinogenic (10).

## NECESSITY OF METABOLIC ACTIVATION FOR MOST CHEMICAL CARCINOGENS

Although there are two major classes of chemicals that induce cancer, direct acting carcinogens (ultimate carcinogens) and indirect carcinogens (procarcinogens) that require metabolic activation by cells, most belong to the latter category. Shown in Table 1 are the chemicals generally recognized as carcinogens in humans and the sites at which they cause tumors. The majority of chemicals listed in Table 1 must be metabolized before they become active. In addition to the chemicals generally recognized as carcinogens in humans as a result of industrial, medical, and societal exposures, a number of other chemicals in the environment, such as aflatoxin $B_1$ and certain N-nitrosamines and N-nitrosamides, are strongly suspected of causing cancer (12,15). It appears likely that

TABLE 1. *Chemicals considered as carcinogens in the human*[a]

| Chemicals | Sites of tumor formation |
| --- | --- |
| Industrial exposures | |
| 2 (or $\beta$)-Naphthylamine | Urinary bladder |
| Benzidine (4,4'-diaminobiphenyl) | Urinary bladder |
| 4-aminobiphenyl and 4-nitrobiphenyl | Urinary bladder |
| Bis(chloromethyl) ether | Lungs |
| Bis(2-chloroethyl) sulfide | Respiratory tract |
| Vinyl chloride | Liver mesenchyme |
| Certain soots, tars, oils | Skin, lungs |
| Chromium compounds | Lungs |
| Nickel compounds | Lungs, nasal sinuses |
| Asbestos | Pleura, peritoneum |
| Asbestos plus cigarette smoking | Lungs, pleura, peritoneum |
| Benzene | Bone marrow |
| Mustard gas | Respiratory system |
| Medical exposures | |
| N,N-Bis(2-chloroethyl)-2-naphthylamine (Chlornaphazine) | Urinary bladder |
| Diethylstilbestrol | Vagina |
| Estrogenic steroids | Breast and uterus |
| Societal exposures | |
| Cigarette smoke | Lungs, urinary tract, pancreas |
| Betel nut and tobacco quids | Buccal mucosa |

[a] Adapted from Miller, ref. 15, and Slaga ref. 27.

additional chemical carcinogens of both natural and synthetic origin will be identified.

The major enzymes that metabolize PAH, drugs, pesticides, and food additives are the microsomal mixed-function oxidases. The enzyme system aryl hydrocarbon hydroxylase is part of the microsomal complex that converts PAH to ultimate carcinogens, which are reactive epoxides. These electrophiles can then be converted to transdihydrodiols by the action of microsomal epoxide hydrases, rearranged spontaneously to phenols, conjugated with glutathione, combined covalently with cellular nucleophiles, or, after conversion to transdihydrodiol, subsequently oxidized to diol-epoxides (1,2,10,16,26). The extent of binding of several types of PAH to mouse skin DNA (2,30) and protein (11) has been reported to correlate with the carcinogenic activity of the hydrocarbon. The Millers (16) have proposed a general theory to explain chemical carcinogenesis that has had a very significant impact on cancer research. They have proposed that all chemical carcinogens that are not themselves chemically reactive must be converted metabolically into a chemically reactive form, and that the activated metabolite is an electrophilic reagent, which reacts with nucleophilic groups in cellular macromolecules to initiate carcinogenesis. The fact that all reactive forms thus far characterized are electrophilic is probably the only connection among the structurally diverse chemical carcinogens.

TABLE 2. *Possible tumor promoters and/or cocarcinogens in man*

Alcohol
Asbestos
Tobacco
High fat, protein, and calorie content of food
Vitamin deficiencies
Unnatural balance of endogenous hormones
Exogenous hormones, diethylstilbestrol (DES)
Diterpenes from plant sources (tea, etc.)
Environmental chemicals, such as hydrocarbons and chlorinated hydrocarbons
Drugs
Radiation
Viruses

## Two-Stage or Multistage Carcinogenesis

Current information suggests that chemical carcinogenesis is a multistage process, with one of the best-studied models in this regard being the two-stage carcinogenesis system using mouse skin. The initiation stage requires only a single application of a direct or indirect carcinogen at a subthreshold dose and is essentially irreversible, whereas the promotion stage is brought about by repetitive treatments following initiation and is initially reversible, later becoming irreversible. Recently, two-stage or multistage carcinogenesis has been shown to exist in a number of systems other than the skin, such as the liver, lung, bladder, colon, esophagus, stomach, mammary gland, and displacenta, as well as in cells in culture (31).

As one might suspect, there is great diversity in promoting agents in the various two-stage systems. Table 2 summarizes the possible tumor promoters and co-carcinogens in human cancers (31). This is not intended to suggest, however, that some of these agents are not carcinogens. Current information suggests that alcohol, tobacco, asbestos, certain diets, and an imbalance in endogenous hormones are associated with a large percentage of cancers in man (44,45).

## Modifiers of Chemical Carcinogenesis

A number of general factors have been shown to play a modifying role in chemical carcinogenesis in experimental animals, and it is very likely that these factors, shown in Table 3 play similar roles in carcinogenesis in man (27). A number of other carcinogens can have an additive, synergistic, or inhibitory effect on the carcinogenic activity of a given carcinogen. Since most chemical carcinogens must be metabolized before they become active, the degree of activation versus detoxification of a particular carcinogen by a target tissue is an important determinant of the carcinogen's potency. Both radiation and viruses have been shown to have an enhancing effect on chemical carcinogenesis (33,35),

TABLE 3. *Factors in or modifiers of chemical carcinogenesis*

| |
|---|
| Other chemical carcinogens |
| Metabolism of chemical carcinogen (activation versus detoxification) |
| Radiation |
| Viruses |
| DNA repair, age, sex, hormones, immunology, trauma, and genetic constitution |
| Diet, nutrition, and life-style |
| Anticarcinogenic chemicals |

as have a number of general factors such as age, sex, hormones, immunological state, trauma, genetic constitution, and DNA repair, exhibiting an enhancing or enhancing effect (28). A discussion of these general factors is obviously beyond the scope of this chapter; however, the roles of diet, nutrition, and life-style in the etiology of cancer are discussed elsewhere in this volume.

As summarized in Table 4, a number of chemicals have been found to have anticarcinogenic activities (27). The anticarcinogenic agents listed inhibit tumor initiation or promotion. In many cases the effect was determined using the mouse skin two-stage carcinogenesis system, but recent reports suggest that this division by effect may also apply to other carcinogenesis systems (27,31). These compounds appear able to inhibit tumor initiation by alteration of the metabolism of the carcinogen (decreased activation or increased detoxification), scavenging of active molecular species of carcinogens to prevent their reaching critical target sites in the cells, or competitive inhibition (28). In addition, chemi-

TABLE 4. *Inhibitors of chemical carcinogenesis*

| |
|---|
| Inhibitors of tumor initiation |
|     Antioxidants: butylated hydroxytoluene (BHT), butylated hydroxyanisole (BHA), selenium, ethoxyquin, and disulfuram |
|     Flavones: 7,8-benzoflavone, 5,6-benzoflavone, and quercetin |
|     Vitamins: A, $B_2$, C, and E |
|     Certain noncarcinogenic polycyclic aromatic hydrocarbons: dibenz(*a,c*)anthracene, benz-(*a*)anthracene, benzo(*e*)pyrene, and pyrene |
|     Environmental contaminants: 2,3,7,8-tetrachlorodibenzo-p-dioxin (TCDD) and polychlorobiphenyls (PCB) |
|     Sulfur mustard |
|     Polyriboinosinic–polyribocytidylic acid (poly I:C) |
|     Anti-inflammatory steroids |
| Inhibitors of tumor promotion |
|     Anti-inflammatory steroids: cortisol, dexamethasone, and fluocinolone acetonide |
|     Retinoids |
|     Protease inhibitors: tosyl lysine chloromethyl ketone (TLCK), tosyl arginine methyl ester (TAME), Tosyl phenylalanine chloromethyl ketone (TPCK), antipain, and leupeptin |
|     Bacillus Calmette-Guerin (BCG) |
|     Polyriboinosinic–polyribocytidylic acid (poly I:C) |
|     Cyclic nucleotides |
|     Dimethylsulfoxide (DMSO) |
|     Butyrate |

TABLE 5. *Classification of intentional food additives*[a]

| | |
|---|---|
| Nutrients | Antioxidants |
| Vitamins | Emulsifiers |
| Minerals | Stabilizers |
| Non-nutritive sweeteners | Thickeners |
| Flavors | Coloring agents |
| Flavor enhancers | Bleaching agents |
| Preservatives | |

[a] Approximately 30 terms are used to describe intentional food additives, most of them cosmetic in nature.

cals have been found that inhibit the promotion or progression of cancer by altering the state of differentiation, inhibiting promoter-induced cellular proliferation, or preventing gene activation by the tumor promoters (28).

## FOOD ADDITIVES AND CONTAMINANTS

A variety of food additives are imposed on mankind daily, intentionally and unintentionally, of which many may represent carcinogenic hazards (Tables 5 and 6). It has been estimated, for example, that approximately 1.1 billion pounds, or 5 pounds per capita, of chemical substances are intentionally added to our food annually (25). These additives are classified in Table 5 (4,46,47). Some, such as nutrients, vitamins, and minerals, are of obvious benefit to man, whereas

TABLE 6. *Unintentional food additives*

Synthetic chemicals
  Agricultural chemicals, pesticides
  Kepone, zineb, endrin, polychlorobiphenyls, DDT, etc.
  Feed additives
  Diethylstilbestrol, ninhydrazone, melangestrol acetate, etc.
  Chemicals migrating from food packaging materials
  Bisphenol, vinyl chloride, etc.
  Chemicals produced by interactions with food additives and other chemicals or food constituents
  Nitrites with primary and secondary amines to yield nitrosamines; diethylpyrocarbonate with ammonia to yield urethan
  Chemicals produced during food processing by heat or ionizing radiation
  Benzo(a)pyrene, anthracene derivatives, acridine derivatives, etc.
  Chemical contamination during food processing
  Asbestos, talc, vinyl chloride, polychlorobiphenyls

Normal constituents of natural food products
  Cycasin, polyaromatic hydrocarbons, safrole

Natural contaminants of natural food products
  Carcinogens from nonmicrobiological sources
  Arsenic, nitrites, nitrosamines
  Carcinogens from microbiological sources
  Ergot alkaloids, pyrrolizidine alkaloids, aflatoxins, etc.

others may be quite hazardous. Suspected of being harmful are the common food coloring agent amaranth FD&C red dye no. 2, which has been shown to be carcinogenic (25), nitrite preservatives, which have been implicated in nitrosamine carcinogenesis (25), and the nonnutritive sweeteners cyclamate and saccharin, which are tumor promoters. Of the many agents that are unintentionally added to the food chain, PAH, pesticides, herbicides, and mycotoxins are known or suspected carcinogens. Another, aflatoxin, has been found to be an extremely potent carcinogen in experimental animals.

Butylated hydroxyanisole (BHA), butylated hydroxytoluene (BHT), and propyl gallate are commonly added to foods to maintain freshness and prevent spoilage by oxidation. They are frequently used in dried cereals, cooking oils, canned goods, and various animal feed, with the average daily intake of phenolic antioxidants by man estimated at 2 mg (5). They are not readily excreted and tend to accumulate in the body (5). Although the phenolic antioxidants are generally recognized as safe by the FDA, there are varying reports as to the effects of these food additives on organisms. It has been reported that BHT decreases cell survival (20), causes chromosomal damage (20), reduces the growth rate of cultured cells (14), and acts as a tumor promoter in the liver and lung (19,43). On the other hand, the phenolic antioxidants, selenium, and vitamins C and E have been shown to protect experimental animals against liver damage, aging, carcinogen-induced chromosomal breakage, and chemical carcinogenesis (3,8,13,24,36–38). Table 7 summarizes some of the beneficial effects of antioxidants.

When added to the diet, BHA, BHT, and ethoxyquin have been found to inhibit the carcinogenic effect of dietary 7,12-dimethylbenz($a$)anthracene (DMBA) or B($a$)P on the forestomach of the mouse and the mammary gland of the rat by 50% or more (37). Addition of BHA to the diet has been shown to protect against pulmonary neoplasms resulting from acute exposures to DMBA, B($a$)P, urethan, or uracil mustard (38). The addition of BHA to diets containing DMBA, 7-hydroxy-12-methylbenz($a$)-anthracene, or dibenz($a,h$)-anthracene was likewise found to inhibit pulmonary tumor formation (38). Intraperitoneal administration of BHA was reported to decrease the number of pulmonary adenomas resulting from subcutaneous administration of diethylnitrosamine and 4-nitroquinoline-N-oxide (36). Selenium and BHT were found to be effective inhibitors of N-2-fluorenylacetamide-induced liver and mammary tumors (3,

TABLE 7. *Beneficial effects of antioxidants*

| |
| --- |
| Maintain freshness and prevent spoilage of food by oxidation. |
| Inhibit toxicity related to some chemicals. |
| Inhibit carcinogenesis (both chemical and ultraviolet radiation). |
| Inhibit carcinogen-induced chromosomal breakage. |
| Inhibit aging of cells in culture and retard aging in mice. |
| Inactivate lipid-containing viruses. |

9,34). BHT was also found to inhibit intestinal carcinogenesis in rats by azoxymethane (42).

When applied to mouse skin, the antioxidants, selenium (22), vitamin E (21,29), and ascorbic acid (23,29) were found to significantly reduce tumor formation by DMBA initiation in a two-stage system of tumorigenesis. Both BHA and BHT were found to significantly inhibit DMBA-initiated tumors in mouse skin, although greater inhibition was noted with BHT (29). When applied topically at a dose of 1 mg six hours prior to, five minutes before, and six hours after DMBA initiation, BHT was found to inhibit tumorigenesis quite effectively (29).

Several investigations have dealt with the possible mechanism of the inhibiting action of antioxidants on chemical carcinogenesis. When applied topically to mice, BHA and BHT were found to inhibit *in vitro* epidermal NADPH-dependent covalent binding of radioactive B(*a*)P and DMBA to DNA (29). In general, BHT was more effective in inhibiting the binding of both B(*a*)P and DMBA to DNA than was BHA (29). This finding of the inhibitory effect of BHT and BHA on binding correlates well with their effect on skin tumorigenesis (29). However, BHA and BHT added *in vitro* were found not to inhibit the epidermal NADPH-dependent covalent binding of radioactive B(*a*)P and DMBA to DNA (29). Even at five times the DMBA or B(*a*)P substrate concentration used in the *in vitro* binding assay, no inhibition was noted. Speir and Wattenberg (32) reported that incubation of radioactive B(*a*)P with DNA with liver microsomes from BHA-fed mice resulted in significantly less covalent binding of B(*a*)P to DNA than B(*a*)P incubated with control microsomes. Thus, it appears that the inhibition of PAH tumorigenesis by antioxidants is related to their ability to prevent the *in vivo* activation of PAH to carcinogenic epoxides or other electrophilic intermediates.

Other antioxidants have been shown to have a protective effect against PAH-, nitrosamine-, and dimethylhydrazine-induced neoplasms. Disulfiram and dimethyldithiocarbamate added to the diet were found to inhibit DMBA-induced mammary tumor formation and adrenal necrosis in female rats (39–41). In the mouse, disulfiram prevented the occurrence of tumors of the forestomach normally caused by the addition of B(*a*)P to the diet (39). Wattenberg (40) showed that disulfiram added to the diet of female mice inhibited large-bowel neoplasia usually produced by repeated subcutaneous administrations of dimethylhydrazine. In general, the antioxidants may protect against chemical carcinogenesis by inhibiting the formation of the carcinogenic electrophile in a number of structurally diverse chemical compounds. Table 8 summarizes the inhibitory effects of antioxidants on a wide range of carcinogens in many different tissues.

Some food preservatives that are not antioxidants have been shown to be hazardous. The dangers to health from nitrites in the environment generally and in processed meat in particular have been established by several investigators. These dangers are associated with the production of nitrous acid in the acid environment of the stomach and the further reaction of this substance with

TABLE 8. *Inhibition of carcinogens by antioxidants*

| Carcinogen | Antioxidant | Species | Site of neoplasm inhibited |
|---|---|---|---|
| BP | BHA, BHT, ethoxyquin, flavones | Mouse | Forestomach, lung |
| BP | BHA, BHT, selenium, vit. C and E, flavones | Mouse | Skin |
| BP | Disulfiram | Mouse | Lung, forestomach |
| DMBA | BHA, BHT, ethoxyquin, flavones | Mouse | Forestomach, lung |
| DMBA | BHA, BHT, ethoxyquin, flavones | Rat | Breast |
| DMBA | BHA, BHT, selenium, vit. C and E, benzoflavones | Mouse | Skin |
| DMBA | Disulfiram, dimethyldithiocarbamate, and benzylthiocyanate | Rat | Breast |
| 7-hydroxymethyl-12-methylbenz-(a)anthracene | BHA | Mouse | Lung |
| Dibenz(a,h)anthracene | BHA | Mouse | Lung |
| Diethylnitrosamine | BHA, ethoxyquin | Mouse | Lung |
| 4-nitroquinoline-N-oxide | BHA, ethoxyquin | Mouse | Lung |
| Uracil mustard | BHA | Mouse | Lung |
| Urethan | BHA | Mouse | Lung |
| N-2-fluorenylacetamide | BHT | Rat | Liver |
| N-hydroxy-N-2-fluorenylacetamide | BHT | Rat | Liver, breast |
| P-dimethylaminoazobenzene | BHT | Rat | Liver |
| Dimethylhydrazine | Disulfiram, BHA | Mice | Colon |
| Azoxymethane | BHT | Rat | Intestine |

naturally occurring and synthetic secondary and tertiary amines to form nitrosamines, which have been shown to be carcinogenic, mutagenic, and cytotoxic (15). Ascorbic acid effectively competes with amines for nitrous acid *in vitro,* and co-administration of ascorbic acid with potentially nitrosatable drugs and foods containing nitrites may reduce the hazards associated with these substances (14). The use of large doses of vitamin C to protect against the common cold, as advocated by Linus Pauling, may also help prevent cancer induction by chemicals. As discussed earlier, other antioxidants have been shown to protect against nitrosamine carcinogenesis.

The nitrofuran food preservative furylfuramide (AF-2) was used widely in Japan for approximately two years until it was found to be mutagenic in bacteria and carcinogenic in mice (18). It is an antimicrobial agent, not an antioxidant. Only time will determine if AF-2 increases the cancer incidence in Japan.

In summary, it is very difficult to determine what effect intentional and unintentional food additives with carcinogenic, co-carcinogenic, and promoting activities will have on the human population. A number of food additives have also been found to have an inhibiting effect on chemical carcinogenesis. Whether these inhibitory agents reach high enough concentrations through dietary intake to counteract the effect of chemicals that may cause cancer in man remains to be established.

## CONCLUSIONS

A. Most human cancers are thought to be chemically induced.

B. All chemical carcinogens that are not electrophilic reactants must be converted metabolically into a chemically reactive form. Chemical carcinogenesis can be divided into at least two stages, initiation and promotion.

C. There are a number of modifiers of chemical carcinogenesis. Some are potent inhibitors of tumor initiation, whereas others selectively inhibit tumor promotion.

D. Food contains both intentional and unintentional additives, of which some have been shown to be carcinogenic and others are suspected of being carcinogenic.

E. The antioxidants BHA and BHT are widely used as food preservatives. These agents, plus selenium and vitamins C and E, have been shown to inhibit skin, lung, mammary, forestomach, colon, and liver cancer in experimental animals exposed to a wide range of carcinogens.

F. These agents appear to inhibit the formation of the carcinogenic electrophile, which has been implicated in the initiation of cancer through alterations of the genetic code.

G. Chemicals in cruciferous plants (brussels sprouts, cabbages, and cauliflower) and citrus fruits are potent inducers of the mixed-function oxidase system. These chemicals have been shown to inhibit carcinogenesis by detoxifying chemical carcinogens.

H. Vitamin A and certain derivatives are potent inhibitors of chemical carcinogenesis by acting on both the metabolism of the carcinogen and the differentiation of the target tissue.

I. Whether these agents reach high enough concentrations through dietary intake to inhibit chemical carcinogenesis in man remains to be determined.

## ACKNOWLEDGMENTS

This research was sponsored jointly by National Institutes of Health Grant CA 20076 and the Office of Health and Environmental Research, U.S. Department of Energy, under contract W-7405-eng-26 with the Union Carbide Corporation.

## REFERENCES

1. Boyland, E. (1950): The biological significance of metabolism of polycyclic compounds. *Biochem. Soc. Symp.,* 5:40–54.
2. Brookes, P., and Lawley, P. D. (1964): Evidence for the binding of polynuclear aromatic hydrocarbons to the nucleic acids of mouse skin: Relation between carcinogenic power of hydrocarbons and their binding to deoxyribonucleic acid. *Nature,* 202:781–784.
3. Cawthorne, R. J., Bunyan, J., Sennitt, M. V., and Green, J. (1970): Vitamin E and hepatotoxic agents. 3. Vitamin E, synthetic antioxidants and carbon tetrachloride toxicity in the rat. *Br. J. Nutr.,* 24:357–384.
4. Code of Federal Regulations 21, Food and Drugs Part 10–199, revised as of April 1, 1975.
5. Collins, A. J., and Sharratt, M. (1970): The BHT content of human adipose tissue. *Food Cosmet. Toxicol.,* 8:409–414.
6. Committee on biologic effects of atmospheric pollutants (1972). Natl. Acad. Sci.
7. Emmett, E. A. (1973): Ultraviolet radiation as a cause of skin tumors. *CRC Cit. Rev. Toxicol.,* 2:211–255.
8. Harman, D. (1968): Free radical theory of aging: Effect of free radical reaction inhibitors on the mortality rate of male $LAF_1$ mice. *J. Gerontol.,* 23:476–482.
9. Harr, J. R., Exon, J. H., Whanger, P. D., and Weswig, P. H. (1972): Effects of dietary selenium on N-2-fluorenylacetamide (FAA)-induced cancer in vitamin E supplemented, selenium depleted rats. *Clin. Toxicol.,* 5:187–194.
10. Heidelberger, C. (1975): Chemical carcinogenesis. *Ann. Rev. Biochem.,* 44:79–121.
11. Heidelberger, C., and Moldenhauer, M. G. (1956): The interaction of carcinogenic hydrocarbons with tissue constituents. IV. A quantitative study of the binding to skin proteins of several $^{14}C$ labeled hydrocarbons. *Cancer Res.,* 16:442–449.
12. IRAC (1972–1977): IARC *Monographs on the Evaluation of Carcinogenic Risk of Chemicals to Man, Vols. 1–15.* International Agency for Research on Cancer, Lyon, France.
13. Jaffe, W. (1946): The influence of wheat germ oil on the production of tumors in rats by methylcholanthrene. *Exp. Med. Surg.,* 4:278–282.
14. Metcalfe, S. M. (1971): Cell culture as a test system for toxicity. *J. Pharm. Pharmacol.,* 23:817–823.
15. Miller, E. C. (1978): Some current perspectives on chemical carcinogenesis in humans and experimental animals: Presidential address. *Cancer Res.,* 38:1479–1496.
16. Miller, E. C., and Miller, J. A. (1966): Mechanisms of chemical carcinogenesis: Nature of proximate carcinogens and interactions with macromolecules. *Pharmacol. Rev.,* 18:805–838.
17. Mirvish, S. S., Wallcave, L., Eagen, M., and shubik, P. (1972): Ascorbate–nitrite reaction: Possible means of blocking the formation of carcinogenic N-nitroso compounds. *Science,* 177:65–68.
18. Nonura, T. (1975): Carcinogenicity of the food additive furylfuramide in foetal and young mice. *Nature,* 258:610–611.
19. Peraino, C., Fry, R. J. M., Staffedt, E., and Christopher, J. P. (1977): Enhancing effects of

phenobarbitone and butylated hydroxytoluene on 2-acetylaminofluorene induced hepatic tumorigenesis in the rat. *Food Cosmet. Toxicol.,* 15:93–96.

20. Sciorra, L. J., Kaufmann, B. N., and Maier, R. (1974): The effects of butylated hydroxytoluene on the cell cycle and chromosome morphology of phytohaemagglutinin stimulated leucocyte cultures. *Food Cosmet. Toxicol.,* 12:33–44.
21. Shamberger, R. J. (1966): Protection against cocarcinogenesis by antioxidants. *Experientia,* 22:116–117.
22. Shamberger, R. J. (1970): Relationship of selenium to cancer. I. Inhibitory effect of selenium on carcinogenesis. *J. Natl. Cancer Inst.,* 44:931–936.
23. Shamberger, R. J. (1972): Increase of peroxidation in carcinogenesis. *J. Natl. Cancer Inst.,* 48:1491–1497.
24. Shamberger, R. M., Boughman, F. F., Kalchert, S. L., Willis, C. E., and Hoffman, G. C. (1973): Carcinogen-induced chromosomal breakage decreased by antioxidants. *Proc. Natl. Acad. Sci. USA,* 70:1461–1463.
25. Shubik, P., (1975): Potential carcinogenicity of food additives and contaminants. *Cancer Res.,* 35:3475–3480.
26. Sims, P., Grover, P. L., Swaisland, A., Pal, K., and Hewer, A. (1974): Metabolic activation of benzo(a)pyrene proceeds by a diol-epoxide. *Nature,* 252:326–327.
27. Slaga, T. J., editor (1979): *Carcinogenesis: A Comprehensive Survey. Modifiers of Chemical Carcinogenesis, Vol. 5.* Raven Press, New York.
28. Slaga, T. J. (1980): Cancer, etiology, mechanisms, and prevention: A summary. In: *Carcinogenesis: A Comprehensive Survey. Modifiers of Chemical Carcinogenesis, Vol. 5,* edited by T. J. Slaga, pp. 243–262, Raven Press, New York.
29. Slaga, T. J. and Bracken, W. M. (1977): The effects of antioxidants on skin tumor initiation and aryl hydrocarbon hydroxylase. *Cancer Res.,* 37:1631–1635.
30. Slaga, T. J., Buty, S. G., Thompson, S., Bracken, W. M., and Viaje, A. (1977): A kinetic study on the *in vitro* covalent binding of polycyclic hydrocarbons to nucleic acid using epidermal homogenates as the activating system. *Cancer Res.,* 37:3126–3131.
31. Slaga, T. J., Sivak, A., and Boutwell, R. K., editors (1978): *Carcinogenesis: A Comprehensive Survey. Mechanisms of Tumor Promotion and Cocarcinogenesis, Vol. 2.* Raven Press, New York.
32. Speir, J., and Wattenberg, L. (1975): Alteration in microsomal metabolism of benzo(a)pyrene in mice fed butylated hydroxyanisole. *J. Natl. Cancer Inst.,* 55:469–472.
33. Tennant, R. W., and Rascati, R. J. (1980): Mechanisms of cocarcinogenesis involving endogenous retroviruses. In: *Carcinogenesis: A Comprehensive Survey. Modifiers of Chemical Carcinogenesis, Vol. 5,* edited by T. J. Slaga, pp. 185–205. Raven Press, New York.
34. Ulland, B., Weisburger, J., Yamamoto, R., and Weisburger, E. (1973): Antioxidants and carcinogenesis: Butylated hydroxytoluene, but not diphenyl-p-phenylene diamine, inhibits cancer induction by N-2-fluorenylacetamide and by N-hydroxy-N-2-fluorenylacetamide in rats. *Food Cosmet. Toxicol.,* 11:199.
35. Ullrich, R. L. (1980): Interactions of radiation and chemical carcinogens. In: *Carcinogenesis: A Comprehensive Survey. Modifiers of Chemical Carcinogenesis, Vol. 5,* edited by T. J. Slaga, pp. 169–184. Raven Press, New York.
36. Wattenberg, L. W. (1972): Inhibition of carcinogenic effects of diethylnitrosamine and 4-nitroquinoline-N-oxide by antioxidants. *Fed. Proc.,* 31:633–636.
37. Wattenberg, L. W. (1972): Inhibition of carcinogenic and toxic effects of polycyclic hydrocarbons by phenolic antioxidants and ethyoxyquin. *J. Natl. Cancer Inst.,* 48:1425–1430.
38. Wattenberg, L. W. (1973): Inhibition of chemical carcinogen-induced pulmonary neoplasia by butylated hydroxyanisole. *J. Natl. Cancer Inst.,* 50:1541–1544.
39. Wattenberg, L. W. (1974): Inhibition of carcinogenic and toxic effects of polycyclic hydrocarbons by several sulfur-containing compounds. *J. Natl. Cancer Inst.,* 52:1583–1587.
40. Wattenberg, L. W. (1975): Inhibition of dimethylhydrazine-induced neoplasia of the large intestine by disulfiram. *J. Natl. Cancer Inst.,* 54:1005–1006.
41. Wattenberg, L. W. (1976): In: *Fundamentals in Cancer Prevention,* edited by P. N. Magee, S. Takayama, T. Sugimura, and T. Matsushima, pp. 153–166. University Park Press, Baltimore.
42. Weisburger, E. K., Evarts, R. P., and Wenk, M. L. (1977): Inhibitory effect of butylated hydroxytoluene (BHT) on intestinal carcinogenesis in rats by azoxymethane. *Food Cosmet. Toxicol.,* 15:139–141.
43. Witschi, H., Williamson, D., and Lock, S. (1977): Enhancement of urethan tumorigenesis in mouse lung by butylated hydroxytoluene. *J. Natl. Cancer Inst.,* 58:301–305.

44. Wynder, E. L. (1976): Nutrition and cancer. *Fed. Proc.,* 35:1309–1315.
45. Wynder, E. L., Hoffmann, D., McCoy, G. D., Cohen, L. A., and Reddy, B. S. (1978): Tumor promotion and cocarcinogenesis as related to man and his environment. In: *Carcinogenesis: A Comprehensive Survey. Mechanisms of Tumor Promotion and Cocarcinogenesis, Vol. 2,* edited by T. J. Slaga, A. Sivak, and R. K. Boutwell, pp. 59–77. Raven Press, New York.
46. Verrett, J., and Carper, J. (1971): *Eating May Be Hazardous to Your Health: The Case Against Food Additives.* Simon & Schuster, New York.
47. Zaratzian, V. L. (1976): Cancer hazards in food. In: *Proc. Symp. on Diet and Cancer,* AAAS, Boston. Feb. 24.

Nutrition and Cancer: Etiology and Treatment,
edited by G. R. Newell and N. M. Ellison.
Raven Press, New York © 1981.

# Alcohol and Carcinogenesis

*Joseph J. Vitale, **Selwyn A. Broitman, and *Leonard S. Gottlieb

*Boston University School of Medicine, Mallory Institute of Pathology, Boston, Massachusetts 02118**; Boston University School of Medicine, Department of Microbiology, Boston, Massachusetts 02118

Although several epidemiological studies (33) suggest that alcohol plays a causative role in carcinogenesis, they are not supported by well-controlled experimental studies. In contrast to epidemiologic data on dietary intake of most nutrients, the reliability of the data on alcoholic beverage or absolute ethanol consumption is even more tenuous. Consequently, interpretation of epidemiological studies relating alcohol consumption to oncogenesis is no more reliable than the data on which the studies are based. Indeed, attempts to derive reliable figures on alcohol ingestion are fraught with more than the usual epidemiologic errors. In the United States, the average consumption of ethanol for each person of drinking age is estimated to be 2.61 gallons of absolute ethanol per year, based on tax-paid withdrawals (35). If one assumes an average daily consumption of 2,500 calories for men and 1,800 calories for women, the caloric contribution of ethanol to the diet of American men and women is approximately 8% and 11%, respectively. The quantity of alcohol consumed that escapes government taxation in this country, and thus is not accounted for in these figures, is probably no less than that sold under governmental sanction. Thus, it is reasonable to estimate that alcohol may contribute as much as 20% to the total calories in the average adult diet in the United States. If one considers that about two-thirds of adults in the U.S. are imbibers of alcohol (60% of women and 77% of men) (35), the average drinker consumes from 13% (tax-paid only) to 26% (tax-paid and illegal) of his or her total daily calories as alcohol![a]

Of the approximately 100 million drinkers in this country, about 10% are chronic alcoholics or alcohol abusers. Although these individuals obviously consume considerably more alcohol than the "average" drinker, it is highly unlikely that this small segment of the drinking population significantly elevates the national average alcohol consumption. The point is that alcohol consumption

---

[a] To provide a perspective for the interested reader, 16% of the total daily caloric intake of 2,500 calories provided as alcohol is easily met by drinking a 6-oz glass (180 ml) of wine (17% alcohol) and a double martini (60 ml of 86 proof gin) daily. Calculations: 17% of 180 ml = 30 ml of alcohol (wine), 43% (gin) of 60 ml = 26 ml of alcohol (gin). Total 56 ml of absolute ethanol times 7 calories per gram of alcohol = 392 calories.

accounts for an alarming proportion of dietary calories in this country and very probably throughout the world. These tend to be "invisible" calories, since they are rarely accounted for in nutritional surveys (36). This is but one reason why it is difficult to delineate precisely the influence of alcohol in geographic epidemiologic studies on a specific disease process.

With regard to the association between nutrition and cancer, the problem of relating alcohol consumption to cancer incidence is even more complex. For example, an estimate of the proportions of fat, carbohydrate, protein, and fiber consumed in any population can be obtained (accepting the limitations of export and import data), since virtually all individuals in a population consume all of these dietary components. Although there is unquestionably significant individual variation in intake, it is possible to estimate the composition of national diets. Thus, for comparative purposes, it can determine whether one country consumes a greater proportion of calories as fat or protein, etc., than another, in order to relate these findings to cancer incidence. This cannot be done as readily with alcohol consumption, since not everyone in a population consumes alcohol, whereas some consume excessive amounts. Relating the national incidence of a disease to the quantity of alcohol consumed can be misleading if only one-half or two-thirds of the population drink alcohol. Furthermore, if a small segment of the population were alcohol abusers and had a high incidence of cancer at a specific organ site, the high incidence of disease in this small group would be obscured by the lower national average.

In addition, it is difficult to obtain reliable ethanol consumption data on a country-by-country basis. In countries where alcoholic beverages are controlled by the government for tax purposes, an indeterminate amount may be consumed without government sanction. Finally, consuming a moderate quantity of alcoholic beverages over a short time period (spree drinking) could have more deleterious effects than consuming a larger quantity over a longer period, particularly by a well-nourished individual. The former might reflect the drinking habits of one segment of a population, but would not be apparent in figures for national average ethanol consumption.

It is of interest that the correlation coefficients between colon cancer and the *total* quantity of alcohol consumed, the absolute alcohol consumed as distilled spirits, and that consumed as wine for the 20 countries in Fig. 1 are 0.359, 0.105, and −0.056, respectively. However, the correlation coefficient between alcohol consumed as beer and colon cancer for those 20 countries is 0.78. These data suggest that there is no association between the consumption of alcohol per se and the death rate from colorectal cancer, whereas the consumption of beer, which contains other constituents besides ethanol, is associated with an increased death rate from colorectal cancer. This observation has also been noted by others (7). However, in view of the extreme limitations in collecting and interpreting alcohol consumption data here and abroad for the reasons alluded to above, it is not now possible to determine the influence of alcohol consumption on colorectal cancer or cancer at other organ sites. Epidemiological

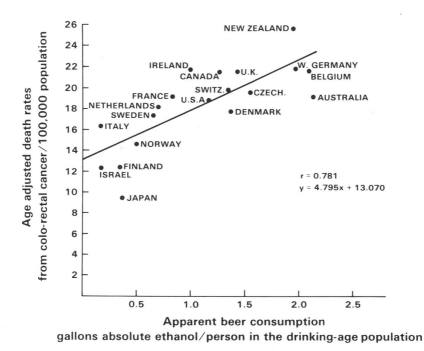

**FIG. 1.** The correlation coefficient between alcohol consumed as beer and colon cancer for 20 countries, based on data for 1966–1970 (35). Age-adjusted death rate from colon cancer from *World Health Statistics Annual, 1970–1971* (43).

studies have suggested that excessive alcohol ingestion is associated with an increased risk of cancer of the head, neck, and lungs (17). In other studies, oropharyngeal and esophogeal cancers have been associated with smoking and drinking (28,45,46), whereas among nonsmokers no apparent correlation between alcohol consumption and laryngeal cancer has been seen (46). It is our perception, based on the epidemiologic data and the lack of experimental data implicating alcohol as a carcinogen, that smoking may be the most important variable in carcinogenesis in these studies.

We know that excessive alcohol ingestion is associated with human liver disease, including cirrhosis, which can be considered a premalignant lesion. On the other hand, the incidence of hepatomas associated with alcoholism is indeed low, and this disease is perhaps not a major health problem, particularly in view of the relatively high consumption of alcohol in this country. In a study at the Boston City Hospital, about 60% of adult patients with hepatocellular carcinoma were found to have a background of alcohol-associated cirrhosis (25). In Africa, in contrast, cancer of the liver occurs usually in patients with hepatitis B-associated cirrhosis. Malignancy of the liver therefore appears to be a result of the cirrhotic lesion and is not directly related to alcohol ingestion.

There is no evidence that alcohol (ethanol) ingestion per se by the well-nourished human or animal results in carcinoma.

## ALCOHOL AS A TOXIN

The controversy persists as to whether alcohol ingestion in the well-nourished individual is cytotoxic, hepatotoxic, biochemically toxic, or harmless (26,27,29). Some observers believe that alcohol is harmful when taken in excessive amounts, regardless of nutritional state. Of approximately 10 million chronic alcoholics in the United States, only 10% develop cirrhosis. Nevertheless, the association between excessive alcohol intake and liver disease or diseases involving other organ systems (e.g., the pancreas) is well established. If one accepts the thesis that alcohol is toxic to cells, then affected cells may be more susceptible to carcinogenic agents, particularly if the alcoholic beverages contain carcinogens, such as nitrosamines, or potential carcinogens.

In excessive amounts, and in subclinically or overtly malnourished individuals, alcohol has been shown to affect the metabolism of various essential nutrients (37). Several nutritional deficiencies, in turn, have been shown to enhance and promote carcinogenesis (38).

## ALCOHOL, NUTRIENTS, AND CANCER

The roles of dietary deficiencies and excesses and of dietary components in oncogenesis are discussed in detail elsewhere in this text. Here we shall provide our own perspective on the role of diet in carcinogenesis and discuss possible interactions between nutrients and alcohol ingestion that may enhance or promote carcinogenesis.

In discussing the role of nutrition in carcinogenesis, it is well to define the terms "nutrition" and "diet." "Nutrition," as used here, refers to the 50 or more known essential nutrients, such as amino acids, iron, zinc, vitamin A, riboflavin, folic acid, and ascorbic acid. Some observers believe that nutrition has never been shown to play the slightest role in carcinogenesis or neoplasia, whereas others believe that it is the most important environmental factor in the causation of almost all major diseases, including coronary heart disease and cancer. "Diet" is another phenomenon. Individuals' diets consist of nutrients and also of additives, preservatives, coloring, residues, fiber, chemicals, and plasticides, fungal, bacterial, and viral contaminants, and perhaps hundreds of additional compounds indicated by "peaks" on a gas chromatogram, any of which may have carcinogenic activity in animals and man. If other internal and external factors are added, such as hormones, steroids, ionizing radiation, and air pollutants, one is hard pressed to know what role nutrients play, directly or indirectly, in carcinogenesis. Since there is little or no evidence of a direct effect of nutrient deficiencies or excesses (save calories) on the formation or promotion of cancer, it is assumed that whatever effect they exert is indirect (38).

A number of vitamin and mineral deficiencies, including protein, are associated with excessive alcohol ingestion (37). Deficiencies of thiamine, folic acid, magnesium, and iron are often exhibited by chronic alcoholics. Other nutritional deficiencies involve pyridoxine, pantothenic acid, riboflavin, zinc, and copper. The correlation between alcoholism and vitamin or mineral nutritional deficiencies may be primary or secondary.

There is evidence that alcohol in excess may produce deleterious nutritional effects by acting directly on tissues and enzyme systems, principally in the liver, which is the major site of both ethanol metabolism and vitamin storage, rather than by simply reducing nutrient intake. Decreased intake of essential nutrients is undoubtedly associated with excessive consumption of calories in the form of alcohol. However, a diseased organ, as a result of nutritional deficiencies or a combination of other factors including alcoholism, can exacerbate a dietary deficiency. This exacerbation comes about as a result of altered absorption of nutrients, decreased storage capacity (in terms of both concentration and functional mass), defective activation of vitamins, or metabolic aberrations in the diseased organ. Thus, when alcoholic subjects are not selected on the basis of hepatic or other diseases, their nutritional status is not markedly different from that of subjects in the same economic class who do not ingest excessive alcohol (39).

Some specific nutrient deficiencies have been identified with excessive alcohol ingestion. Among the more serious diseases of alcoholism is Wernicke's encephalopathy, which is associated with acute, severe thiamine ($B_1$) deficiency (39). Thiamine deficiency or excess has not been implicated in carcinogenesis, nor has it been shown to play a significant role in immunocompetency.

Pyridoxine (vitamin $B_6$) deficiency has been associated with alcohol ingestion. Although $B_6$ deficiency can cause several clinical disorders, including peripheral neuropathy, convulsions, and sideroblastic anemia, as well as liver disease, it has not been related to development of cancer. On the other hand, in experimental studies vitamin $B_6$ has been shown to play a very important role in the production of antibodies to various antigens (3).

Evidence elucidating the mechanisms of folate deficiency in chronic alcoholism is somewhat equivocal. However, it appears that folate deficiency is usually secondary to liver disease (in terms of increased release of folic acid or possible decreased affinity for folate) and changes in absorption (which are most notable following a concentrated drinking spree), rather than to a primary dietary deficiency. Other inconclusive evidence suggests that alcohol reversibly suppresses the hematopoietic response to folic acid in anemic folate-deficient patients, and that malabsorption of folic acid cannot completely account for the effect (39).

Folic acid deficiency has been shown, however, to impair both humoral and cellular immunity (20,39). Furthermore, the adverse effects of folic acid deficiency on the hematopoietic system, as well as on the gastrointestinal tract, are well known. Whether these morphological changes associated with folic acid deficiency enable chemicals or other carcinogenic agents to become reactive is not known. Indeed, folic acid deficiency could be expected to suppress oncogenesis, for its association with decreased cell turnover is the basis for its use in cancer chemotherapy regimens.

Excretion of magnesium is usually enhanced by alcohol ingestion, and magnesium deficiency signs and symptoms are common in alcoholic patients (14,21). However, although these signs and symptoms are associated with cardiovascular, renal, and neurological changes, there is little evidence that magnesium deficiency promotes carcinogenesis or affects immune function in host defense systems.

Alcohol probably increases the excretion of electrolytes, such as zinc, cadmium, molybdenum, and copper, and perhaps a number of other trace minerals, but the role of these electrolytes in carcinogenesis is not clear. Nonetheless, several epidemiological studies have reported changes in the concentrations of several trace elements in the blood or serum of cancer patients (21).

Alcoholic patients also may have severe long-standing iron deficiency, and the role of iron in carcinogenesis may be very significant. There is abundant evidence that iron deficiency without anemia produces profound defects in cell-mediated immunity (39). Apparently iron deficiency does not affect the humoral arm. Chronic prolonged and severe iron deficiency does produce gastric atrophy in rats (39). Recent studies from Colombia and our own laboratory and reports from the National Cancer Institute Epidemiological Section indicate that iron deficiency may play a role in the etiology of gastric cancer. There is evidence from our own studies that chronic severe iron deficiency, in the absence of other clinical manifestations, produces atrophy and intestinalization of the stomach, a premalignant condition (39). In Colombia, the gastric cancer rate is four times higher than that in the United States.

Others have suggested that chronic iron deficiency and chronic riboflavin deficiency enhance the development of the Plummer–Vinson syndrome (43), which is associated with an increased risk of cancer of the upper alimentary tract in women (19,47).

### Vitamins A and E

Low blood or serum levels of vitamins A and E in alcoholic patients (16,23,31) have been reported, but it is often difficult to interpret these findings. Poorly nourished individuals can be expected to have low levels of most nutrients, and whether the effect is due primarily to alcohol ingestion per se or to caloric restriction is not clear. Obviously, diseases of the liver or gastrointestinal tract would be expected to produce defects in retinal binding protein or other carrier proteins, or malabsorption of fats and fat-soluble vitamins, resulting in low blood levels of several nutrients. However, one report indicates that acute alcohol administration results in a lowered vitamin A level (1). Vitamin A clearly plays some role in cell differentiation (39), and deficiency states have been shown to enhance or promote the induction of pulmonary (11,13,30), bladder (10), colon (24), and cervical tumors (9). Several epidemiologic studies support the experimental data and suggest an association between relatively low dietary intakes of vitamin A and a relatively high incidence of lung cancer in Norway (5). A study several years ago (40) suggested an association between vitamin A and oropharyngeal cancer.

Vitamin E is a known antioxidant, and it and other antioxidants, such as butylated hydroxytoluene, have been shown to reduce the incidence of some chemically induced tumors (15,34,41). Vitamin E, considered by some to be a nutrient "looking for a role in human disease," may eventually be shown to have an important function in the prevention of oncogenesis.

## ALCOHOL AND IMMUNOCOMPETENCY

Depressed immune response and oncogenesis are not necessarily causally related. We need to ask How depressed a "depressed" immune system is. A five-or tenfold decrease in antibody production or in T-cell response to a mitogen does not necessarily render a host immunoincompetent. Immune responses are normally exaggerated, and what may be considered a depressed response in a sick patient or in an *in vitro* system may have little to do with eventual response to an infectious agent, a "transformed" cell, or a chemical carcinogen. The immune system is multifaceted; depression in one component may well be compensated for by another component, leaving the host well protected.

A number of studies indicate that alcohol in moderate to excessive amounts may have adverse effects on peripheral T-and B-lymphocytes. Many of these studies suffer, however, from the fact that they were carried out in patients with alcoholic cirrhosis or alcoholic hepatitis. One must distinguish between the effect of alcohol ingestion on T- and B-cell numbers and function and the effect of the disease process itself on these same parameters. Nevertheless, a number of studies have concluded that T- and B-cells may be reduced in number and function in the patient with alcoholic liver disease or cirrhosis (20).

The studies of Brayton et al. (6) are significant, since those authors used normal human volunteers exposed to alcohol to measure diminished leukocyte mobilization. They also noted that human polymorphonuclear leukocytes obtained after alcohol ingestion or exposure to alcohol *in vitro* showed no decrease in ability to phagocytize or kill ingested bacteria. Still, alcohol may diminish leukocyte mobilization, thus contributing to increased susceptibility to infection in patients who have been drinking. Furthermore, there is little evidence that an increased incidence of infection is related to an increased risk of malignancy.

Nonetheless, cogent arguments can be made for and against a role for alcohol in producing nutritional imbalances which, in turn, promote carcinogenesis by altering immune function. Observations from human studies strongly suggest that loss of function and defects in cell-mediated immunity are associated with carcinogenesis (e.g., use of immunosuppressive agents and the increased incidence of neoplasia), and that spontaneous remission of many tumors is associated with the return of normal cell-mediated immune function. The observation by some that immunosuppression correlates better with myeloproliferative diseases than with other types of neoplasia does not negate the strong circumstantial evidence, both clinically and experimentally derived, that the immune system plays some role in the pathogenesis of carcinoma. Animal studies support the observation that depressed cell-mediated immunity is associated with tumorigenesis. Several essential nutrient deficiencies, including vitamin A, methionine, choline, folic acid (or folic acid antagonists), vitamin C, and protein, have been shown to adversely affect immune response and to enhance experimental chemical carcinogenesis (38,39).

## ALCOHOL AS AN INDUCER OF ENZYME SYSTEMS INVOLVED IN CARCINOGENESIS

Most procarcinogens do not result in tumors at the site of application, but require activation by various enzyme systems found in most tissue, including liver (4,12,18), lymphocyte (42), skin (22), lung (32), and colon (2). Alcohol is known to stimulate microsomal enzyme systems involved in both the activation and inactivation of potential carcinogens (21). One cannot be certain ingestion of alcohol with a given carcinogen will activate or deactivate that carcinogen. Thus, one could even envision beneficial effects of ethanol consumption. The route of activation or deactivation depends on the chemical composition or structure of the carcinogen.

For the purposes of this discussion, let us select a chemical that may be activated by those enzyme systems that convert procarcinogens into carcinogens. The activated procarcinogen or carcinogen can diffuse into the bloodstream and affect various target organs or the site at which the procarcinogen is activated. Depending on the route taken by the carcinogen or the site at which activation takes place, any organ or organ system might be susceptible to the development of tumors. It seems reasonable, therefore, to assume that if the colon is exposed to a carcinogen, and not the lungs or other organs, tumors would develop in the colon.

How, then, does alcohol theoretically affect carcinogenesis? In the jargon of the oncologist, alcohol has never been shown to be an *initiator* of cancer. Furthermore, there are those who might object to the use of the word "promoter," since there is no convincing evidence that, once initiated, a tumor develops faster or bigger or metastasizes more readily after alcohol ingestion. Clearly, alcohol could be expected to enhance oncogenesis only in the presence of an activated carcinogen. Alcohol diffuses through the body fluids readily and every organ system is exposed to it. Depending upon an individual's predisposition to a disease (e.g., pancreatitis or hepatitis), alcohol might enhance the progression of that disease.

In the case of the liver, the lesions associated with choline deficiency in the experimental animal can be "promoted" by the ingestion of alcohol. Cirrhosis develops sooner with alcohol ingestion in a choline-deficient animal, as does hepatic cancer, even in the absence of known carcinogens. If one were to expose a choline-deficient animal that has been given alcohol to a liver carcinogen, experimental studies suggest that the induction of tumors in the liver would be very rapid and pronounced (28,29,31).

Another example can be cited: vitamin A deficiency and iron deficiency are associated with epithelial metaplasia. Either deficiency in the absence of a carcinogen has never been shown to initiate cancer, but either will promote existing oncogenesis (38). Vitamin A deficiency, for example, results in epithelial metaplasia of the colon, and carcinogenesis could be expected to occur in the colon if the activated carcinogen were to localize in that organ. On the other hand, if the epithelial metaplasia caused by vitamin A deficiency occurred in the lung, then the carcinogen could be expected to produce cancer in the lung rather than in the colon, at least initially. The ingestion of alcohol, which can activate procarcinogens, could be expected to promote oncogenesis in the colon, the lung, or both, in the host with vitamin A deficiency.

It may be that ethanol is neither a promoter nor an initiator of oncogenesis in most individuals, and perhaps promotes or initiates only in those with a genetic predisposition to cancer. However, from what is known about its relationship to nutrients and its enhancement of nutritional deficiency, alcohol may indeed be an "enhancer" of carcinogenesis. It seems likely, also, that what alcoholic beverages contain may be at least as important as ethanol consumption per se. This is illustrated in Fig. 1, in which the correlation between the ingestion of beer and colon cancer was shown to be better than the reported association between colon cancer and breast cancer or between either of these cancers and fat intake (8).

## SUMMARY

The available data suggest that excessive alcohol ingestion coupled with some carcinogenic insult (e.g., smoking) enhances or promotes tumorigenesis. There is no evidence that alcohol is an initiator of cancer. However, alcoholic beverages may serve as carriers of carcinogens. There are several ways by which chronic alcohol ingestion may promote or enhance the onset of neoplasia or metastases. Chronic alcoholism, particularly in the marginally nourished individual, can result in the loss of various essential nutrients, precipitating nutritional deficiencies. Such deficiencies have been shown to promote experimentally induced tumors in animals and to depress immune function. Thus, chronic alcoholism may promote carcinogenesis only in the marginally or poorly nourished host.

## ACKNOWLEDGMENT

The authors would like to acknowledge the support of Grant No. CA-16750 from the National Large Bowel Project of the National Cancer Institute, National Institutes of Health.

## REFERENCES

1. Althausen, T. L., Uyeyama, K., and Loran, M. R. (1960): Effects of alcohol on absorption of vitamin A in normal and gastrectomized subjects. *Gastroenterology,* 38:942–945.
2. Autrup, H., Harris, C. C., Stoner, G. D., Jesudason, M. L., and Trump, B. F. (1977): Binding of chemical carcinogens to macromolecules in cultured human colon. *J. Natl. Cancer Inst.,* 59:351–354.
3. Axelrod, A. E., and Trakatellis, A. C. (1974): Relationship of pyridoxine to immunologic phenomenon. *Vitam. Horm.,* 2:591.
4. Billing, B. A., and Black, M. (1971): The action of drugs on bilirubin metabolism in man. *Ann. NY Acad. Sci.,* 179:403–410.
5. Bjelke, E. (1975): Dietary vitamin A and human lung cancer. *Int. J. Cancer,* 15:561–565.
6. Brayton, R. G., Stokes, P. E., Schwarts, M. S., and Louria, D. B. (1970): Effect of alcohol and various diseases on leukocyte mobilization, phagocytosis and intracellular bacterial killing. *N. Engl. J. Med.,* 282:123–128.
7. Breslow, N. E., and Enstrom, J. E. (1974): Geographic correlations between cancer mortality rates and alcohol–tobacco consumption in the U.S. *J. Natl. Cancer Inst.,* 53:613–618.
8. Carroll, K. K., and Khor, H. T. (1975): Dietary fat in relation to tumorigenesis. *Prog. Biochem. Pharmacol.,* 10:308–353.
9. Chu, E. W., and Malmgren, R. A. (1965): Inhibitory effect of vitamin A on the induction of tumors of forestomach and cervix in the Syrian hamster by carcinogenic polycyclic hydrocarbons. *Cancer Res.,* 25:884–895.
10. Cohen, S. M., Wittenberg, J. F., and Bryan, G. T. (1974): Effect of hypo- and avitaminosis A on urinary bladder carcinogenicity of N-[4-(5-nitro-2-fur1)2-thiazolyl]formamide. *Fed. Proc.,* 33:602.
11. Cone, M. V., and Nettesheim, P. (1973): Effects of vitamin A on 3-methylcholanthrene induced squamous metaplasias and early tumors in the respiratory tract of rats. *J. Natl. Cancer Inst.,* 50:1599–1606.
12. Davies, D. S., and Thorgeirsson, S. S. (1971): Mechanism of hepatic drug oxidation and its relationship to individual differences in rates of oxidation in man. *Ann. NY Acad. Sci.,* 179:411–420.
13. DeLuca, L., Maestri, N., Bonanni, F., and Nelson, D. (1972): Maintenance of epithelial cell differentiation: The mode of action of vitamin A. *Cancer,* 30:1326–1331.
14. Fink, E. B. (1969): Therapy of magnesium deficiency. *Ann. NY Acad. Sci.,* 162:901–905.
15. Harman, D. (1961): Prolongation of the normal lifespan and inhibition of spontaneous cancer by antioxidants. *J. Gerontol.,* 16:247.
16. Insunza, I., and Ugarte, G. (1970): Esteatorrea en alcoholicos con y sin cirrosis hepatica. *Rev. Med. Chile,* 98:669–673.
17. Jensen, O. M. (1979): Cancer morbidity and causes of death among Danish brewery workers. *Int. J. Cancer,* 23:454–463.
18. Kuntzman, R., Mark, L. C., and Brand, L. (1966): Metabolism of drugs and carcinogens by human liver enzymes. *J. Pharmacol. Exp. Ther.,* 152:151–156.
19. Larsson, L. G., Sandstrom, A., and Westling, P. (1975): Relationship of Plummer–Vinson disease to cancer of the upper alimentary tract in Sweden. *Cancer Res.,* 35:3308–3316.
20. Leevy, C. M., and Zetterman, R. (1974): Malnutrition and alcoholism: An overview. In: *Alcohol and Abnormal Protein Synthesis,* edited by M. Rothschild, M. Oratz, and S. Schrieber, pp. 3–15. Pergamon Press, New York.
21. Lieber, C. S., Seitz, H. K., Garro, A. J., and Worner, T. M. (1979): Alcohol-related disease and carcinogenesis. *Cancer Res.,* 39:2863–2886.
22. Levin, W., Conney, A. H., and Alvares, A. P. (1972): Induction of benzo($\alpha$)pyrene hydrolase in human skin. *Science,* 176:419–420.
23. Losowsky, M. S., and Leonard, P. J. (1967): Evidence of vitamin E deficiency in patients with malabsorption or alcoholism and the effects of therapy. *Gut,* 8:539–543.
24. Newberne, P. M., and Rogers, A. E. (1973): Rat colon carcinomas associated with aflatoxin and marginal vitamin A. *J. Natl. Cancer Inst.,* 50:439–448.
25. Purtilo, D. T., and Gottlieb, L. S. (1973): Cirrhosis and hepatoma occurring at Boston City Hospital (1917–1968). *Cancer,* 32:458–462.
26. Rogers, A. E., Newberne, P. M., Vitale, J. J., and Gottlieb, L. S. (1974): Alcohol cirrhosis in baboons. *N. Engl. J. Med.,* 290:910–911.

27. Rogers, A. E., Fox, J. G., Whitney, K., Lenhart, G., Wallstrom, A., and Gottlieb, L. S. (1979): Acute and chronic effects of ethanol in nonhuman primates. In: *Primates in Nutritional Research,* edited by K. C. Hayes, pp. 249–289. Academic Press, New York.

28. Rothman, K., and Keller, A. (1972): The effect of joint exposure to alcohol and tobacco on risk of cancer of the mouth and pharynx. *J. Chronic Dis.,* 25:711–716.

29. Rubin, E., and Lieber, C. S. (1974): Fatty liver, alcohol hepatitis and cirrhosis produced by alcohol in primates. *N. Engl. J. Med.,* 290:128–135.

30. Saffiotti, U., Montesano, R., Sellacumar, A. R., and Borg, S. A. (1967): Studies on experimental lung cancer: Inhibition by vitamin A of the induction of tracheobronchial squamous metaplasia and squamous cell tumors. *Cancer,* 20:857–864.

31. Smith, F. R., and Lindenbaum, J. (1974): Human serum retinol transport in malabsorption. *Am. J. Clin. Nutr.,* 27:700–705.

32. Stoner, G. D., Harris, C. C., Autrup, H., Trump, B. F., Kingsbury, E. W., and Myers, G. A. (1978): Explant culture of human peripheral lung. I. Metabolism of benzo($\alpha$)pyrene. *Lab. Invest.,* 38:685–695.

33. Tuyns, A. J. (1979): Epidemiology of alcohol and cancer. *Cancer Res.,* 39:2840–2843.

34. Ulland, B. M., Weisburger, J. H., Yamamoto, R. S., and Weisburger, E. K. (1973): Antioxidants and carcinogenesis: Butylated hydroxytoluene, but not diphenly-p-phenylenediamine, inhibits cancer induction by N-2-fluorenylacetamide and by N-hydroxy-N-2-fluorenylacetamide in rats. *Food Cosmet. Toxicol.,* 11:199–207.

35. U.S. Department of Health, Education and Welfare, Public Health Service (1971): *Alcohol and Health.* (HSM) 72-9099. U.S. Government Printing Office, Washington, D.C.

36. U.S. Department of Health, Education and Welfare, Public Health Service (1979): *Dietary Intake Source Data, United States, 1971–1974.* (PHS) 79-1221. U.S. Government Printing Office, Washington, D.C.

37. Vitale, J. J., and Coffey, J. (1971): Alcoholism and vitamin metabolism. In: *The Biology of Alcoholism, Vol. 1, Biochemistry,* edited by B. Kissen and H. Begleiter, pp. 327–352. Plenum Press, New York.

38. Vitale, J. J. (1975): Possible role of nutrients in neoplasia. *Cancer Res.,* 35:3320–3325.

39. Vitale, J. J. (1979): Deficiency diseases. In: *Pathologic Basis of Disease,* edited by S. L. Robbins and R. S. Cotran, pp. 483–520. W. B. Saunders Co., Philadelphia.

40. Wahi, P. N., Bodkhe, R. R., Arora, S., and Srivastava, M. C. (1962): Serum vitamin A studies in leukoplakia and carcinoma of the oral cavity. *Indian J. Pathol. Bacteriol.,* 5:10–16.

41. Wattenberg, L. W. (1972): Inhibition of carcinogenic and toxic effects of polycyclic hydrocarbons by phenolic antioxidants and ethoxyquin. *J. Natl. Cancer Inst.,* 48:1425–1430.

42. Whitlock, J. P., Jr., Cooper, H. L., and Gelboin, H. V. (1972): Arl hydrocarbon (benzopyrene) hydrolase is stimulated in human lymphocytes by mitogens and benz($\alpha$)anthracene. *Science,* 177:618–619.

43. World Health Organization (1974): *World Health Statistics Annual, 1970–1971: Vital Statistics and Causes of Death,* ISBN 92-4-067711-9. World Health Organization, Geneva.

44. Wynder, E. L. (1977): Nutritional carcinogenesis. *Ann. NY Acad. Sci.,* 300:360–378.

45. Wynder, E. L., Bross, I. J., and Feldman, R. M. (1957): A study of the etiological factors in cancer of the mouth. *Cancer,* 10:1300–1323.

46. Wynder, E. L., Covey, L. S., Mabuci, K., and Muslumski, M. (1976): Environmental factors in cancer of the larynx: A second look. *Cancer,* 38:1591–1601.

47. Wynder, E. L., Hultberg, S., Jacobson, F., and Bross, I. J. (1957): Environmental factors in cancer of the upper alimentary tract: Swedish study with special reference to Plummer–Vinson syndrome. *Cancer,* 10:470–487.

*Nutrition and Cancer: Etiology and Treatment,*
edited by G. R. Newell and N. M. Ellison.
Raven Press, New York © 1981.

# Nutritional Problems Associated with Cancer Chemotherapy

## Stephen K. Carter

*Northern California Cancer Program, Palo Alto, California 94304*

The nutritional state of a patient interacts significantly with cancer chemotherapy. Many patients with cancer suffer from cachexia and malnutrition. Inanition and weight loss are often seen, as is anorexia. The nutritional status of the patient is an important prognostic variable for response to chemotherapy, as well as to other types of cancer treatment. On the other hand, cancer drugs can cause toxic side effects that can significantly affect the patient's nutritional status. Side effects, such as nausea, vomiting, stomatitis, diarrhea, fever, and chills, can further decrease appetite and physical activity, with resultant increased weight loss. This chapter will attempt to review the basic principles of cancer chemotherapy and then describe the interaction between nutrition and the use of anticancer drugs.

## PRINCIPLES OF CANCER CHEMOTHERAPY

The goal in using drugs to treat cancer is to selectively kill tumor cells. This goal is pursued by implementing the principles of the "cell-kill hypothesis," as elucidated by Skipper and his colleagues (40). Those principles are as follows: (a) the survival of an animal (with L1210 leukemia) is inversely related either to the number of leukemic cells inoculated or to the number remaining after treatment; (b) a single leukemic cell is capable of multiplying and eventually killing the host; (c) for most drugs, a clear relationship exists between the dose given and the drug's ability to eradicate tumor cells; and (d) a given dose of a drug kills a constant fraction of cells, not a constant number, regardless of the cell number present at the time of therapy. The fourth principle means that cell destruction by drugs follows first-order kinetics. The clinical implication of first-order cell destruction is that, in order to eradicate a tumor population effectively, it is necessary either to increase the dose to the maximum limits tolerated by the host or to start treatment when the number of cells is small enough to allow destruction of the tumor at doses that are reasonably well-tolerated.

The logical conclusion derived from the above hypothesis is that the maximum opportunity for achieving cure exists during the early disease stage. It is more difficult to eradicate disseminated disease than localized cancer, and much easier to control small tumors than larger ones.

According to the experimental model view, the growth curve of a cancer follows a Gompertzian function. This means that growth is always exponential, but with a growth constant that is simultaneously slowing exponentially. Therefore, as tumor mass increases, its mass-doubling time becomes progressively longer. The Gompertzian aspect of tumor growth is recognizable only when a tumor is measured in its clinically palpable range. In the clinically undetectable period, the growth is assumed to be exponential. Although this may be true in rodent models, there is no evidence that it obtains in humans.

If the Gompertzian model were clinically relevant, it would have significant clinical implications. The assumption that it is relevant has guided a good deal of clinical chemotherapy research over the last decade. As a mass responds to treatment, i.e., becomes smaller, it is assumed that the doubling time increases as a consequence of a greater number of cells moving into cycle. This larger percentage of metabolically active cells should increase the sensitivity of the neoplastic population to cell cycle-specific agents. This reasoning has led to the sequential use of cell cycle nonspecific agents, such as cyclophosphamide, to reduce the mass, followed by cell cycle-specific agents, such as Ara-C or methotrexate. Although these sequential combinations are theoretically attractive, none has proved clearly superior to other approaches in clinical trials.

Another implication of the Gompertzian growth concept is that metastases should be more sensitive to chemotherapy in general, and to cell cycle-specific agents in particular, than the primary tumor from which they arise. The smaller the metastatic focus, the greater the differential sensitivity should be. Therefore, the insensitivity of a primary tumor to a given drug regimen might not predict the response of its metastases to the same regimen. This theoretical construct has made "adjuvant" chemotherapy highly attractive.

A *sine qua non* of the cell-kill hypothesis and the Gompertzian growth concept is the inverse relationship between sensitivity to chemotherapy and tumor burden. This is based not only on a purely kinetic construct but on the basis of biochemical resistance as well. This means that the larger the total malignant mass, the higher will be the proportion of variants permanently resistant to a given compound or regimen. This has been estimated to be one in $10^6$ to $10^7$ cells by Hutchinson and Schmid (14). Hutchinson and Schmid have shown that it takes only five or six doses of cyclophosphamide to induce a significant resistance in L1210, and Skipper et al. (40) have data indicating that as few as two or three doses of methyl-CCNU do the same in rodent solid tumors.

A third factor, besides kinetics and resistance, that can explain clinical results differing from experimental models is pharmacology. The higher the cell number, the greater is the chance that sites exist, either within the tumor or in selected organs, at which tumor cells are protected from efficient exposure to cytotoxic drugs.

In experimental systems, a steep dose–response curve has been observed with most anticancer drugs. In these systems, the maximum dose of drug compatible with host survival appears to achieve maximum reduction of the tumor cell population. For many agents, twice the dose that kills 10% of the animals ($LD_{10}$) is lethal to 90% ($LD_{90}$).

Skipper and his colleagues (40) have reported that high-dose intermittent drug treatment with almost all antitumor agents is substantially more effective than low-dose, equitoxic daily treatment. As a result of studies such as these, most cytotoxic drug treatments in the U.S. use high-dose intermittent scheduling. However, the superiority of this scheduling is not clearly established by existing clinical data.

### Mechanism of Action of Antineoplastic Drugs

In the past 25 years, the cancer therapist has acquired several classes of antineoplastic drugs: cytotoxic agents, such as antimetabolites, alkylating agents, antitumor antibiotics, and mitotic inhibitors, and a miscellaneous group of synthetic agents, enzymes, and hormones.

Cytotoxic drugs, like ionizing rays, do not kill tumor cells directly, but prevent cell division and thereby cell proliferation. A number of fundamental molecular processes must continue to take place for cells to proliferate. The genetic material, DNA, must be replicated without error once every cycle. This requires an adequate supply of purine and pyrimidine nucleotides as building blocks, the enzyme DNA polymerase, and, last, an intact DNA template to direct the synthesis of new DNA. DNA also acts as a template for the synthesis of complementary RNA, a process catalyzed by RNA polymerase. RNA is then translated into proteins through a complex polymerization reaction that takes place on the ribosomes in the cell cytoplasm. The sequence of nucleotides of the messenger RNA determines the sequence in which amino acids, attached to their specific transfer RNA, are positioned in the growing protein. After the cells have replicated their DNA, thereby acquiring a double complement of genetic material, they undergo mitosis. The various chemotherapeutic agents interfere with one or the other of these essential cellular processes.

### Effects on Cellular Processes

Antimetabolites interfere with the synthesis of building blocks for nucleic acids. Methotrexate (a folic acid antagonist), 6-mercaptopurine and 6-thioguanine (purine analogs), and 5-fluorouracil and cytarabine or cytosine arabinoside (pyrimidine analogs) are the best-known examples. Cytarabine is also a competitive inhibitor of DNA polymerase. Imidazole carboxamide is a structural analog of 5-aminoimidazole-4-carboxamide, a precursor in the *de novo* synthesis of purine bases. Other agents besides purine and pyrimidine analogs can inhibit the synthesis of these bases or their nucleotides. Hydroxyurea may interfere with conversion of ribonucleotides into deoxyribonucleotides. The nitrosoureas BCNU (carmustine), CCNU (lomustine), and methyl-CCNU interfere with the insertion of carbon fragments in the purine ring. Procarbazine can inhibit biosynthesis of DNA, RNA, and protein.

Alkylating agents contain highly reactive alkyl groups and have a complex action. They damage the DNA template and cross-link the two strands of the double helix, preventing replication. The most common of these drugs in clinical use are nitrogen mustard, chlorambucil, cyclophosphamide, melphalan, triethylene thiophosphoramide (Thiotepa®), and busulphan. Some agents have complex modes of action, one of which is alkylation—mitomycin C, nitrosoureas, and imidazole carboxamide.

Many of the "antibiotic" type antitumor agents bind selectively with DNA, forming complexes that block the formation of DNA-dependent RNA, e.g., actinomycin D, daunorubicin, Adriamycin®, and mithramycin.

The enzyme L-asparaginase causes depletion of endogeneous asparagine. This amino acid is nonessential for normal cells, but some malignant cells require an exogenous source of asparagine for protein synthesis.

The principal mitotic inhibitors are the *Vinca* alkaloids, vincristine and vinblastine, and the semisynthetic epipodophylotoxin derivatives, VM-26 and VP-16213. They produce metaphase arrest by acting against the microtubules of the mitotic spindle apparatus.

Hormones may inhibit cancers originating in organs that are normally sensitive to their suppressant action or their maturing effect. They may also have an indirect effect through inhibition of certain pituitary secretions that may stimulate the growth of malignant lesions derived from tissues sensitive to pituitary hormones. Corticosteroids inhibit poorly differentiated lymphoid cells, probably by a direct action. They retard the growth of breast cancers, most likely through inhibition of pituitary secretions. By similar mode of action, androgens may be effective against breast cancer in premenopausal women. Estrogens also cause tumor regressions in prostatic carcinoma by a double mechanism of direct tumor inhibition and indirect pituitary influence. The maturing effect of progesterone on the normal endometrium and the sensitivity of this tissue to hormonal stimuli prompted the use of progestagens in the treatment of advanced endometrial carcinoma.

## FACTORS AFFECTING CHOICE OF CHEMOTHERAPY

Factors affecting the choice of chemotherapy include general sensitivity of the tumor type to chemotherapy, specific sensitivity of the individual's tumor to individual agents, the likelihood of response and clinical improvement versus serious toxicity (assessment of therapeutic index), and whether chemotherapy is to be used as a single modality against advanced disease, in a combined modality setting (e.g., with radiation therapy for regional disease), or in the adjuvant setting after potentially curative surgery.

Since acute leukemia, lymphomas, pediatric solid tumors, breast and ovarian cancer, and small-cell lung cancer are generally sensitive to chemotherapy, the choice of antineoplastic drug treatment is generally appropriate, even if the patient is bedfast from his disease. On the other hand, the relative chemoinsensitivity of renal, pancreatic, esophageal, colorectal, non-small-cell lung cancer, and melanoma, coupled with the negative effect of adverse performance status on the likelihood of a meaningful response, is such that most medical oncologists prefer to avoid the toxicity of presently available chemotherapy in nonambulatory patients with these diseases. Whether the ambulatory patient with dissemination of one of these cancers should be treated depends on several factors, including the patient's informed desire for treatment, the availability of adequate facilities, and the possibility of contributing toward an eventual solution through involvement in a therapeutic research protocol.

The ability to determine the specific sensitivity (or lack of it) of an individual patient's tumor to chemotherapeutic agents is a long-sought-after, but frustratingly distant goal. Discovery of the influence of the estrogen receptor content of a mammary tumor on the effectiveness of endocrine therapy is the most significant advance yet made (26). Recent work establishing the effects of chemotherapeutic agents on clonability of human tumor cells *in vitro* (37) and on the labeling index of tumor cells *in vitro* (24) is promising, but still not of routine clinical usefulness.

Assessments of therapeutic index may vary greatly. For example, a 60-year-old debilitated man with head and neck cancer is a less suitable candidate for *cis*-platinum (II) therapy than a relatively healthy 30-year-old woman with ovarian cancer. Although the likelihood of a partial response may be the same, the latter individual is much less likely to have disastrous side effects.

The setting in which chemotherapy is to be used is an extremely important variable. In disseminated breast cancer, many oncologists would choose Adriamycin® as a component of initial treatment. Its use in simultaneous combination with radiation therapy to the chest wall in a patient with Stage III disease can produce severe local toxic effects, and militates toward at least a reduction in dosage. In dealing with disease that may have been eradicated by surgery, surgeons in many communities are unwilling to expose patients to the risks of even a "low dose" of Adriamycin®.

## CHEMOTHERAPY TOXICITY AND ITS NUTRITIONAL IMPACT

Cancer chemotherapeutic effectiveness depends on selective toxicity, on cancer cells being eradicated to a greater degree than normal cells. This involves an interaction of host–tumor–drug relationships. Theoretically, if an antitumor agent were nontoxic to the host, the dosage could be increased indefinitely until total eradication of the tumor cells occurred. This has never been achieved with existing agents, since all are limited by host toxicity.

Toxicity is an essential and unavoidable aspect of current cancer chemotherapy. The tenets of the cell-kill hypothesis imply that the higher the dose that can be administered, the greater the degree of cell kill achievable. What limits the dose, and theoretically the cell-kill achievable, is toxicity to normal host-tissue. Because of this, the achievement of low-level toxicity becomes a touchstone of an adequately administered dose level. For orally administered compounds, the establishment of low-level toxicity can be viewed as a poor man's pharmacology for adequate systemic absorption. For this reason, determining the maximum tolerated dose (MTD) is the major goal of the Phase I studies of new anticancer compounds. This MTD becomes the dose used in the efficacy-seeking Phase II and III trials (6).

The major toxicity of cancer chemotherapy is in the bone marrow (7). This can be manifested by leukopenia, thrombocytopenia, or anemia. Of the three, leukopenia has the highest incidence and is the most common dose-limiting toxic effect with cytotoxic drugs. If severe leukopenia results, then infection becomes a risk. Infection is accompanied by fever, chills, anorexia, and increased energy consumption. All can lead to a deterioration in the nutritional state of the patient.

The frequency of infection with cancer chemotherapy is inversely related to the level of circulating neutrophils. Bodey et al. (2) have shown that in acute leukemia no increased frequency of infection is seen unless the neutrophil count is less than $1,000/mm^3$. In their experience, infection occurred in every patient who had fewer than 100 neutrophils/$mm^3$ for more than three weeks. If the neutrophil count remained above $2,000/mm^3$, the frequency of infection was only 2%. When it fell to less than $100/mm^3$, the frequency rose to 28%.

The fatality rate for major organ infection was also related to fluctuations in the neutrophil count. The fatality rate was 80% among patients whose neutrophil counts remained below $100/mm^3$ during the first week of infection. Among patients who had an initial neutrophil count of fewer than $1,000/mm^3$, the fatality rate was 60% if the neutrophil count decreased further, but only 27% if the count increased to more than $1,000/mm^3$.

Because infection can disseminate very rapidly in the neutropenic patient, it is of critical importance to institute treatment at the first sign of infection. Fever may be the only such sign because these patients cannot produce an adequate inflammatory response and may have extensive infection with none of the usual clinical signs and symptoms.

The lining of the gastrointestinal tract is a highly vulnerable target for cytotoxic drugs, probably because of the rapid turnover of cells in the mucosa. Rapid cell division deep in mucosal crypts produces cells that are pushed up the crypt wall. The squamous mucosa of the oral pharyngeal and esophageal surfaces also display more rapid turnover of cells than does the skin. Toxic effects on the mucosal linings can include oral ulceration, cheilosis, glossitis, and pharyngitis, and are often called stomatitis. Drugs that may be dose-limited by oral mucosal toxicity include actinomycin D, methotrexate, and methyl glyoxal bis-guanylhydrazone. Severe oral toxicity has been reported after Adriamycin®, daunomycin, 5-fluorouracil, and azeserine (27). When 5-fluorouracil is given by continuous infusion, stomatitis may be the dose-limiting toxic effect.

Early oral ulceration caused by methotrexate may be responsive to the administration of citrovorum factor (calcium leukovorin) as a mouthwash without compromising systemic drug effectiveness (4), at least with high methotrexate doses. Ulcerations due to other causes are best treated by discontinuation of the offending agent(s) until the ulcerations have cleared completely, good oral hygiene, and liberal use of viscous xylocaine. If the lips are the major site of involvement, it is better to apply the viscous xylocaine as an ointment; if the oral pharynx, to use a mouthwash containing viscous xylocaine with or without other ingredients, such as diphenhydramine (Benadryl®) and magnesium–aluminum hydroxide antacids.

Esophagitis is rarely seen with any drug used alone, unless generalized mucositis is present or there is concomitant radiation therapy to a field involving the esophagus. Under these circumstances, Adriamycin® may be a particular offender (11). Methyl glyoxal bis-guanylhydrazone (MGBG, methyl GAG) is an exception; esophagitis may be the only manifestation of drug toxicity (19). The treatment of esophagitis is similar to that of stomatitis involving the oral pharynx. It is well to remember that pain on swallowing can also be due to Candidal esophagitis, especially in the leukemic patient; a barium swallow and/or esophagoscopy may be indicated to rule out this possibility.

Like esophagitis, symptomatic proctitis is rarely seen in the absence of generalized mucositis or concomitant local radiation therapy unless 5-FU and the other fluorinated pyrimidines have been administered. There is no useful local therapy other than stool softeners and good anal care.

Under some conditions, mucositis is an indication for hospitalization, especially if there is associated leukopenia: the combination of the two increases the likelihood of sepsis from the patient's own gut flora. The conditions include confluent oral ulceration, with or without oral bleeding or fever; inability to swallow liquids (in general, these patients also handle their secretions poorly); and loose stools six or more times per day with or without bloody diarrhea or prolapsed hemorrhoids associated with proctitis. Intravenous fluids and close monitoring of vital signs and electrolytes are indicated in all such patients. Such toxic effects prevent patients from ingesting nourishment orally and so can lead to dehydration and a deterioration in nutritional status.

Among the most ubiquitous toxic effects of cancer chemotherapy are nausea and vomiting. These effects are generally thought to be mediated by the chemoreceptor trigger zone, which is located in the fourth ventricle. The drugs that can cause these effects (Table 1) encompass all the major classes. Nausea and vomiting, along with concomitant anorexia, result in diminished oral intake, fluid and electrolyte imbalance, general weakness, and weight loss (5).

Sedation before and during chemotherapy administration may be useful in some patients, particularly those who have developed vomiting as a conditioned response to the sight of the offending drug. The use of intravenous hyperalimenta-

TABLE 1. *Chemotherapeutic agents with emetic side effects*

I. *Uniformly associated with emesis (moderate to severe)*
Nitrogen mustard
BCNU
CCNU
Methyl-CCNU
Streptozotocin
Dacarbazine
*Cis*-platinum
Cyclophosphamide
Actinomycin D
Hexamethylmelamine
5-azacytidine

II. *Commonly associated with emesis (mild or moderate)*
Phenylalanine mustard
Chlorambucil
5-fluorouracil
Methotrexate
Vinblastine
Adriamycin®
Daunomycin
Procarbazine

tion has, among other things, been reported to reduce the frequency and severity of nausea and vomiting (15). This requires further evaluation, as does the possible use of enteral alimentation with a continuous infusion rather than a bolus approach (32). Although glucocorticoids should generally be avoided, they can reverse anorexia and produce appetite stimulation in some terminal patients, and many oncologists employ them judiciously in this setting.

One drug, vincristine (and occasionally its relative, vinblastine), produces constipation by acting on the autonomic nervous system rather than the gastrointestinal tract directly. This constipation is best treated by prophylaxis with a stool softener, a bulk laxative such as methyl cellulose (Metamucil®) or milk of magnesia, at bedtime. If high colonic impaction with obstipation develops, the patient may require hospitalization and supportive care.

L-asparaginase is the only chemotherapeutic agent that produces pancreatitis. The pancreatitis is usually symptomatic and frequently hemorrhagic; it may be fatal (41). Routine monitoring of serum amylase is indicated in all patients receiving L-asparaginase. The drug should be discontinued if the amylase level becomes abnormal or if the patient develops symptoms of pancreatitis. Immediate hospitalization and care, as for any other form of acute pancreatitis, are indicated.

Cyclocytidine, an analog of cytosine arabinoside, produces transient jaw pain associated with sialadenitis. The same symptom (although probably not from the same cause) is occasionally seen with the *Vinca* alkaloids. No specific therapy is indicated.

Hepatitis of clinical significance is, fortunately, an unusual complication of chemotherapy for cancer, although many of the agents produce transient, mild elevation of liver enzymes shortly after administration. In patients with preexisting serious liver disease, methotrexate can rarely produce fatal hepatitis. The cirrhosis that develops in some patients on long-term, daily methotrexate is a complication of chronic use (36). Thiopurines and the sex steroids may produce jaundice, usually of the self-limited, cholestatic type. Although Adriamycin® is not hepatotoxic, its use in combination with thiopurines such as 6-mercaptopurine may produce serious hepatic damage (28). The same observation has been made for the combination of two nitrosoureas that normally produce only "chemical" hepatitis, streptozotocin and BCNU (25).

Diarrhea could be considered part of a general mucosal toxic effect. Among the agents that can cause severe diarrhea are 5-fluorouracil, actinomycin D, methotrexate, hydroxyurea, 5-azacytidine, and the nitrosoureas. Other drugs cause it occasionally (Table 2). Severe diarrhea can cause dehydration, electrolyte imbalance, inanition, and ultimately malnutrition.

Central nervous system (CNS) toxicity can lead to mental obtundations or disorientations, which result in diminishment of oral intake, thus accelerating malnutrition. Vincristine, which usually causes only peripheral neuropathy, can at high doses cause weakness, insomnia, confusion, disorientation, and hallucination (8,12,39). Although 5-fluorouracil (28,29,30,35) only occasionally causes cerebellar ataxia, a new drug, ftorafur, which acts as a prodrug for 5-fluorouracil, at high doses causes a whole range of CNS toxic effects. L-asparaginase can cause unpredictable lethargy, depression, disorientation, confusion, and hallucination (31,32). *Cis*-platinum is still another drug that can lead to confusion and increased cerebrospinal fluid pressure.

When drugs are combined, the toxicologic impact can be magnified. Ideally, all chemotherapy, whether single-agent or combination, is titrated to a maximum

TABLE 2. *Chemotherapeutic agents that can cause diarrhea*

|  |
|---|
| I. *Prominent* |
| 5-fluorouracil |
| Actinomycin D |
| Methyl glyoxal bisguanylhydrazone |
|  |
| II. *Commonly Occurs* |
| Methotrexate |
| Hydroxyuria |
| BCNU |
| CCNU |
| Methyl-CCNU |
| 5-azacytidine |
|  |
| III. *Occasionally Occurs* |
| 6-mercaptapurine |
| Cyclophosphamide |
| Procarbazine |
| Vincristine |

tolerated dose. With combinations of drugs, more organ systems may be damaged. In general, combination chemotherapy is more aggressive than single-agent therapy and carries with it greater risks. This is particularly true when salvage of extensive disease is a possibility, as it is in malignant lymphomas, oat-cell lung cancer, and testicular tumors.

One highly effective and highly toxic regimen is the three-drug combination used in testicular cancer involving *cis*-diamminedichloro-platinum, vinblastine, and bleomycin. Einhorn and Donohue (10) have reported that in 47 evaluable patients with metastatic testicular carcinoma this regimen achieved a 100% overall response rate, with a complete response rate of 70%. Many of these patients have been disease-free for prolonged periods, and cure is a reasonable assumption. This highly effective, curative regimen is also significantly toxic, with a definite impact on the nutritional status of the patients.

Einhorn and Donohue have attributed the toxic effects of the regimen to the individual drugs. The platinum caused moderate to severe nausea and vomiting in all patients. In addition, most patients had a 25% to 50% decrease in creatinine clearance, with three patients experiencing significant azotemia. The bleomycin produced fever, chills, and cutaneous striae in all patients. The vinblastine produced myalgia in half of the patients; in some, this was severe enough to require narcotic analgesia. Leukopenia was seen in all, with nadir usually being $1,000/mm^3$ between days 7 and 14. Eighteen patients required hospitalization for presumed sepsis with granulocytopenic fever. Seven of these had documented gram-negative sepsis. As could be expected, this wide range of toxic side effects had a nutritional impact. The average weight loss in these patients was 20 pounds. Since most were otherwise healthy young men, they did not require hyperalimentation.

Successful therapy in small-cell lung cancer involves a combination of multiple drugs with irradiation. One of the common regimens involves Adriamycin®, cyclophosphamide, and vincristine, followed by irradiation, and then drugs again. Einhorn and Donohue (9) have reported that in 55 patients this regimen achieved a 89% response rate, with 48% of the patients having a complete disappearance of all clinically evident disease. The median duration of complete remission was 78 weeks. Again, there was a significant toxic cost to be paid for this successful therapy. Alopecia, nausea, vomiting, and myelosuppression were seen in all patients. The median nadir of the granulocyte count was $1,100/mm^3$ 1 to 2 weeks after chemotherapy. Five patients developed granulocytopenic infections requiring hospitalization and antibiotics. When the X-ray treatment was begun, all patients suffered lethargy and anorexia. The nutritional impact was an average weight loss of 7 kg.

## NUTRITIONAL STATUS AS A PROGNOSTIC INDICATOR

When a patient's prognosis is evaluated, four major factors must be studied: the stage of the tumor or its extent in anatomic tumors; the biological characteris-

TABLE 3. *Situations in which optimal chemotherapy dose should be diminished by 50%*

Age over 65 years
Prior radiation therapy to bone marrow-producing areas
Prior chemotherapy
Poor performance status
Weight loss >10%
Temperature >101°
Major organ dysfunction that would affect drug pharmacology, e.g.,
    bilirubin >3 and creatinine >1.5 (mg%)
WBC <3,000/mm³
Platelets <100,000/mm³

tics of the tumor, as reflected in its growth rate and properties of invasion; the basic health of the host, including age, nutritional status, organ function, and immunologic reactivity; and the sensitivity or responsiveness of the tumor to therapeutic modalities.

Host factors are critical to prognosis in general and chemotherapy responsiveness in particular. The host factor of major importance is performance status, which is a quantitative translation of the presence of symptoms and functional ability. Regardless of the intrinsic sensitivity of a tumor to drugs, patients who are cachectic and bedridden, with poor performance status, respond poorly to drugs. This is in large part caused by their inability to tolerate the usual drug doses needed to achieve response (Table 3).

Weight loss is a prominent effect of disseminated cancer, and many patients undergoing chemotherapy must deal with this problem. The incidence of weight loss prior to chemotherapy, in a large series of cancer patients at the time of entry into chemotherapy protocols, ranged from 40% for patients with breast cancer, acute myelocytic leukemia, and sarcoma to more than 80% in patients with cancer of the pancreas and stomach (40).

Weight loss prior to entry into chemotherapy study is a poor prognostic sign. In most studies in which this has been examined, patients with weight loss have had a shorter survival and lower response rate than those without this prognostic variable.

Nutritional status is not routinely measured in patients prior to institution of chemotherapy. It is generally understood that patients with a poor nutritional status tolerate drugs poorly and have a low response rate. This lack of measurement is partially the result of a lack of an established methodology for reporting nutritional status. In some studies, weight loss has been shown to be an important prognostic variable, but it may not fully correlate with nutritional status. Weight loss is usually recorded over some finite period of time. It is conceivable that a patient without significant weight loss could be in a poor nutritional state. It is also conceivable that a patient could have lost in excess of 10 to 20 pounds and still be in a good nutritional state.

The prognostic variable that is commonly used and that probably encompasses some of the impact of the nutritional status is performance status. Performance

TABLE 4. *Karnofsky performance status*

| | | |
|---|---|---|
| 100% | Normal, NED | Able to carry on normal activity; no special care needed. |
| 90% | Able to carry on normal activity, minor symptoms or signs of disease | |
| 80% | Normal activities with effort, some symptoms or signs of disease | |
| 70% | Cares for self, unable to carry on normal activity or do active work | Unable to work, able to live at home; cares for most of personal needs; varying assistance is needed. |
| 60% | Requires occasional assistance, but is able to care for most of needs | |
| 50% | Requires considerable assistance and frequent medical care | |
| 40% | Disabled; requires special medical care and assistance | Unable to care for self; requires hospital or institutional care; disease may be progressing rapidly. |
| 30% | Severely disabled, hospitalization indicated although death not imminent | |
| 20% | Very sick, hospitalization necessary; active supportive Rx needed | |
| 10% | Moribund, fatal | |
| 0% | Dead | |

status is a discrete measure of a patient's ambulatory functioning; it is most often defined on a 10-point scale originally devised by Karnofsky et al. (18) (Table 4).

The importance of the ambulatory status of patients can be seen in the survival of males with adenocarcinoma of the lung reported in a study by the Eastern Cooperative Oncology Group (Table 5) (21). The median survival time varied from 11 to 34 weeks, depending on the patient's performance status and extent of disease at the start of treatment.

The impact of performance status can be demonstrated in results with chemotherapy for head and neck cancer. In a recent study at Wayne State University (1) the prognostic variables affecting drug response were analyzed. In 74 patients with a Karnofsky performance status of >70%, the response rate was 32%, with a median survival of 28 weeks. In 38 patients with a performance scale of <40%, only 13% responded and the median survival was nine weeks.

TABLE 5. *Estimated survival time for males with inoperable adenocarcinoma of the lung*[a]

| Initial performance status | Extent of disease | Median survival (weeks) | Probability of surviving 36 weeks |
|---|---|---|---|
| Ambulatory | Limited | 34 | .48 |
| Ambulatory | Extensive | 22 | .30 |
| Nonambulatory | Limited | 17 | .19 |
| Nonambulatory | Extensive | 11 | .06 |

[a] Adapted from Lagakos, ref. 21.

Moertel et al. (30) have reported a strong relationship between performance status and response to 5-fluorouracil in gastrointestinal cancer. Kansal et al. (17) have done the same with disease remission and survival in patients with acute myelogenous leukemia. In Hodgkin's disease, Jones et al. (16) have shown that performance status predicted achievement of complete response at higher significance levels than did stage, symptoms, or presence of bone marrow disease. Performance status has also been shown to predict response to chemotherapy in ovarian carcinomas (3), head and neck cancer (13), and other tumors. Zelen (42) has demonstrated a striking relationship between performance status at presentation and survival in lung cancer patients treated with a placebo. At Stanford (20), Karnofsky status has been shown to be an excellent predictor of serious toxic effects among patients with testicular cancer treated with *cis*-platinum, vinblastine, and bleomycin. With a performance score of 60 to 100, performance status was a more accurate predictor of serious toxic effects than were prior chemotherapy or radiation and interval since previous therapy.

There is mounting evidence that good nutritional status can favorably influence the results of therapy. Striking improvement in performance status has been shown to result from aggressive nutritional support in cancer patients (33). Since performance status predicts response rates, toxic effects, and survival rates, nutritional support may prove to be an important adjunct to cancer chemotherapy. It has not yet been proven in a randomized prospective trial that aggressive measures to improve nutritional or performance status increase response or survival rates. Several promising pilot experiences do exist (23,34). At M. D. Anderson Hospital, an increased rate of response to an aggressive combination including bleomycin, cyclophosphamide, vincristine, methotrexate, and 5-fluorouracil has been reported in debilitated patients with lung cancer who were given intravenous hyperalimentation.

## REFERENCES

1. Amer, M. H., Al-Sarraf, M., and Valtkevicius, V. K. (1979): Factors that affect response to chemotherapy and survival of patients with advanced head and neck cancer. *Cancer,* 43:2202–2206.
2. Bodey, G. P., Buckley, M., Sathe, Y. S., and Freireich, E. J. (1966): Quantitative relationships between circulating leukocytes and infections in patients with acute leukemia. *Ann. Intern. Med.,* 64:328–340.
3. Bonomi, P., Marrin, B., Wilbanks, J., and Slayten, R. (1978): Phase II trial of hexamethylmelamine in ovarian carcinoma after alkylating agent failure. *Proc. Am. Assoc. Cancer Res.,* 19:335.
4. Bruckner, H. W., and Bertino, J. R. (1975): Absorption of leucovorin from a "mouthwash." *Cancer Chemother. Rep.,* 59:575.
5. Brunner, K. W., and Young, C. W. (1965): A methylhydrazine derivative in Hodgkin's disease and other malignant neoplasms: Therapeutic and toxic effects studied in 51 patients. *Ann. Intern. Med.,* 63:69–86.
6. Carter, S. K. (1977): Clinical trials in cancer chemotherapy. *Cancer* 40(suppl.):544–557.
7. Carter, S. K., Bakowski, M., and Hellmann, K. (1977): *Chemotherapy of Cancer.* John Wiley & Son, New York.
8. Casey, E. S., Jellife, A. M., LeQuesne, M., et al. (1973): Vincristine neuropathy: Clinical and electrophysiologic observations. *Brain,* 96:69–86.

9. Einhorn, L. H., and Donohue, J. (1977): Cis-diammine dichloroplatinum, vinblastine and bleomycin combination chemotherapy in disseminated testicular cancer. *Ann. Intern. Med.,* 87:293–298.

10. Einhorn, L. H., and Donohue, J. P. (1979): Combination chemotherapy in disseminated testicular cancer: The Indiana University experience. *Semin. Oncol.,* 6:87–93.

11. Greco, F. A., Brereton, H. D., Kent, H., Zimbler, H., Merrill, J., and Johnson, R. E. (1976): Adriamycin and enhanced radiation reaction in normal esophagus and skin. *Ann. Intern. Med.,* 85:294.

12. Holland, J. F., Scharlow, C., Gailani, S., et al. (1973): Vincristine treatment of advanced cancer: A cooperative study of 392 cases. *Cancer Res.,* 33:1258–1264.

13. Holoye, P. Y., Goepfert, H., and Samuels, M. L. (1978): Combination chemotherapy of head and neck carcinoma. *Proc. Am. Assoc. Cancer Res.,* 19:358.

14. Hutchinson, D. J., and Schmid, F. A. (1973): In: *Drug Resistance and Selectivity,* edited by E. Mihich, pp. 73–126. Academic Press, New York.

15. Issell, B. F., Valdivieso, M., Zaren, H. A., Copeland, E. M., and Bodey, G. P. (1978): Protection of chemotherapy toxicities by intravenous hyperalimentation. *Proc. Am. Assoc. Cancer Res.,* 19:149.

16. Jones, S. E., Coltman, C. A., and Fisher, R. (1978): Comparison of 3 combination drug programs for advanced Hodgkins disease. *Proc. Am. Assoc. Cancer Res.,* 19:333.

17. Kansal, V., Omura, G. A., and Soong, S. (1976): Prognosis in adult acute myelogenous leukemia related to performance status and other factors. *Cancer,* 38:329–334.

18. Karnofsky, D. A., Abelmann, W. H., Craver, L. F., and Burchenal, J. E. (1948): The use of nitrogen mustard in the palliative treatment of cancer. *Cancer,* 1:634–656.

19. Knight, W. A., and Livingston, R. B.: *Manuscript in preparation.*

20. Krikorian, J. G., Daniels, J. R., Brown, B. W., and Humis, (1978): Variables for predicting serious toxicity (vinblastine dose, performance status and prior therapeutic experience) (1978): Chemotherapy for metastatic testicular cancer with cis-dichloroplatinum (II), vinblastine and bleomycin. *Cancer Treat. Rep.,* 62:1455–1463.

21. Lagakos, S. W. (1977): Prognostic factors for survival time in inoperable lung cancer. In: *Lung Cancer: Clinical Diagnosis and Treatment,* edited by M. Straus, pp. 271–280. Grune and Stratten, New York.

22. Land, V. J., Sutow, W. W., Fernbach, B. J. (1972): Toxicity of L-asparaginase in children with advanced leukemia. *Cancer,* 30:339–347.

23. Lanzotti, N. J., Copeland, E. M., George, S. L. (1975): Cancer chemotherapy response and intravenous hyperalimentation. *Cancer Chemother. Rep.,* 59:436–439.

24. Livingston, R. B.: *Unpublished observations.*

25. Lokich, J. J., Drum, D. E., and Kaplan, W. (1974): Hepatic toxicity of nitrosourea analogues. *Clin. Pharmacol. Ther.,* 16:363.

26. McGuire, W. L.: Hormone receptors: Their role in predicting prognosis and response to endocrine therapy. *Semin. Oncol.* (in press).

27. Middleman, E., Luce, J., Frei, E., III (1971): Clinical trials with Adriamycin. *Cancer,* 28:844.

28. Minow, R. A., Stern, M. H., Casey, J. H., Rodriguez, V., and Luna, M. A. (1976): Clinical pathologic correlation of liver damage in patients treated with 6-mercaptopurine and adriamycin. *Cancer,* 38:1524.

29. Moertel, C. G., Reitermeier, R. J., and Bolton, C. F. (1964): Cerebellar ataxia associated with fluorinated pyrimidine therapy. *Cancer Chemother. Rep.,* 41:15–16.

30. Moertel, C. G., Schutt, A. J., Hahn, R. G., and Reitmeier, R. (1974): Effects of patient selection or results of phase II chemotherapy trials in gastrointestinal cancer. *Cancer Chemother. Rep.,* 58:257–259.

31. Ohnuma, T., Holland, J. F., and Freeman, A. (1970): Biochemical and pharmacological studies with L-asparaginase in men. *Cancer Res.,* 30:2297–2305.

32. Page, C. P., Ryan, J. A., Jr., and Haff, R. C. (1976): Continual catheter administration of an elemental diet. *Surg., Gynecol. Obstet.,* 142:184.

33. Pariera, M. D., Conrad, E. J., Hicks, W., and Elman, R. (1955): Clinical response and changes in nitrogen balance, body weight, plasma proteins and hemoglobin following tube feeding in cancer cachexia. *Cancer,* 8:803–808.

34. Phillips, T. L., Wharam, M. D., and Margolis, L. W. (1975): Modification of radiation injury to normal tissues by chemotherapeutic agents. *Cancer,* 35:1678–1684.

35. Reihl, J. L., and Brown, W. J. (1964): Acute cerebellar syndrome secondary to 5-fluorouracil therapy. *Neurology (Minneap.)*, 14:254.
36. Roenigk, H. H., Bergfeld, W. F., St. Jacques, R., Ownes, F. J., and Hawk, W. A. (1971): Hepatotoxicity of methotrexate in treatment of psoriasis. *Arch. Dermatol.*, 103:205.
37. Salmon, S. E., Hamburger, A. W., Soehnlen, B., Durie, B. G. M., Alberts, D. S., and Moon, T. E. (1978): Quantitation of differential sensitivity of human-tumor stem cells to anticancer drugs. *N. Engl. J. Med.*, 298:1321.
38. Samuels, M. L., Leary, W. B., Alexanian, R. (1967): Clinical N-isopropyl-$\alpha$($\alpha$-methylhydrazine)-p-toluamide hydrochloride in malignant lymphoma. *Cancer*, 20:1187–1194.
39. Sandler, S. G., Tubin, W., and Henderson, E. S. (1969): Vincristine induced neuropathy: A clinical study of fifty leukemic patients. *Neurology (Minneap.)*, 19:367–374.
40. Skipper, H. E., Schabel, F. M., and Wilcox, W. S. (1964): Experimental evaluation of potential anticancer agents XIII on the criteria and kinetics associated with curability of experimental leukemia. *Cancer Chemother. Rep.*, 35:1–111.
41. Whitecar, J. P., Bodey, G. P., Harris, J. E., and Freireich, E. J. (1970): L-asparaginase. *N. Engl. J. Med.*, 282:732.
42. Zelen, M. (1973): Keynote address on biostatistics and data retrieval: First international workshop for therapy of lung cancer. *Cancer Chemother. Rep.*, 4:431–442.

*Nutrition and Cancer: Etiology and Treatment,*
edited by G. R. Newell and N. M. Ellison.
Raven Press, New York © 1981.

# Nutritional Problems Associated with Radiation Therapy

## Sarah S. Donaldson

*Department of Radiology, Division of Radiation Therapy, Stanford University School of Medicine, Stanford, California 94305*

An important determinant of cachexia and malnutrition experienced by the majority of cancer patients is the toxicity and morbidity of the treatment itself. At present, the armamentarium to fight malignancy successfully includes powerful tools and aggressive philosophies. Consequently, the effects of these therapies are visible in normal cell populations as well as in malignant cell populations. Present cancer treatment modalities are not confined exclusively to malignant cell populations; thus, the ratio of benefit of treatment to complications resulting from treatment is not ideal. As greater emphasis has been placed on means of destroying neoplastic cells, proportionately less attention has been directed at the general and nutritional consequences of such treatments. The nutritional problems associated with radiation therapy are well known, and correlate with the clinical manifestations and pathophysiology of radiation injury. There is an understandable reluctance on the part of many physicians to acknowledge iatrogenic normal tissue damage, particularly when it involves tissue injury leading to nutritional sequelae, among patients undergoing radiation therapy, with or without chemotherapy.

Radiation therapy delivered to any portion of the gastrointestinal tract may create nutritional disorders, either directly or indirectly, by its effect on the tumor or on adjacent normal tissues. These disorders may develop acutely during therapy, or may progress and become chronic after the completion of irradiation. Thus, the nutritional consequences of radiotherapy are related to the location of the tumor and the region being irradiated (for example, the oral cavity and pharynx, the esophagus, the stomach, the small and large bowel, and special organs such as the liver and pancreas). Table 1 lists some of the more common problems caused by radiation therapy that may contribute to nutritional problems. Mucositis, stomatitis, gingivitis, and esophagitis resulting from radiation to the upper gastrointestinal tract lead to a decreased oral intake. Radiation alterations of the taste sensors affect feeding behavior and have a great impact on a patient's appetite and eating. Xerostomia resulting from radiation effects on the major and minor salivary glands intensifies difficulty in eating and contrib-

TABLE 1. *Localized effects of radiotherapy leading to alterations in nutritional status*

| Region | Acute | Chronic |
|---|---|---|
| Oral cavity and pharynx | Sore throat<br>Dysphagia<br>Xerostomia<br>Mucositis<br>Anorexia<br>Alteration in smell<br>Loss of taste | Ulcer<br>Xerostomia<br>Dental caries<br>Osteoradionecrosis<br><br>Trismus<br>Altered taste |
| Esophagus | Dysphagia | Fibrosis<br>Stenosis<br>Fistula |
| Stomach, small and<br>  large intestine | Anorexia<br>Nausea<br>Vomiting<br>Diarrhea<br>Acute enteritis<br>Acute colitis | <br>Ulcer<br>Malabsorption<br>Diarrhea<br>Chronic enteritis<br>Chronic colitis |
| Liver and pancreas | Anorexia<br>Nausea<br>Vomiting | Ascites<br>Jaundice |

utes to dental decay, further complicating eating habits. Dysphagia, anorexia, nausea, and vomiting result in decreased food intake. Radiation enteritis may lead to malabsorption, obstruction, fistula, stricture, ulceration, or perforation, and in this way affect a patient's nutritional balance.

Radiosensitivity varies from cell to cell and from tissue to tissue. This variation depends on multiple factors involving the cells and their environment, perhaps the most important of which is the phase of the cell within the reproductive cycle (13). Table 2 lists radiation tolerance doses for various regions, as described by Rubin and Casarett (32). These are listed as minimum tolerance doses, i.e., doses that are predicted to result in a 5% incidence of severe complications within 5 years after completion of treatment. The predicted long-term injury may directly interfere with adequate nutrition, as will be detailed under each organ system. Although irradiation can kill cells in all phases of their cycle, in most cell lines $G_2$ and M phases are more sensitive than $G_1$. Populations in which most cells are in $G_2$ and M are more radiosensitive than populations in which most cells are in $G_1$. Therefore, cells that are actively dividing are more sensitive than those that divide only occasionally or that cannot divide (13). This and other known factors, useful in radiobiology of pure cell symptoms, are difficult to apply to tissues and organs because of the complexity of the various cell symptoms that compose them. Histopathologic correlations of chronic (post-treatment) histologic lesions are difficult, as the lesions observed by a pathologist may not occur in the most radiosensitive cells of the organ. For example, in the small intestine, the most radiosensitive are the epithelial

TABLE 2. *Radiation tolerance dose* [a]

| Organ | Injury at 5 Years | TD 5/5[b] |
|---|---|---|
| Skin | Ulcer, severe fibrosis | 5,500 |
| Oral mucosa | Ulcer, severe fibrosis | 6,000 |
| Salivary gland | Xerostomia | 5,000 |
| Esophagus | Ulcer, stricture | 6,000 |
| Stomach | Ulcer, perforation | 4,500 |
| Intestine | Ulcer, stricture | 4,500 |
| Colon | Ulcer, stricture | 4,500 |
| Rectum | Ulcer, stricture | 5,500 |
| Liver | Liver failure, ascites | 3,500 |

[a] From Rubin and Casarett ref. 32, with permission.
[b] TD 5/5: Minimal tolerance dose. The dose that, when applied to a given population of patients under standard treatment conditions, results in no more than a 5% severe complication rate within 5 years after treatment. Standard conditions refer to megavoltage therapy (1–6 MeV), fractionation of 1,000 rads/week, five daily fractions.

cells of the crypts, which are destroyed within three days after irradiation. However, by the time the pathologist may examine the intestine, in cases that develop clinical lesions several months or years later, the initially damaged epithelium has been replaced many times. The visible alterations are primarily in the submucosa and vessels, often with secondary ulcerations caused not by the initial epithelial injury but by ischemia. In spite of this complexity, it is also obvious that tissues and organs do vary in radiosensitivity as a whole, and this is generally so because of the variation in radiosensitivity in one or more cell systems within each organ (13,33).

It is the purpose of this chapter to review nutritional problems associated with tissue injury accompanying radiation therapy and/or combined modality radiation–chemotherapy, and to provide a rational therapeutic approach for these specific nutritional problems. There have been several recent reviews of this subject (8,9). This chapter will emphasize the problems resulting from radiotherapy.

## ORAL CAVITY AND PHARYNX

### Clinical Course and Pathophysiology

The soft tissues of the mouth and pharynx are relatively responsive to irradiation and, therefore, may present potential complications of radiation injury when treated with high doses. Such complications may be manifest by nutritional sequelae. These cavities are lined by nonkeratinizing, stratified squamous epithelium. The epithelial cell renewal rate is somewhat higher than that of the skin, and thus its radiosensitivity is greater. The submucosa consists of vascular connective tissue in which a variety of other structures of different radiosensitivities are present. The numerous minor salivary glands are largely of the mucous type and are more radioresistant. Radiation changes seen in the skeletal muscle of the tongue are thought to be the result of vascular insufficiency rather than of direct muscle cell injury. Posteriorly, in the oral cavity, the submucosa contains abundant lymphatic tissue of Waldeyer's ring, the cells of which are highly radiosensitive but capable of rapid repopulation (3).

A radiomucositis or radiation reaction in normal tissues, as seen among patients with head and neck cancer, runs a predictable course. The severity of the mucositis is directly proportional not only to the dose but also to the volume irradiated. Most epidermoid carcinomas of the mouth and pharynx are treated with total radiation doses of between 6,000 and 7,000 rads delivered at a rate of 180–200 rad/day, 5 times/week. The symptoms that can be expected from such treatment include sore throat, pain on swallowing, dry mouth, lack of appetite, and altered taste. Physical examination may reveal a spectrum of findings ranging from erythema, edema, and patchy mucositis to a confluent mucositis. With conventional radiotherapy, some degree of mucositis is usually noted between the third and fifth week of treatment. The mucositis may progress from a denudation of epithelial tissues to the formation of a pseudomembrane, superficial ulceration, and bleeding. This is caused by failure of regeneration of the epithelium lost by desquamation. A very severe acute response can result in a chronic radiation ulcer. However, by the end of a 6 to 8 week course of therapy regeneration usually begins to replace the thinned or denuded mucosa. The squamous epithelium is usually completely restored, though thinner than normal, 4 to 6 weeks after therapy has been completed. Repopulation of lymphatic tissue in Waldeyer's ring in adults may occur within months of completion of treatment, with prominent islands of lymphocytes in the tongue and pharyngeal tonsil. However, children show a relative atrophy of lymphatic tissue, as if normal lymphoid involution had been prematurely induced by irradiation. Skeletal muscle of the tongue is markedly radioresistant to direct effects of radiation, presumably because its cells are not dividing (3).

Of all nutritional effects, the alterations of taste have perhaps the greatest impact on a patient. Changes in taste experienced by cancer patients have been observed as unequal alterations in taste sensitivity, both suppressed and heightened sensations. Bitter and acid tastes are most susceptible to impairment; salty and sweet tastes are less influenced. Quantitative tests of taste threshold to sucrose, hydrochloric acid, and quinine before, during, and after oral pharyngeal irradiation reveals the loss of taste to be exponential and rapid (5). Differential taste sensations are concentrated in different areas of the mouth, i.e., sweet mostly in the anterior portion, sour mostly in the middle, and bitter posteriorly; changes may thus be detected according to which area is irradiated. Conger (5) describes full recovery of taste to pre-irradiation acuity within 60 to 120 days of completion of treatment, and ascribes the mechanism of taste alteration to radiation-induced damage of the microvilli of the taste cells or their surfaces.

The olfactory system has been studied in experimental animals and found to be highly radioresponsive, even in fairly low doses and dose rates (6). Radiation appears to have its major effects on the peripheral olfactory apparatus, rather than on the olfactory bulb.

⌊Exposure of salivary glands during irradiation to the head and neck results in decreased salivation⌋ The volume of salivary secretion declines, while the quality changes to a viscid, acid mixture with abnormally high amounts of organic material. Thus, a change in the character of saliva occurs, from a clear watery secretion to a tenacious semiopaque substance, resulting in dysphagia. An increase in salivary amylase production, indicating acinar cell damage, has been demonstrated within hours following single fractions of 1,000 rads (23). There does not appear to be a critical dose level associated with diminished salivary secretion. Multiple factors, such as age, method of collection, time of day, presence of cancer, and administration of drugs, influence the salivary flow rate (40). The rate of recovery of salivary function is variable; however, even pronounced disturbances appear to show ultimate recovery after high doses of fractionated radiotherapy (12). The irradiation of salivary glands and resultant changes in the quality and quantity of saliva, as well as radiation reaction of the mucosa, are general factors in the origin of dental caries in these patients. The decrease of salivation causes an alteration in the composition of oral bacterial flora which, in turn, promotes caries formation. The teeth, which are ordinarily protected by salivary flow, become covered by the sticky material which provides an excellent substrate for bacterial attack. Intraoral acid pH levels are associated with a higher incidence of caries. Cariogenic microorganisms resulting from altered dietary habits and salivary changes appear before the onset of dental caries, regardless of whether or not a topical fluoride gel is used to prevent caries. As salivary flow decreases, the volume and concentration of salivary albumin, IgG, and lysozymes increase. Among 30 patients undergoing radiotherapy for head and neck cancer, a net immunoprotein deficit has been observed, in which the increased concentration of salivary immunoproteins was offset by a reduction of more than 93% in output of saliva (4).

A serious late complication affecting nutrition is the development of ulceration, which can occur from one month to more than one year after completion of therapy. Some of these ulcers are associated with and are secondary to osteoradionecrosis. Ulcerations, when not associated with adjacent osteonecrosis, generally heal with only supportive care. Those associated with osteonecrosis are more refractory to treatment. Radionecrosis of oral tissue can result from combinations of trauma and infection superimposed on tissues irradiated to levels of tissue tolerance. Radiation has a potential to affect developing teeth by direct cellular damage, as well as to produce a change in the mitotic stage of development, and, in fully formed teeth, to denature their organic components. This is of particular concern when administering radiation to a young child, whose permanent teeth have not yet fully developed. These changes can be magnified by the decline in salivation. Patients may experience an increased sensitivity of their teeth to cold, heat, and sweets.

An analysis of the percentage change in weight during a course of head

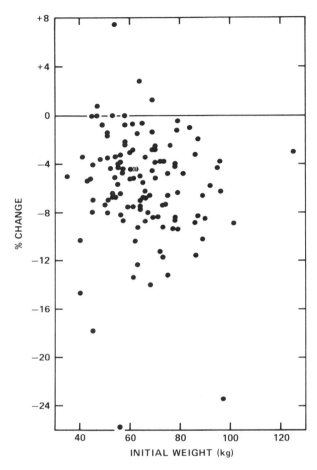

**FIG. 1.** Percentage of weight change as a function of initial weight during a course of radiation therapy among 122 adults with squamous-cell carcinoma of the oral cavity, oropharynx, or hypopharynx.

and neck radiation serves as a simple and direct measure of the nutritional effects of head and neck radiotherapy. One hundred twenty-two patients with squamous cell carcinoma of the oral cavity, oropharynx, and hypopharynx undergoing high-dose radiation with curative intent at Stanford University Medical Center were analyzed for their percentage weight change during a 6 to 8 week course of external beam radiotherapy (Fig. 1). No specific dietary therapy was administered to these patients. There was no direct correlation between percentage weight loss and age of patient or dose of radiation received (8). Figure 1 demonstrates that only four of these patients actually gained weight during the course of treatment; four patients maintained a stable weight. Overall, 114 of 122 patients (93%) lost weight even during a short course of treatment, with an average loss of 3.7 kg. Fourteen of the 22 patients (8.7%) lost more than 10% of their body weight between initiation and completion of their course of radiotherapy. Many patients had a chronic nutritional problem prior to the diagnosis. Of these 122 adult patients, 64% weighed less than 70 kg at the initiation of radiotherapy.

### Therapeutic Management

Management of the symptoms resulting from treatment is usually supportive, with intent to relieve symptoms and prevent further complications. If infection is to be prevented, good oral hygiene is essential. This can be achieved by frequent oral irrigations of 3% hydrogen peroxide (⅔ cup) mixed with lukewarm water (1-⅓ cup) or ½ teaspoon salt and 1 teaspoon baking soda mixed with one quart of water. Because undiluted hydrogen peroxide or concentrated salt and soda can be painful when applied to irradiated tissues that have desquamated, careful attention must be paid to the concentration of the solution. Expensive commercial mouthwashes are often astringent, causing a burning sensation, and may upset the balance of oral flora, thereby predisposing to a fungal infection. In general, such preparations should be avoided. Use of gravity drainage and a Water Pik is helpful in performing optimal oral irrigations. Oral hygiene with daily alkalinization of the mouth is essential in avoiding posttreatment dental caries, since the acidic pH of postradiation saliva may be the most important factor in postradiation dental caries. Alcohol and tobacco use should be avoided, to prevent further irritation to sensitive tissues. Unfortunately, their use is exceedingly common in patients with head and neck cancers and is virtually impossible to reduce.

Xerostomia creates difficulties in eating, swallowing, and talking. Sugarless gum and/or sugarless lemon drops may help stimulate saliva. Various salivary substitutes and artificial saliva have been tried without uniform success. The degree of xerostomia is directly related to the subsequent degree of dental caries. Oral hygiene may be effective in preventing these caries. Attention should be given to prophylactic dental care. All patients should be evaluated by a dentist regarding the status of the teeth, i.e., the need for extraction and for fluoride treatment prior to radiation therapy. It was once recommended that all teeth be removed prior to radiation; however, many workers have shown that only nonsalvageable teeth need to be extracted prior to therapy. With proper oral care, periodontal disease, periapical abscess, and osteonecrosis should not be of greater frequency. Indeed, Bedwinek et al. (1) have demonstrated a greater incidence of osteonecrosis in patients whose teeth were extracted prior to irradiation. The teeth should be kept clean by brushing and frequent use of dental floss. Daily fluoride treatments by mouthwash or gel should be continued after completion of radiotherapy and as follow-up treatment at home.

In case of intraoral infections, cultures should be taken, with prompt administration of appropriate antibiotics. Routine use of oral penicillin throughout the course of radiotherapy has been advocated, although its benefits have not yet been established.

Trismus can result from tumor infiltration or postradiation fibrosis of the masseter and pterygoid muscles of mastication. In such an event, the patient should routinely exercise with increasing numbers of wooden tongue blades between the teeth or should wear an appliance to increase the vertical dimension of the occlusion. In the event of osteoradionecrosis, a conservative approach to treatment should be vigorously employed.

Continual attention must be given by the radiotherapist to field size and beam geometry. They may be build-up of radiation dose from 109% to 170% in the area immediately adjacent to dental silver amalgams or gold fillings (14). Individualized cerrobend fields and beam-shaping devices are essential in sparing adjacent normal tissues when planning head and neck radiotherapy.

For patients with head and neck cancer, a well-balanced diet is essential. In patients experiencing intraoral pain, the consistency of food may have to be adjusted to facilitate swallowing. Tube feedings, defined formula diets, or intravenous hyperalimentation have all been tried as means of treating the inevitable malnutrition. Patients undergoing a protracted course of radiation therapy for head and neck cancer have been shown to gain weight during treatment when hyperalimentation was used routinely and to experience minimal radiation reaction during intensive radiotherapy. Studies are now under way to evaluate the role of optimal nutritional support in head and neck cancer patients at the onset of radiotherapy, to prevent complications of radiation that ultimately lead to poor nutrition. At a minimum, all head and neck patients should be seen by a clinic nutritionist prior to radiotherapy for nutritional assessment, evaluation, and consultation regarding specific nutritional needs before, during, and after a planned course of radiotherapy.

## ESOPHAGUS

### Clinical Course and Pathophysiology

Radiation administered to portions of the thorax, including the lung and mediastinum, or to the vertebrae often results in alterations in nutrition directly caused by esophageal irritation. Esophageal squamous epithelium has about the same radiosensitivity as the oral mucosa. It is predictable that the submucosa will respond to radiation initially by edema and vascular dilatation and then by progressive fibrosis with telangiectasia. The esophageal epithelium is moderately radiosensitive but usually regenerates rapidly. Subacute and chronic ulcerations may persist even in the absence of tumor, but are unusual. Narrowing of the lumen as the result of submucosal fibrosis is rare. Damage to the smooth muscle may be caused not only by interstitial fibrosis but by homogenization of the collagen fibers (3). Functional abnormalities may result from injury and/

or fibrosis of the muscular nerve plexus. Vascular injury may occur but is less prominent than in other areas of the gastrointestinal tract.

Complaints of dysphagia in a normal esophagus exposed to radiation usually occur after 2 to 3 weeks of therapy at doses of approximately 3,000 rads, and generally last for two weeks after a course of thoracic irradiation. The tolerance dose for chronic injury to the esophagus is about 6,000 rads at a dose of 1,000 rad/week. Radiation to a diseased esophagus may result in fistulae, sinus tract formation, or ulceration, with possible perforation. Such complications are invariably the result of tumor necrosis.

The enhancement of radiation effects by certain chemotherapeutic agents, specifically Adriamycin® and daunorubicin, has recently been observed, with esophageal complications of enhanced esophagitis and dermatitis (18) and of esophageal stricture (20). Thus, there is good evidence that chemotherapeutic agents, particularly the anthracyclines, reduce the tolerance level to conventional radiation, and that increased complications can be anticipated when chemotherapy is given as adjuvant treatment to radiotherapy in the region of the esophagus.

## Therapeutic Management

Prevention of the esophageal irritation by lead shielding from direct exposure to the X-ray beam is the most reliable method of preventing the esophagus from radiation injury. Topical anesthetics, such as viscus Xylocaine®, Chloroseptic®, and Oxaine M® may provide topical relief and prove effective prior to eating. Analgesics may be required. A soft, bland diet is helpful, and ethanol intake should be restricted. Radiation injury with fibrosis leading to stenosis can create nutritional difficulties initially with solid foods, so that a soft and ultimately a liquid diet may be necessary for a given patient. For chronic problems, temporary or permanent feeding tubes may be necessary to provide optimal nutritional support.

## STOMACH AND SMALL AND LARGE INTESTINE

### Clinical Course and Pathophysiology

Gastric radiation is capable of reducing gastric acidity at low levels, i.e., approximately 2,000 rads given in a fractionated course. Higher doses, i.e., 4,500 rads and over, have been associated with ulcer formation. After gastric doses of 5,500 rads or more, 50% of patients will develop clinical evidence of gastric mucosal injury (33). The proliferative zone of the two mucosal areas of the stomach lies in the isthmus of the glands and the contiguous portion of the base of the gastric gland pits. This proliferative zone and the surface epithelium of the stomach are most likely to show the acute effects of radiation injury, whereas the convoluted gastric glands with their parietal and chief cells are more resistant to irradiation changes (3). Radiation ulcers are usually solitary, are not of the "peptic-acid" type, and do not respond to diet or antacids. Gastric acidity is low or absent. Severe loss of appetite and weight may follow gastric ulcer formation. In addition to symptomatic ulcer, hemorrhage may complicate high-dose irradiation to the stomach.

The symptom complex of nausea, vomiting, and diarrhea frequently accompanies radiation to the small and large bowel. The symptoms may occur with initiation of gastrointestinal irradiation and may persist throughout therapy, thus resulting in weight loss and malnutrition. Acute symptoms from radiation begin with frequent watery bowel movements, associated with intermittent cramps. A picture of delayed radiation-induced enteritis may occur at any time following a course of high-dose gastrointestinal irradiation, and may present either as chronic diarrhea or as a partial or complete bowel obstruction. Bowel ulceration, stricture, or fistulae may result. The dose at which enteric injury becomes significantly frequent is approximately 4,500 rads, but it varies considerably with the patient and the fractionation scheme. Following 5,000 to 6,000 rads, from 25% to 50% of patients will have some clinical pathologic small intestinal lesions (31). Below 4,000 rads this injury is uncommon. Important in determining the effects of abdominal radiation in the small intestine is the mobility of, or, in contrast, the fixation of the small intestine. The entire duodenum and upper jejunum at the ligament of Treitz are fixed in place, as is the terminal ileum by its attachment to the usually immobile cecum. The motility of the intervening small intestines during the weeks of fractionated radiation therapy may protect against a critically high dose. Thus, the terminal ileum is the portion most often involved in radiation injury. However, if therapeutic radiation were applied as often to the upper abdomen as it is to the lower, the relatively immobile duodenum and upper jejunum would probably have as frequent radiation injury as the terminal ileum, because mucosal cell replication rates are essentially equally rapid in all portions of the small intestine. If preexisting peritoneal adhesions from any source attach loops of small intestine within the field of irradiation, these loops may receive greater cumulative radiation doses and suffer greater damage (7).

The pathophysiology of radiation enteritis can be partially explained by morphological changes, alterations in cell kinetics, decreases in enzyme activities, disturbances in absorption, and vascular abnormalities. Radiographic studies of the irradiated bowel demonstrate nonspecific findings consistent with chronic inflammation or fibrosis. Whole-abdominal irradiation may result in malabsorption of glucose, fats and electrolytes. Reeves et al. (30) demonstrated alterations in fat absorption by using $^{131}$I-labeled glycerol trioleate in patients undergoing radiation. In those patients who showed a definite decrease to low-normal levels of blood radioactivity, and an associated high fecal fat level, clinical diarrhea was evident. Reeves et al. (29) also reported that 77% of all patients that were undergoing abdominal or pelvic $^{60}$Co teletherapy demonstrated some degree of altered absorption of neutral fat with $^{131}$I. The resulting high fecal fat levels correlated with clinical diarrhea. A decrease in both disaccharide (36) and peptidase (22) enzymes has been observed in the mucosa after exposure to radiation therapy. Protein losses secondary to radiation-induced malabsorption have been reported (11). This protein loss appears to be dose-related (38) and may occur within dose ranges commonly used in clinical practice. Hypoproteinemia has been attributed to protein leakage through damaged mucosal cells (29). Radiation of rats, in fractions as low as 300 rads, increases the 24-hr loss of intravenously injected radioactive-labeled protein from the bowel from 4% in controls to 20% to 30% in irradiated animals (39). Goodner et al. (17) reported a net movement of sodium and water from blood into the gut lumen of rats subjected to radiation therapy. In both acute and chronic radiation damage of the terminal ileum, bile salt absorption from the ileum may be impaired. The increased bile salt accumulation in the lumen of the colon leads to failure of water and salt reabsorption in the colon and to diarrhea.

The epithelial cells of the small intestine have the most rapid cell turnover of the alimentary tract. Cell kinetics studies have shown a high turnover rate of the small intestinal mucosa, with a subsequent interference in cell division by radiation, followed by rapid recovery. The epithelium of the intestinal crypts and villi is completely replaced in 3 to 6 days, a rate of cell turnover equaled only by rapidly growing tumors. Since ionizing radiation preferentially affects intermitotic cells with short reproductive cycles, the enteric mucosa is one of the most radiosensitive mammalian tissues. Most of the acute and some of the delayed changes of radiation enteropathy depend on these cytokinetics. Trier and Browning (38) have demonstrated shortening of intestinal villi in the irradiated small intestine as early as the second week of X-ray exposure. These authors documented mucosal changes at maximal doses of 3,000 rads/4 weeks in asymptomatic patients. In their study, a reduction of mitoses preceded reduction of surface epithelium during X-ray therapy, and recovery of mitotic activity preceded the return of epithelial surface to normal when exposure to X-ray was stopped. Histologic examination of the mucosal lesions showed normal mitoses within three days and normal villi within 2 weeks after cessation of treatment, with minimal coexistent gastrointestinal symptoms of the histologic lesion (38).

Chronic radiation changes may include ulceration, perforation, telangiectasia, vascular thromboses, submucosal fibrosis, and hyalinization. Alterations in the composition of the gastrointestinal flora, with bacterial overgrowth, may contribute to chronic radiation injury (25). The late manifestations, although less frequent than the acute ones, are expressions of severe chronic reaction to injury that often requires surgical resection and may be life-threatening. These late effects may produce signs and symptoms 6 weeks to 10 years after completion of radiation. In most patients, there is a latent asymptomatic period of varying time between acute and late reactions.

Radiation enteritis, with its nutritional consequences, is a syndrome well-recognized by the radiotherapist. The incidence is not well-known, as often iatrogenic complications either are not carefully reported or are misdiagnosed as manifestations of the underlying malignant disease. To know the magnitude of the problem of radiation enteritis, we have only retrospective studies and personal experiences upon which to rely. The incidence of small intestinal injury varies at any given radiation dose with the presence or absence of adhesions which may fix loops of intestine in the field of irradiation. More than 50% of the small-bowel specimens that come to a surgical pathologist with a history of radiation show evidence of previous intraperitoneal disease (3). In addition, there is individual variation in susceptibility to chronic radiation injury. Although many patients undergoing similar radiation regimens have acute symptoms, only a portion progress to chronic disease, even though all the factors seem otherwise equal. Among a series of 384 patients undergoing radiation for carcinoma of the bladder, 8% were found to have severe bowel complications (15). The incidence was even higher (11%) when wide-field, whole-pelvic radiation was used, a treatment program commonly utilized for patients with advanced bladder cancer. A consecutive series of 129 patients undergoing radiation for ovarian cancer showed that almost 30% of patients suffered symptoms of radiation enteritis lasting more than eight weeks beyond completion of radiation (19). For half of these patients, the symptoms were severe, requiring either systemic corticosteroids or surgical intervention for alleviation of symptoms. A review of all children receiving whole-abdominal radiation as part of their treatment for malignant disease at Institut Gustave-Roussy revealed an incidence of acute radiation enteritis, defined as nausea, vomiting, and diarrhea, with a need for intravenous infusion, in 70% of children (10). More than half of these children had weight loss during therapy as a clinical indicator of poor nutritional status, which served as an important parameter in assessing fluid and electrolyte status. Thirty-six percent of the children in this series developed delayed radiation enteritis, manifest as bowel obstruction, which required dietary management to reverse their symptoms. The addition of chemotherapy, particularly actinomycin D, was felt to augment the bowel toxicity from radiotherapy in this study. Others have also observed that the addition of chemotherapy to radiation therapy may potentiate mucosal injury to the bowel (34).

Although the basic structure of the colon is similar to that of small intestine, certain differences exist which may alter the relative radiation sensitivity of these organs. The large intestine is much less mobile, especially at either end, than the small intestine, and because of such fixation it may receive greater doses of radiation than comparable lengths of small intestine during the therapeutic course. Furthermore, the rectosigmoid is located in close proximity to organs commonly irradiated, i.e., the ovaries, uterus, bladder, and prostate. Thus, radiation proctitis is a very common, although not often serious, acute complication of radiation therapy. Chronic injury from radiation occurs in the large bowel with a clinical frequency about equal to or even in excess of that of the small intestine (7). Although radiation colitis and/or proctitis are not uncommon, they are seldom a major factor in nutritional abnormalities related to radiotherapy. Severe colon and rectum injury may require surgical decompression and/or bypass procedures, but usually are associated with minimal nutritional sequelae.

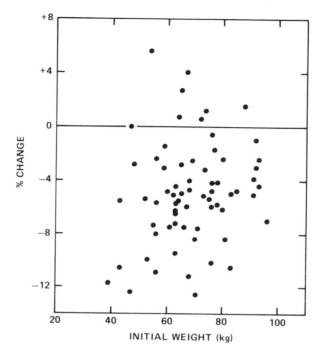

**FIG. 2.** Percentage of weight change as a function of initial weight during a course of abdominal–pelvic radiation therapy among 67 adults with non-Hodgkin's lymphoma.

Although the nutritional consequences of abdominal–pelvic radiation are well-recognized, precise data concerning their severity are difficult to obtain. An assessment of weight change during radiotherapy is a simple and seemingly accurate measure of nutritional status. Figure 2 shows an analysis of weight change during a course of whole-abdominal–pelvic radiation as a function of initial weight among 67 adults with non-Hodgkin's lymphoma irradiated with curative intent at Stanford University Medical Center. Fifty-nine of the 67 patients (88%) suffered a weight loss during the approximate six-week course of therapy. The average weight loss among this group was 3.4 kg. Nine of the 67 patients (13%) suffered a loss of more than 10% body weight during the course of this treatment. Forty of the 67 adults (59%) weighed less than 70 kg at the time of initiation of radiation. None of these patients had specific dietary therapy during their course of radiation.

## ✳ Therapeutic Management ✳

The traditional therapy for radiation-induced gastrointestinal injury has been supportive medical management in an attempt to minimize symptoms caused by anticancer therapy. This can often be achieved by administration of antiemetics, antispasmodics, anticholinergic compounds, and antidiarrheal drugs. Tranquilizers are sometimes used. Careful attention to fluid and electrolyte balance, to avitaminosis, and to signs of infection is mandatory, as these conditions are readily reversible by appropriate medical management. Gastric irritation may respond to a bland diet. Corticosteroid therapy is contraindicated, for it might lead to peptic ulcer rather than protection against radiation injury. Surgery may be necessary, as in therapy for peptic ulcer, if the patient fails to respond to medical management. Small-bowel injury may be treated by systemic corticosteroids; hydrocortisone enemas and/or suppositories may relieve symptoms of colitis and/or proctitis. Such efforts to avoid, minimize, or effectively medically treat this radiation complication are greatly needed, since surgical intervention is often associated with complication or failure (26).

Careful attention to the time, dose, and fractionation of radiation therapy, use of multiple fields, and calculation of radiation dose to be administered are the safest ways to minimize the risk of radiation bowel damage. Often, modification of the details of radiation, such as alteration of beam direction or patient positioning following localization of small intestinal loops by pretreatment roentgenograms, can minimize the risk of radiation injury. Successful protection of the small bowel and proximal colon has been achieved in laboratory animals by using a selective superior mesenteric artery infusion of a vasoconstrictor (Pitressin®) during abdominal irradiation (35).

Specific medications, such as tetracycline or cholestyramine, may be useful in patients demonstrating abnormal glycine [1-$^{14}$C]cholate breath tests (27) and in those shown to have cholerheic enteropathy, by binding excess bile salts (2). The suggestion has been made that gastrointestinal syndrome following radiotherapy may be related to an excessive production of prostaglandins, and that acetylsalicylate, a prostaglandin-synthetase inhibitor, may effectively control diarrhea, pain, and flatulence experienced by patients undergoing pelvic radiotherapy (24). The anti-inflammatory drug salicylazosulfapyridine, conventionally used in the treatment of idiopathic inflammatory bowel disease, has been reported to cause striking and radiographical improvement in four patients with severe chronic radiation enteritis and/or colitis. This suggests that chronic radiation effects may be suppressed by anti-inflammatory therapy (16). Phenothiazine antiemetics are sometimes useful. Diarrhea often responds well to Lomotil® or deodorized tincture of opium.

Recently, attention has been given to specific dietary therapy in the management of radiation damage to the bowel. A specific low-residue, low-fat diet, free of gluten and free of milk and milk products has been shown to be therapeutically effective in children who developed delayed radiation enteritis or small-bowel obstruction (10). These treated children had radiographic and histological reversal of severe bowel damage coincident with specific dietary therapy alone. Although few published data are available on the prophylactic administration of dietary therapy used specifically to prevent the onset of late complications, ongoing clinical studies at the Institut Gustave-Roussy (Villejuif, France) suggest that dietary therapy during abdominal radiation can prevent significant bowel injury. Since the institution of "prophylactic" dietary therapy in children receiving whole or hemiabdominal therapy, there have been no cases of severe acute radiation enteritis and no cases of delayed radiation enteritis. Prior to the routine administration of dietary management, the incidence of acute radiation enteritis was 70% and that of delayed enteritis was 36% of that institution.

Long-term nutrition with a defined formula diet during or following abdominal–pelvic radiation has been demonstrated to offer protection against radiation enteropathy, with prevention of diarrhea and with weight gain. Hyperalimentation is now being widely used as supportive nutritional therapy in cancer patients. Poor-risk, nutritionally depleted patients have been shown to improve symptomatically, gain weight, and tolerate full courses of radiation therapy. Patients with enteric fistulae can effectively be treated preoperatively with intravenous hyperalimentation to initiate positive nitrogen balance and anabolism. Our present experience with nutritional support for cancer patients undergoing radiation to the abdomen and pelvis is based upon retrospective data. Prospective randomized trials are now underway to evaluate critically the role of optimal nutritional support in this group of patients.

## LIVER

### Clinical Course and Pathophysiology

Radiation injury to the liver is now well described (21) and is understood to be distinct from hepatitis from other causes. The tolerated dose when the entire liver is irradiated is in the range of 3,000 to 3,500 rads/21 to 18 days (21) in adults, but less in children, ranging from 1,200 to 2,500 rads, in face of chemotherapy (37). Regenerating liver, after partial hepatectomy, is even less tolerant to irradiation.

The clinical syndrome most commonly appears 2 to 6 weeks after completion of therapy, and is associated with hepatomegaly, weight gain, ascites, jaundice, and elevation of serum alkaline phosphatase. The syndrome can be associated with thrombocytopenia, and is greatly enhanced by the concomitant administration of actinomycin D (37). The clinical and histologic picture is one of veno-occlusive disease, and resembles the Budd–Chiari syndrome.

### Therapeutic Management

The nutritional impact of radiation hepatitis is similar to that of hepatitis from other causes. Patients with hepatitis have profound anorexia, nausea and vomiting, and abdominal distention and discomfort related to ascites and hepatomegaly. They are best managed by general supportive measures, as radiation hepatitis is usually transient. Patients with radiation injury to the liver need careful nutritional counseling so that protein, carbohydrate, and fat intake can be well monitored.

## PANCREAS

### Clinical Course and Pathophysiology

Both the exocrine and endocrine cells of the pancreas are postmitotic with low turnover rates; the pancreas has therefore been considered to be radioresistant. There are, however, very few studies of radiation injury to the pancreas.

With the increased use of whole-abdominal radiation, as in therapy for the malignant lymphomas, there are greater opportunities to observe radiation effects on the pancreas. The potential use of heavy particle radiation, such as neutrons or negative pi meson therapy, intraoperative radiation, and/or interstitial therapy for carcinoma of the pancreas, will increase opportunities to study the radiation response of the human pancreas.

Laboratory studies have shown a temporary decrease in enzyme production and pancreatic secretion following radiation (28). Clinical experience with large numbers of patients has shown no change in serum amylase following 4,000 rads to the upper abdomen for the treatment of lymphoma. In addition, we have successfully treated an entire pancreas with 4,000 rads in a child with juvenile diabetes mellitus and Hodgkin's disease, with no subsequent abnormalities in serum or urine glucose or in insulin requirements.

### Therapeutic Management

Upper-abdominal irradiation may be associated with symptoms such as anorexia, nausea and vomiting, and diarrhea, as has previously been mentioned, which respond to supportive medical management. Specific abnormalities of exocrine or endocrine pancreatic dysfunction related to radiation can be expected to be rare.

## THOUGHTS FOR THE FUTURE

Present cancer treatment modalities, including irradiation, are not confined exclusively to malignant cell populations. Morbidity to normal tissues, ultimately affecting the nutritional status, must be considered when such therapy is prescribed. It is essential to weigh the potential benefit of treatment against the complications resulting from such therapy. If the nutritional sequelae from irradiation can be effectively prevented and/or treated by attention to nutritional support before, during, or following radiotherapy, such aggressive forms of therapy are justified.

A serious drawback within the field of nutrition and cancer has been the lack of prospective, randomized clinical trials designed to investigate the impact of nutritional problems associated with current cancer therapy, such as radiation therapy. Such clinical trials require long-term follow-up and large patient numbers to provide significant data. Important questions to be answered by well-constructed prospective randomized clinical trials should include:

   A. What is the effect of nutritional support on the neoplasm?

   B. To what degree, if any, does nutritional support improve the patient's tolerance to treatment?

   C. What is the duration of this response?

   D. Can nutritional support prevent and/or protect against radiation-associated normal tissue injury?

We must continually be aware of the potential importance of evaluating radiation therapy patients for their nutritional needs and must be alert to possible prevention of radiation injury by nutritional awareness.

## ACKNOWLEDGMENTS

This research was supported in part by US PHS Research Grant CA-05838 from the National Cancer Institute, and Contract #N01-CP-65825 from the Diet, Nutrition, and Cancer Program, National Cancer Institute, National Institutes of Health, Bethesda, Maryland.

The author thanks Ms. Marie Graham for her help in preparing the chapter.

## REFERENCES

1. Bedwinek, J. M., Shukovsky, L. J., Fletcher, G. H., and Daley T. E. (1976): Osteonecrosis in patients treated with definitive radiotherapy for squamous cell carcinoma of the oral cavity and naso- and oropharynx. *Radiology,* 119:665–668.
2. Berk, R. N., and Seay, D. G. (1972): Cholerheic enteropathy as a cause of diarrhea and death in radiation enteritis and its prevention with cholestyramine. *Radiology,* 104:153–156.
3. Berthrong, M., and Fajardo, L. F. (1981): Radiation injury in surgical pathology. Part II. *Am. J. Surg. Pathol. (in press).*
4. Brown, L. R., Dreizen, S., Rider, L. J., and Johnston, D. A. (1976): The effect of radiation-induced xerostomia on saliva and serum lysozyme and immunoglobulin levels. *Oral Surg.,* 41:83–92.
5. Conger, A. D. (1973): Loss and recovery of taste acuity in patients irradiated to the oral cavity. *Radiat. Res.,* 53:338–347.
6. Cooper, G. P. (1968): Receptor origin of the olfactory bulb response to ionizing radiation. *Am. J. Physiol.,* 215:803–806.
7. DeCosse, J. J., Rhodes, R. S., Wentz, W. B., Reagan, J. W., Dworken, H. J., and Holden, W. D. (1969): The natural history and management of radiation-induced injury of the gastrointestinal tract. *Ann. Surg.,* 170:369–384.
8. Donaldson, S. S. (1977): Nutritional consequences of radiotherapy. *Cancer Res.,* 37:2407–2413.
9. Donaldson, S. S., and Lenon, R. A. (1979): Alterations of nutritional status. Impact of chemotherapy and radiation therapy. *Cancer,* 43:2036–2052.
10. Donaldson, S. S., Jundt, S., Ricour, C., Sarrazin, D., Lemerle, J., and Schweisguth, O. (1975): Radiation enteritis in children. A retrospective review of clinicopathologic correlation and dietary management. *Cancer,* 35:1167–1178.
11. Duncan, W., and Leonard, J. C. (1965): The malabsorption syndrome following radiotherapy. *Q. J. Med.,* 34:319–329.
12. Eneroth, C. M., Henrikson, C. O., and Jakobsson, P. A. (1972): Effect of fractionated radiotherapy on salivary gland function. *Cancer,* 30:1147–1153.

13. Fajardo, L. F., and Berthrong, M. (1978): Radiation injury in surgical pathology. Part I. *Am. J. Surg. Pathol.*, 2:159–199.
14. Gibbs, F. A., Palos, B., and Goffinet, D. R. (1976): The metal/tissue interface effect in irradiation of the oral cavity. *Radiology*, 119:705–707.
15. Goffinet, D. R., Schneider, M. J., Glatstein, E., Ludwig, H., Ray, G. R., Dunnick, R., and Bagshaw, M. A. (1975): Bladder cancer: Results of radiation therapy in 384 patients. *Radiology*, 117:149–153.
16. Goldstein, F., Khourey, J., and Thornton, J. J. (1976): Treatment of chronic radiation enteritis and colitis with salicylazosulfapyridine and systemic corticosteroids. *Am. J. Gastroenterol.*, 65:201–208.
17. Goodner, C. J., Moore, T. E., Bowers, J. Z., and Armstrong, W. D. (1955): Effects of acute whole-body X-irradiation on the absorption and distribution of $Na^{22}$ and $H^3OH$ from the gastrointestinal tract of the fasted rat. *Am. J. Physiol.*, 183:475–484.
18. Greco, F. A., Brereton, H. D., Kent, H., Zimbler, H., Merrill, J., and Johnson, R. E. (1976): Adriamycin and enhanced radiation reaction on normal esophagus and skin. *Ann. Intern. Med.*, 85:294–298.
19. Hintz, B., Fuks, Z., Kempson, R., Eltringham, J., Zaloudek, C., Williamson, T., and Bagshaw, M. A. (1975): Results of postoperative megavoltage radiotherapy of malignant surface epithelial tissues of the ovary. *Radiology*, 114:695–700.
20. Horwich, A., Lokich, J. J., and Bloomer, W. D. (1975): Doxorubicin, radiotherapy, and oesophageal stricture. *Lancet*, 2:561–562.
21. Ingold, J. A., Reed, G. B., Kaplan, H. S., and Bagshaw, M. A. (1965): Radiation hepatitis. *Am. J. Roentgenol.*, 93:200–208.
22. Jervis, H. R., Donati, R. M., Stromberg, L. R., and Sprinz, H. (1969): Histochemical investigation of mucosa of exteriorized small intestine of the rat exposed to X-radiation. *Strahlentherapie*, 137:326–343.
23. Kashima, H. K., Kirkham, W. R., and Andrews, J. R. (1965): Postirradiation sialadenitis: A study of the clinical features, histopathologic changes and serum enzyme variations following irradiation of human salivary glands. *Am. J. Roentgenol.*, 94:271–291.
24. Mennie, A. T., Dalley, V. M., Dinneen, L. C., and Collier, H. O. J. (1975): Treatment of radiation-induced gastrointestinal distress with acetylsalicylate. *Lancet*, 2:942–943.
25. Mitchell, G. W., Bardawil, W. A., and Bloedorn, F. G. (1972): The effect of irradiation on gastrointestinal tract. *Clin. Obstet. Gynecol.*, 15:674–691.
26. Morgenstern, L., Thompson, R., and Friedman, N. B. (1977): Modern enigma of radiation enteropathy: Sequelae and solutions. *Am. J. Surg.*, 134:166–172.
27. Newman, A., Katsaris, J., and Blendis, L. M. (1973): Proceedings: Small bowel injury following pelvic irradiation: A common complication of radiotherapy. *Gut*, 14:826.
28. Pieroni, P. L., Rudick, J., Adler, M., Nacchiero, M., Rybak, B. J., Perlberg, H., and Dreiling, D. A. (1976): Effect of irradiation on the canine exocrine pancreas. *Ann. Surg.*, 184:610–614.
29. Reeves, R. J., Cavanaugh, P. J., Sharpe, K. W., Thorne, W. A., Winkler, C., and Sanders, A. P. (1965): Fat absorption studies and small bowel X-ray studies in patients undergoing $Co^{60}$ teletherapy and/or radium application. *Am. J. Roentgenol.*, 94:848–851.
30. Reeves, R. J., Sanders, A. P., Isley, J. K., Sharpe, K. W., and Baylin, G. J. (1959): Fat absorption from the human gastrointestinal tract in patients undergoing radiation therapy. *Radiology*, 73:398–401.
31. Roswit, B. (1974): Complications of radiation therapy: The alimentary tract. *Semin. Roentgenol.*, 9:51–63.
32. Rubin, P., and Casarett, G. W. (1972): A direction for clinical radiation pathology: The tolerance dose. In: *Frontiers of Radiation Therapy and Oncology, Vol. 6*, edited by J. Vaeth, pp. 1–16. University Park Press, Baltimore.
33. Rubin, P., and Casarett, G. W. (1968): *Clinical Radiation Pathology, Vol. 1*, pp. 1–517. W. B. Saunders, Philadelphia.
34. Schenken, L. L., Burholt, D. R., Hagemann, R. F., and Lesher, S. (1976): The modification of gastrointestinal tolerance and responses to abdominal irradiation by chemotherapeutic agents. *Radiology*, 120:417–420.
35. Steckel, R. J., Snow, H. D., Collins, J. D., Barenfus, M., and Patin T. (1974): Successful radiation protection of the normal intestinal tract in the dog. *Radiology*, 11:451–455.
36. Tarpila, S. (1971): Morphologic and functional response of human small intestine to ionizing irradiation. *Scand. J. Gastroenterol.*, 6 (suppl. 12):1–52.

37. Tefft, M., Mitus, A., Das, L., Vawter, G. F., and Filler, R. M. (1970): Irradiation of the liver in children: Review of experience in the acute and chronic phases, and in the intact normal and partially resected. *Am. J. Roentgenol.*, 108:365–385.
38. Trier, J. S., and Browning, T. H. (1966): Morphologic response of the mucosa of human small intestine to X-ray exposure. *J. Clin. Invest.*, 45:194–204.
39. Vatistas, S., and Hornsey, S. (1966): Radiation-induced protein loss into the gastrointestinal tract. *Br. J. Radiol.*, 39:547–550.
40. Wescott, W. B., Mira, J. G., Starcke, E. N., Shannon, I. L., and Thornby, J. I. (1978): Alterations in whole saliva flow rate induced by fractionated radiotherapy. *Am. J. Roentgenol. Radium Ther. Nucl. Med.*, 130:145–149.

*Nutrition and Cancer: Etiology and Treatment,*
edited by G. R. Newell and N. M. Ellison.
Raven Press, New York © 1981.

# Daily Nutritional Care For Cancer Patients[a]

*Ernest H. Rosenbaum, †Carol A. Stitt, **Harry Drasin,
and Isadora R. Rosenbaum

*Mount Zion Hospital and Medical Center, San Francisco, California 94115; ** University
of California at San Francisco, San Francisco, California 94143; † Washoe Medical Center
Reno, Nevada 89502*

Maintaining good nutrition is a particular problem for cancer patients because cancer and cancer therapy (surgery, radiotherapy, or chemotherapy) often cause a loss of appetite. Many cancer patients lose great amounts of weight, 15 to 30 lb, or more. These patients become malnourished to the point of starvation, setting up a vicious cycle: decreased appetite and weight loss result in fatigue and depression; progressive weakness results in less activity, depression, and even less appetite; further weight loss and weakness result in reduced resistance to disease and a poorer prognosis.

Physicians can foster in cancer patients an awareness of the importance of adequate protein and calorie intake and can reinforce the idea that adequate nutrition is an integral part of anticancer therapy, without which other treatment modalities are less likely to succeed. Patients often must take a new approach to eating; food must be thought of as medicine on which their health, in no small way, depends. With good nutrition, patients heal better after surgery, experience fewer unpleasant side effects from radiotherapy and chemotherapy, such as nausea or vomiting, need fewer interruptions of radiotherapy, tolerate more chemotherapy, and perhaps have less immune suppression (that part of which is due to malnutrition alone). Most important, patients feel better physically and mentally and are more active.

The daily nutritional care of cancer patients must take several factors into account: the protein and calorie content of a well-balanced diet, based on adult nutritional requirements; the increased energy requirements caused by the tumor, infection, anemia, and other factors (12); and the effects of both tumor and therapy that make it difficult for the patient to eat.

---

[a] Adapted from: *Nutrition for the Cancer Patient,* by Ernest H. Rosenbaum, M.D., et al. Bull Publishing, Palo Alto, California, 1980.

## BASIC NUTRITION

Certain essential food nutrients—proteins, fats, carbohydrates, vitamins, and minerals—are vital for normal body functioning, repair of body tissues, energy, and metabolic resources. More than 50 different nutrients have been identified as needed for optimal health, with considerable question as to how much of each is required. Nutritionists have developed a general guide for daily use in choosing a good diet, the most widely used being the Basic Four Plan.

In the Basic Four Plan, foods are divided into four groups—protein, milk, vegetable–fruit, and bread–cereal—and minimum numbers of servings from each have been established. These minimum daily requirements are based on the assumption that the person is in good health. Illness, fever, surgery, or weight loss increase these requirements.

The *protein group* consists of dried beans and peas, eggs, fish, meat (beef, lamb, liver, pork, veal), nuts, peanut butter, poultry, tofu (soybean curd), and other soybean products. Foods in this group are the main sources of protein and also supply B vitamins and iron. Two servings a day are needed. One serving consists of: 1 cup of cooked beans, 2 eggs, 2 to 3 oz of meat, poultry, or fish, or 4 tablespoons of peanut butter.

The *milk group* consists of all forms of milk: buttermilk, cheese, cottage cheese, dry milk, evaporated milk, fortified soy milk, ice cream, skim milk, whole milk, and yogurt. Foods in this group are important sources of vitamins A, B, and D, and calcium, as well as protein. Two servings a day are needed. One serving consists of: 1 oz of cheese, 3 oz of cottage cheese, ½ cup of evaporated milk, 1½ cups of ice cream, 1 cup of milk, or 1 cup of yogurt.

The *vegetable–fruit group* consists of all fruits and vegetables, including juices and dried fruits. Foods in this group provide vitamins and minerals. Four servings a day are needed, including one citrus fruit (orange or grapefruit) for vitamin C and one dark green or deep yellow vegetable for vitamin A. One serving consists of: ½ cup of fruit, 1 medium-sized fresh fruit, ½ cup of juice, or ½ cup of vegetables.

The *bread–cereal group* consists of bread and cereal products, such as baked goods, cereal, crackers, flour, pasta, and rice. Foods in this group provide carbohydrates, B vitamins, and iron. Four servings a day are needed. One serving consists of: 1 slice of bread, ¾ cup of cooked cereal, 1 cup of dry cereal, 2 graham cracker squares, ½ cup of cooked noodles, macaroni, or rice, or 5 saltines.

In addition to the Basic Four, 3 to 4 tablespoons of *fats and oils* (butter, cream, margarine, mayonnaise, salad dressing, or vegetable oil) should be included daily to provide calories and vitamin E and to avoid burning body fats.

Much attention has recently been focused on *megavitamin therapy* for cancer; however, there is no reliable scientific evidence of the effectiveness of large amounts of vitamins or minerals in treatment of human cancers, and responsible recommendations for the use of vitamins or minerals in treatment cannot be made at this time.

A balanced diet will make vitamin and mineral supplements unnecessary for most patients. (In some cases, vitamin and mineral supplements may be needed because of the side effects of certain types of cancer or of therapy, which may result in vitamin and mineral losses or increased requirements.) Vitamin and mineral supplements may be needed by patients who are unable to eat a balanced diet, those who have anorexia, malabsorption, or weight loss, or who drink or smoke excessively.

### Protein and Calorie Requirements

The cancer patient must be concerned with obtaining a sufficient amount of protein and calories to repair body tissues and maintain a normal weight. The physician or dietitian should determine the desirable normal weight for each patient, and, using this figure as a point of reference, determine the protein and calorie requirements necessary to obtain or maintain this weight.

An adult has a daily nutritional requirement of approximately 0.5 g of protein per pound of desirable body weight. Extra protein is needed to accelerate recovery from illness or surgery. If the patient is already malnourished, an even greater amount of protein (0.7 to 0.9 g/pound of desirable body weight) will be needed.

To use protein for tissue repair instead of energy, the body must have enough calories. Sex, age, and activity affect the number of calories needed. The average daily calorie requirement for men is 18 calories per pound; for women, 16 calories per pound. The cancer patient who is already malnourished will need an increased number of calories (20 calories per pound for men; 18 calories per pound for women).

We have found it helpful for patients to determine whether they are meeting their daily protein and calorie requirements by weighing themselves daily and keeping a list of foods they eat. Using a simple table of protein and calorie contents of common foods (9), the protein and calorie intake can be calculated each day. The patient is thus put in control of regulating his or her diet to meet nutritional needs.

## COMMON PROBLEMS: A DIETARY APPROACH

Many common problems secondary to cancer and cancer therapy, such as anorexia, nausea, vomiting, or diarrhea, can affect the patient's diet, making it difficult to maintain adequate nutrition. The reverse is also true: the patient's diet can affect the problem by further aggravating preexisting difficulties. We have found that specific dietary approaches to each problem, when combined with medication as necessary, can help minimize the severity of many common side effects of cancer and cancer therapy and enable patients to eat better.

In addition to the specific dietary approaches outlined below, we have found the general recommendation of taking frequent small meals, as opposed to three large meals a day, to be a most important factor in helping the patient who has difficulty in tolerating food, for whatever reason. In addition, high-protein, high-calorie diet supplements should be recommended whenever the patient is unable to maintain an adequate nutritional intake.

## Anorexia

Anorexia is one of the major unresolved dietary problems and one of the most common side effects of cancer and cancer therapy. "Feeling full" is a common factor contributing to progressive anorexia. Depression, stress, and anxiety may also cause a loss of appetite. Anorexia leads to major problems and sets up a self-perpetuating cycle.

When appetite no longer motivates the patient to eat, an entirely new approach to eating must be learned. The physician must encourage the idea that food is a necessary part of therapy. The patient must be taught to follow a planned nutritious diet, to select foods that give maximum nutrient return, and to follow suggestions for making the eating experience more attractive, thereby enhancing appetite. He or she should be encouraged to eat frequent, small meals and to snack between meals. If possible, a third of the daily protein and calorie requirements should be taken at breakfast. Exercising for 5 to 10 min one-half hour before meals will help stimulate appetite. Stress at mealtimes should be avoided. Foods should appeal to the sense of smell. Eating with family or friends, setting an attractive table, and trying for variety in foods will all help make food more appealing.

## Bloating

Bloating may occur after eating just a few bites. It can be caused by the inability of the stomach and intestines to digest food properly or by decreased transit time of food in the intestines. The latter may be caused by nervousness and tension, certain anticancer drugs, narcotics, lack of adequate exercise, or constipation. Bloating may also be related to the type of food eaten; fatty, fried, and greasy foods tend to remain in the stomach for longer periods of time. Carbonated beverages, gas-producing foods, and milk may also cause bloating.

Frequent small meals are recommended instead of three large meals a day. Sitting up or walking around after meals will aid digestion. A fat-restricted diet should be followed, with emphasis on sweet or starchy foods and low-fat protein foods. The following foods should be avoided: fatty, fried, and greasy foods, gas-forming vegetables (broccoli, brussels sprouts, cabbage, cauliflower, corn, cucumber, beans, green peppers, rutabagas, sauerkraut, and turnips), carbonated beverages, chewing gum, and milk.

## Colostomy

The colostomy patient can eat a normal diet, although he or she may want to avoid foods that produce gas or odor or cause irritation. Foods should be chewed slowly and thoroughly; swallowing air should be avoided, since it can lead to gas formation. Plenty of fluids are advised to prevent dehydration. The following foods may present problems for the colostomy patient:

Foods that may cause irritation are nuts, popcorn, skins on fruits and vegetables (such as apples and corn), foods with seeds (such as strawberries, raspberries, and tomatoes), and certain fresh vegetables, such as coleslaw, salads, and coconut. Foods that may produce gas include cabbage, brussels sprouts, green pepper, cucumber, onions, dried beans or peas, and beer. Foods that may produce odor are onions, eggs, and fish. To help control odor, yogurt, buttermilk, and cranberry juice have proved effective.

## Constipation

Constipation can be caused by a lack of high-fiber or bulk-forming foods in the diet, narcotics, lack of exercise, or emotional stress. It is often accompanied by decreased appetite and a bloated feeling.

The diet should contain foods that are high in fiber and bulk, such as fresh fruits and vegetables, dried fruit, whole-grain breads and cereals, and bran. Bran should be added gradually, starting with 2 teaspoons per day. This amount can gradually be increased up to 4 to 6 teaspoons per day. Too rapid an increase may cause diarrhea and bloating. Fluid intake of 4 to 6 glasses per day should be encouraged. A glass of prune juice or hot lemon water taken in the morning may also help.

Laxatives and enemas should be prescribed as needed. Patients requiring narcotics should not take bulk-forming laxatives, because the combination itself causes constipation; instead, stool softeners may be used. Certain other laxatives, when used on a continuous basis, cause irritation of the digestive tract and often make it difficult to regain normal bowel habits once they are discontinued. Patients should therefore be cautioned against self-prescribing when laxatives are required.

## Dehydration

Dehydration may occur after surgery, radiotherapy, or chemotherapy, or because of diarrhea, sweating, fever, nausea, or an inability to drink fluids. Frequent feedings of liquids or foods that become liquid at room temperature are recommended: juice, fruit ades (Kool-Aid; Gatorade, etc.), punch, soft drinks, tea, milk, milkshakes, ice cream, eggnogs, soup, broth, fruits with a high fluid content, such as grapes or watermelon, Jello, sherbet, fruit ices, and popsicles.

## Dental Problems

Although some cancer patients will experience dental problems from disease or therapy, for the most part these problems are preventable or can be managed. A dentist should be consulted by all patients with tumors of the head and neck; dental prophylaxis can help minimize or avoid oral problems during and after treatment. Radiotherapy to the head and neck area causes the teeth to become susceptible to decay. Patients should try to avoid foods and drinks that leave sugar on teeth. The teeth should be cleaned thoroughly after eating; a fluoride mouth rinse should also be used daily.

## Diarrhea

Diarrhea can be caused by chemotherapy, radiotherapy to the abdomen, or surgery to the bowel. It may also be the result of bacterial overgrowth, malabsorption of fats, sensitivity to a specific food or group of foods, food allergy, or emotional or psychological problems.

At first, the diet should consist solely of fluids, to allow the bowel to rest. Mild liquids should be taken: fruit ades (Kool-Aid, Gatorade, etc.), ginger ale, peach or apricot nectar, water, and weak tea. Liquids should be taken warm or at room temperature, because cold or hot foods may aggravate the diarrhea. Carbonated beverages should be allowed to lose their "fizz" before being consumed. Foods low in roughage and bulk should be gradually added to the diet; steamed rice, cream of rice, bananas, applesauce, mashed potatoes, dry toast, and crackers, eaten warm or at room temperature. Frequent small meals will be easier to tolerate. As diarrhea decreases, the patient can progress to a low-residue or soft diet. A low-residue oral nutritional supplement, such as Citrotein or Precision LR Diet, may be indicated.

Fluid intake should be encouraged to replace the fluid lost in diarrhea. The following fluid electrolyte replacement formula can be flavored to taste: 1 quart of boiled water, 1 teaspoon of salt, 1 heaping teaspoon of baking soda, and 4 teaspoons of sugar. Potassium loss must also be replaced. Foods high in potassium include bananas, apricot and peach nectars, potatoes, and milk. A potassium supplement will be needed if diarrhea persists.

The types of foods apt to aggravate diarrhea include fatty, greasy, and spicy foods, coffee, regular (non-herbal) teas, carbonated beverages containing caffeine, citrus juices (orange, grapefruit), foods high in bulk and fiber (bran, wholegrain cereals and breads, popcorn, nuts, and raw vegetables and fruits, except apples), and hot or cold beverages. An anti-diarrhea medication such as Lomotil or Imodium may need to be prescribed.

## Dry Mouth

Radiotherapy to the head and neck area causes a decrease in saliva production, resulting in a dry mouth. Soft, bland foods are recommended, especially cool or cold foods with a high liquid content, such as ice cream, popsicles, puddings, watermelon, and grapes. Solid foods can be made easier to swallow by adding gravies, sauces, melted butter, broths, mayonnaise, yogurt, or salad dressing. Dunking bread and other baked foods in milk, tea, or coffee will make them easier to swallow. If solid foods are too difficult to swallow, a pureed diet or a full liquid diet should be tried. A liquid high-protein supplement is recommended to ensure adequate nutrition.

Sucking on sugar-free hard candy or popsicles or chewing sugar-free gum may help to stimulate saliva production. Since tooth decay is a major problem for patients receiving radiotherapy to the head and neck area, the use of sugar-free products is advised. "Artificial saliva" can be purchased commercially or prepared by a pharmacist.

Hot, spicy, or acid foods may be irritating, and should be eaten with caution.

### Dysphagia

Swallowing difficulty may occur because of radiotherapy to the mouth or neck area, surgery of the mouth or throat, cardiovascular disease, or generalized weakness. Difficulties may range from problems of temporary discomfort caused by pain, swelling, or dryness of the mouth or throat to more severe problems requiring supplementation by tube feeding, intravenous fluids to prevent dehydration, and retraining of swallowing reflexes.

If swallowing difficulties are not severe, the following approach should be helpful: Frequent small meals are recommended. Solid foods should be soft and cooked until tender. They should be cut into bite-sized pieces and moistened with liberal amounts of gravies, mayonnaise, salad dressing, sauces, sour cream, or yogurt. Hard or dry foods, such as crackers, nuts, popcorn, potato chips, pretzels, and raw vegetables, should be avoided.

A pureed diet may be necessary. A liquid diet is not recommended because it is easy for liquids to be aspirated. Beverages of a thick milkshake consistency are safer than thin liquids. A liquid high-protein diet supplement, thickened with ice cream if necessary, will help ensure an adequate protein and calorie intake. Custard and pudding are easy to swallow and make good protein and calorie supplements. For those with more severe swallowing difficulties, a swallowing training program (9) may be needed to teach the patient how to swallow safely and comfortably.

### Edema

Water retention may occur in the arms or legs because of removal of or radiation to lymph glands. It may also occur in the abdomen, chest, head, or neck because of cancer therapy or the cancer itself. Hormonal drugs also cause water retention.

Salt intake should be decreased. A low-salt diet restricts salt intake to about

3 to 4 g a day (the equivalent of 1½ teaspoons). No salt should be added to food while it is being cooked, and at most only a very small amount to food at the table. Salt substitutes, such as Co-Salt or Adolph's Salt Substitute, will help satisfy the need for salty taste. Various herbs and spices can also take the place of salt.

In addition to restricting the amount of salt added to food, foods of naturally high salt content should be avoided, such as bouillon and canned soups, canned herring and sardines, canned, cured, and dry meat (such as bacon, cold cuts, corned beef, frankfurters, ham, luncheon meats, and sausage), potato chips and corn chips, salted crackers, nuts, and snack foods, soy sauce, catsup, barbecue sauce, and hard cheese.

A more restricted diet limits salt intake to about ½ g (¼ teaspoon) per day and requires the use of special milk, bread, and other food products low in salt. The physician should provide a special diet if he feels the patient requires this much salt restriction.

If diuretics are prescribed, potassium balance should be considered. The patient should be instructed to try to eat foods high in potassium, such as apricots, bananas, cantaloupe, dates, figs, milk, orange juice, prunes, potatoes, raisins, tangerine juice, and tomato juice. A commercial potassium supplement may also be needed.

## Esophagitis

Esophagitis may occur as a side effect of chemotherapy or radiotherapy to the head and neck area or may occasionally be caused by infection. The recommended dietary approach is similar to that used with a sore or ulcerated mouth or throat.

Gargling and swallowing an analgesic solution, such as Xylocaine, before meals will lessen irritation. Such a solution can also be made by dissolving 1 to 2 tablespoons of baking soda and 1 teaspoon of salt in 1 quart of warm water. Two or four tablespoons should be used before meals. Another solution can be made by mixing 1 tablespoon of sour cream with either 1 tablespoon of liquid Tylenol or 1 tablespoon of Benalyn. Systemic analgesics, such as Tylenol with codeine or other narcotics, may also be needed to relieve pain.

## Heartburn

Keeping the stomach full by eating frequent small meals will help neutralize stomach acids. A bland diet may be temporarily necessary. The patient should be instructed not to lie down for two to three hours after meals. If he must stay in bed, or if heartburn persists after lying down, the head and chest should be elevated with pillows or by putting six-inch bed blocks under the head of the bed.

Hot, spicy foods, coffee, liquor, smoking, and stress, which stimulate increased acid output by the stomach, should be avoided. An antacid taken one or two hours after meals and at bedtime may provide relief.

## Indigestion

Indigestion is usually caused by overeating or by foods that are too spicy or fatty. Indigestion may also accompany constipation, bloating, forced feeding, or stress. Frequent small meals and a bland diet can be helpful. Overeating and foods found to cause indigestion should be avoided. An antacid taken one or two hours after meals may help relieve discomfort.

Milk and milk products, such as ice cream, cottage cheese, and cheese, should be avoided. Butter, cream, and sour cream may also be difficult to digest. If the patient is especially sensitive to milk, he may need to avoid packaged foods containing milk. Buttermilk or yogurt are usually well tolerated, as well as many processed cheeses.

Lactose-free milk substitutes, such as Mocha Mix, Dairy Rich, and other soy-milk products, are recommended. Some lactose-free substitutes for other milk products are also available, such as IMO—an imitation sour cream—and Cool Whip or Party Whip nondairy whipped toppings.

Lact-Aid (available without prescription in health food and drug stores), a lactase tablet, can be added to milk 24 hours prior to use to make it lactose-free. Lact-Aid should not be added to cream, ice cream, sour cream, cottage cheese, or diet supplements.

## Nausea and Vomiting

Nausea and vomiting are common side effects of chemotherapy and radiotherapy and may also be caused by intestinal obstruction. Continued vomiting makes it impossible to eat; thus, the effort should be to try to reduce nausea before vomiting occurs. If the patient vomits after chemotherapy or radiotherapy, he or she should avoid eating for several hours before therapy; however, some patients who experience "dry heaves" may be able to get relief by eating lightly before therapy.

Food and drink should be taken slowly. Foods should not be forced past the point of tolerance. Small, frequent meals and rest after eating are recommended. A clear liquid diet may be best at first, especially apple and cranberry juice, fruit ades (Kool-Aid, Gatorade, etc.), ginger ale and 7-Up, Jello, tea, or iced tea. It may be helpful to take beverages chilled. Popsicles, salty foods, soda crackers, and toast are often well tolerated.

If nausea occurs in the morning, techniques used for morning sickness during pregnancy—such as eating melba toast, dry toast, or crackers first thing in the morning—may also be helpful. Overly sweet, greasy, hot, or spicy foods and foods with strong odors should be avoided. Cold foods may be more appealing because they have less odor.

Compazine or Dramamine 30 to 60 minutes before meals may be prescribed. For morning nausea, medication should be taken on awakening 15 to 30 minutes before getting out of bed, to get maximum effectiveness before breakfast. With vomiting, a Compazine or Dramamine suppository may be indicated.

The use of marijuana to reduce nausea is generally effective for many people (8). It can be smoked, taken in suppositories, ingested in capsules, or included in food. Because of the legal ramifications and the care needed to get maximum benefit, the patient and physician should have good background information before using marijuana for nausea.

### Pain

The control of pain is a dietary problem because pain can cause anorexia and seriously limit the patient's ability to eat. The physician should prescribe appropriate medication and instruct the patient in its proper scheduling for maximum relief. The patient can also be helped by special pain control techniques, such as self-hypnosis, relaxation (6), and stress reduction (4).

### Stomatitis

A sore or ulcerated mouth or throat is a frequent side effect of chemotherapy or radiotherapy to the head and neck area. This condition will usually clear up in a few days unless recovery is slowed by malnutrition.

The diet should consist of soft, bland foods. Solid foods should be soft and cooked until tender. A full liquid diet or a pureed diet may be needed if solid food is too irritating. Frequent small meals served cold or at room temperature will help make foods more tolerable. Foods especially well tolerated are applesauce, cold liquids, cooked cereal, strained cream soup, custard, soft-cooked eggs, plain ice cream, Jello, milkshakes, mashed potatoes, popsicles, pudding and sherbet.

Anesthetic gels such as Xylocaine Viscous, mouth sprays, lozenges, or systemic analgesics such as Tylenol with codeine may be needed to help relieve pain. Medications such as milk of magnesia (1 tablespoon swished around the mouth), Orabase, or a methylcellulose solution (e.g., Cologel), will stick to ulcerations and give them a protective coating. Liquid Xylocaine or a mouth wash of 1 to 2 tablespoons of baking soda and 1 teaspoon of salt dissolved in 1 quart of warm water, used before meals, will lessen irritation. Cool yogurt may also be soothing.

If brushing the teeth is painful, they can be cleaned with a cotton swab and a 3% solution of hydrogen peroxide diluted to half strength with warm water. Sponge-tipped swabs (Toothettes) impregnated with dentrifice are also available. The mouth can also be cleaned and freshened with a solution of equal part of Cepacol mouthwash, hydrogen peroxide, and water or 1 to 2 tablespoons of baking soda and 1 teaspoon salt in a quart of warm water.

Supportive mouth care and a continued high-protein, balanced diet will help accelerate healing of mouth and tongue sores.

## Taste Blindness

"Taste blindness" refers to a loss of taste or a change in the way foods taste. It may occur temporarily as a side effect of chemotherapy, radiotherapy (especially to the head and neck area), or because of the cancer itself. Foods may taste bitter or rancid, and the patient may develop aversions to eggs, fish, meat, poultry, fried foods, tomatoes, and tomato products.

Since taste blindness commonly includes aversions to several of the most popular protein foods, it is important to find alternatives that are more palatable and also good sources of protein, such as milk, ice cream, bland cheeses, cottage cheese, and peanut butter.

Frequent small meals are recommended, as well as a liquid high-protein diet supplement. Fresh fruits, gelatin salads, and lettuce have been found appealing to patients with taste blindness. Zinc deficiency can alter taste, and taste abnormalities may be improved in some patients by a zinc supplement.

## Weight Loss

Weight loss results from calorie deficiency. It can be the ultimate result of bloating, constipation, diarrhea, vomiting, and poor digestion or poor absorption of food; it can also occur secondary to surgery. The key is to try to maintain adequate calorie intake. Cancer patients (like patients suffering from burns, stress, or infections) may need up to 25% *more* calories than normal. Frequent small meals, between-meal snacks, and a high-protein, high-calorie diet supplement will help maintain calorie intake.

Extra calories and protein can be added to daily cooking by using: cream, evaporated milk, or fortified milk in making cooked cereal, cream sauces, puddings, or soups; sour cream on baked potatoes and in cream soups; high-calorie gravies and sauces on meats and vegetables; extra butter or margarine with cooked cereal, noodles, rice, sauces, soups, and vegetables; cheese or hard-cooked eggs with casseroles, noodles, rice, or sauces; and peanut butter on apple wedges or celery, and in cookies, frostings, and sandwich fillings.

## DIET SUPPLEMENTS

Cancer patients have an increased need for calories. For the patient with weight loss or anorexia, standard diets may be insufficient. Dietary supplementation is needed when calorie intake is insufficient to attain or maintain desirable weight. Oral supplementation should be utilized if 5% or more of desirable weight has been lost. Tube or intravenous feedings may be necessary, in addition to oral feedings, if more than 10% of desirable weight has been lost.

TABLE 1. *Supplemental dietary preparations*

*Elemental diets (chemically defined)*

| | |
|---|---|
| Flexical | Vivonex |
| Precision LR | Vivonex HN high nitrogen diet |
| Precision high-nitrogen | Vital |
| Precision isotonic | |

*Supplemental Formulas*

| | |
|---|---|
| Instant Breakfast | Sustacal |
| Ensure | Sustagen |
| Ensure Plus | |
| Meritene liquid or powder | |
| Nutri-1000 | |

*Modular Feedings*

| *Fat* | *Protein* | *Carbohydrate* |
|---|---|---|
| Medium-chain triglycerides | Liquid predigested protein | Controlyte |
| | | Hycal |
| | | Polycose |

A large variety of diet supplements is available to increase protein and calorie intake (Tables 1 and 2). Further discussions of these products can be found in the literature (2,3,5,11). Taste comparisons of some products are also available (1,10). Selection of a diet supplement must be coordinated with any special medical problems, such as lactose intolerance or the need for a low-residue diet. Factors to be considered in selection of a supplement include digestibility, lactose, osmolality, calories, fat, protein, viscosity, residue, taste, and price.

In addition to the supplements listed in Table 1, many other brands of protein drinks and protein powders are available in supermarkets, drug stores, and health food stores. One should compare other products to those listed to make sure comparable amounts of protein and calories are provided.

Elemental or chemically defined diets are recommended when a clear liquid diet must be the sole source of nutrition. All are low-residue and lactose-free and have minimal to low amounts of fat. The nutrients are easily digested and absorbed. Invariably, they are hyperosmolar and generally contain 1 cal/ml. Their cost is generally high, and they are used only in special circumstances, such as the inability of the gastrointestinal tract to tolerate or absorb complex formulas. Tube feedings are preferred over oral feedings, as taste is often poorly tolerated. Further information on their use can be found elsewhere (1,10).

Supplemental formulas are used as protein and calorie supplements or as complete feedings. Their composition demands a high level of gastrointestinal function able to tolerate high-fat content, whole proteins and complex carbohydrates. They are generally somewhat hyperosmolar, but far less so than the elemental products. Calorie content is generally around 1 cal/ml. Taste is generally well tolerated, and comparisons are available. Prices are less than those for elemental products.

TABLE 2. Basic qualities of some commonly used supplements (not a complete list)

| | Protein g/liter | Protein composition | Cal/ml | OSM | Volume for 100% RDA | Lactose | Taste |
|---|---|---|---|---|---|---|---|
| **Chemically defined** | | | | | | | |
| Vivonex | 20.4 | Crystalline amino acids | 1.0 | 500–678 (flavored) | 1,800 cc | 0 | Poor |
| **Low-residue** | | | | | | | |
| Precision LR | 26 | Egg-white solids | 1.1 | 525 | 1,710 cc | 0 | Fair |
| **Standard** | | | | | | | |
| Ensure | 37 | Na + Ca caseinate soy | 1.0 | 450 | 1,920 cc | 0 | Very good |
| Meritene | 60 (Liquid) | Skim milk, no caseinate | 1.0 | 560–617 | 1,200 cc | Yes | Good |
| Sustacal | 60 (Liquid) | Na + Ca caseinate soy | 1.0 | 625 | 1,080 cc | 0 | Good |

Modular feedings are specific nutrients that do not constitute a complete feeding. Three types are available, depending on the need for replacement of fat, carbohydrate, or protein. Recipes for their use are available from the manufacturer. Liquid predigested protein (cherry flavor is tolerated best) can supply 60 g of protein daily when 30 cc are taken four times a day.

## DAILY NUTRITIONAL MANAGEMENT

Whether the patient is at home or in the hospital, a planned approach to eating will aid in nutrition. We have found the following techniques to be helpful.

While the patient is still in the hospital, he or she should have the opportunity to consult with the hospital dietitian. The dietitian can help the patient plan a balanced daily menu that includes the proper amounts of protein and calories, advise the patient on management of any eating problems, and plan a home nutrition program. A high-protein or high-calorie diet supplement should be added to the menu. The dietitian should discuss the various diet supplements and may be able to let the patient taste-test different brands.

Frequent small meals are the best way to ensure that the patient gets enough food, and can be especially helpful if anorexia is present. The patient should be given snacks between meals, such as high-protein diet supplements, milk-shakes, eggnogs, puddings, or sandwiches. If a meal must be interrupted or missed because of a test, therapy, or an examination, the patient's food should be saved in a warmer or ordered on return to the room.

The daily menu should be filled out when the patient is feeling well enough to plan his meals imaginatively. He or she should have help if necessary and should order favorite foods. Protein and calorie values should be considered, but thought should be given to eye appeal and aroma so that the food will be as appetizing as possible. Giving variety to the menu will improve the appetite. The patient may want to save some of the menus to use as examples for home meal planning.

Having favorite foods brought from home will often improve appetite. In some hospitals, families are allowed to use the ward kitchen to prepare special food or to warm up food brought from home. Food may also be ordered from a restaurant. Mealtime atmosphere is important. Flowers and pictures can brighten the hospital room. Eating with family, friends, or other patients, or turning on the radio, television, or music for company will make mealtime more pleasant.

Specific relaxation exercises before meals may be helpful in reducing tension and may improve appetite (6). For some patients, a glass of wine or beer before meals is relaxing and stimulating to the appetite. Light exercise for five to ten minutes approximately one-half hour before meals may help in stimulating appetite.

In addition to the suggestions applicable to both hospital and home, there are some techniques to keep in mind when the hospital facilities and staff are no longer available.

The daily menu should be planned in advance to include the proper number of servings from the Basic Four and the necessary amounts of protein and calories. In addition to planning the foods to be eaten, it can be helpful to plan the times for eating.

Help in preparing meals is sometimes necessary for the patient who must do his or her own cooking. A friend or relative may be able to help by preparing foods in advance. Home aid in preparing meals is also available in many communities. A nutritious diet can also be planned using canned, packaged, and frozen foods.

Having small portions of food in containers ready to serve diminishes the problem of figuring out what to eat at a time when appetite may be poor or the patient does not feel like cooking. A microwave oven may be a practical investment in order to heat small portions of food quickly.

Extra protein can be added to the diet by using fortified milk (1 cup of nonfat dry milk solids added to 1 quart of whole milk) for drinking and in all recipes calling for milk. Peanut butter, cheese, cottage cheese, and chopped hard-boiled eggs are high-protein snacks and can also be added to recipes.

Extra calories can be added to the diet by adding cream or butter to soups, cooked cereals, and vegetables. Gravies, sauces, and sour cream can be added to vegetables, meat, poultry, and fish. A high-calorie diet supplement can be added to normal recipes.

An attractive table setting and foods with eye appeal can also make a difference in appetite. Garnishes such as parsley, lemon wedges, olives, cherry tomatoes, or shredded raw vegetables add interest. A small plate makes small portions of food seem more attractive.

Appealing to the sense of smell will improve appetite. Gravies and sauces are aromatic and enhance the taste of food; they also add calories and make swallowing easier.

Desserts are an appealing part of the meal and are a good way to add calories to the diet. Ice creams and puddings are soft and easy to swallow.

It is important for the cancer patient to feel free to follow his or her own preferences in eating and not feel confined to a rigid and unappealing dietary regimen. The most important consideration in the cancer patient's diet is that he or she be educated to be able to choose foods that can be tolerated so that an adequate protein and calorie intake may be maintained, thereby avoiding the all too common problem of progressive malnutrition.

## ACKNOWLEDGMENTS

We wish to thank Mary Ann Stewart for invaluable help in editing this chapter and Virgilia F. Mapa for typing.

## REFERENCES

1. Bury, K. D., Stephens, R. V., Cha, C. J., and Randall, H. T. (1974): Chemically defined diets. *Can. J. Surg.,* 17:124–134.
2. Coubrough, H. (1977). A trial of elemental diets in a surgical ward. *J. Hum. Nutr.,* 31:367–369.
3. DeWys, W. D., and Herbst, S. H. (1977): Oral feeding in the nutritional management of the cancer patient. *Cancer Res.,* 37:2429–2431.
4. Doolittle, M. J. (1979): Stress and cancer: New directions in treatment. In: *A Comprehensive Guide for Cancer Patients and Their Families,* edited by E. H. Rosenbaum, and I. R. Rosenbaum, pp. 3-1–3-13. Bull Publishing Co., Palo Alto, Calif.
5. Drasin, H., Rosenbaum, E. H., Stitt, C. A., and Rosenbaum, I. R. (1979): The challenge of nutritional maintenance in cancer patients. *West. J. Med.,* 130:145–152.
6. Fink, D. H. (1962): *Release from Nervous Tension.* Simon and Schuster, New York.
7. Heymsfield, S. B., Bethel, R. A., and Ansley, J. D., et al. (1979): Enteral hyperalimentation: An alternative to central venous hyperalimentation. *Ann. Int. Med.,* 90:63–71.
8. Raffman, R. (1979): *Using Marijuana in the Reduction of Nausea Associated with Chemotherapy.* Murray Publishing Co., Seattle.
9. Rosenbaum, E. H., and Rosenbaum, I. R. (1979): *A Comprehensive Guide for Cancer Patients and Their Families,* pp. 4-30–4-36, 4-100–4-105. Bull Publishing Co., Palo Alto, Calif.
10. Russell, R. I. (1975): Elemental diets. *Gut.,* 16:68–79.
11. Shils, M. E., Bloch, A. S., and Chernoff, R. (1976): Liquid formulas for oral and tube feeding. *Clin. Bull.,* 6:151–158.
12. Warnold, I., Lundholm, K., and Schersten, I. (1978): Energy balance and body composition in cancer patients. *Cancer Res.,* 38:1801–1807.

*Nutrition and Cancer: Etiology and Treatment,*
edited by G. R. Newell and N. M. Ellison.
Raven Press, New York © 1981.

# Anorexia and Cachexia in Malignant Disease

## Daniel L. Kisner and William D. DeWys

*Division of Cancer Treatment, National Cancer Institute, Bethesda, Maryland 20205*

Malnutrition and wasting are frequently associated with malignant disease and often represent the cancer patient's most debilitating problems. This malignant cachexia is an important factor in cancer morbidity and mortality. It is caused by the combined effects of decreased nutrient intake and accelerated nutrient utilization. The increased utilization results from the superimposition of tumor metabolism upon host metabolism. Anorexia (appetite loss) is the most common cause of decreased nutrient intake, but treatment-related gastrointestinal tract symptoms or anatomical changes may also play a role.

In patients with advanced cancer, malnutrition is almost universal. Nixon et al. (34) recently surveyed the nutritional status of 54 hospitalized cancer patients, using anthropometrics, creatinine–height index, and serum albumin level. Virtually all patients exhibited loss of adipose tissue, visceral protein, or skeletal muscle. The creatinine–height index was less than 80% of standard in 88% of the patients.

The incidence of weight loss in a large series of cancer patients at the time of entry into chemotherapy protocols ranges from 40% for patients with breast cancer, acute myelocytic leukemia, and sarcoma to more than 80% in patients with cancer of the pancreas and stomach (12). About 60% of patients with carcinoma of the lung, colon, or prostate have experienced weight loss prior to entering a phase III chemotherapy protocol (12).

Pretreatment weight loss is associated with a decreased median survival and frequency of response to chemotherapy. The effect of weight loss before beginning chemotherapy on subsequent survival for patients entering 12 protocols of the Eastern Cooperative Oncology Group is shown in Table 1 (11,12). Patients were divided into two groups according to whether or not they had pretreatment weight loss. For nine of the 12 protocols, survival was significantly longer in patients who had not lost any weight, and in many protocols the median survival for the no-weight-loss patients was twice as long as that for patients with weight loss. This effect of weight loss on survival was seen within performance-status and disease-extent groupings (12). The effect of pretreatment weight loss on response to chemotherapy was most clearcut for breast cancer patients. Patients with no weight loss had a 61% response rate (complete plus partial), whereas only 44% of patients with weight loss responded (P < 0.01) (12). Patients

TABLE 1. *Effect of pretreatment weight loss on survival*

| Tumor type | No. of patients | Median survival (weeks) | | p Value |
| --- | --- | --- | --- | --- |
| | | No weight loss | Weight loss | |
| Favorable non-Hodgkin's lymphoma | 290 | * | 138 | <0.0001 |
| Breast | 289 | 70 | 45 | <0.01 |
| Acute nonlymphocytic leukemia | 129 | 8 | 4 | NS** |
| Sarcoma | 89 | 46 | 25 | <0.001 |
| Unfavorable non-Hodgkin's lymphoma | 311 | 107 | 55 | <0.0001 |
| Colon | 307 | 43 | 21 | <0.0001 |
| Prostate | 78 | 46 | 24 | <0.04 |
| Lung, small-cell | 436 | 34 | 27 | <0.02 |
| Lung, non-small-cell | 590 | 20 | 14 | <0.0001 |
| Pancreas | 111 | 14 | 12 | NS |
| Nonmeasurable gastric | 179 | 41 | 27 | <0.05 |
| Measurable gastric | 138 | 18 | 16 | NS |

* Only 20 of 199 have died, so median survival cannot be estimated.
** NS = not significant.

with no weight loss also had a higher response rate for colon (16% versus 8%) and lung cancer (14% versus 9%), but these differences were of borderline statistical significance.

The impact of malnutrition is being assessed as a prognostic factor more routinely in clinical trials. The data indicating malnutrition to be an independent prognostic factor are growing and may soon justify the use of malnutrition as a stratification factor in randomized studies of chemotherapy for some tumor types.

## DECREASED NUTRIENT INTAKE

Reduced calorie intake should be analyzed from the perspective of our current understanding of normal food intake control mechanisms. Davis and Levine (8) have proposed an integrated model for the control of food ingestion, based on two premises. One is that chemoreceptors in the mouth and nose serve a gating function (selecting foods of high nutritive value), as well as an important motivational or excitatory role in driving the central nervous system mechanisms that control the rate of eating. The second premise is that the accumulation of ingested substances in the intestinal tract counteracts the excitatory efforts of gustatory stimulation, resulting in an inhibition of intake. Positive signals from oronasal stimulation and negative signals from gastrointestinal distention are evaluated and integrated in the central nervous system and control food intake. Psychological, metabolic, and hormonal factors also influence eating via this integration center.

Abnormalities of taste or smell may occur in cancer patients (10,13) and may be associated with reduced calorie intake (9). The most frequently reported abnormality is an elevation of the recognition threshold for sweet substances. This would be expected to decrease the stimulus for further eating normally derived from pleasant tastes in food. Less frequent abnormalities include an elevated threshold for salt or sour and a lower threshold for bitter. The latter would provide a negative stimulus to the eating control center. These abnormalities in taste sensation correlated with patient symptoms, extent of disease, and reduced calorie intake, and were reversible with response of the tumor to antitumor therapy (10).

The frequent symptom of a sense of fullness or early satiety by anorectic cancer patients suggests the importance of inhibitory signals from the gastrointestinal tract in limiting their food intake. Several factors might contribute to reduced eating by their effects on visceral sensing systems. Abnormalities in taste could result in decreased digestive secretions (20), which could then lead to delayed digestion and more prolonged stimulation of gastrointestinal volume sensors. Secondly, atrophic changes that occur in the mucosa of the small intestine in cancer patients (1) may delay digestion and assimilation of nutrients, but gross malabsorption does not develop in most cancer patients. Similar atrophic changes occur in other wasting illnesses, so one should not view this enteropathy as specific to malignant disease. Barry (1) concluded that these epithelial changes were the result of weight loss, not a cause of it. However, once such atrophic changes have developed, they may contribute to a perpetuation of weight loss.

A third change in the gastrointestinal tract that may affect visceral sensing is wasting of the muscle wall of the stomach. This process parallels wasting of skeletal muscle in an experimental animal model (DeWys, W. D., unpublished observation). Decreased digestive secretions, atrophic changes in the mucosa, and decreased muscle in the stomach wall could result in delayed digestion and assimilation of food, prolonged stimulation of gastrointestinal volume sensors, and suppression of subsequent eating.

Another factor in appetite control involves the modulation of central nervous system synthesis and subsequent brain levels of the neurotransmitter serotonin (4,29). Serotonin is known to stimulate the satiety center and reduce calorie intake in animals. The amino acid precursor of serotonin is tryptophan. Unbound tryptophan is transported across the blood–brain barrier by a mechanism common to the branched-chain amino acids, leucine, isoleucine, and valine (16,29). A meal high in carbohydrates would result in a rise in plasma insulin levels, leading to lower levels of the branched-chain amino acids as the result of increased peripheral utilization. This would allow successful tryptophan competition for the transport mechanism, increased brain tryptophan levels, and subsequent serotonin synthesis.

Circulating tryptophan is bound to albumin and competes with the fatty acids for albumin binding sites (7). A fatty meal results in displacement of tryptophan, with rising free plasma levels and greater transport into the brain, again promoting serotonin synthesis (16). Krause et al. (23) have reported increased brain serotonin levels in tumor-bearing rats that displayed reduced food intake. This was accompanied by increased levels of free plasma tryptophan, caused by lowered albumin levels and increased plasma fatty acid levels. The reduced calorie intake in this animal model was reversed with intracisternal (but not oral) administration of the serotonin antagonists, methylsergide and cyproheptidine. Those authors postulate a relationship between tryptophan–serotonin metabolism and anorexia in tumor-bearing animals. No reports of related work in humans exist to date. This work raises the fascinating possibility that appetite in cancer patients may be stimulated by administering branched-chain amino acids to depress transport of tryptophan into the central nervous system. Research in this area is ongoing at the present time.

Hormonal changes in cancer patients may influence eating. One example is the insulin resistance reportedly present in cancer patients who are losing weight (21,22,28). The result is glucose intolerance. The prolonged postprandial elevation of blood glucose may then suppress appetite (31).

There are several possible mechanisms by which psychologic factors may influence appetite (18). In a depressed patient, a pleasant taste may generate a less positive stimulus for eating. Stress in a cancer patient may cause release of catecholamines, which could depress eating by effects on hypothalamic centers.

Antineoplastic therapy may also play a role in the reduction of calorie intake. Specific toxic effects, such as mucositis, nausea and vomiting, enteritis, radiation-related mouth "blindness", or short-bowel syndromes secondary to surgical procedures, may be important in some patients. These treatment-related problems will be dealt with elsewhere. In addition, there is evidence that treatment may affect food intake by psychological conditioning. Bernstein (2) has demonstrated that learned aversion to a specific food occurs in pediatric patients when that food is consumed shortly before or after chemotherapy administration. Learned aversions to a variety of foods have been demonstrated in animals treated with radiotherapy (39). This is a histamine-mediated phenomenon and can be blocked in rats with antihistamines (26). This area is being studied further in cancer patients.

Clearly, the reduced nutrient intake seen in cancer patients is only partially understood. Further research directed at basic pathophysiologic considerations is needed so that rational specific therapy for this problem can be developed.

## ACCELERATED NUTRIENT REQUIREMENTS: HOST–TUMOR METABOLISM

The precise extent to which the presence of a malignant tumor increases host nutrient utilization and contributes to weight loss is somewhat controversial, and probably varies from patient to patient. However, there is little doubt that aberrant metabolism plays some role in most patients.

Costa et al. (6) recently reported on a small series of patients with non-small-cell lung carcinoma, with recurrent metastatic disease who were followed with careful dietary intake studies. They demonstrated that patients who lost weight did not have a lower dietary intake than those whose weight remained stable. Barring unexplained malabsorption, it is likely that in some patients accelerated nutrient utilization was the cause of weight loss.

A second study that attempted to put the relative roles of increased calorie demand and decreased calorie intake into quantitative perspective has been reported by Warnold et al. (44) (Table 2). In ten cancer patients, energy expenditure per 24 hours was calculated from oxygen consumption and heart rate data, and energy intake was calculated from records of food intake and standard food composition tables. The results in the cancer patients were compared with similarly obtained data in a series of nine hospitalized controls. The results showed both decreased calorie intake and increased energy expenditure in the cancer patients, as compared with controls (Table 2). Omission of data on two cancer patients receiving parenteral nutrition leads to a mean daily caloric intake of 1,340 kcal for cancer patients and 1,420 kcal for controls. Also instructive are the results with one patient who was studied preoperatively and 20 weeks after surgical removal of a 4.5-kg tumor (Table 3). If this patient is considered as his own control, his initial study showed an intake deficit of 880 kcal, whereas his energy expenditure was excessively by 1,140 kcal. This suggests that decreased calorie intake and increased energy expenditure were nearly equal in importance in his negative calorie balance. However, five of the ten cancer patients had calorie intakes, on initial study or follow-up study, below the range of calorie intakes recorded in the control group, reemphasizing the role of reduced calorie intake in the pathogenesis of weight loss in cancer patients.

These data and a variety of other known metabolic events serve to differentiate the malignant cachexia syndrome from uncomplicated starvation. Reduction of calorie intake in a normal person results in decreased ATP requirement, decreased oxygen consumption, increased mobilization of fatty acids from adipose tissue, and decreased gluconeogenesis from amino acids. Conservation of amino acids is necessary for synthesis of key enzymes for survival. This normal decrease in oxidative metabolism does not occur in cancer patients (15,46,47).

TABLE 2. *Caloric intake and expenditure (kcal/24 hr) in cancer patients and controls* [a]

|                 | Intake | Expenditure |
| --------------- | ------ | ----------- |
| Controls        | 1,470  | 1,420       |
| Cancer patients | 1,340  | 1,980       |

[a] Adapted from Warnold et al., ref. 44.

TABLE 3. *Daily energy intake, expenditure, and calculated balance in a patient before and after removal of a 4.5-kg tumor* [a]

|  | Energy intake kcal/24 hr | Energy expenditure kcal/24 hr | Energy balance kcal/24 hr |
|---|---|---|---|
| Tumor present | 1,390 | 3,330 | −1,940 |
| 20 weeks after tumor removal | 2,270 | 2,190 | +80 |
| Difference | 880 | 1,140 |  |

[a]Data from patient 3 in Warnold et al., ref. 44.

Energy expenditure, basal oxygen consumption, and $CO_2$ production are all inappropriately high for the nutritional status of the cancer patient (46). Cancer patients also have accelerated gluconeogenesis at a slightly faster rate than that of a control group (46). These events will be discussed below in further detail.

By what mechanisms does a malignant tumor increase the utilization of energy and nutrients by its host? Energy requirements within a tumor include the energy required for active transport of nutrients and ions. The maintenance of electrochemical gradients, such as the transport of sodium and potassium in tumor cells, has been estimated to account for 85% of their energy metabolism (25). However, other investigators place this estimate lower (17).

A second category of energy requirement is the energy necessary for tumor growth, which includes the requirement for the substrates that form the components of the new tissue and the extra energy needed for synthetic processes. The energy for synthesis is required primarily for protein deposition. The reported values for energy requirements for growth of normal cells are between 0.7 and 1.85 KJ heat/KJ protein deposition. Thus, the energy cost of 1 g of protein deposition is 4 kcal for substrate plus 3.0 to 7.9 kcal for synthetic processes (32). Each 10 g of tumor protein deposited would require about 70 to 119 kcal of energy. The energy needed to meet the metabolic cost of growth translates into heat production, and heat production by growing tumors is well described (24).

The fuel consumption by a tumor, including active transport and synthesis of both tumor and stromal proteins, may be expected to result in an increased resting metabolism in cancer patients, which has indeed been observed (3,33, 38,42,46,47,50) (Table 4). If we accept +15% as the upper limit of normal basal metabolism (BMR), based on data by Boothby and Sandiford (3), then the frequency of abnormal BMR pooled from several studies (3,35,40,44,48, 49,52) (Table 4) ranges from +35% for patients with carcinomas to +74% for patients with leukemia. In two series the ranges of abnormal values were reported (33,38), and the average degree of elevation was +30% to +35%. The degree of elevation of BMR and the correlation of increased BMR with increased heart rate are similar in patients with leukemia and patients with hyperthyroidism (33).

TABLE 4. *Frequency and range of values for elevated basal metabolism rate (BMR) in cancer patients*

| Tumor type | Frequency of elevated BMR[a] | Range of values | Average BMR |
|---|---|---|---|
| Leukemia | 99/133 | −8 to +91 | +35 |
| Myeloma | — | +14 to +60 | +28 |
| Lymphoma | 2/4 | +11 to +65 | +38 |
| All other malignant diseases | 11/31 | +6 to +57 | +29 |

Data in columns 2 and 3 are overestimates because patients with normal values are excluded from the report of Silver et al. (38).

[a] Based on pooled data of references (3,33,38,42,46,47,50), with numerators being patients with BMR +15% or greater and denominators patients reported.

The cancer patient's metabolism is adjusted in several ways to meet the energy demand of the malignant lesion. Most notably, carbohydrate metabolism is affected. Cancer patients who are losing weight are glucose-intolerant when given an oral or parenteral glucose load (21,30,37,46). This glucose intolerance has been shown to be secondary to a systemic insulin resistance (22,30,32,39) that is not explained by simple starvation. The glucose intolerance in these patients may be the result of decreased peripheral glucose uptake or of increased glucose production. Lundholm et al. (28) have reported reduced glucose uptake in isolated forearms of cancer patients in response to an insulin challenge. In this same study, they demonstrated depressed incorporation of glucose carbon into glycogen and carbon dioxide in isolated skeletal muscle fibers in response to insulin stimulation, as compared to controls. Thus, peripheral insulin resistance (with regard to glucose utilization) resulting in reduced glucose clearance was a factor in these patients. However, accelerated glucose production via gluconeogenesis has also been repeatedly documented in cancer patients (19,32,45) and contributes to glucose intolerance.

Anaerobic utilization of glucose by glycolytic pathways has long been known to be characteristic of the neoplastic cell (15,43). Each mole of glucose completing glycolysis in malignant tissue yields 2 moles of ATP *to the tumor*. Lactic acid produced in this process is transported to the liver and kidney for resynthesis to glucose via gluconeogenesis, requiring expenditure of 6 moles of ATP for each mole of glucose produced, for a net loss of 8 moles of high-energy phosphates to the patient. This cyclic pathway is known as the Cori cycle. Increased Cori cycle activity has been documented in patients with cancer (19,45). In analyzing the quantitative importance of this cycle, Young (51) has estimated from the data of several studies (19,35,45) that less than 10% of the daily total energy expenditure in cancer patients can be accounted for by lactate recycling. However, this does not account for the fact that if the lactate had undergone oxidative metabolism in the liver via the Krebs cycle, it would have yielded 30 moles of ATP for each mole of lactate. The overall importance of the Cori cycle must be regarded as unsettled, but it is of interest that Holroyde et al. (19)

observed the greatest Cori cycle activity in patients with the highest total energy expenditure and this correlated with weight-loss status. The increased or poorly regulated hepatic gluconeogenesis in cancer patients might be caused by a specific end-organ insulin resistance in the liver, similar to that documented in peripheral tissues (28). Seemingly against this hypothesis would be the recent report of Waterhouse et al. (48) demonstrating normal suppression of gluconeogenic conversion of labeled alanine to glucose in cancer patients in response to a glucose infusion. Unfortunately, conversion of lactate to glucose was not also measured, leaving open the possibility that gluconeogenesis may simply have continued unimpeded, with a shift to lactate as the predominant substrate.

Another possible consequence of hepatic insulin resistance might be depressed glycogen synthesis or increased degradation, similar to that seen in peripheral tissues (28). Depressed glycogen stores might make the cancer patient intolerant of intermittent fasting, with a resultant increased utilization of amino acids and fatty acids for energy production.

Lipid metabolism is also somewhat aberrant in patients with malignant disease. Waterhouse and Kemperman (49) have demonstrated a less-than-expected suppression of radiolabeled free fatty acid oxidation after glucose loading in patients with advanced cancer. Oxidized fatty acids have been shown to stimulate hepatic gluconeogenesis (36). One mechanism involved in this process is the resulting increased levels of acetyl-CoA and NADH, which inhibit pyruvate dehydrogenase, thereby blocking pyruvate oxidation and making more pyruvate available for resynthesis to glucose (36). Thus, poorly regulated fatty acid metabolism could play some role in the accelerated gluconeogenesis seen in cancer patients.

There is no solid evidence that cancer patients have accelerated lipolysis. Fasting free fatty acid levels are usually normal (19,21,37), and fall appropriately with glucose administration and rising insulin levels (28,37). In an isolated forearm study, cancer patients and controls had similar levels of free fatty acids, acetoacetate, and glycerol in response to an insulin challenge (28). Fatty acid oxidation in isolated skeletal muscle is also similar for cancer patients and normal subjects (28). It is difficult to know whether poorly regulated fatty acid oxidation is important in the fat wasting so commonly seen in cancer patients. More likely, fat mobilization occurs largely during fasting, although at accelerated rates because of greater overall energy expenditure in cancer patients.

Protein metabolism is also altered in cancer patients. Forced-feeding studies in cancer patients reveal increased calorie and nitrogen requirements to achieve nitrogen balance (46). Synthesis of albumin is less than normal (40). The studies of Toporek (41) suggest that a factor in the blood of the tumor-bearing host may suppress albumin synthesis. Diminished concentrations of many enzymes, particularly in liver, suggest less than optimal synthesis of protein in general. Some or all of this decrease in protein synthesis may be the result of protein or caloric deficiency.

An apparent exception to decreased protein synthesis is the preservation of immunoglobin production. Serum immunoglobin levels in patients with solid tumors are usually normal or elevated (46).

In contrast to the decreased protein synthesis in the host is the continued protein synthesis in the tumor at the expense of host nitrogen balance, the so-called "nitrogen trap" concept (15). Muscle catabolism is one source for this body nitrogen depletion. Ekman et al. (14) have recently reported increased peripheral muscle activities of the catabolic enzymes cathepsin-D and $\beta$-glucuronidase in skeletal muscles of tumor-bearing animals, compared to pair-fed controls. This indicates that these changes are not caused only by reduced caloric intake, but also by the presence of a malignant lesion.

Increased utilization of amino acids for conversion to glucose has been demonstrated in cancer patients (48), but appears to be normally suppressed by glucose administration. Lundholm et al. (27,28) have examined muscle metabolism in muscle biopsies from cancer patients. Protein synthesis was reduced and protein breakdown increased in cancer patients, as compared with metabolically healthy controls (27,28). Protein synthesis in muscle from cancer patients could be increased by the addition to the medium of high levels of amino acids or insulin. This suggests that, in the cancer patient, there is a reduction in the efficiency of amino acid utilization for muscle protein synthesis, but that this is overcome by raising the supply of amino acids or insulin. The predominance of degradation over synthesis may explain the muscle loss that is a prominent part of the weight loss of the cancer patient, and may contribute to the decreasing activity level of the advanced cancer patient.

## CONCLUSIONS

We have attempted to address metabolic disturbances present in cancer patients caused by reduced nutrient intake and altered host metabolism induced by the malignant lesion. In all likelihood, these two phenomena rarely exist in isolation in a single patient. Rather, the cancer patient usually suffers reduced intake and is unable to adapt with the usual mechanisms to preserve lean tissue mass and reduce gluconeogenesis (5).

Future research efforts should be aimed at further delineating host–tumor metabolic relationships, with the development of specific forms of biochemical or dietary intervention as the ultimate goal.

## REFERENCES

1. Barry, R. E. (1974): Malignancy, weight loss and the small intestinal mucosa. *Gut,* 15:562–570.
2. Bernstein, I. L. (1978): Learned taste aversions in children receiving chemotherapy. *Science,* 200:1302–1303.
3. Boothby, V. M., and Sandiford, I. (1972): Summary of the basal metabolism data on 8,614 subjects with especial reference to the normal standards for the estimation of the basal metabolic rate. *J. Biol. Chem.,* 54:783–803.

4. Breisch, S., Zemlan, F., and Hoebel, B. (1976): Hyperphagia and obesity following seratonin depletion by intraventricular p-chlorophenylalanine. *Science,* 192:382–385.
5. Brennan, M. (1977): Uncomplicated starvation versus cancer cachexia. *Cancer Res.,* 37:2359–2364.
6. Costa, G., Vincent, R., Aragon, M., Tracy, P., and Homan, P. (1979): Weight loss and cachexia in lung cancer. *Proc. Am. Soc. Clin. Oncol.,* 20:387.
7. Curzon, G., Friedel, J., and Knott, P. J. (1973): The effect of fatty acids on the binding of tryptophan to plasma protein. *Nature,* 242:198–200.
8. Davis, J. D., and Levine, M. W. (1977): A model for the control of ingestion. *Psychol. Rev.,* 84:379–412.
9. DeWys, W. D. (1977): Taste and feeding behavior in patients with cancer. In: *Nutrition in Cancer, Vol. 5, Current Concepts in Nutrition,* edited by M. Winick, pp. 131–136. John Wiley & Sons, New York.
10. DeWys, W. D. (1978): Changes in taste sensation and feeding behavior in cancer patients: A review. *J. Hum. Nutr.,* 32:447–453.
11. DeWys, W. D., and Begg, C. (1978): Comparison of adriamycin and 5-fluorouracil in advanced prostatic cancer. *Proc. Am. Soc. Clin. Oncol.,* 19:331.
12. DeWys, W. D., Begg, C. B., Lavin, P., *et al.* (1980): Prognostic effects of weight loss prior to chemotherapy in cancer patients. *Am. J. Med. (in press).*
13. DeWys, W. D., and Walters, K. (1975): Abnormalities of taste sensation in cancer patients. *Cancer,* 36:1888–1896.
14. Ekman, L., Karlberg, I., Edstrom, S., Lundholm, K., and Schersten, T. (1979): Different mechanisms behind increased lysosomal enzyme activities in insufficient nutrition and cancer cachexia. Paper presented at the First European Congress on Parenteral and Enteral Nutrition, September, 1979.
15. Fenniger, L. D., and Mider, G. B. (1954): Energy and nitrogen metabolism in cancer. *Adv. Cancer Res.,* 2:229.
16. Fernstrom, J., and Wurtman, R. (1971): Brain serotonin content: Physiological dependence on plasma tryptophan levels. *Science,* 173:147–151.
17. Himms-Hagen, J. (1976): Cellular thermogenesis. *Annu. Rev. Physiol.,* 38:315.
18. Holland, J. C. B. (1977): Anorexia and cancer: Psychological aspects. *Cancer,* 27:363–367.
19. Holroyde, C. P., Gabuzda, T. G., Putnam, R. C., Paul, P., and Reichard, G. A. (1975): Altered glucose metabolism in metastatic carcinoma. *Cancer Res.,* 35:3710.
20. Kare, M. R. (1969): Digestive function of taste stimuli. In: *Olfaction and Taste,* edited by C. Pfaffman, pp. 586–592. Rockefeller University Press, New York.
21. Kisner, D., Haller, D., Blecher, M., Hamosh, M., Peterson, B., and Schein, P. (1980): Insulin resistance in malignant cachexia. *Cancer Treatment Reports (in press).*
22. Kisner, D., Hamosh, M., Blecher, M., Haller, D., Jacobs, E., Peterson, B., and Schein, P. (1978): Malignant cachexia: Insulin resistance and insulin receptors. *Proc. Am. Assoc. Cancer Res.,* 19:199.
23. Krause, R., James, H., Humphrey, C., Greep, J., and Fischer, J. (1979): Cancer anorexia: A plasma amino acid-mediated phenomenon. Paper presented at the First European Congress on Parenteral and Enteral Nutrition, September, 1979.
24. Lawson, R. N., and Chughtai, M. S. (1963): Breast cancer and body temperature. *Can. Med. Assoc. J.,* 88:68–70.
25. Levinson, C., and Hemping, H. G. (1967): The role of ion transport in the regulation of respiration in the Ehrlich mouse ascites-tumor cell. *Biochim. Biophys. Acta,* 135:306.
26. Levy, C. J., Carroll, M. E., Smith, J. C., and Hofer, K. G. (1974): Antihistamines block radiation-induced taste aversion. *Science,* 168:1044–1045.
27. Lundholm, K., Bylund, A. C., Holm, J., and Schersten, T. (1976): Skeletal muscle metabolism in patients with malignant tumor. *Eur. J. Cancer,* 12:465–473.
28. Lundholm, K., Holm, G., and Schersten, T. (1978): Insulin resistance in patients with cancer. *Cancer Res.,* 33:4665–4670.
29. Madras, B. K., Cohen, E. L., and Messing, R. (1974): Relevance of free tryptophan in serum to tissue tryptophan concentrations. *Metabolism,* 23:1107–1116.
30. Marks, P., and Bishop, J. (1957): The glucose metabolism of patients with malignant disease and of normal subjects as studied by means of an intravenous glucose tolerance test. *J. Clin. Invest.,* 36:254.

31. Mayer, J. (1955): Regulation of energy intake and the body weight: The glucostatic theory and the lipostatic hypothesis. *Ann. NY Acad. Sci.,* 63:15–43.
32. Millward, D. J., and Garlick, P. J. (1976): The energy cost of growth. *Proc. Nutr. Soc.,* 35:339–349.
33. Minot, G. R., and Means, J. H. (1924): The metabolism–pulse ratio in exophthalmic goiter and leukemia. *Arch. Intern. Med.,* 33:576–580.
34. Nixon, D., Heymsfield, S., Cohen, A., Jutner, M., Ansley, J., Lawson, D., and Rudman, D. (1980): Protein–calorie undernutrition in hospitalized cancer patients. *Am. J. Med. (in press).*
35. Reichard, G. A., Jr., Moury, N. F., Hochella, N. J., Putnam, R. C., and Weinhouse, S. (1964): Metabolism of neoplastic tissue XVII blood glucose replacement rates in human cancer patients. *Cancer Res.,* 24:71.
36. Ruderman, E., Toews, C., and Shafrin, E., (1969): Role of free fatty acids in glucose homeostasis. *Arch. Intern. Med.,* 123:299.
37. Schein, P., Kisner, D., Haller, D., Blecher, M., and Hamosh, M., (1979): Cachexia of malignancy: Potential role of insulin in nutritional management. *Cancer,* 43:2070.
38. Silver, S., Poroto, P., and Crohn, E. B. (1950): Hypermetabolic states without hyperthyroidism (nonthyrogenous hypermetabolism). *Arch. Intern. Med.,* 85:479–482.
39. Smith, J. C. (1971): Radiation: Its detection and its effects on taste preferences. *Prog. Physiol. Psychol.,* 4:53–118.
40. Steinfield, J. L. (1960): $I^{131}$-albumin degradation in patients with neoplastic disease. *Cancer,* 13:974–984.
41. Toporek, M. (1971): Effect of albumin fraction from blood of tumor-bearing rats on serum protein production by isolated perfused normal rat livers. *Cancer Res.,* 31:1962–1967.
42. Torepka, A. R., and Waterhouse, C. (1956): Metabolic observations during forced feeding of patients with cancer. *Am. J. Med.,* 20:225–238.
43. Warburg, O. (1930): *Metabolism of Tumors.* Constable & Co., Ltd., London.
44. Warnold, I., Lundholm, K., and Schersten, T. (1978): Energy balance and body composition in cancer patients. *Cancer Res.,* 38:1801–1807.
45. Waterhouse, C. (1974): Lactate metabolism in patients with cancer. *Cancer,* 33:66.
46. Waterhouse, C. (1974): How tumors affect host metabolism. *Ann. NY Acad. Sci.,* 230:86–93.
47. Waterhouse, C. L., Fenninger, L. D., and Keutmann, E. H. (1951): Nitrogen exchange and caloric expenditure in patients with malignant neoplasm. *Cancer,* 4:500–514.
48. Waterhouse, C., Jeanpretre, N., and Keilson, J. (1979): Gluconeogenesis from alanine in patients with progressive malignancy. *Cancer Res.,* 39:1969–1972.
49. Waterhouse, C., and Kemperman, J. (1971): Carbohydrate metabolism in subjects with cancer. *Cancer Res.,* 31:1273–1278.
50. Watkin, D. M. (1961): Nitrogen balance as affected by neoplastic disease and its therapy. *Am. J. Clin. Nutr.,* 9:446–460.
51. Young, V. R. (1977): Energy metabolism and requirements in the cancer patient. *Cancer Res.,* 37:2336.

*Nutrition and Cancer: Etiology and Treatment,*
edited by G. R. Newell and N. M. Ellison.
Raven Press, New York © 1981.

# Enteral Hyperalimentation of the Cancer Patient

## *William P. Steffee and **Susanna H. Krey

*Boston University School of Medicine, University Hospital, Boston, Massachusetts 02118;
**Clinical Nutrition Unit, University Hospital, Boston, Massachusetts 02118

The ability to intervene nutritionally in nearly every patient in need has provided the therapist with the tools to prevent wastage of lean body mass in the host while mounting intensive efforts against the tumor. This is not to imply that all cancer patients should receive optimal nutritional support, since if a terminal state exists, malnutrition is not an unreasonable way to die. Unfortunately, in many instances, the terminal state itself *is* malnutrition, often when efforts directed towards the tumor have been almost totally successful.

Attempts to overcome anorexia by encouraging the patient to consume adequate amounts of nutrients by the usual oral route can become a burden that many seriously ill patients cannot, and should not, tolerate. The recent development of enteral hyperalimentation as a means of nutritional intervention has been dramatic. Solutions are available that allow the therapist to support nearly every patient in need. These range from palatable supplements to special formulations designed to manipulate metabolism at a biochemical level. The development of small, comfortable nasogastric and nasojejunal tubes provides an acceptable alternative to death by starvation. Enteral hyperalimentation should be a therapeutic modality of every physician, whether or not he deals with cancer patients.

## HISTORICAL PERSPECTIVE

Many physicians regard the products utilized in enteral hyperalimentation as a blending of common foodstuffs that has undoubtedly evolved from the kitchens of home economists. Such assumptions cannot be further from the truth. In fact, perhaps the most useful formulas, those of an elemental nature, are spinoffs of the space program. Important to early space travelers were problems associated with the disposal of human waste products during confinement to small spacecraft. Urine presented few difficulties, but such was not the case for fecal material. A potential solution arose from two sources: emerging studies that demonstrated nearly complete absorption of nutrients from the first portion of the jejunum, and ongoing investigations conducted by the National Cancer Institute concerning the effect of synthetic amino acid diets on cell growth.

Physiological considerations of nutrient digestion and absorption must be understood if clinicians are to make appropriate use of modern formulations. Although significant insight was gained before 1950, an accurate assessment of the rapidity of digestion and absorption could not be made until the development of modern multilumen tubes. Even with the requirement for pancreatic exocrine activities, only 50 to 100 cm of small bowel were found necessary for complete digestion and absorption (2). If the need for digestion were to be eliminated and only "elemental" products infused, absorption of nutrients, particularly single amino acids, would begin in the duodenum and proceed to completion in the first few centimeters of jejunum. In fact, the only organ required under such artificial circumstances is a very short segment of jejunum.

Ongoing studies of peptide transport, recently reviewed by Mathews and Adibi (10), are accumulating evidence to suggest alternative means of amino acid absorption. Although these studies are still incomplete from a clinical perspective, investigations concerning separate transport mechanisms for di- and tripeptides show promise that they, too, may provide complete support for endogenous protein synthesis by use of only a small segment of jejunum.

Those involved with solving the early astronaut's dilemma reached similar conclusions. An obvious way to deal with bowel movements was to eliminate the need for them. The goal was to deliver to the jejunum a nutrient solution that would not require digestion and would be completely absorbed high in the gastrointestinal tract. If nothing reached the colon, there would be no need for bowel movements. The formulation would be "elemental"; single amino acids and sugars, essential micronutrients, and absolutely no residue. One of the most difficult problems concerned the requirement for amino acids that were not readily available in the crystalline form. However, Greenstein and colleagues (8) from the National Cancer Institute had considerable experience and interest in the nutritive qualities of these amino acids and agreed to work with NASA contractors. The result was a concentrated solution ($\pm$ 2200 mOsm/liter), a cubic foot of which was calculated to nourish an astronaut for nearly a month (16).

Unfortunately, the lessons learned thus far about the ability of the gut to handle a hyperosmolar load were not yet fully understood. Initial administration of the solution to volunteers resulted in explosive diarrhea and vomiting, symptoms also experienced by the astronauts. These effects negated further efforts directed towards space travel; however, the clinical applications of a nutrient solution requiring absolutely no digestion and only a few inches of jejunum for absorption were recognized. That is, one need not have a stomach, pancreatic exocrine function, bile acids, ileum, colon, etc. Feedings could be administered above and below fistulae, inflamed bowel, obstructed pancreatic and bile ducts, and other pathologic states. One of the major applications would be in cases of short-bowel syndrome, from whatever cause. In fact, one of the early studies was entitled, "Use of the Space Diet in the management of a patient with extreme short bowel syndrome," by Thompson and colleagues (15). Solutions currently available to the physician include not only this first formulation (Vivonex), but also a rapidly growing variety of other products that provide the tools required to treat nearly all patients in need.

## FORMULATION OF ENTERAL PRODUCTS: NUTRIENT SOURCES

When considering any nutritional product for enteral hyperalimentation, it is important to understand the composition or formulation of the product in order to use it optimally and appropriately. For proper application, all such products should be evaluated for their protein sources, carbohydrate and fat content, and mineral and vitamin fortification.

### Protein Sources

Protein or amino acid sources are usually in one of five forms: (a) intact protein in the form of pureed beef, fish concentrate, eggs, or milk; (b) protein isolates from milk (casein), soybeans, or egg white; (c) hydrolyzed protein (casein) with added amino acids to make a complete amino acid mix; (d) di- and tripeptides with additional crystalline amino acids; and (e) purified free crystalline amino acids.

It is important to know the chemical form of the protein to determine how much physiological digestion will be necessary for optimal absorption, particularly when dealing with an impaired gut. As indicated above, in the healthy intestine, protein digestion occurs in the first 50 to 100 cm of the jejunum, and hence a wide variety of formulas can be used. However, as a general rule, the more dysfunctional the gut, the more defined a formula should be. For example, if the gut has undergone shortening from any cause, disuse atrophy, or exposure to chemotherapy or extensive radiation, the more elemental formula may be better absorbed, utilized, and tolerated.

If whole proteins are used, it is important to know the source of the protein to evaluate its protein quality, as this determines the value of the protein for tissue repair, growth, and maintenance. Hence, the biological value and digestibility of the protein of the formula becomes an important consideration. There is a wide range of biological values for protein sources; however, among animal protein sources eggs have the highest biological value, followed by milk protein, fish, and meat. Plant proteins can provide an adequate supply of essential amino acids, but only if ingested in amounts greater than those of animal proteins, and in combinations that include all essential amino acids.

Digestibility of proteins follows a trend similar to the biological value of proteins. Although animal proteins have both an adequate supply of essential amino acids and high digestibility, individual plant proteins tend to be low in one or more essential amino acids and have a lower digestibility. Most crystalline amino acid formulas requiring absolutely no digestion are patterned after high biologic value proteins, most often egg albumin.

## Carbohydrate Sources

The highest percentage of calories typically comes from carbohydrates. The form of the carbohydrate is important, as it is the largest contributing factor to solution osmolarity. Earlier formulations, particularly those of an elemental nature, used glucose or sucrose as the primary fuel substrate. Their use led to osmolarities often exceeding 1200 mOsm/liter, which resulted in diarrhea. In more recent formulas, starches, dextrins, and glucose oligosaccharides have been substituted as the carbohydrate source, in an effort to decrease the osmolar load. Glucose oligosaccharides are soluble polymers of glucose, containing five or more glucose molecules, that can be hydrolyzed by the enzymes in the intestinal mucosa without the need for pancreatic amylase. Since oligosaccharides are longer chain carbohydrates, they are not sweet, and hence can be easily mixed with beverages and foods containing glucose and sucrose without drastically increasing sweetness, should the oral route be chosen.

## Fat Sources

Fat content and source vary from product to product. Fat may contribute from less than 1% to as much as 47% of total calories in currently available commercial formulas, and has little effect on product osmolarity. Fat is found primarily as long-chain fats—corn, soy, or safflower oils. Some products contain medium-chain triglycerides (MCT), usually in combination with other long-chain fats. Since there are ample data (13) indicating that MCT is more easily absorbed than long-chain fats, products containing MCT may be useful when significant maldigestion or malabsorption is present.

## Vitamin and Mineral Content

With few exceptions, almost all nutritional formulas provide complete nutrition. In most cases, 2,000 calories of the product will either meet or exceed the National Research Council Recommended Dietary Allowance (5). Trace elements have also been supplemented; however, since the micronutrient requirements of the stressed patient generally are unknown, the clinician must be alert to the development of deficiency states. This is particularly true when the more chemically defined formulas are utilized.

## TYPES OF FORMULAS

There are essentially seven categories of enteral products. These categories are an arbitrary classification by the authors, based upon product composition, and include: general, milk-base, lactose-free, chemically defined, elemental, special formulations, and caloric additives or supplements (Table 1).

## General Formulas

These formulas are either home (kitchen) blenderized tube feedings or commercially prepared blenderized formulas. They are nutritionally complete, contain intact protein and milk, and have moderate to high residue. A blenderized diet is appropriate for the patient with an anatomically intact and functionally sound intestinal tract. The advantages of these feedings are that they are readily available, include trace elements and micronutrients normally found in intact food, and restore normal bowel movements, at a minimal cost. Disadvantages include the requirement for bowel movements, a high viscosity making it difficult for them to flow through small feeding tubes, and the necessity for complete digestive capabilities. Table 2 gives a diet prescription for a home-prepared blenderized diet, as this formula is less expensive than the commercial formula (7).

## Milk-base Formulas

There is a wide variety of products that rely on milk for the base and therefore contain lactose. All are nutritionally complete products, containing a generous amount of protein. They are most useful as an oral nutritional supplement for patients who, for many reasons, have difficulty in meeting their full nutritional requirements through normal oral intake. There are many advantages in using these relatively inexpensive products, including an excellent taste and strong acceptance by patients for oral supplemental use. The chief disadvantage is that they contain lactose. Frequently, the critically ill patient begins to develop dysfunction caused by lactase deficiency secondary to brush-border atrophy and/or damage. In many cases, the classic symptoms of lactose intolerance—diarrhea, abdominal bloating, and cramping—are often confused with more serious or unresolved pathologic states. Failure to recognize the true nature of the complaints will result in unnecessary delay in the implementation of the metabolic support process.

## Lactose-free Products

Products in this category are most often the "ideal" tube-feeding formulas; they are nutritionally complete products of low cost, create few osmolar problems, are lactose-free, and offer a broad range of choices relative to protein source, fat, and carbohydrate content. Most of these products have been designed specifically for tube feedings; however, many with added flavors are suitable for oral use. Products such as Ensure Plus and Magnacal, which are higher in osmolarity than other formulas in this group, are more calorically dense (1.5 and 2.0 cal/cc, respectively) and hence can provide more nutrition in less fluid volume.

TABLE 1. *Enteral hyperalimentation chart*

| | General | | | Milk-base | | |
|---|---|---|---|---|---|---|
| | Formula 2® | Compleat-B® | Vitaneed® | Meritene® | Carnation Instant Breakfast® | Nutri 1000® |
| Calories/cc | 1 | 1 | 1 | 1 | 1 | 1 |
| Carbohydrate source | Lactose sucrose | Maltodextrin lactose, sucrose | Corn syrup solids maltodextrins | Lactose, corn syrup, sucrose | Sucrose, corn syrup, lactose | Sucrose, lactose corn syrup solids |
| Protein source | Wheat, beef, egg, milk | Beef, skim milk, vegetable | Beef, calcium, caseinate | Skim milk | Milk, sodium caseinate, soy protein isolate | Skim milk |
| Fat source | Egg yolk, corn oil, beef fat | corn oil, beef fat | Soy oil soy lecithin | corn oil | whole milk | Corn oil |
| Protein gram/liter | 38 | 40 | 35 | 60 | 58 | 40 |
| Fat gram/liter | 40 | 40 | 40 | 33 | 31 | 55 |
| Carbohydrate gram/liter | 123 | 120 | 130 | 115 | 135 | 101 |
| mOsm/kg | 435–510 | 390 | 400 | 550 | — | 500 |
| Na/K mEq/liter | 26/45 | 68/33 | 24/32 | 40/42 | 41/70 | 23/39 |
| Residue | High | High | High | Med. | Med. | Med. |
| Vitamin content | yes | yes | yes | yes | yes | yes |
| Cost/1000 Kcal[b] | B | C | B | B | A | A |
| Producer | Cutter | Doyle | Organon | Doyle | Carnation | Cutter |
| Flavors[c] | Orange | Natural flavor | Natural flavor | Varied | Varied | Chocolate, vanilla |
| Form | Ready to use | Ready to use | Ready to use | Ready to use | Powder | Ready to use |
| Uses/features | Blenderized tube feeding requires digestion & absorption | Blenderized tube feeding, requires digestion & absorption | Blenderized tube feeding requires digestion & absorption, low Na, lactose free | High protein, supplemental, tube feeding, requires digestion & absorption | Supplemental, easily available, requires digestion & absorption | Supplemental, tube feeding, requires digestion & absorption |

a) Unflavored
b) Key: A = <$2.00; B = $2.00–4.00; C = $4.01–6.00; D = $6.01–8.00; E = $8.01–10.00; F = >$10.00. Price is dependent on many factors: method of purchase, region, etc. Prices within each defined group are competitive.
c) Flavors may change values
© 1980, Clinical Nutrition Unit, University Hospital, Boston, Mass. Comprehensive listing is not intended in this chart.

TABLE 1. Continued

Lactose-free

| | Sustacal® | Citrotein® | Nutri 1000 LF® | Isocal® | Osmolite® | Renu® | Ensure® | Ensure Plus® | Magnacal™ |
|---|---|---|---|---|---|---|---|---|---|
| Calories/cc | 1 | .66 | 1 | 1 | 1 | 1 | 1 | 1.5 | 2 |
| Carbohydrate source | Sucrose, corn syrup | Sucrose, Maltodextrin | Sucrose corn syrup | Glucose oligosaccharides | Corn syrup | Corn syrup solids Maltodextrins | Corn syrup sucrose | Corn syrup sucrose | Corn syrup solids maltodextrins, sucrose |
| Protein source | Calcium & sodium caseinates & soy protein isolates | Egg albumin | Calcium & sodium caseinates soy protein isolates | Calcium & sodium caseinate soy protein isolate | Calcium & sodium caseinate, soy protein isolate | Calcium caseinate, soy protein isolate | Sodium & calcium caseinate, soy protein isolate | Sodium & calcium caseinate, soy protein isolate | Calcium caseinate |
| Fat source | Partially hydrogenated soy oil | Partially hydrogenated soybean oil | Corn oil | Soy oil MCT oil | MCT oil, corn oil, soy oil | Soy oil soy lecithin | Corn oil | Corn oil | Soy oil soy lecithin |
| Protein gram/liter | 60 | 43 | 40 | 34 | 35 | 33 | 37 | 55 | 70 |
| Fat gram/liter | 23 | 2 | 55 | 44 | 34 | 40 | 37 | 53 | 80 |
| Carbohydrate gram/liter | 138 | 129 | 101 | 130 | 138 | 130 | 145 | 197 | 250 |
| m Osm/kg | 625[a] | 496 | 380 | 300 | 300 | 330 | 450[a] | 600[a] | 520 |
| Na/K mEq/liter | 39/53 | 31/19 | 23/39 | 22/33 | 22/23 | 22/32 | 32/32 | 46/48 | 43/32 |
| Residue | Low | Low | Low | Low | Low | Low | Low | Low | Low |
| Vitamin content | yes | yes | yes | yes | yes | yes | yes | yes | yes |
| Cost/1000 Kcal[b] | B | C | A | B | B | A | A | B | A |
| Producer | Mead Johnson | Doyle | Cutter | Mead Johnson | Ross | Organon | Ross | Ross | Organon |
| Flavors[c] | Varied | Orange, grape | Chocolate, vanilla | Unflavored | Unflavored | Vanilla | Varied | Varied | Vanilla |
| Form | Ready to use | Powder | Ready to use | Ready to use | Ready to use | Ready to use | Ready to use | Ready to use | Ready to use |
| Uses/features | High protein, supplemental, tube feeding, requires digestion & absorption | Supplemental, lactose, gluten, cholesterol free, clear liquid supplement | Supplemental, tube feeding, lactose free, low Na, requires digestion & absorption | Tube feeding, requires digestion & absorption, low Na, lactose free | Supplemental, tube feeding lactose free, low Na, requires digestion & absorption | Supplemental, tube feeding, requires digestion & absorption, low Na, lactose free | Supplemental, tube feeding, lactose free, requires digestion & absorption | Supplemental, tube feeding, lactose free, requires digestion & absorption | Supplemental, tube feeding, lactose free, requires digestion & absorption, high calorie, high protein |

TABLE 1. *Continued*

| | Chemically defined formulas | | | | | Elemental | | |
|---|---|---|---|---|---|---|---|---|
| | Precision isotonic® | Precision LR® | Precision HN® | Flexical® | Vital® | Vivonex® | Vivonex HN® | Vipep™ |
| Calories/cc | 1 | 1 | 1 | 1 | 1 | 1 | 1 | 1 |
| Carbohydrate source | Glucose oligosaccharides sucrose | Maltodextrin sucrose | Maltodextrin sucrose | Corn syrup, modified tapioca starch | Glucose oligo- + poly saccharides | Glucose oligosaccharides | Glucose oligosaccharides | Corn syrup, sucrose corn starch |
| Protein source | Egg albumin | Egg albumin | Egg albumin | Casein hydrolysate crystalline amino acids | Whey soy + meat protein hydrolysate, free essential amino acids | L-Amino acids | L-Amino acids | Peptides of 2–4 amino acid units, 4–14 amino acid units, free amino acids |
| Fat source | Soybean oil | Soy oil | Soy oil | Soy oil MCT oil | Sunflower oil | Safflower oil | Safflower oil | MCT oil, corn oil |
| Protein gram/liter | 30 | 26 | 44 | 23 | 42 | 21 | 42 | 25 |
| Fat gram/liter | 31 | 0.8 | 0.5 | 34 | 10 | 1 | 1 | 25 |
| Carbohydrate gram/liter | 150 | 249 | 218 | 152 | 185 | 226 | 210 | 176 |
| mOsm/kg | 300 | 525 | 557[a] | 550[a] | 450 | 550[a] | 844[a] | 520 |
| Na/K mEq/liter | 35/26 | 30/22 | 43/23 | 15/32 | 17/30 | 37/30 | 34/18 | 33/22 |
| Residue | Low | Low | Low | Low | Low | Low | Low | Low |
| Vitamin content | yes | yes | yes | yes | yes | yes | yes | yes |
| Cost/1000 Kcal[b] | C | B | D | C | C | B | E | B |
| Producer | Doyle | Doyle | Doyle | Mead Johnson | Ross | Eaton | Eaton | Cutter |
| Flavors[c] | Vanilla, orange | Varied | Citrus | Varied | Varied | Varied | Varied | Varied |
| Form | Powder | Powder | Powder | Powder | Powder | Powder | Powder | Powder |
| Uses/features | Supplemental, tube feeding, lactose free, isotonic, absorbed in upper gut | Supplemental, tube feeding, lactose free, absorbed in upper gut | Supplemental, tube feeding, lactose free, absorbed in upper gut, high protein | Supplemental, tube feeding, lactose free, absorbed in upper gut | Supplemental, tube feeding, absorbed in upper gut, Low Na | Supplemental, tube feeding, lactose free, no pancreatic stimulus, absorbed in upper gut | Supplemental, tube feeding, lactose free, absorbed in upper gut, high protein | Supplemental, tube feeding, uses free amino acid peptide carrier system, lactose free, absorbed in upper gut |

TABLE 1. *Continued*

| | Special formulations | | | | Caloric additives | | |
|---|---|---|---|---|---|---|---|
| | Amin-Acid® | Hepatic-Aid™ | Microlipid® | Controlyte® | Polycose® | Sumacal® | Sumacal Plus® |
| Calories/cc | 1.9 | 1.6 | 4.5 | 5 cal/gm 2 cal/cc | 4 cal/gm 2 cal/cc | 2 | 2.5 |
| Carbohydrate source | Maltodextrose, sucrose | Maltodextrins, sucrose | — | Corn starch | Hydrolysis of corn starch | Glucose syrup solids Maltodextrins | Maltodextrins glucose syrup solids |
| Protein source | Crystalline essential amino acids | Branch chain and aromatic amino acids | | | | | |
| Fat source | Partially hydrogenated soybean oil | Soybean oil, lecithin mono + diglycerides | Safflower oil Soy lecithin | Vegetable oil | | | |
| Protein gram/liter | 19 | 43 | — | trace | — | — | — |
| Fat gram/liter | 66 | 36 | 500 | 96 | — | — | — |
| Carbohydrate gram/liter | 330 | 287 | — | 286 | 500 | 500 | 625 |
| m Osm/kg | 900[a] | 900 | 32 | 5390[a] | 850 | 680 | 890 |
| Na/K mEq/Liter | <8/<8 | — | —/— | 2.6/0.4 | 27 | 9/6 | 9/8 |
| Residue | Low | Low | Low | Low | Low | Low | Low |
| Vitamin content | no | no | no | no | no | no | no |
| Cost/1000 Kcal[b] | E | F | A | A | A | B | A |
| Producer | McGaw | McGaw | Organon | Doyle | Ross | Organon | Organon |
| Flavors[c] | Varied | Varied | Unflavored | Unflavored | Unflavored | Cherry, lemon & lime | Unflavored |
| Form | Powder | Powder | Ready to use | Powder | Powder / Liquid | Ready to use | Ready to use |
| Uses/features | Supplemental, tube feeding, low electrolytes, essential amino acids, lactose free, indicated for renal disease | Supplemental, tube feeding, high branch chain amino acid formula, low electrolytes, lactose free, indicated for liver disease | Supplemental, pure fat emulsion, low osmolarity, low electrolytes, lactose free | Supplemental, low electrolytes, low protein, lactose free | Supplemental, lactose free | Supplemental, lactose free | Supplemental, lactose free |

TABLE 2. *Formulation of blenderized diet for home use*[a]

| Ingredients | Amount |
|---|---|
| Farina, cooked enriched | 1 cup |
| Eggs, hard-cooked | 3 |
| Skim milk powder | 4 tablespoons |
| Ground lean beef, cooked (preferably ground round) | 7 oz = ½ cup |
| Carrots, canned | ½ cup |
| Wax beans, canned | ½ cup |
| Corn oil | ¼ cup |
| Orange juice | 1½ cup |
| KARO syrup, dark | ½ cup |
| Salt | ½ teaspoon |
| Water and juice from canned vegetables | 2 cups |
| Vitamin supplement | 1 |

Total volume = 2,000 cc
Carbohydrate: 122 g/liter
Protein: 47 g/liter
Fat: 725 g/liter
Calories/cc: 1
Na: 44 mEq/liter
K: 31 mEq/liter

[a] Adapted from Goodhardt and Shils, ref. 7.

There are very few specific disadvantages of these products; however, caution must be maintained when using these more calorically dense formulas. Their high osmolarity, without additional free water, may lead to the development of a hyperosmolar syndrome.

## Chemically Defined Formulas

Chemically defined diets are formulations that are less "natural" but not completely elemental. They require a minimal amount of digestion. For example, those products containing egg albumin still require pancreatic enzyme activity prior to absorption. These products are high in carbohydrate, variable in protein, and low in fat. Requiring very little digestion, they are virtually bulk-free. The low fat content makes them suitable for conditions associated with fat malabsorption.

The advantages of these products are that they can be used under conditions in which an only minimal digestion is possible and, because of their low fat and residue content, can also be used to supplement clear liquid diets. The disadvantages are that they are relatively expensive, can create osmolar complications because they are relatively high in osmolarity, and are generally poor in taste, resulting in poor acceptance by patients if administered by mouth. The specific use of chemically defined diets for placing the pancreas "at rest" by delivering intact proteins intrajejunally (1) is not compatible with the absorption of the amino acids required to establish adequate nutritional support.

## Elemental Diets

An elemental diet can be defined as a formula that delivers to the intestinal absorptive surface a complex mix of nutrients that can be absorbed with little or no additional activity required of gut and appended organs. To date, in the authors' opinions, only three products meet this strict definition. They are primarily composed of simple sugars and crystalline L-amino acids. One product contains crystalline amino acids as well as di- and tripeptides. As discussed earlier, there is some evidence in the literature that these short peptide chains are absorbed by transport mechanisms different from those that transport single amino acids. The optimal form of protein in these formulas has yet to be established.

The main advantage to these diets is that virtually no digestion is necessary. It is most likely that these diets cause minimal stimulation of pancreatic, biliary, and small-intestinal secretions. They can therefore be used in conditions such as pancreatitis and gastrointestinal fistula, where bowel rest is desired. Whether stimulation of these secretions occurs or not, the important nutritional consideration is that they are not necessary. The therapist need not be concerned about optimal pancreatic exocrine function, since only modest absorptive capabilities must be intact. This is of concern in patients undergoing chemotherapy or radiation therapy, in whom extensive mucosal damage is undoubtedly present. In addition, these diets are nonallergenic, and are thus potentially useful in cases of food allergies.

The disadvantages to these formulas are similar to those of chemically defined diets, in that they are expensive, can create osmolar complications and are poor in taste, thus reducing oral acceptance by patients. In general, the oral use of elemental diets must be discouraged. It is highly unlikely that any patient suffering from disease for which their use is indicated will tolerate the amounts required over the period of time necessary for healing to be accomplished.

## Special Formulations

The two products in this category are designed for specific organ failures. Amin-Aid (McGaw) is designed for patients with renal failure and Hepatic-Aid (McGaw) is designed for patients experiencing hepatic encephalopathy.

Amin-Aid is an essential amino acid formula designed to limit the delivery of nonessential nitrogen while supporting anabolism. It is a calorically dense supplement (1.9 cal/cc) which can be used orally or by tube feeding to provide nutritional support in patients with acute renal failure, or in end-stage kidney disease, prior to achievement of optimal dialysis. This formula is essentially free of sodium and potassium.

Hepatic-Aid is a product containing both essential and nonessential amino acids, with carbohydrate and fat, in a readily digestible form. The amino acid composition is unique in that it is relatively high in branched-chain amino acids (valine, leucine, and isoleucine) and low in aromatic amino acids (phenylalanine, tyrosine, and tryptophan). The rationale for this formulation is based on recent studies suggesting that an imbalance of plasma amino acids contributes to the clinical expression of hepatic encephalopathy in patients with liver failure. It is suggested that Hepatic-Aid can reverse this imbalance towards normal, thus leading to clinical improvement. However, prospective, randomized, controlled studies have yet to be reported.

### Supplements (Caloric Additives)

Nutritional supplements are designed to augment other intake, and should not be used as meal replacements because they are nutritionally incomplete. Most are caloric supplements, and include carbohydrates: Polycose (Ross), Hycal (Beecham), Calpower (General Mills), and fats: Medium Chain Triglycerides (Mead Johnson), Microlipid (Organon). Protein supplements include Susta-Protein (Mead Johnson), Casec (Mead Johnson), and EMF (Control Drug).

These module products have a broad range of use. They can be used to increase various components of oral or formula diets. They can be combined to meet specific patient requirements, or to adapt an already existing commercial formula. Whenever these products are used, it is important to note changes in caloric density and in osmolarity, especially with the high-carbohydrate products. In some instances, particularly when caloric supplements are used to enhance the caloric density of other formulas in cases requiring fluid and/or protein restriction, so little of the base formula may be administered that inadequacies in vitamin and trace nutrient delivery may result. In general, however, these products are a useful adjunct to enteral hyperalimentation.

### Therapeutic Placement of Enteral Products

Therapeutic placement of the products mentioned is reasonably clear if one considers the functional capacity of the gut (Table 3). If complete digestive and absorptive capacities are intact, formulas high in fiber and complete "natural" products can be used. If the gut is totally afunctional, intervention by parenteral nutrition techniques is obviously indicated. Understanding the composition of formulas will allow for appropriate placement as the gastrointestinal tract progressively loses functional capacity. Eventually, elemental diets can be absorbed through a short segment of jejunum, with no requirements for stomach, pancreas, or hepatic activities, a fact that will enable the knowledgeable therapist to employ enteral hyperalimentation in many instances in which more expensive parenteral methods are currently utilized.

TABLE 3. *Therapeutic placement of formulas*

| | | | Enteral hyperalimentation | | |
|---|---|---|---|---|---|
| | Formula | | | | |
| General | Milk base | Lactose free | Chemically defined | Elemental | Parenteral |
| Blenderized Compleat B Formula 2 Vitaneed | Meritine Nutri 1000 Carnation Instant Breakfast | Ensure Ensure + Isocal Nutri 1000 LF Sustacal Citrotein Osmolite Renu Magnacal | Precision LR Precision HN Precision Isotonic Flexical Vital | Vivonex Vivonex HN Vipep | TPN Peripheral Systems |

FUNCTIONAL GUT

AFUNCTIONAL GUT

MALNUTRITION⟶

## Physiologic Conditions Effecting Choice of Nutrient Solution
### Gastrointestinal Function

A statement often heard in nutrition circles is, "if the gut works, use it." However, it should be obvious that a spectrum of gut function exists, ranging from maintenance of complete facilities for ingestion, digestion, and absorption of intact nutrients to total dysfunction.

Obstruction of the gastrointestinal tract is usually obvious, and in many instances can be overcome. Lesions of the oropharynx and esophagus that functionally will not allow passage of food will sometimes allow the passage of small feeding tubes. In most instances, the disorder is such that a temporary or permanent operative gastrostomy or jejunostomy should be considered. Obstruction in the gastroduodenal area is less receptive to tube passage; however, endoscopic approaches can be utilized before operative jejunostomy is attempted. If exploratory laparotomy is indicated, insertion of a small polyvinyl tube via needle jejunostomy may be the most appropriate means of maintaining enteral hyperalimentation. Obstruction of the ileum and lower GI tract is usually not responsive to therapy by the enteral route. It is feasible, although as yet untested, to insert a double lumen tube, instill an elemental diet high in the jejunum, and aspirate at a more distal point just proximal to the obstruction. However, in most cases, it would be prudent to intervene nutritionally by the parenteral route if at all possible.

Dysfunction resulting from adynamic ileus is common, particularly after surgical intervention. There is growing evidence that the main reason for limiting ingestion of food during the immediate postoperative period is dysfunction of the stomach and colon, and that there is a relatively early return of small-bowel peristaltic activity, at least to a degree to accommodate an elemental diet. This is the basis for the interest in the needle jejunostomy approach for early postoperative feeding, as reported by Page (12).

Interference with optimal digestive and absorptive capabilities of an otherwise intact gut is common in the hospitalized patient and should be considered to influence the choice of nutrient solution. This is particularly true because the therapist now has the ability to eliminate digestive requirements and need be concerned only with absorption. Pancreatic exocrine function may be limited as the result of excision or destruction of pancreatic mass by tumor, inflamation, or obstruction. Obstruction of the bile ducts may occur and can lead to fat malabsorption caused by the inability to create micelles, etc. Mucosal digestive capacity may be limited. Primary lactase deficiency is thought to be present as a genetic trait in a high percentage of blacks and other ethnic groups. Secondary lactase deficiencies, as described above, can occur over short periods of time, and may influence symptoms of many hospitalized individuals subjected to intensive refeeding regimens.

It is common knowledge that mucosal regeneration is influenced by many chemotherapeutic agents and by external irradiation, both of which interfere with protein synthesis. It should be apparent that, at some point, nutritional delivery via the gut can be maintained by taking advantage of those solutions requiring no terminal digestion. Since we do not know exactly at which point the use of an elemental diet becomes mandatory, especially when dealing with questionable digestive capacities, the slow 24-hour delivery of an elemental diet to the remaining absorptive area can be effective in maintaining nutritional status.

The therapist should keep in mind that a major cause of mucosal atrophy is malnutrition itself, perhaps reducing the margin of safety from chemotherapeutic agents and irradiation mentioned above. Malnutrition has been documented to affect nearly all aspects of digestion and absorption (14). Since many of the patients seen by a nutrition support service have not benefited from prior intervention, such considerations are important and may perhaps be an indication for earlier trials with elemental formulas. This is particularly true if severe malnutrition coexists with other causes of gut dysfunction, such as short-bowel syndrome of any etiology. Another dysfunction that should not be overlooked is simply the very sick patient's inability to utilize the bathroom. It may be a distinct advantage for such a patient to be fed and yet not require frequent encounters with a bedpan.

## Pancreatic Endocrine Function

Many patients seen by a nutrition support service experience glucose intolerance secondary either to primary diabetes mellitus or to stress, sepsis, pancreatic destruction, etc. Failure to recognize inadequacy of insulin response can lead to the development of a hyperosmolar state that can potentially be lethal. A knowledge of the calorie source in nutrient solutions is mandatory for optimal delivery of enteral hyperalimentation. Most elemental solutions, in an effort to decrease pancreatic lipase requirements, provide nearly all calories in the form of glucose or short-chain glucose polymers. Other solutions attempt to avoid total reliance upon glucose by adding medium-chain triglycerides as a fuel substrate. These artificial fats have a considerably greater affinity for pancreatic lipase and, in fact, can be almost completely prepared for absorption by the activity of brush-border lipases. Recognition of this effect suggests that near-elemental formulations can be used to advantage in cases of marked glucose intolerance. In all instances, insulin must be administered in amounts necessary to enable optimal delivery of nutrients. Nutrients should not be withheld in attempts to minimize insulin delivery.

## Renal and Hepatic Dysfunction

Many patients who require nutritional intervention suffer from multi-organ dysfunction which, in many instances, includes the liver and/or kidneys. This review cannot fully develop the hypothesis and rationale for the use of commercially available special formulations containing essential amino acids or branched-chain amino acids. However, it should be obvious that renal or hepatic failure places significant constraints on the delivery of enteral hyperalimentation, particularly with regard to limitations of protein, fluid, and electrolytes. Although wide variation exists, most commercial solutions provide protein in a ratio of 1 g nitrogen to approximately 150 cal, the amount believed necessary to support the patient under stress. This can result in the delivery of more than 100 g of protein daily, clearly more than the amount recommended for patients with nitrogen retention disorders who are not undergoing dialysis.

Fluid delivery, particularly in the acute state, is often the most limiting factor. Although newer solutions of high caloric concentration are becoming available, in most instances powdered calorie sources can be added to commercial formulas to decrease both fluid and protein delivery relative to caloric density.

Electrolyte concentrations may be significant, particularly in patients with renal failure. It may be necessary to restrict delivery of potassium, phosphorus, and magnesium in many patients, making knowledge of formula content mandatory. The therapist must be cautioned, however, that renal dysfunction is primarily a problem of regulation. In some instances, arbitrary restriction of electrolytes can result in severe imbalance.

It should be recognized that many solutions designed for specific therapy of renal and hepatic failure may not be nutritionally complete (see Special Formulation in Table 1).

## Cardiac Dysfunction

The ability of the cardiovascular system to handle the influx of nutrients and accompanying water and electrolytes must be assessed in all patients before intervention is considered. Clearly, in many patients with preexisting cardiovascular dysfunction, fluid restrictions become the most limiting factor. This is particularly true if the large amounts of priority solutions necessary to maintain cardiac function are delivered.

## ASSESSMENT OF NUTRITIONAL REQUIREMENTS

The three primary goals for the prevention of body mass wastage during times of stress are:

(A) Define and meet the energy requirements of each patient so that no deficit exists.

(B) Supply protein and amino acids in amounts necessary to support optimal rates of protein synthesis.

(C) Administer vitamins, minerals, and other trace nutrients in quantities required during stress.

It should be obvious that an exact prescription to meet these needs is nearly impossible because of our lack of understanding of the requirements of stressed patients, particularly those with cancer.

### Calories

Calorie requirements of the cancer patient undergoing therapy are undoubtedly greater than those required to maintain basal function. Most clinicians recognize that these requirements may exceed 200% of basal energy expenditure, particularly if complicated surgery and/or sepsis compounds requirements already increased as the result of a large tumor burden. It is most reasonable to initiate therapy with the goal of attaining an intake approximately twice basal energy expenditure, and then to adjust using clinical judgment. Estimates of basal expenditure are easily determined using readily available nomograms (3), or by use of formulas in computer-based models (6). Using this approach, it can be seen that a small, elderly woman will rarely require more than 2,400 cal/day. However, such an amount may clearly be inadequate for a young man with a large tumor burden.

### Protein

We have little knowledge of protein requirements of the tumor-bearing host. In addition to the requirements induced by stress, there is general agreement that the tumor mass exhibits some priority for amino acids. Such an effect has been described as a "nitrogen trap" (9) or "one-way passage" for nitrogen. It is probable that a rapidly growing tumor, like any normally growing tissue, will exhibit increased amino acid requirements. The exact amount required is unknown. The usual amounts of protein found in enteral solutions for therapeutic use having a gram nitrogen to calorie ratio of 1:150 are probably adequate if amounts required to meet caloric demands are delivered. Therapists should be aware that some solutions are designed for maintenance and not for therapeutic use. In those instances, the N/cal ratio is in the range of 1:300. As discussed above, protein delivery may need to be restricted if nitrogen retention disorders coexist.

### Vitamins and Other Trace Nutrients

Here, as with calories and protein, we have little understanding of the requirements of the tumor and the stressed tumor-bearing host. In almost all instances, a "shotgun" approach is utilized, in which nearly all known requirements are delivered in excess. Considerations relative to whether additional trace elements should be added or removed to retard tumor growth are beyond the scope of this chapter.

## DELIVERY SYSTEMS FOR ENTERAL PRODUCTS

### Oral Intake

Because of the problems associated with anorexia, it is very difficult to provide nutritional support for a cancer patient by oral intake alone. At times, however, patients will refuse more aggressive modes of nutritional support, leaving the therapist with the necessity to increase the calorie and protein content in the patient's daily meals and snacks. Such an effort is indeed a challenge. In these circumstances, enteral products are important as nutritional supplements to daily intake. When used in this way, three basic characteristics of the formula should be noted: high calorie and protein content; lactose content; and patient acceptance. Perhaps the primary consideration is taste, a sensation that may be significantly disturbed, particularly in patients with cancer.

The oral intake of the cancer patient can be improved by creative approaches that include alternatives to food aversions, increased seasoning, use of wine, and making breakfast the main meal of the day. Enhanced social stimulation, such as eating in group settings and eating with family, is of equal importance. Behavior modification techniques with respect to food preferences, along with persistent, gentle encouragement to continue efforts to improve nutrition, are significant contributions. Despite the rewards of successfully meeting this challenge, in most instances, especially with the hospitalized patient, nutritional intervention techniques must be employed if the requirements of the stressed patient are to be met.

### Feeding Tubes

One of the most rapidly expanding areas in the field of enteral hyperalimentation is the evolution of feeding tubes that offer significant advantage for nutrient delivery and patient comfort. The following discussion is not meant to be complete, but will provide the reader with sufficient knowledge to meet almost all clinical situations. The reader is referred to standard surgical texts for descriptions of usual gastrostomy and jejunostomy procedures.

Three basic types of tubes are generally available: polyvinyl chloride, silastic, and polyurethane derivatives. Standard nasogastric suction tubes are made from polyvinyl chloride. They are rigid, inflexible, uncomfortable, and prone to cause mechanical erosion of mucosal surfaces if they remain in place for extended periods of time. In general, they should not be used for enteral hyperalimentation. Even small "pediatric" tubes create sufficient discomfort, by comparison with newer tubes, to make their use inappropriate. Some novel approaches, such as those proposed by Moss (11), use large, multilumen polyvinyl chloride tubes. However, efforts to combine simultaneous esophogeal suction, occlusion of the gastroesophageal junction, gastric suction, and duodenal delivery of nutrients require further definition of their clinical advantage by well-controlled prospective trials before patients should be submitted to their routine use.

Silastic tubes have recently been introduced, with the primary advantage of relative softness and flexibility. They tend to stretch during the process of swallowing, so that patients are usually not irritated by their presence in the sensitive pharyngeal area. Some of these tubes are very small (6 French), and although they may be useful in selected cases of severe pharyngitis, their general use should be discouraged because of difficulties in aspirating the stomach to ensure uncomplicated delivery (see below). Silastic tubes are usually weighted with mercury at the tip; they are available in lengths and designs that permit transduodenal passage and nasojejunal delivery of solutions (see discussion of complications).

Tubes made from polyurethane materials are also available and, in general, have a design similar to those made of silastic. One model is impregnated with a hydrophilic substance on the insertion end and inside the tube. When exposed to water, the tip becomes exceedingly slippery without added lubricant. A stainless steel stylet of a size to create sufficient rigidity can be inserted into the tube, making insertion easier in uncooperative and/or comatose patients. The stylet is easily removed, even with some tortuosity of the tube. Of course, proper placement of the tube must be confirmed by the usual methods of aspiration and/or air insufflation, as well as by abdominal auscultation. If any question exists as to appropriate placement, particularly in the comatose individual, an X-ray is mandatory. The mercury tips of newer tubes facilitate X-ray interpretation.

Some mention should be made of the use of needle jejunostomy, which can be performed at time of surgery. This approach, using a 16-gauge 36-inch polyvinyl chloride catheter, has been described in detail (12). It makes enteral hyperalimentation possible for almost all patients who have sufficient jejunal absorptive surface despite gastrocolic dysfunction. It should be stressed that we do not know how far below the ligament of Treitz complex nutrients can be delivered intrajejunally and still stimulate the secretion of pancreatic enzymes necessary for their digestion prior to absorption. It appears that the use of elemental diets in these instances might offer significant advantage, in that they require no pancreatic secretion. In addition, in situations in which short segments of bowel are available or desirable for absorption, the demonstrated lack of pancreatic secretion when these solutions are delivered intrajejunally should help to decrease intrajejunal volume and increase transit time, thereby enabling more complete absorption of nutrients. Such a consideration is also valid when nasojejunal tubes, described above, are utilized.

### Administration of Tube Feedings

The secret to successful administration of enteral hyperalimentation is controlled delivery. There are a variety of methods of delivering enteral solutions; however, the protocol outlined in Table 4 will minimize the all too common

TABLE 4. *Example of orders required for the safe delivery of enteral hyperalimentation*

| Solution | Hours infused | Rate (ml/hr) | Strength (percent) |
|---|---|---|---|
| For day 1 Vivonex HN | 24.00 | 50.0 | 25.0 |
| For day 2 Vivonex HN | 24.00 | 50.0 | 50.0 |
| For day 3 Vivonex HN | 24.00 | 75.0 | 50.0 |
| For day 4 Vivonex HN | 24.00 | 75.0 | 75.0 |
| For day 5 Vivonex HN | 24.00 | 100.0 | 100.0 |

On subsequent days, continue as on the last day above.

Add a liquid vitamin qd on days 1 to 4.

Aspirate feeding tube for residual every 4 hr. If more than 100 cc found, hold infusion for 1 hr and restart. If residual over 100 cc repeatedly, reduce rate by one-half and notify responsible physician.

Check urine sugar and ketones q6h. If positive, notify responsible physician.

Maintain head of bed elevated to 30°.

Weigh patient daily and record in chart.

Maintain accurate daily intake and output, please.

Please keep record of solution administration separate.

Thank you.

                    Signed             Date:

complications of tube feeding that lead to unsuccessful delivery and inadequate nutrition.

Continuous enteral infusion is by far the preferred method of delivering tube feedings. The continuous-drip method decreases the risk of aspiration and makes it more likely that the patient will obtain the appropriate volume. A continuous feeding can usually be delivered by gravity drip. For optimal control of delivery, the formula can be infused by pump.

Bolusing of enteral solutions is not recommended for the hospitalized patient. Bolusing the formula through the tube by syringe, or any rapid administration of the formula, can lead to aspiration, dumping syndrome secondary to osmolarity of solutions, diarrhea, and general intolerance of the formula by the patient. Bolusing is acceptable for well, stable patients on home tube feedings who are not bedridden. However, great care must be given when administering these feedings.

The start-up chart in Table 4 is an ideal demonstration of how infusion rate and concentration of solution are manipulated to deliver the desired nutrients with the least degree of intolerance. The product used in the example, an elemental diet, is a hyperosmolar solution, and hence is started at a low concentration (25% strength) and at a low infusion rate (50 cc/hr). Both rate and concentration are slowly increased over a five-day period until appropriate levels of each are achieved. Solutions that are isotonic, or almost isotonic, can be advanced more quickly than hyperosmolar solutions. These solutions are typically begun at 50% strength with a low rate for 24-hours and then advanced to full strength, increasing the rate until desired volume is obtained. In general, concentration should be increased before rate. An exception to this is in jejunostomy feedings, during which the dilution capacity of the stomach is bypassed. In such instances, it appears useful to increase rate before concentration.

If diarrhea is a problem despite appropriate management of solution concentration and infusion rate, an antidiarrheal agent, such as deodorized tincture of opium, can be added, usually 10 drops per liter of solution. If diarrhea persists, the enteral solution should be reevaluated. Typically, a more defined formula is appropriate.

It is obvious from the start-up chart in Table 4 that complete nutrition is not provided until day three or four (depending on solution used) because of the slow advancement of the solution to full strength concentration. It is therefore necessary to add a liquid vitamin on days one to four, as indicated in the chart, so that vitamin needs will be met.

Regular checking of residual stomach contents while a patient is on enteral hyperalimentation is a precautionary measure to decrease risk of aspiration. The residual volume is an indicator of gastric retention and overall tolerance of formula by the patient. With new small-bore feeding tubes, this often becomes a tedious nursing task; however, smaller syringes tend to alleviate the nuisance problem of collapsing tubes with aspiration. Also, if the patient is tolerating the formula, the amount aspirated should not be thrown away but reinfused in the tube. A second precautionary measure to avoid aspiration is that the bed should be elevated so that the patient's head and shoulders are at a 30-degree angle.

Any patient on enteral hyperalimentation should have urine sugars and ketones monitored every 6 hours. Glucosuria is an indicator of the patient's inability to tolerate the carbohydrate load of the formula, and the patient may therefore require insulin coverage. Urine sugars should be correlated with the patient's blood sugar to establish renal threshold, and the patient should then be placed on a sliding scale of crystallin zinc insulin dosage based on urine sugars. For example:

$$
\begin{array}{ll}
0 \ -1+ & \text{no coverage} \\
1+ -2+ & \text{5 units} \\
2+ -3+ & \text{10 units} \\
3+ -4+ & \text{15 units}
\end{array}
$$

Additionally, every patient on enteral hyperalimentation should be weighed daily. This is of extreme importance when a patient is receiving a hyperosmolar formula. Continued glucosuria with simultaneous weight loss and negative fluid balance, as indicated by accurately kept intake and output sheets, are strong warnings of hyperosmolar syndrome.

These simple procedures of continuous drip, appropriate management of solution concentration and infusion rates, checking residuals, checking urine sugars and ketones, weighing patients, and maintaining accurate intake and output sheets, can prevent many of the complications often associated with enteral hyperalimentation. Following these procedures and monitoring the patient accordingly leads to safe administration of enteral hyperalimentation and successful nutritional support of the patient.

### Combined Enteral and Parenteral Nutrition

In many cases, particularly in those patients with multi-organ dysfunction requiring elemental diets, the gut may be dysfunctional to a degree that limits the achievement of nutritional adequacy within a reasonably short time. Should this situation be anticipated, it is most effective to intervene parenterally using the relatively noninvasive techniques of the peripheral "lipid system" (4). Recent advances in solution preparation have made compatible solutions routinely available on any hospital floor, at any time of day, without the requirement for compounding by pharmacy. If the patient has adequate venous access, can tolerate the fluid load, and has no contraindication to fat emulsion delivery, he can be maintained nutritionally after a brief 24- to 36-hour adjustment period. As documented evidence of successful enteral hyperalimentation is obtained, the lipid system can gradually be tapered. If the gut proves to be afunctional, nutritional support by standard central procedures is indicated.

## COMPLICATIONS

Complications arising from nutritional intervention by enteral hyperalimentation can be placed in two broad categories. The first category includes those that can be avoided by considering the impact of the various solutions on other organ systems, as discussed above. Fluid overload, congestive heart failure, pulmonary edema, and excessive azotemia all fall into this category. Those of the second category are preventable providing the procedure is delivered under optimal control conditions. These relate primarily to three broad areas: pulmonary aspiration, gastrointestinal effects, and metabolic disturbances.

### Pulmonary Aspiration

Pulmonary aspiration is perhaps the most lethal complication associated with enteral hyperalimentation. The etiology is quite obvious; either infused solution delivered directly to the bronchial tree as the result of tube misplacement, or else regurgitated stomach contents are aspirated into the lungs. Correct initial placement of the tube must be confirmed by techniques described above before initiating infusion. If any question exists, X-ray confirmation of placement is mandatory. Tubes must be checked daily by the nursing staff to ensure that they have not migrated up from the stomach with resultant pharyngeal delivery of solutions.

Vomiting per se cannot be prevented in patients undergoing enteral hyperalimentation, since many individuals are nauseated for reasons related either to disease or to therapy. It is mandatory, however, that the volume of solution remaining in the stomach at any time be kept at an absolute minimum so that, should regurgitation occur, the effects on the lung are minimized. Most important, failure to monitor stomach contents can result in large accumulations if an organic or functional gastric emptying defect is present. This will result in regurgitation of large volumes, which in the seriously ill or obtunded patient invariably leads to aspiration.

Continuous controlled delivery of nutrients over 24-hour periods, and frequent scheduled monitoring of stomach contents by testing for residual volumes, must be part of any enteral hyperalimentation protocol. Should evidence of delayed gastric emptying be present, such disabilities can in many instances be circumvented by the insertion of a nasal jejunal tube with resultant delivery beyond the pylorus and ligament of Treitz. In such instances, nutrient delivery can be maintained while at the same time the stomach is emptied by secondary nasogastric suction.

### Gastrointestinal Complications

Gastrointestinal complications are primarily of three types: mechanical, gastric retention, and diarrhea.

Mechanical complications are usually related to mucosal erosions secondary to the prolonged use of large polyvinyl chloride tubes. Such problems have been minimal in our experience since the introduction of smaller silastic and polyurethane tubes. Even patients with the most severe erosive pharyngitis appear to tolerate a small silastic tube. Experience with silastic tubes in patients with esophogeal varices is limited, and recommendations for their use must be left to individualized clinical judgment.

Gastric retention, as indicated above, is common in patients undergoing enteral hyperalimentation. There is some evidence that bolus feeding, particularly of the elemental diets, can create gastric retention. Such effects are eliminated by continuous infusion. Should minor difficulties develop, it is important to remember the physiologic effect of fats in the stomach, which cause delayed gastric emptying. It may be advantageous for the therapist to change to non-fat-containing solutions if problems exist that are not clearly anatomical in nature. These considerations are also important when reinstituting oral intake; ingested fat causes gastric retention. In many instances, transition to oral intake may be best accomplished by delivering enteral hyperalimentation during nocturnal hours, while encouraging oral intake at usual meal times.

Diarrhea is a common problem in enteral hyperalimentation and has the potential of arising from several sources. Perhaps the most common is related to the various medications that invariably are administered by tube once it has been placed for feeding purposes. It is important to remember that the gut itself, and particularly the activities of the digestive enzymes of the brush border (which undergo rapid turnover), are especially susceptible to protein malnutrition. One of the early enzyme activities to become impaired is that of lactase, which is undoubtedly the reason why most therapists avoid milk-based formulas as enteral hyperalimentation solutions. It has been our experience that the delivery of almost any solution to a patient with severe protein malnutrition will result in some initial malabsorption. For this reason, it is reasonable to begin any formula slowly and at half-strength concentration.

Perhaps the most common cause of diarrhea has an osmotic basis. If solutions of high osmolarity are introduced into the intestinal lumen, and if the ability of gut mucosa to absorb those nutrients quickly is impaired by either disease or malnutrition, water will move into the lumen to satisfy the osmotic gradient faster than the solutes can be transported into the intestinal mucosal cell. The result is a rapidly increased volume within the lumen which quickly takes the form of watery diarrhea. Such effects can be avoided by delivering solutions initially at a hypo-osmolar concentration and gradually increasing both rate and concentration. It is important to realize that if intrajejunal feeding is used the initial diluting capacity of the stomach is eliminated. In such cases, it is usually prudent to increase volume first and then concentration. The industry is making major efforts to provide many solutions in an isotonic state. If such solutions are used, it is certainly not essential, from an osmotic point of view, to start with the very dilute solutions that are required for elemental diets.

Diarrhea can generally be avoided by adherence to the above principles; however, in many instances, particularly when rapid transit time is evident as the result of disease or therapy, it is important to make an effort to control gut motility. This is most conveniently accomplished by the use of deodorized tincture of opium, which can be added initially in a concentration of 10 drops/liter of solution; dosage can then be titrated, depending upon effect. The therapist must realize that excessive amounts of DTO will have a central nervous system effect and can lead to obtundation and respiratory depression. It must be used with caution in older individuals, particularly those with central nervous system dysfunction.

## Metabolic Complications

Almost every metabolic complication that has been noted to occur with total parenteral nutrition can occur with enteral hyperalimentation. Such complications include electrolyte disturbances, mineral deficiencies, vitamin inadequacies, and others. Perhaps the most lethal, and avoidable, is hyperosmolar coma, which in the older literature has been described as *tube feeding syndrome*. Its development relates to a rise in blood glucose concentrations above the renal threshold, glucosuria, and resultant free-water loss accompanying an osmotic diuresis. This is particularly true when high glucose-containing solutions, such as are currently found in available elemental diets, are delivered to patients with either diabetes mellitus or syndromes expressed as *insulin resistant*. This complication is entirely preventable if attention is paid to blood sugar levels, the presence of glucosuria, and close monitoring of body weight. It must be stressed that daily weights are essential in monitoring of fluid balance, but have little to do with the reversal of weight loss resulting from illness or disease, an event that occurs with uncommonly low frequency in the stressed hospitalized patient.

Nutritional support is not withheld because of hyperglycemia; insulin is delivered in amounts appropriate to meet the demands of the stressed individual. Insulin coverage should be via frequent subcutaneous injections of regular insulin. Long-acting insulins must be avoided, since it is undoubtedly true that tube malfunction or displacement will occur at times of peak activity of insulin delivered in quantities required for coverage of administered glucose. Reactive hypoglycemia will most certainly result in such instances. In a severely stressed individual, continuous intravenous delivery of regular insulin at a rate calculated to maintain optimal blood sugar concentrations can be accomplished provided adequate nursing care is available by individuals who understand the potentially disastrous effects of sudden cessation of nutrient delivery in the face of ongoing insulin activity.

The amount of free water required to prevent dehydration can usually be found in the most commonly administered solutions that have a caloric density of one cal/ml. More concentrated formulas can be of distinct advantage in treating patients with significant fluid overload. However, the use of such highly concentrated solutions in a marginally dehydrated individual can lead to progressive dehydration, hypertonicity, and death. Again, such problems can be avoided by understanding the fluid requirements of the individual, closely monitoring intake and output, and meticulous determination and recording of daily weights.

## SUMMARY

A broad perspective of enteral hyperalimentation has been presented, with the goal of enabling the therapist to intervene nutritionally in a safe and effective manner. By understanding the basic principles of solution formulation, therapeutic placement, clinical application, and controlled delivery, this therapeutic modality can be utilized to prevent wastage of body mass in almost every patient undergoing therapy for cancer. The use of enteral hyperalimentation as an alternative to intervention by total parenteral nutrition must not be overlooked.

## REFERENCES

1. Blackburn, G. L., Williams, L. F., Bistrian, B. R., Stone, M. S., Phillips, E., Hirsch, E., Clowes, G. H., and Gregg, J. (1976): New approaches to the management of severe acute pancreatitis. *Am. J. Surg.*, 131:114–124.
2. Borgström, B., Dahlqvist, A., Lundh, G., and Sjövall, J. (1957): Studies of intestinal digestion and absorption in the human. *J. Clin. Invest.*, 36:1521–1536.
3. Committee on Dietetics of the Mayo Clinic (1971): *Mayo Clinic Diet Manual.* W. B. Saunders Co., Philadelphia.
4. Deitel, M., and Kaminsky, V. (1974): Total nutrition by peripheral vein—the lipid system. *Con. Med. Assoc. J.*, 111:152–154.
5. Food and Nutrition Board, National Research Council (1979): *Recommended Dietary Allowances.* Natl. Acad. Sci., Washington, D.C.
6. Geller, R. J., Blackburn, S. A., Glendon, D. H., Henneman, W. H., and Steffee, W. P. (1979): Computer optimization of enteral hyperalimentation. *J. Parent. Ent. Nutr.*, 3:79–83.
7. Goodhart, R. S., and Shils, M. E., editors (1973): *Modern Nutrition in Health and Disease.* Lea & Febiger, Philadelphia.
8. Greenstein, J. P., Birnbaum, S. M., Winitz, M., and Otey, M. C. (1957): Quantitative nutritional studies with water-soluble, chemically defined diets. *Biochem. Biophys. Res. Commun.*, 72:396–416.
9. Henderson, J. F., and Lepage, G. A. (1959): The nutrition of tumors: A review. *Cancer Res.*, 19:887–902.
10. Matthews, D., and Adibi, S. (1976): Progress in gastroenterology—peptide absorption. *Gastroenterology*, 71:151–161.
11. Moss, G., (1979): Postoperative ileus is an avoidable complication. *Surg. Gynecol. Obstet.*, 148:81–82.
12. Page, C. P., Ryan, J. A., and Haff, R. C. (1976): Continual catheter administration of an elemental diet. *Surg. Gynecol. Obstet.*, 142:184–188.
13. Senior, J. R., editor (1968): *Medium Chain Triglycerides.* University of Pennsylvania Press, Philadelphia.
14. Suskind, R. M. (1975): Gastrointestinal changes in the malnourished child. *Pediatr. Clin. North Am.*, 22:873–883.
15. Thompson, W. R., Stephens, R. V., Randall, H. T., and Bowen, J. R. (1969): Use of the "Space Diet" in the management of a patient with extreme short bowel syndrome. *Am. J. Surg.*, 117:449–459.
16. Winitz, M., Graff, J., Gallagher, N., Narkin, A., and Seedman, D. (1965): Evolution of chemical diets as nutrition for man-in-space. *Nature*, 205:741–743.

*Nutrition and Cancer: Etiology and Treatment,*
edited by G. R. Newell and N. M. Ellison.
Raven Press, New York © 1981.

# Parenteral Hyperalimentation of the Cancer Patient

Edward M. Copeland, III, John M. Daly, and Stanley J. Dudrick

*The University of Texas Medical School at Houston, The University of Texas System Cancer Center, M. D. Anderson Hospital and Tumor Institute, Houston, Texas 77030*

The importance of the relationship between nutrition and cancer has been recognized for many years, but not until the successful clinical application of intravenous hyperalimentation (IVH) and enteral chemically defined diets did the physician have the proper tools to improve this relationship in the seriously ill patient. Nutritional replenishment is now possible to some degree in almost all patients, and the significant roles played by adequate building blocks in the form of carbohydrates, amino acids, vitamins, minerals, and fats in the management of acute and chronic illnesses are being recognized and appreciated. The importance of nutritional rehabilitation and maintenance of the cancer patient before, during, and after treatment is now being evaluated with controlled clinical trials using IVH. Intravenous nutritional replenishment has interrupted the vicious cycle created by malnutrition, adequate nutrients are provided to the patient as adjunctive support during therapy, and, if the cancer responds to treatment, appetite returns and weight gain is maintained.

Cancer cachexia should no longer be a contraindication to adequate oncologic therapy. Nutritional replenishment can be undertaken prior to the indicated antineoplastic therapy, and nutritional restoration has not been observed clinically to stimulate tumor growth. Nutrients supplied in excess of the needs of the cancer should be available for use by the host to heal wounds, repair immunologic mechanisms, replenish protein stores, phagocytize cancer cells, and restore enzyme systems to normal. Cachexia is harmful to cancer patients because the malnourished patient has a narrow safe therapeutic margin for most radiation therapy and chemotherapy. The tumoricidal doses of these agents may be much closer to the lethal dose for normal tissues in malnourished patients than in well-nourished ones. Physicians should be alert for the signs and symptoms of malnutrition and should be prepared to individualize nutritional therapy for each patient.

Absorption of food stuffs via a functional gastrointestinal tract is the best means of maintaining adequate nutrition; however, delivery of adequate nutrients to the gut does not always result in adequate nutritional restoration of the starving patient. In the severely malnourished individual, the gastrointestinal columnar mucosal cells become cuboidal and the brush border is reduced in height. Decreased production of mucosal cells and decreased migration from the crypts occur, gastrointestinal motility diminishes, and overgrowth of facultative and anaerobic bacteria results. These environmental, absorptive, and morphologic abnormalities of the gastrointestinal tract in the malnourished patient are reversible following protein–calorie replenishment. However, the process is slow because adequate enteral nutrients are initially partially malabsorbed, and uncomfortable symptoms of nausea, diarrhea, abdominal pain, and bloating limit the patient's desire to eat or obtain nutrients via nasogastric, gastrostomy, or jejunostomy feeding tubes. Similarly, nutritional supplementation via the gastrointestinal tract can be time consuming, and the operative insertion of feeding tubes can impose on the patient an acute surgical stress that further delays nutritional restoration. Thus, intravenous hyperalimentation has become an extremely useful tool when the gastrointestinal tract is unavailable for nutrient administration or when nutritional replenishment via the gut may not be rapid enough to achieve adequate nutritional restoration before the patient must undergo oncologic therapy.

There are many tests for evaluating nutritional status, and most tests for nutritional assessment can be correlated with somatic compartments. The fat compartment can be evaluated by measuring the triceps skinfold thickness, the visceral protein compartment by measuring serum albumin concentration and by skin testing for delayed hypersensitivity, and the skeletal muscle compartment by measuring upper arm circumference and creatinine–height index. Although our team uses all available nutritional tests, and each is important, the practicing physician, without the aid of an organized nutritional support service, cannot always perform all available tests. Our team defines malnutrition as a recent, unintentional loss of 10% or more of body weight, a serum albumin concentration of less than 3.4 g/100 ml, and/or a negative reaction to a battery of recall skin test antigens. Patients who satisfy two of these three criteria and who have a reasonable chance of responding to appropriate oncologic therapy are candidates of IVH. Also, patients who cannot maintain adequate enteral nutrition because of malnutrition associated with previous cancer therapy are candidates for nutritional rehabilitation with IVH, as are nutritionally healthy patients whose treatment plan requires multiple courses of chemotherapy, possibly combined with surgery or radiation therapy, if maintenance of optimum nutrition during therapy is considered important to maximize the chance for response to treatment, to reduce complications of oncologic therapy, and to improve quality of life.

## INTRAVENOUS HYPERALIMENTATION: TECHNIQUES

Intravenous hyperalimentation at most institutions should be the responsibility of a team of people, including a physician team leader, registered nurses, dietitians, pharmacists, and rehabilitation therapists. Solutions for IVH generally contain 20% to 30% dextrose and 3.5% to 5% amino acids. The osmolarity of this solution is between 1800 and 2400 mOsm, necessitating infusion via a large-bore central vein rather than a peripheral vein. Most often, the subclavian vein is catheterized percutaneously via the infraclavicular approach so that the tip of the feeding catheter can be directed into the middle of the superior vena cava, where rapid dilution of the nutrients takes place with less risk of thrombophlebitis than if the infusion were administered through a smaller vessel, such as the internal jugular vein. Accurate positioning of the catheter tip within the middle of the superior vena cava is verified by obtaining a chest roentgenogram prior to beginning infusion of the hypertonic IVH solutions.

The IVH delivery system should not be used indiscriminately, and blood, blood by-products, and medications should be administered via an alternate vein whenever possible. A simultaneous peripheral intravenous infusion is often necessary to administer antibiotics, supplemental fluids, or chemotherapeutic agents. The incidence of catheter-related sepsis in our series of patients has ranged from 1% to 6%, with the highest rate of sepsis occurring in patients with cancer of the head and neck, who generally have open wounds or tracheostomy or pharyngostomy stomas nearby that may constantly contaminate the catheter dressings. A recent addition to parenteral infusion equipment is the long silastic catheter, the tip of which can be directed percutaneously through a vein in the anticubital space to lie in the middle of the superior vena cava. Thus, the catheter–skin entrance site is removed to an area distant from the head and neck region. Preliminary results with the use of this catheter for the infusion of IVH solutions have been acceptable, and sepsis has been minimized by meticulous catheter care identical to that followed for catheters inserted through the infraclavicular area. At present, our group continues to use the standard infraclavicular approach to the subclavian vein unless the potential for infection in this area dictates that an alternate site be selected.

The IVH solutions should be given at constant rate to promote proper use of the administered glucose, amino acids, minerals, and vitamins. Initially, 1,000 ml is delivered in 24 hours to confirm the patients ability to metabolize the infused glucose effectively. In the absence of glycosuria and hyperglycemia, the flow rate may be increased to 1,000 ml every 12 hours. Pancreatic islet cells will again need the opportunity to adapt with an increased insulin output in response to the increased glucose infusion, but within three to five days the average adult will usually tolerate a daily ration of 3,000 ml of IVH solution. Extremely malnourished patients, however, may tolerate only 2,000 ml/day until partial nutritional rehabilitation has been achieved, and attempts to give more initially may result in cardiac decompensation. The abrupt cessation of IVH may lead to insulin shock or reactive hypoglycemia. For this reason, IVH should be tapered off during the 24 to 48 hr prior to completely discontinuing it. Generally, the patient is expected to gain five to ten pounds during a three-week period of IVH. The initial three- to four-pound weight gain will be rehydration, but then the patient should gain lean body mass at a rate of about one-half pound per day. Body weight gain greater than one pound per day should be considered fluid retention, and the IVH delivery rate should be decreased or a diuretic administered.

During treatment with IVH, the patient's metabolic status should be reviewed frequently to detect any need to alter the flow rate or composition of the nutrient solution. Important factors to examine on a regular basis are fractional urine sugar concentration every six hours, daily weights, daily intake and output, serum electrolytes, blood urea nitrogen, and blood sugar levels three times a week, serum levels of albumin, magnesium, phosphorus, clacium, and creatinine once a week, liver function tests, coagulation parameters, and complete blood count once a week, and frequent patient reevaluation for any temperature elevation.

The nurse assigned to the hyperalimentation team changes the patient's catheter dressing and IVH delivery tubing three times a week, each time repreparing the skin with acetone or ether and an antiseptic solution. An antimicrobial ointment and a sterile dressing are reapplied to cover the catheter–skin entrance site. If proper technique is always used, a single feeding catheter can remain in place for long periods of time without complications.

The patient who develops a febrile episode during IVH is presumed to have catheter-related sepsis unless another primary focus of infection can be identified. Diagnosis of catheter-related sepsis is confirmed by a blood culture and a catheter culture positive for the same organism. The catheter should be removed immediately, and temperature will usually return to normal within 24 to 48 hr if the catheter was the source of infection. If a primary focus of infection other than the catheter is apparent and blood cultures are negative, the primary focus should be treated appropriately and the catheter can be left in place. A positive blood culture, however, is an unequivocal indication for catheter removal. Catheter reinsertion into the superior vena cava, usually through the opposite subclavian vein, is considered safe 24 to 48 hr after temperature has returned to normal and blood cultures have become negative.

Intravenous fat solutions are now available in the United States for parenteral use. Although they are isotonic, 290 mOsm/L, and can be infused via a peripheral vein without fear of inducing thrombophlebitis, their primary role in intravenous nutritional therapy currently is to provide the essential fatty acid, linoleic acid. The fatty acid fraction of the commercially available fat preparations is approximately 54% linoleic acid, adequate quantities of which can be delivered by the twice-weekly administration of one 500-ml bottle of the fatty acid solutions. The fat should be infused through a peripheral vein; it should not be mixed with IVH solution, since the two mixtures are not miscible. Delivery of the fatty acid solution via the Y-connector of the IVH delivery system has proved safe; nevertheless, peripheral administration remains our current recommendation.

The potential toxicity of polyunsaturated fatty acids has been recently noted. Mertin and Hughes (23) reported that the addition of the polyunsaturated fatty acids, linoleic acid and arachadonic acid, to *in vitro* human lymphocyte cultures significantly reduced blastogenic transformation to phytohemagglutinin (PHA), indicating a reduction in immunological reactivity of the lymphocytes. To date, however, the exact role of linoleic acid in the immunological mechanism remains unclear. In our laboratory, Ota et al. (26) evaluated the effects of Intralipid on *in vitro* Varidase and PHA lymphocyte blastogenesis. Physiologic and pharmacologic concentrations of Intralipid in culture media increased Varidase lymphocyte transformation by an average of 11.3% and 18.9%, respectively, compared with Varidase lymphocyte transformation in culture media alone. These same concentrations also increased PHA lymphocyte blastogenesis by an average of 8.2% and 18%, respectively. Contrary to previous reports, these data demonstrated that Intralipid significantly enhanced Varidase and PHA lymphocyte transformation; consequently, Intralipid added to a parenteral nutrient regimen might enhance rather than suppress immunocompetence. Theoretically, essential fatty acid deficiences should be more deleterious to the cancer patient than any potential suppression of immunological reactivity secondary to the administration of small doses of linoleic acid.

## POTENTIAL FOR SEPSIS AND FOR STIMULATION OF TUMOR GROWTH

Prior to 1972, IVH had not been applied to the treatment of a large number of cancer patients because of two potential problems: (a) septic complications might have resulted from the use of the indwelling superior vena cava catheters necessary for the administration of IVH in patients who had depressed leukocyte counts associated with chemotherapy or radiotherapy and depressed immunocompetence secondary to oncologic treatment, malnutrition, or tumor burden; and (b) tumor growth might have been stimulated by the potent nutritional solutions. Wilmore and Dudrick (34) had previously shown that proper aseptic management of the indwelling catheter and the IVH delivery system and aseptic mixing of the IVH solutions by the pharmacist minimized septic complications secondary to IVH in noncancer patients, and in 1972 our group speculated that similar results could be obtained in cancer patients. At that time there were a number of cachectic cancer patients in our institution, who were not considered candidates for adequate oncologic therapy because of fear of complications that result from the use of antineoplastic agents in malnourished patients. These patients would have been denied adequate oncologic treatment without nutritional replenishment by IVH. Enteral replenishment had failed already. Under these circumstances, the potential stimulation of tumor growth by nutritional replenishment was an academic question, and the possible risk of infection secondary to the indwelling subclavian vein catheter was acceptable.

Intravenous hyperalimentation was initially used to treat 93 cachectic cancer patients with a wide variety of malignant diseases (3). The average period of IVH was 24.8 days. One-half of the patients in the study received chemotherapy and had leukocyte counts below 2,500 cells/mm³ for an average of 7.2 days. No organisms were grown from catheters in place for less than 10 days, and eight positive cultures (7.3%) were obtained from catheters in place for longer than 10 days. The catheter could be incriminated as a source of infection only in two patients (2.2%), both of whom had *Candida albicans* cultured from the catheter and bloodstream. Patients tolerated a therapeutic course of radiation therapy or chemotherapy or a major surgical procedure that could have been potentially fatal without nutritional rehabilitation with IVH.

An additional factor in the low rate of observed catheter sepsis may have been a return of the immune mechanism to normal function. Cell-mediated immunity can be divided into two broad categories: primary and initiated by contact with a new antigen, or established in the past, capable of immediate recall, and demonstrable by response to skin-test antigens. Short-term chemotherapy will suppress primary cell-mediated immunity, but should have no effect on established immunity. Malnutrition suppresses established cell-mediated immunity. Both types of immunity are important in preventing sepsis during chemotherapy; if the patient becomes malnourished during chemotherapy or is malnourished at the outset of treatment, he may have minimal immunological defenses against infection and increased susceptibility to sepsis.

The potential for acceleration of tumor growth during nutritional repletion has been shown in studies done in animals. Cameron and Pavlat (2) and Steiger et al. (32) suggested that nutritional therapy in tumor-bearing malnourished rats stimulates tumor growth; in studies in our laboratory, this possibility has also been identified in some (9) but not all (10) tumor models. Daly et al. (10) designed an experimental protocol to mimic the clinical situation often seen in human cancer patients, by using malnourished, immune-incompetent animals with a viable neoplasm. Purified protein derivative (PPD)-reactive rats bearing transplanted Morris hepatomas were protein depleted by ingesting a high-carbohydrate, protein-free diet for two weeks. At this point PPD reactivity was lost. Next, the rats were randomized to receive continuation of the high-carbohydrate, protein-free diet, normal rat chow, or IVH. After one week, no animals continuing the high-carbohydrate, protein-free diet regimen regained PPD reactivity, whereas almost all animals receiving the IVH or regular diet became PPD-reactive. Tumor-weight to body-weight ratios were not significantly different in all groups, although tumors in the nutritionally replenished animals were somewhat larger. Tumor growth had not been stimulated out of proportion to host nutritional replenishment by either IVH or the normal diet, and nutritionally replenished animals were immunocompetent. Although certain malignant neoplasms might produce a substance that is directly immunosuppressive, in this experimental model PPD reactivity could be correlated with dietary intake and was restored by proper nutritional repletion.

Although significant stimulation of growth of the Morris hepatoma was not noted with seven days of nutritional replenishment, Daly and co-workers have identified both stimulation and retardation of growth of the Walker 256 carcino-sarcoma in Sprague–Dawley rats during nutritional manipulation (9). If nutritional replenishment can stimulate tumor cell replication and metabolism, there may be an optimal time period during early nutritional replenishment when tumor cell growth and division are maximal and the tumor is most susceptible to antimetabolites, such as methotrexate. In the experiments of Daly et al., acceleration of tumor growth in transplanted Walker 256 carcinosarcomas began within 48 hours of nutritional replenishment, and within six days was similar to tumor growth patterns in well-nourished animals that had never undergone a period of protein depletion. Reynolds et al. (27), using the same experimental protocol, gave animals methotrexate two or six days after protein replenishment had begun. These times were chosen to correspond with the period of rapid tumor growth after nutritional replenishment identified by Daly. Methotrexate administration had no effect on tumor or carcass weight if a protein-free diet was continued. The greatest inhibition of tumor growth occurred in rats that were switched from a protein-free to a regular diet and were treated with methotrexate two days after nutritional replenishment had begun. The greatest reduction in tumor weight compared with the greatest gain in carcass weight also occurred in these rats. Since methotrexate inhibits DNA synthesis, Reynolds et al. concluded that the good response to methotrexate after nutritional replenishment had begun was secondary to an increase in tumor-cell replication stimulated by feeding the regular diet. Conversely, they concluded that the poor response to methotrexate in rats continued on the protein-free diet was secondary to depressed tumor-cell metabolism and replication coincident with minimal carcass weight gain in these animals.

Thus, acceleration of tumor growth in animals by nutritional manipulation depends upon the animal–tumor model used, the period of prior nutritional deprivation, and the time and method of nutritional replenishment. Stimulation of tumor growth by nutritional replenishment of human patients has not been identified; nevertheless, results from rat experiments suggest that this possibility exists in the mammalian species, and that appropriate antineoplastic therapy should be instituted early in nutritional rehabilitation. Data in rats, however, cannot be applied directly to malnourished cancer patients, since doubling times of human malignant tumors are measured in days or weeks and the cancer may not kill the patient until several years after the initial clone of malignant cells has developed. The doubling time of animal tumors can often be measured in hours, and this relatively rapid growth can result in death of the animal within five to seven weeks of initial tumor inoculation. Dietary protein depletion or repletion would be expected to have a more obvious and measurable effect on a tumor such as a Walker 256 carcinosarcoma because of its rapid growth. Also unlike tumors in rats, tumors in cachectic human beings receiving nutritional therapy have not been noted to be more responsive to DNA-specific chemotherapeutic agents.

## CLINICAL MATERIAL

Observations in animals and man suggest that the application of IVH as adjunctive nutritional therapy for the cancer patient is safe and nutritionally efficacious. Since the initial report of our experience with IVH and cancer patients in 1972, Solassol and Joyeux (30), Filler et al. (16), Harvey et al. (19), and van Eys (35) have reported large series of patients nutritionally replenished with IVH without an increase in septic complications over those observed in noncancer patients and with no evidence of tumor growth stimulation. These reports are often criticized because the analyses were not done in a prospective and randomized fashion; nevertheless, they represent data from more than 2,000 patients who have received IVH with no indication that tumor growth was increased by the use of the nutritional solutions.

At our instiutions, more than 1,500 patients have received IVH and nutritional support for oncologic therapy during the last seven years. Our group evaluated the results of IVH as treatment for 406 consecutive cancer patients suffering from a wide variety of malignant diseases (6). The treatment categories were chemotherapy (43%), general and thoracic surgery (24%), head and neck surgery (10), radiation therapy (10%), fistulas (6%), and supportive care (7%). Response to chemotherapy or radiation therapy was defined as 50% or greater reduction in measurable tumor mass. Hyperalimentation was used for an average of 23.9 days, and average weight gain in these 406 patients during IVH was five pounds.

Intravenous hyperalimentation was used for an average of 22.8 days during 260 courses of chemotherapy in 175 patients. Depression of leukocyte counts below 2,500 cells/mm$^3$ occurred in 51.5% of patients and lasted for an average of 7.7 days. Only four pathogenic organisms were grown from cultures of 212 consecutive subclavian vein catheters, and only three patients had simultaneous positive blood and catheter cultures (an incidence of catheter-related sepsis of 1.4%). Tumor response was obtained in 27.8% of patients who completed a planned course of chemotherapy. This response rate reflects our ability to select patients for IVH and chemotherapy, rather than an overall percentage response of a patient group to a particular drug protocol. Many of these 175 patients had relapsed after initial response to chemotherapy and were being treated with a different drug regimen that was known to have limited effectiveness. Gastrointestinal symptoms of nausea, vomiting, and diarrhea were reduced or better tolerated if IVH was used with chemotherapy, and patients were not required to eat in order to maintain body composition.

The concept of increased tolerance for 5-fluorouracil (5-FU) during nutritional maintenance with IVH was initially tested in animals (31). Rats that nourished themselves *ad libitum* with ordinary rat chow were compared with animals nourished entirely by IVH. Both groups received a daily intraperitoneal dose of 5-FU, 15 mg/kg/day, for seven days. Eighty percent of animals eating *ad libitum* died within 10 days of initiation of 5-FU injections, whereas only 30% of animals nourished by IVH died during the 10-day period. This experience was extrapolated to human patients suffering from malnutrition and metastatic colon cancer. Sixteen patients who had lesions evaluable for chemotherapeutic response were placed on IVH for seven days prior to beginning treatment with 5-FU (15 mg/kg/day diluted in 50 ml of 5% dextrose in water and delivered intravenously during a one-hour period). Ten malnourished patients with metastatic colon cancer who did not receive IVH during 5-FU administration served as controls. In the IVH group, five patients (31%) responded with a greater than 50% reduction in measurable tumor volume and received a total dose of 7.4 g 5-FU over an average of 8.6 days. Only one control patient (10%) responded to an average total dose of 3.8 g 5-FU given over an average of only 4.4 days. The control group lost an average of 4.2 lb during the study, whereas the IVH group gained weight. These data are similar to those of Moertel et al. (24), who had previously reported that patients with gastrointestinal cancer and a good performance status have a better response to 5-FU than patients with similar disease processes and a poor performance status. Whether the increased response in nutritionally healthier patients was secondary to nutritional repletion or to tolerance of a larger dose of 5-FU remains to be determined.

The studies currently sponsored by the Diet, Nutrition, and Cancer Program of the National Cancer Institute are nearing completion. At present, neither response rate nor survival has been improved in patients receiving IVH (14). In many of these studies, patients with only minimal degrees of malnutrition were entered into the randomization process. Little if any documentation of differences in response rate would be expected unless patients with severe malnutrition were selected for study. From the ethical standpoint, most investigators are reluctant to deny patients suffering from severe degrees of malnutrition access to nutritional rehabilitation either enterally or parenterally to obtain randomized, prospective data.

In a pilot study by Isell et al. (21), 26 patients undergoing oncologic therapy with Adriamycin, Ifosfamide, and *Corynebacterium parvum* were randomized to receive either IVH for 10 days prior to chemotherapy and 31 days through the first course of chemotherapy or conventional enteral or intravenous methods of nutrition and fluid and electrolyte maintenance. During the first course of chemotherapy, the IVH group experienced less nausea and vomiting and had a significant improvement in anthropometric measurements compared to the non-IVH control group. A response to chemotherapy was identified in four patients in the IVH group and in only one patient in the conventional therapy group. These results are preliminary, but support retrospective data previously reported by Lanzotti et al. (22) and Copeland et al. (4). Based on studies to date, both retrospective and prospective, IVH should be used in cancer patients as a means of nutritional rehabilitation when such a goal is desirable to optimize response to chemotherapy and to minimize complications from the antineoplastic agents, and when this goal cannot be attained by enteral means.

Seniukov et al. (29) recently reported an evaluation of the efficacy of the postoperative use of IVH in malnourished patients with carcinoma of the larynx.

Seventy patients received IVH and 90 patients were fed via a nasogastric feeding tube. The two groups were carefully matched for stage of disease and dose of preoperative radiation therapy. Primary wound healing occurred in 75% of the parenterally fed group and 40% of the enterally fed group. Ten percent of patients in the parenteral group developed pharyngeal fistulas, compared to 29% of patients in the enteral group. This study suggests that patients who are given their nutrient mixture by vein and are thereby guaranteed a certain calorie intake have significantly better postoperative wound healing than those who are fed via the gastrointestinal tract and are possibly malabsorbing a portion of the supplied nutrients.

Dionigi and co-workers (15) compared 98 patients with surgically resectable gastrointestinal malignancies treated with IVH pre- and postoperatively to 94 surgical patients with similar tumors treated with conventional fluid therapy. The IVH group had better nitrogen balance, significantly greater weight gain, improved general well-being, better wound healing, and an average hospital stay of 18 days, compared to 25 days for the control patients.

In our series (6), 100 patients received IVH as nutritional support for a general or thoracic surgical procedure. Fifty-two patients underwent curative resections that included esophagectomies, gastrectomies, and abdominal–perineal resections. Although this group of patients was reported retrospectively, recovery from these surgical procedures would have been doubtful without IVH. IVH was used for an average of 24.2 days, and the patients gained an average of 4.2 lb. In those who received IVH pre- and postoperatively, weight gain and a rise in serum albumin concentration were obtained almost entirely during the preoperative period. Weight and serum albumin concentration were maintained during the postoperative period, but no increase in either occurred. Those individuals receiving IVH only postoperatively usually had developed one of the complications of prolonged inanition, such as paralytic ileus, wound dehiscence, or wound infection, before IVH was begun. Weight gain in these patients was difficult to achieve, probably because of increased energy expenditure secondary to the surgical complications. In contrast, those who received IVH preoperatively had virtually no postoperative complications and were often eating within five days of bowel resection. Based on the comparative data of Seniukov and Dionigi and the retrospective data reported by our group, we recommend that a malnourished patient be nutritionally replenished preoperatively, rather than waiting for some catastrophic postoperative complication to occur.

Three patients had pharyngeal incompetence after head and neck surgical procedures, and the incompetence was thought to be secondary to muscle weakness and reversible muscle injury. Nutritional rehabilitation was begun with IVH, and deglutitory muscular rehabilitation was accomplished. In addition to return of general body muscle strength and tone, swallowing function returned after 18 to 48 days of IVH. Patients with malignant neoplasms of the oropharyngeal area often present a special nutrition problem because of their previous heavy alcohol intake and consequent dietary indiscretions. These patients are frequently undernourished and have vitamin deficiencies when an oropharyngeal malignancy develops, and malnutrition is increased if the cancer produces obstruction or pain on eating. Nutritional assessment becomes particularly important in this group, and the intensity of preoperative nutritional replenishment must be carefully matched to the degree of malnutrition and the magnitude of anticipated oncologic therapy (8).

Thirty-nine malnourished patients required IVH to complete a planned course of radiotherapy (6,7). Radiation therapy to the gastrointestinal tract had resulted in severe and dose-limiting acute radiation enteritis or stomatitis. These patients ingested almost no food and were unable to digest and absorb those few nutrients that did reach the small intestine. IVH was used for an average of 37.6 days, and the average weight gain was 7.8 lb. Anorexia, nausea, and vomiting disappeared during IVH unless the patients attempted to eat, in which case all symptoms recurred. The average dose of radiotherapy delivered during IVH was 3,827 rads in an average of 3.5 weeks. Ninety-five percent of the patients completed the planned course of radiotherapy and improved symptomatically. Fifty-four percent responded with a greater than 50% reduction in tumor size. Those patients responding to radiotherapy were able to maintain the weight gained during IVH after it was discontinued, but nonresponding patients promptly lost weight. Responding patients gained an average of $13.0 \pm 6.5$ lb during IVH and radiotherapy, whereas nonresponding patients gained only $4.9 \pm 8.8$ lb during a similar treatment course. Serum albumin rose from 3.1 g/100 ml to 3.5 g/100 ml during treatment of responding patients, but did not rise significantly from 3.1 g/100 ml in nonresponding patients. Intravenous hyperalimentation allowed a planned course of radiation therapy to be delivered to a group of poor-risk, malnourished cancer patients. Symptoms of radiation stomatitis and enteritis were reduced or eliminated as long as bowel rest was maintained, and a correlation between tumor response and improvement in nutritional status was identified.

Twenty-four cachectic patients with enterocutaneous fistulas were treated with IVH. Such fistulas presented unique problems because they often involved areas of irradiated bowel or abdominal wall or the patient's life expectancy was considered so short that the referring physician did not think the time required to treat the fistulas was justified. Nevertheless, 44% of the fistulas closed spontaneously and 28% were successfully closed surgically. Those patients in whom fistula closure was achieved returned home and were able to lead productive lives for at least a short period of time. In two patients, spontaneous fistula closure occurred even though gastrointestinal cancer was present in biopsy specimens from the fistula tract.

Our results for spontaneous closure of enteric fistulas arising from irradiated bowel were uniformly poor (7). Although spontaneous closure was achieved in several patients, each fistula eventually reopened, and the patient died or required operation. We recommend that patients who have radiation-related fistulas of the gastrointestinal tract be considered surgical candidates and, if malnourished, be prepared for an appropriate surgical procedure by administration of IVH for 10 to 21 days preoperatively to stimulate anabolism and weight gain.

Attempts at enteral nutritional repletion failed in 28 patients who required admission to the hospital specifically for IVH. The gastrointestinal tract was functional in more than half of these patients; nevertheless, they had little desire to eat and were often depressed. Seventeen patients had received prior chemotherapy or radiation therapy as outpatients and were unable to recover from the inanition that occurred during treament. Seven patients had not recovered sufficiently from a major abdominal surgical procedure before their hospital discharge, and could not regain their weight on an outpatient dietary regimen. Each of these patients improved symptomatically during IVH and was released from the hospital on an enteral diet after an average of 13.4 days of IVH. The vicious cycle of malnutrition, anorexia, and further malnutrition had been interrupted by nutritional replenishment with IVH, and psychological support relieved much of the depression initially identified in these patients. Possibly the gastrointestinal digestive and absorptive processes were improved along with nutritional state; it is even more likely that the patients were psychologically better motivated to eat because of improvement in strength and general well-being. In anorectic cancer patients, Russ and DeWys (28) have correlated taste abnormalities with malnutrition, and a better appetite might have been a manifestation of an improvement in taste sensation. Nevertheless, anorexia disappeared, hunger returned, and patients noted an improvement in general well-being and looked forward to meals.

## NUTRITION AND IMMUNOLOGY

Cancer and malnutrition are thought to be singularly immunosuppressive. Anesthesia, operative treatment, radiation therapy, and chemotherapy also can depress host immunocompetence. The relative extent to which malnutrition contributes to immune incompetency during oncologic therapy is unknown. Cancer patients who are immunologically incompetent have been shown to have a poor response to radiation therapy and chemotherapy and to have an abbreviated disease-free interval. The response of the immune system to the effects of chemotherapy is both dose- and time-related. Intensive intermittent drug therapy, for example, has been shown by Hersh et al. (20) to be less immunosuppressive and more oncolytic than continuous chemotherapy. The nutritional status of patients in these studies was not reported. Hersh and his group did suggest that recovery of the host immune response and regression of cancer might be related in a cause-and-effect manner, and that this relationship might be responsible for prolonged survival in patients who were immunologically competent. Those patients who received intermittent chemotherapy may have maintained a better nutritional status, which may have contributed to the competency of the immune system.

Chronic protein deprivation appears to depress T-cell-mediated cellular immunity more than humoral immunity of B-cell origin. Experimentally, we showed that nutritional deprivation depressed *in vivo* skin-test reactivity and that nutritional restoration resulted in weight gain and return of skin-test reactivity to normal (11). In similar animal models, Floyd et al. (17) recently reported that malnutrition also inhibits lymphocyte function *in vitro* and that this function can be restored by proper nutritional replenishment. Haffejee and Angorn (18) studied 20 patients with carcinoma of the esophagus and found that nutritional replenishment with reversal of negative nitrogen balance resulted in a significant increase in total lymphocyte counts, percent of T-lymphocytes, and blastogenic response to PHA prior to therapeutic reduction in tumor bulk. Harvey et al. (19) studied 68 sequential cancer patients receiving nutritional therapy and found that 84% of those who initially had negative skin-test reactions became immunocompetent and had a significantly lower complication rate than did patients who were initially immunocompetent and became anergic. Thus, attempts to improve and maintain host immune function in cancer patients seem justified.

In an attempt to define the contribution of malnutrition to the suppression of immunocompetence associated with malignant disease and with oncologic therapy, 160 patients who were malnourished or whose treatment would ordinarily result in malnutrition were tested with a battery of five recall skin-test antigens at 10- to 14-day intervals throughout antineoplastic therapy and nitritional rehabilitation with IVH (12). Skin tests were read 48 hours after intradermal injection and a reaction to any one of the five antigens consisting of 10 mm of induration was considered a positive result. Originally negative tests were interpreted as having converted to positive if at least 10 mm of induration existed at one or more antigen sites and a 100% increase in the diameter of induration was obtained compared to the pre-IVH reaction. Ninety patients initially had negative reactions to the battery of five recall skin-test antigens; 51% of these patients converted at least one skin-test reaction to positive. Seventy patients initially were positive reactors, and 85% of these remained so throughout nutritional and oncologic treatment.

Forty-five of 76 chemotherapy patients were initially negative reactors, and 25 (56%) converted their skin-test reactions to positive in an average of 18.8 ± 2.5 days of IVH. Patients whose skin tests converted to positive received IVH for a total of 30.4 ± 3.3 days, whereas patients who remained skin-test negative received IVH for an average of 26.2 ± 3.9 days. A response to chemotherapy was obtained in 38% of evaluable patients who maintained positive reactions or converted from negative to positive. Only 20% of patients whose skin-test reactions remained negative or converted from positive to negative had a tumor response to chemotherapy. However, there was no significant difference in tumor response rate between patients whose tests remained negative, remained positive, or converted from negative to positive. The uneven distribution of tumor sites and histologic morphologies in these three groups eliminated any statistically significant correlation between sequential skin-test results, response to chemotherapy, weight gain, or increase in serum albumin concentration. Nevertheless, no patient whose skin-test reactions converted from positive to negative had a tumor response to chemotherapy.

In the surgery group, skin tests for 36 patients remained positive or converted from negative to positive. Twenty-five percent of these patients had a significant postoperative complication. In 13 patients, skin test reactions remained negative or converted from positive to negative during IVH. Nine of these 13 patients (69%) had significant postoperative complications, and seven died, most of an overwhelming infection. Thus, there was a significant increase in morbidity and mortality among patients whose skin-test reactions remained negative or converted from positive to negative, compared to patients whose skin tests remained positive or converted from negative to positive.

Of the 20 patients in the radiation therapy group, skin-test reactions for nine failed to convert from negative to positive or to remain positive during radiotherapy. These patients were usually receiving radiation therapy to T-cell-bearing areas, such as the thymus or large areas of bone marrow, and the number or efficacy of circulating T-lymphocytes that are responsible for delayed cutaneous hypersensitivity may have been reduced. Although positive skin-test reactivity was often difficult to achieve in this group, there were few complications secondary to radiotherapy, and nutritional rehabilitation was considered adequate. In the 15 patients who received IVH for nutritional supportive care, 56% of the negative reactors converted to positive reactors in an average of 11.6 days of IVH and gained an average of 5.8 lb during this time. For patients whose skin-test responses remained or converted to positive during treatment with IVH, subsequent oncologic therapy was usually uncomplicated.

Intravenous hyperalimentation was responsible for nutritional repletion in each of these 160 patients, and was probably responsible for, or at the very least was associated with, return of positive skin-test reactivity in most negative reactors. Radiotherapy, certain chemotherapeutic drugs, and the physiologic events associated with anesthesia and operative intervention may be immunosuppressive; nevertheless, this study indicates that at least a portion of the immune depression associated with antineoplastic therapy is secondary to malnutrition and is not necessarily the result of a direct suppressor effect on the immune system by the oncologic treatment regimen or by a circulating substance liberated by the neoplasm. The report on these 160 patients represents an expansion of a study of 47 patients recently evaluated to determine the effect of IVH on established cell-mediated immunity in the cancer patient (35). The following conclusions of the initial study remain justified and consistent with the additional patient information: (a) immune depression attributed to chemotherapy may, in part, be secondary to malnutrition; (b) skin-test reactivity, in general, was depressed during radiation therapy, even though nutrition was estimated to be adequate; and (c) surgical patients with negative skin-test reactions had significantly greater postoperative morbidity and mortality than patients with positive skin tests.

## CONCLUSIONS

Brennan (1) postulates that cancer patients are less well adapted to respond to the added insult of starvation than are noncancer patients. Normal homeostatic mechanisms exist to conserve lean tissue mass and total body protein. The cancer patient seems less able to use these lean tissue-conserving mechanisms and to decrease gluconeogenesis from protein stores in the presence of starvation. Thus, Brennan postulates that the loss of lean tissue mass continues unabated in the malnourished cancer patient. He agrees, however, that these observations in the tumor-bearing host are inevitably compounded by decreases in intake and a decrease in the efficient use of ingested nutrients. Theologides (33) is a proponent of the theory that cancers produce peptides and other small molecules that modify the activity of host enzymes that in turn, modulate the metabolism of many compounds potentially responsible for maintenance of host nutritional homeostasis. We continue to believe that most cases of malnutrition encountered in cancer patients are secondary to a decrease in nutritional intake related to the anatomical location of the neoplasm or to the adverse gastrointestinal or general systemic effects of oncologic therapy. Certainly our explanation seems plausible in mammalian species with small volumes of malignant tissue. Daly et al. (13) recently reported the effects of nutritional repletion of malnourished rats with small (5% carcass weight) or large (25% carcass weight) tumor burdens. The presence of a small tumor did not affect protein repletion in host liver or muscle when an adequate diet was provided, whereas the presence of a large tumor significantly inhibited host nutritional replenishment. In human beings, our experience has been that patients with small tumor burdens are nutritionally replenished rapidly when supplied with adequate building blocks in the form of amino acids, minerals, vitamins, and glucose. Studies by Nixon et al. (25) in patients with advanced cancer indicate that there is a retardation of nutritional repletion in patients with large tumor burdens. The data of these investigators indicate a block in the repletion of lean body mass but not adipose tissue in advanced cancer patients with protein–calorie malnutrition and suggest that current techniques of IVH cannot be expected to result in rapid nutritional repletion in such patients.

The data obtained in human beings by Nixon and his group (25) are remarkably similar to data obtained in animals with small and large tumor burdens. Once malignant disease has advanced to a certain stage, it may be difficult to achieve adequate nutritional replenishment with any techniques currently available. Repletion becomes almost impossible when cachexia is superimposed on a history of multiple courses of chemotherapy and maximally tolerated doses of radiation therapy. There are, however, terminal cancer patients who will respond to treatment with IVH with improvement in weight and a feeling of general well-being. Occasionally our group has begun IVH only to find that the patient has a metastatic malignant process for which there is no remaining treatment. In such a situation, we attempt to nourish the patient by enteral means and discontinue IVH. Forced enteral nutritional replenishment of terminal cancer patients has been reported to improve the quality of remaining life, and our group has made similar observations using IVH in patients with metastatic malignant disease who are not extremely cachectic and have not received multiple courses of chemotherapy or radiation therapy. We continue, however, to recommend that IVH not be used for patients who have been treated with all possible modalities of oncologic therapy and are dying of the combined effects of malnutrition and progressive cancer growth. These patients' nutritional state should be maintained as adequately as possible using all available enteral diets, but at present IVH is not often indicated. Prolongation of pain for the patient and anguish for the family do not seem to justify the use of IVH in cancer patients.

For those patients in whom oncologic therapy is a reality, cancer cachexia should no longer be a contraindication to treatment. Adequate nutritional replenishment should be undertaken prior to the indicated antineoplastic therapy. Attention to proper metabolic, physiologic, and nutritional repletion and maintenance can minimize the complications from all modalities of oncologic therapy. An enlightened approach to the management of the malnourished cancer patient is to rehabilitate him nutritionally with intravenous hyperalimentation before, during, and/or after all forms of therapy whenever this goal cannot be accomplished by enteral means. Nutritional repletion has resulted in a return of immunocompetence and has been associated with a reduction in sepsis and proper wound healing, and possibly with an increase in tumor response to chemotherapy. If these observations are related as cause and effect, then a method of restoring and maintaining adequate nutrition should be added to the armamentarium of the oncologist.

## REFERENCES

1. Brennan, M. F. (1977): Uncomplicated starvation versus cancer cachexia. *Cancer Res.,* 37:2359–2364.
2. Cameron, I. L., and Pavlat, W. A. (1976): Stimulation of growth of a transplantable hepatoma in rats by parenteral nutrition. *J. Natl. Cancer Inst.,* 56:597–602.
3. Copeland, E. M., MacFadyen, B. V., Jr., McGown, C., and Dudrick, S. J. (1974): The use of hyperalimentation in patients with potential sepsis. *Surg. Gynecol. Obstet.,* 138:377–380.
4. Copeland, E. M., MacFadyen, B. V., Jr., Lanzotti, V., and Dudrick, S. J. (1975): Intravenous hyperalimentation as an adjunct to cancer chemotherapy. *Am. J. Surg.,* 129:167–173.
5. Copeland, E. M., MacFadyen, B. V., Jr., and Dudrick, S. J. (1976): Effect of intravenous hyperalimentation on established delayed hypersensitivity in the cancer patient. *Ann. Surg.,* 184:60–64.
6. Copeland, E. M., and Dudrick, S. J. (1976): Nutritional aspects of cancer. *Curr. Probl. Cancer,* 1:1–51.
7. Copeland, E. M., Souchon, E. A., MacFadyen, B. V., Rapp, M. A., and Dudrick, S. J. (1977): Intravenous hyperalimentation as an adjunct to radiation therapy. *Cancer,* 39:609–616.
8. Copeland, E. M., Daly, J. M., and Dudrick, S. J. (1979): Nutritional concepts in the treatment of head and neck malignancies. *Head Neck Surg.,* 1:350–363.
9. Daly, J. M., Reynolds, H. M., Rowlands, B. J., Baquero, G. E., Dudrick, S. J., and Copeland, E. M. (1978): Nutritional manipulation of tumor-bearing animals: Effects on body weight, serum protein levels, and tumor growth. *Surg. Forum,* 29:143–144.

10. Daly, J. M., Copeland, E. M., and Dudrick, S. J. (1978): Effects of intravenous nutrition on tumor growth and host immunocompetence in malnourished animals. *Surgery,* 84:655–658.
11. Daly, J. M., Dudrick, S. J., and Copeland, E. M. (1978): Effects of protein depletion and repletion on cell-mediated immunity in experimental animals. *Ann. Surg.,* 188:791–796.
12. Daly, J. M., Dudrick, S. J., and Copeland, E. M. (1980): Intravenous hyperalimentation: Effect on immunocompetence in cancer patients. *Ann. Surg.,* 192:587–592.
13. Daly, J. M., Copeland, E. M., Dudrick, S. J., and Delaney, J. M. (1980): Nutritional repletion of malnourished tumor-bearing and non-tumor bearing rats: Effects on body weight, liver, muscle and tumor. *J. Surg. Res.,* 28:507–518.
14. DeWys, W. D., and Kisner, D. (1979): Maintaining caloric needs in the cancer patient. *Contemp. Surg.,* 15:25–30.
15. Dionigi, R., Guaglio, R., Bonera, A., Cerri, M., Rondanelli, R., and Campani, M. (1979): Clinical–pharmacological aspects, application and effectiveness of total parenteral nutrition in surgical patients. *Int. J. Clin. Pharmacol. Biopharm.,* 17:107–118.
16. Filler, R. M., Jaffe, N., Cassady, J. R., Traggis, D. G., and Das, J. B. (1977): Parenteral nutritional support in children with cancer. *Cancer,* 39:2665–2669.
17. Floyd, C., Ota, D., Corriere, J. N., Dudrick, S. J., and Copeland, E. M. (1979): Effect of protein depletion on serum factors for lymphocyte transformation. *Surg. Forum,* 30:57–60.
18. Haffejee, A. A., and Angorn, I. B. (1979): Nutritional status and the nonspecific cellular and humoral immune response in esophageal carcinoma. *Ann. Surg.,* 189:475–479.
19. Harvey, K. B., Bothe, A., and Blackburn, G. L. (1979): Nutritional assessment and patient outcome during oncologic therapy. *Cancer,* 43:2065–2069.
20. Hersh, E. M., Whitecar, J. P., McCredie, K. B., Bodey, G. P., and Freireich, E. J. (1971): Chemotherapy, immunocompetence, immunosuppression, and prognosis in acute leukemia. *N. Engl. J. Med.,* 285:1212–1216.
21. Issell, B. F., Valdivieso, M., Zaren, H. A., Dudrick, S. J., Freireich, E. J., Copeland, E. M., and Bodey, G. P. (1978): Protection against chemotherapy toxicity by IV hyperalimentation. *Cancer Treat. Rep.,* 62:1139–1143.
22. Lanzotti, V. C., Copeland, E. M., George, S. L., Dudrick, S. J., and Samuels, M. L. (1975): Cancer chemotherapeutic response and intravenous hyperalimentation. *Cancer Chemother. Rep.,* 59:437–439.
23. Mertin, J., and Hughes, T. (1975): Specific inhibitory action of polyunsaturated fatty acids on lymphocyte transformation induced by PHA and PPD. *Int. Arch. Allergy Appl. Immunol.,* 48:203–208.
24. Moertel, C. G., Schutt, A. J., Hahn, R. G., and Reitemeier, R. J. (1974): Effects of patient selection on results of phase II chemotherapy trials in gastrointestinal cancer. *Cancer Chemother. Rep.,* 58:257–260.
25. Nixon, D., Rudman, D., Heymefield, S., Ansley, J., and Kutner, M. (1979): Abnormal hyperalimentation response in cachectic cancer patients. *Proc. Am. Assoc. Cancer Res.,* 20:173.
26. Ota, D. M., Copeland, E. M., Corriere, J. N., Ritchie, E., Jacobson, K., and Dudrick, S. J. (1978): The effects of a 10% soybean oil emulsion on lymphocyte transformation. *J. Parent. Ent. Nutr.,* 2:112–115.
27. Reynolds, H. M., Daly, J. M., Rowlands, B. J., Dudrick, S. J., and Copeland, E. M. (1980): Effects of nutritional repletion on host and tumor response to chemotherapy. *Cancer,* 45:3069–3074.
28. Russ, J., and DeWys, W. D. (1977): Correction of taste abnormality of malignancy with intravenous hyperalimentation. *Arch. Intern. Med.,* 138:799–803.
29. Seniukov, M. V., Khmelevskii, I. M., Zubov, O. G., Sloventantor, V. I., and Kaplan, N. A. (1978): Parenteral feeding of patients with cancer of the larynx undergoing combination therapy. *Vestn. Otorhinolaryngol.,* 2:66–72.
30. Solassol, C., and Joyeux, H. (1980): Artificial gut with complete nutritive mixtures as a major adjuvant therapy in cancer patient's treatment. Proceedings of the International Society of Parenteral Nutrition, Rio de Janiero, Brazil, August 28, 1979. *Acta Chir. Scand.,* Suppl. 494, 186–188.
31. Souchon, E. A., Copeland, E. M., Watson, P., and Dudrick, S. J. (1975): Intravenous hyperalimentation as an adjunct to cancer chemotherapy with 5-fluorouracil. *J. Surg. Res.,* 18:451–454.
32. Steiger, E., Oram-Smith, J., Miller, E., Kuo, L., and Voss, H. M. (1975): Effects of nutrition on tumor growth and tolerance to chemotherapy. *J. Surg. Res.,* 18:455–461.

33. Theologides, A. (1979): Cancer cachexia. *Cancer,* 43:2004–2012.
34. Wilmore, D. W., and Dudrick, S. J. (1969): Safe long-term venous catheterization. *Arch. Surg.,* 98:256–258.
35. van Eys, J. (1979): Malnutrition in children with cancer: Incidence and consequence. *Cancer,* 43:2030–2035.

*Nutrition and Cancer: Etiology and Treatment,*
edited by G. R. Newell and N. M. Ellison.
Raven Press, New York © 1981.

# Malnutrition in Pediatric Oncology

## Jan van Eys

*The University of Texas System Cancer Center, M. D. Anderson Hospital and Tumor
Institute, Houston, Texas 77030*

Nutrition in pediatric oncology is separate from the general problems encountered in the interrelationships between nutrition and cancer. Many of the factors of diet and dietary contaminants in the etiology of adult cancer pertain only in a very special way to the pediatric age group. Many of these factors require prolonged exposure before the harmful effect is realized. Therefore, such putative oncogens must begin their effect at the very early formative moments when teratogenesis and oncogenesis are most marked. One deals, therefore, with the physiology of placental transfer. In the search for the etiology of pediatric cancer, genetic factors loom relatively large, probably because age and environmental exposure do not overshadow the contribution of genetics. The primary problem in pediatric oncology, therefore, is that of malnutrition.

Cancer in children is quantitatively and qualitatively different from cancer in adults. It is quantitatively different because the overall incidence is lower, and because the relative incidence of various cancers is unique among children. Leukemia ranks first in incidence, with central nervous system malignancies second. Among solid tumors, sarcomas predominate, whereas carcinomas are rare (Table 1) (41). The diseases are qualitatively different because many are peculiarly pediatric. Wilms' tumor, neuroblastoma, and childhood null-cell acute lymphocytic leukemia are almost exclusively limited to the pediatric age range.

Childhood cancer is, however, not rare, and one in 600 children will be affected. Since our current cure rate approximates 60%, in a few years, one in 1,000 young adults will have had cancer as a child (31). The course of cancer, its treatment, and the side-effects of such treatment are enormous public health concerns. This chapter will deal primarily with the effect of nutrition on the course of cancer in childhood. Because childhood cancer care is in a state of rapid evolution, no summary will be given of the current mode of therapy for specific diseases, since such a summary would be out of date before this book is in print. It is sufficient to point out that much of the success of pediatric cancer care is the result of chemotherapy. Children have tumors that are chemotherapy-sensitive, and they tolerate chemotherapy better than do adults. Cancer cure in children can be achieved by chemotherapy only, as demonstrated for acute lymphocytic leukemia (23).

TABLE 1. *Relative frequency of major histologic categories of malignant neoplasms in the United States for children under 15 years of age*[a]

| Histologic Category | White | | Black | |
|---|---|---|---|---|
| | Rank order | Percent of total | Rank order | Percent of total |
| Leukemia | 1 | 33.8 | 1 | 24.9 |
| Central nervous system | 2 | 19.2 | 2 | 24.4 |
| Lymphoma | 3 | 10.6 | 3 | 14.2 |
| Sympathetic nervous system | 4 | 7.7 | 5 | 7.1 |
| Soft-tissue sarcoma | 5 | 6.8 | 7 | 4.0 |
| Kidney tumors | 6 | 6.3 | 4 | 8.0 |
| Bone tumors | 7 | 4.5 | 6 | 4.9 |
| Retinoblastima | 8 | 2.7 | 8 | 3.1 |
| Gonadal and germ cell tumors | 9 | 1.8 | 9 | 2.7 |
| Liver tumors | 10 | 1.5 | 10 | 0.4 |
| Teratoma | 11 | 0.3 | 11 | 0.4 |
| Miscellaneous | — | 4.9 | — | 5.8 |

[a] Adapted from Sutow, (41).

Much of chemotherapy is nutritional therapy (46). Chemotherapeutic agents are often antimetabolites to dietary elements, the best example being the antifolate methotrexate. Nevertheless, the problem of nutrition and cancer in children is still very basic. Malnutrition is very common, especially in children with metastatic or recurrent disease. Morbidity and mortality from malnutrition is a serious problem. We must view nutrition as a basic problem and not one hopelessly intertwined with cancer.

## ASSESSMENT OF THE NUTRITIONAL STATE IN CHILDHOOD

The nutritional status of children is a major public health preoccupation. Major national decisions rest on the assertions of whether given population groups are adequately or inappropriately fed. To this end, survey methodology that can assess nutritional status with simple clinical, anthropometric, and clinical laboratory parameters has been developed. Such methodology must be simple so that large population groups can be evaluated by paramedical personnel. Samples of body fluids must either be amenable to laboratory testing under field conditions or they must be transportable to a central laboratory.

Public health information was obtained from such surveys. In addition, some insight into nutritional status, as diagnosable from survey methodology, was gained. However, such surveys largely ignored concomitant diseases in the survey population. The ten-state nutrition survey spent little time on the effect of various disease stages on the obtained information (22,26). Even more limited surveys with a specific population in mind rarely assumed that the subset of surveyed populations might have peculiar diseases. The survey of the Navajo Indian children is a specific case in point (12).

Alternately, the survey was conceived as a method of testing an *a priori* hypothesis of the relationship of a specific abnormality to the lack of adequate nutrition. Investigation of the relationship between nutrition and mental development is a classical example of such research. There are ample data correlating clinical, biochemical, and developmental parameters of specific nutrients and their related deficiency diseases. Since "pure" single-nutrient malnutrition is very rare indeed, the data of micronutrient assays are usable in overall nutritional evaluation, but their expense and degree of complexity have precluded large-scale survey applications.

The current interest in the relationship between diet, nutrition, and cancer has suddenly created a recognition of a void in knowledge that is all the more surprising because the void was assumed not to exist. There are very few data on medical parameters that allow general early malnutrition to be diagnosed before it becomes clinically obvious. Almost all information assumes that malnutrition can be diagnosed, and uses such assumptions to ascertain the extent of the problem. When one is dealing with a basically healthy (i.e., nondiseased) approximation, this is possible (60), but the parameters used are sketchy. When the subset of population to be surveyed is a group of children with cancer, there are absolutely no data that guarantee that parameters used for healthy children are applicable to the child with cancer. Utilization of the parameters used for healthy children are open to question.

### Effects of Growth and Development

The specific standards for assessing the nutritional state of children are complicated by the child's growth and development (60). Definitions of malnutrition in adulthood are usually based on weight loss. This standard cannot be used for children because a lag in expected growth may be the only early sign of protein–calorie inadequacy. Unfortunately, serial observations are not always available. Calorie requirements do vary widely with age. Table 2 shows the recommended daily allowance for calories and protein with increasing age (32). Furthermore, anthropometric measurements of muscle mass, triceps skinfold, midarm circumference, and other measures have few standard values for children below certain ages. The effect of growth is therefore one of relative increased requirements and poor standards. In children who have cancer, there is the further tendency to think that height and weight are proportionately changing when the disease process or the degree of food intake limits further growth; however, this is not true (53) (Fig. 1).

Additional complications are the different norms for biochemical parameters that pertain to children, as compared to those for adults. There is still a major need for nutritional descriptive research to set standards for normal children. This is specifically different from applying preconceived standards to normal children, as is done in surveys. The Department of Agriculture has instituted

TABLE 2. *Food and Nutrition Board, National Academy of Sciences–National Research Council: recommended daily dietary allowances*

|  | Age (years) | Weight (kg) | Height (cm) | Energy (kcal) | Protein g |
|---|---|---|---|---|---|
| Infants | 0.0–0.5 | 6 | 60 | kg × 117 | kg × 2.2 |
|  | 0.5–1.0 | 9 | 71 | kg × 108 | kg × 2.0 |
| Children | 1–3 | 13 | 86 | 1,300 | 23 |
|  | 4–6 | 20 | 110 | 1,800 | 30 |
|  | 7–10 | 30 | 135 | 2,400 | 36 |
| Male | 11–14 | 44 | 158 | 2,800 | 44 |
|  | 15–18 | 61 | 172 | 3,000 | 54 |
|  | 19–22 | 67 | 172 | 3,000 | 54 |
|  | 23–50 | 70 | 172 | 2,700 | 56 |
|  | 51+ | 70 | 172 | 2,400 | 56 |
| Female | 11–14 | 44 | 155 | 2,400 | 44 |
|  | 15–18 | 54 | 162 | 2,100 | 48 |
|  | 19–22 | 58 | 162 | 2,100 | 46 |
|  | 23–50 | 58 | 162 | 2,000 | 46 |
|  | 51+ | 58 | 162 | 1,800 | 46 |

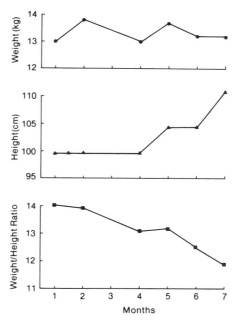

**FIG. 1.** Weight and height in a child with neuroblastoma, who received intensive chemotherapy with little response. His weight remained stable but he experienced significant linear growth, resulting in objective criteria for severe malnutrition. From van Eys, ref. 53, with permission.

human nutrition laboratories, one of which is devoted to the study of human infant nutrition, to establish national standards.

## ASSESSMENT OF MALNUTRITION

### Height and Weight Standards

The eighth report of the FAO/WHO Expert Committee on Nutrition (30) emphasized the importance of measurements of height as well as weight. It was thought that the extent of height deficit in relation to age could be regarded as a measure of the duration of malnutrition. More important, the expression of weight-for-height gives a measure of the nutritional status, which is, to a degree, independent of age and age-related external standards. With regard to height, one could consider weight-for-height an index for current nutritional status. The standards used for weight-for-height are usually derived from the health examination survey data from the National Center for Health Statistics (28). The data have recently been updated (27).

The adequacy of a patient's nutrition is best expressed by a quantitative number that is the percent of weight-for-height of the 50th percentile for age (57). Eighty percent of the 50th percentile can be used as the cutoff point of severe and overt malnutrition. With such data, a graph can be constructed illustrating

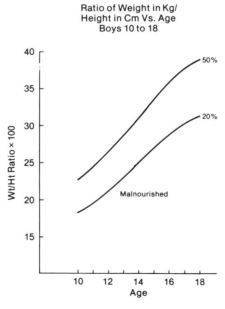

**FIG. 2.** Height and weight charts for age. The line for malnutrition reports the 80% of the 50th percentile mark. From van Eys, ref. 53, with permission.

the relationship of weight-for-height versus age, and the definition of malnutrition. As will be illustrated later, there is a relationship between this percentage of the 50th percentile and the relative nutritional state. No standards exist to utilize this measure for the diagnosis of marginal malnutrition, although the weight–height ratio and skinfold thickness correlate well with socioeconomic class (22). Thus, the relationship of weight-for-height and nutritional state is not quantized but is a continuum.

### Biochemical Parameters

There is no biochemical parameter or group of parameters that can be used to assess individual malnutrition. Children have higher nutrient requirements than do adults, when expressed per unit of body weight. Therefore, stores are more readily exhausted, and deficiencies quickly become apparent. However, the majority of malnutrition is global malnutrition, in which individual nutrients are rarely uniquely deficient. Although there is value in determining micronutrients, these by themselves are static measures of a process. Therefore, the relationships between degree of malnutrition and degree of measured abnormality are not simple.

In general, three biochemical measures are used for childhood nutrition evaluation: serum albumin, serum iron, iron-binding capacity, and percent saturation. These measures are refined by the measurment of transferrin. Serum amino acids are used to assess protein malnutrition.

The most reliable and common indicator of protein inadequacy is the measure of serum albumin. Normal values depend on age, and as a strict definition of value, 3.0 g/dl is usually taken as evidence of malnutrition. This is a strict criterion, and marginal inadequacy probably exists when the patient is below 3.5 g/dl. Interestingly, there is no clear relationship between the weight-for-height ratio and serum albumin in children with cancer (16,42). This must indicate that malnutrition in children with cancer is primarily calorie and not protein–calorie malnutrition.

The deficiency of any blood component is a balance of synthesis and loss. To use a biochemical parameter as a measure of nutrition implies that insufficient substance is available for synthesis. Serum albumin is significantly susceptible to low blood values resulting from excessive renal or serosal surface loss; however, a well-nourished patient is frequently able to compensate for this loss in serum albumin. In cases in which hypoalbuminemia with third-space loss is present, there is clearly inadequacy of albumin biosynthesis as well as excessive loss. Until proved otherwise, malnutrition is a factor in such instances.

Iron is generally designated as the most freuently observed specific nutritional deficiency in North America (59). The diagnosis of iron deficiency is simple in principle. Serum iron, serum transferrin saturation, and the measurement of serum ferritin (the storage form of iron) will document the biochemical iron deficiency seen with iron-deficiency anemia. The use of hypochromic anemia as a measure in the child with cancer is somewhat dangerous. Anemia can arise secondary to marrow invasion or a chemotherapeutically induced marrow depression, so that anemia per se does not indicate iron deficiency. Furthermore, many patients with malignant disease have had frequent transfusions, again negating the direct relationship of serum hemoglobin concentrations and iron status. There are other reasons for hypochromic anemia, the most common in children being lead poisoning and thalassemia syndromes. In a specific well infant, the best measure of iron deficiency is a clinical response to iron; however, in an acute single-evaluation setting, this is not practical. Since iron deficiency is so common in the general population, it is a necessary evaluation in the child with cancer, but it does not specifically point to a direct relationship between this form of malnutrition and the presence of cancer. However, iron deficiency is aggravated by gastrointestinal loss. This is seen in the general population because of gastrointestinal reaction to cows' milk. In many instances, a protein-losing enteropathy develops in children with malignant diseases. Under such circumstances, gastrointestinal iron loss is also aggravated. Finally, there is significant blood loss in the child with cancer as the result of our diagnostic zeal. Therefore, iron is not directly reliable as a measure of overall protein-calorie nutrition.

Data for normal subjects in hemoglobin and selected iron-related findings have been published by the National Center for Health Statistics (29). The mean levels for hemoglobin, serum iron, and percent transferrin saturation were collected from the Health and Nutrition Examination Survey (HANES).

Serum amino acid levels change in the development of protein–energy malnutrition. In severe protein–energy malnutrition, the total plasma amino acid concentration may be reduced to half the normal value. This is especially true for the essential amino acids, most markedly so in the case of branched-chain amino acids and free amine. Lysine and phenylalanine are somewhat less affected. Alanine, on the other hand, may be elevated in early kwashiorkor. It has been suggested that the serum amino acid pattern can be used to quantitate malnutrition. The ratio of the sum of lysine, serine, glutamine, and taurine over the sum of valine, leucine, isoleucine, and methionine could be used to characterize early malnutrition. In normal children, the mean value is around 1.5, whereas in subclinical malnutrition the values range between 2.0 and 4.0; in frank kwashiorkor, they are higher yet. However, the amino acid pattern is much less affected by energy starvation without a low protein/carbohydrate ratio. Since in children with cancer the protein malnutrition is least striking, the serum amino acid patterns may not be applicable to the state of cancer and malnutrition. The subject of amino acid patterns in malnutrition has been reviewed extensively by Alleyne et al (1).

## Other Anthropometric Measurements

The anthropometric measurements generally used in adults are the triceps skinfold to evaluate fat stores, the arm muscle circumference, and creatinine–height index to evaluate lean body mass. As mentioned before, there simply

TABLE 3. *Total number of patients below 50% RDA*[a]

| | | |
|---|---|---|
| Calories | 11 | 16% |
| Protein | 2 | 3% |
| Vitamin A | 10 | 15% |
| Thiamin | 5 | 7% |
| Riboflavin | 4 | 6% |
| Niacin | 7 | 10% |
| Vitamin C | 5 | 7% |
| Calcium | 13 | 19% |
| Phosphorus | 4 | 6% |
| Iron | 15 | 22% |

[a] The numbers reflect percent of patients of the total sample of patients
surveyed.

are not enough standards to utilize these measures for children with cancer, at the present time.

### Dietary History

The usual concept is that dietary histories are unreliable. They are indeed so for precise evaluation of the intake of specific nutrients. However, for gross evaluation of dietary intake of calories and major nutrients, the dietary history is a valid approach to assessment. In our experience, there is a high correlation between the physical parameters and the dietary history. Table 3 indicates the results of an evaluation of children with newly diagnosed cancer. It confirms the anthropometric and biochemical observation that the primary deficiency in intake is in calories and iron rather than protein. The accuracy of dietary history has been greatly helped by the development through the Diet, Nutrition, and Cancer Program of specific dietary diaries and programming to translate the actual diary into food intake.

## THE CONSEQUENCE OF MALNUTRITION IN CHILDREN

### Kwashiorkor and Marasmus

The primary consequence of severe protein–energy malnutrition is a pair of syndromes that are generally called kwashiorkor and marasmus. In addition, there is a mixed presentation, usually designated as marasmic kwashiorkor. Kwashiorkor is found predominantly in older infants and young children whose requirements for protein and energy have not been met for a prolonged period of time. These children are apathetic, irritable, weak, and inactive. They often have peripheral edema and an enlarged fatty liver. There is almost always a weight deficit. They may be hypothermic, and there are changes in the hair and the skin. Low serum albumin and anemia are always present. The skin changes usually involve hypopigmentation, with areas of hyperpigmentation. There is often desquamation of skin. The hair is thin, often sparse, deeply pigmented, dry, and brittle. Marasmus is more likely to be found in infancy and is character-ized by wasting of muscle and subcutaneous tissues, with stunting of growth. Hypothermia, motor retardation, and listlessness are present. The skin changes are not as striking as those found in kwashiorkor. There is, by definition, no edema. The children are irritable and fretful, apathetic, and inactive. The appetite may actually be diminished.

In either disease, once an overt state has been reached, the mortality is high. These children are extremely susceptible to infection, as will be discussed later. The acute calorie deficiency, without a relatively equally severe protein deficiency, will lead to marasmus. Kwashiorkor, on the other hand, is more classically a major protein deficiency. Marasmus is more frequently seen than kwashiorkor in children with malignancies.

## Nutrition and Immunity

The relationship between nutrition and immunity has been reviewed many times. It is clear that this relationship is clinically highly significant. Table 4 illustrates data from observations on pediatric patients with cancer. In this series of patients, all of whom had metastatic disease to and from bone, the number of infections was scored. When the incidence of infections was compared between well-nourished and malnourished patients, there was a highly significant difference, in that 83% of malnourished children had infectious episodes, whereas only 36% of well-nourished children had such episodes (52). The objective evaluation of the consequence of dietary deficiencies on the immune system has been reviewed frequently (24,34,35,39). The interaction of nutrition and infection is seen outside the setting of cancer. The most seriously affected element of immunity is the cell-mediated immune response. It is also important that

TABLE 4. *Presence of infections in children with metastatic cancer*[a]

|  | Infectious Episodes | | |
|  | Yes | No | Total |
| --- | --- | --- | --- |
| Well-nourished | 13 | 23 | 36 |
| Malnourished | 19 | 4 | 23 |
| Total | 32 | 27 | 59 |

[a] The difference between well-nourished and malnourished is sta-tistically significant, with $P < 0.002$. The tabulation represents patients enrolled on a specific chemotherapy protocol. All chemo-therapy protocols were pushed to hematologic toxicity. When an episode of infection was present, it was scored as yes; when no infection occurred, it was scored as no.

iron deficiency may depress bactericidal activity of leukocytes. On the other hand, iron-binding proteins, such as lactoferrin and transferrin, inhibit microbial growth by reducing the availability of iron. Excessive saturation of these proteins with iron will, in fact, cause potentially overwhelming infection. This can be aggravated if transferrin is diminished in a greater degree than is iron. This subject has been extensively reviewed by Pearson and Robinson (33).

There may be a special role for zinc in the development of immune deficiency (24,35). Human zinc deficiency does occur endemically in certain areas of the world. More important, prolonged intravenous hyperalimentation can cause zinc deficiency if not supplemented by that metal.

The association between nutrition and immunity, especially cell-mediated immunity, is so clear that it is customary to use the evaluation of the immune system through skin tests as a measure of nutritional adequacy. In children, this presents difficulties, since they have unformed immune systems, and one cannot be certain that exposure to the common antigens is indeed taking place. Nevertheless, even in children with cancer there is a strong correlation between malnutrition and positive skin tests (43). In adult patients, a circulating peripheral lymphocyte count is also used as a measure of nutritional adequacy. This cannot be used for children with cancer, except during initial evaluations, because therapy itself will severely modify the number of circulating lymphocytes. It must be pointed out, however, that the anamnestic response to antigens to which the host was previously immunized remain after chemotherapy, although the degree of response may be diminished (5,38).

### Malnutrition and Mental Development

There is a complex relationship between nutrition and behavior. As already mentioned, severe protein–calorie malnutrition and nutritional marasmus are associated with behavioral alterations. More important, severe undernutrition in early life can affect structural and biochemical development of the central nervous system (11,58). The current high rate of cure associated with pediatric cancer makes the consideration of defective brain development after malnutrition an extra impetus toward early nutritional intervention.

## MARGINAL MALNUTRITION

### The Problem of Definition

The standards of overt malnutrition are rigidly set; however, there is a state in which the body's reserves are insufficient to cope with the extra demands imposed by serious illness, malignancy, and other stresses, even though biochemical and anthropologic measurements do not support the diagnosis of overt malnutrition. There is, at present, no overt measurement that will enable the objective diagnosis of marginal malnutrition to be made; however, there is a relationship between the number that can be derived from the percent of weight-for-height of the 50th percentile which allows a continuing relationship between nutritional state and outcome. At the present time, there is an intensive effort to evaluate and validate various methodologies for their applicability to pediatric and adult cancer patients. One of the potential areas of evaluation is the immunologic system, which is relatively undeveloped in children but forms a very high percentage of the body economy (53).

### Acute Versus Chronic Onset

Malnutrition in patients with cancer is of relative acute onset. There is, however, one situation in which marginal malnutrition can be diagnosed. Children who were overtly malnourished and who have recently been rehabilitated will have a period during which the criteria for overt malnutrition have disappeared although a marginal malnutrition is still present. It is common experience that after intensive rehabilitation with intravenous hyperalimentation patients will lose weight as soon as the infusion is discontinued, even if there is adequate oral intake of calories.

## MALNUTRITION AND CANCER IN CHILDREN

### Overt Malnutrition

The incidence of overt malnutrition in patients with cancer is significant. It is highest in children who have metastatic or progressive disease (47,48). In children enrolled in a study for evaluation for hyperalimentation, all of whom had tumor metastatic to and from bone, the incidence of malnutrition was in excess of 40% (47,48). Even in newly diagnosed patients, a significant number of children are overtly malnourished (14,16). Our current prospective studies of evaluating all patients corroborate observations. However, malnutrition is not evenly distributed among all patients with cancer. The percentage of malnourished children is highest among those with Ewing's sarcoma and neuroblastoma, whereas in osteosarcoma malnutrition is relatively rare. This was confirmed by evaluating two separate studies, a study of the value of hyperalimentation in children with malignancies to and from bone, and a Southwest Oncology Group study of the use of Adriamycin/DTIC (47,48) (Table 5).

### Marginal Malnutrition

As has already been mentioned, marginal malnutrition cannot be objectively diagnosed. Patients who do not meet the criteria for overt malnutrition may nevertheless become overtly malnourished with very little insult. This is most readily seen in patients in whom overt malnutrition has only recently been reversed. Such patients readily slip back into the malnourished state. This is

TABLE 5. *Effect of diagnosis on nutrition, metastatic pediatric solid tumors*[a]

| Diagnosis | Total | Overtly malnourished |
|---|---|---|
| Neuroblastoma (stage III & IV) | 28 | 15 (53.6%) |
| Ewing's sarcoma | 12 | 6 (50.0%) |
| Wilms' tumor (stage IV or metastatic) | 9 | 6 (66.6%) |
| Gliomas plus retinoblastoma, metastatic | 6 | 3 (50.0%) |
| Osteosarcoma | 9 | 2 (22.2%) |
| Rhabdomyosarcoma | 15 | 2 (13.3%) |
| Other tumors | 21 | 5 (23.8%) |
| Total | 100 | 39 (39.0%) |

[a] From van Eys, (48), with permission.

most frequently observed in patients brought to improved nutritional state with intravenous hyperalimentation, which then is stopped, without stopping the stresses on the body from chemotherapy or other tumor manipulations. If the sudden onset of overt malnutrition is a retrospective clue to past marginal malnutrition, then one can generate predictors of marginal malnutrition in pediatric cancer. These are: (a) when diseases are present that are accompanied by a high incidence of overt malnutrition, such as Ewing's sarcoma and neuroblastoma; (b) when there has been inadequate food intake in the face of active disease; and (c) when there has recently been intensive therapy, such as abdominal irradiation or high doses of systemic chemotherapy (48). It is therefore quite feasible to diagnose marginal malnutrition on clinical grounds. Objective criteria will, we hope, be soon available.

## The Consequences of Malnutrition in Children with Cancer

The consequences of malnutrition in children with cancer are multiple. There is the danger of the development of overt marasmus or kwashiorkor. It has already been mentioned that among the symptoms of protein–energy malnutrition are listlessness and depression. This is an early sign. Malnourished children simply do not feel well. They are listless, depressed, and often uncooperative with parents and medical team alike.

A second major consequence of malnutrition lies, of course, in the depression of the immune system. It has already been mentioned that the incidence of infection is high in malnourished children with cancer, as compared to children who are well nourished.

A third consequence is the poor tolerance to chemotherapy seen in children with malnutrition. It is customary, in studies of new drugs, to divide patients into good- and poor-risk categories on the basis of bone marrow reserve, as evidenced by peripheral blood counts. There is a very high correlation of poor risk with the diseases that have a high risk of nutritional inadequacy, as tabulated in Table 5. Table 6 illustrates this correlation (48).

TABLE 6. *Correlation between chemotherapeutic and nutritional risk*[a]

| | Bone marrow reserve | | |
| --- | --- | --- | --- |
| | Good risk | Poor risk | Total |
| High nutritional risk[b] | 40 | 15 | 55 |
| Minimal nutritional risk[b] | 44 | 1 | 45 |
| Total | 84 | 16 | 100 |

[a] From van Eys, (48), with permission.
[b] High and minimal nutritional risk is defined by the diagnosis as tabulated in Table 3. Those diseases that have a 50% or higher incidence of malnutrition are called "high nutritional risk"; those that have a 25% or lower incidence are called "minimal nutritional risk."

Without being able to pinpoint the direct route by which cause and effect occur, malnutrition is in and of itself a poor prognostic criterion in newly diagnosed cancer patients (16). There was a significant correlation between the number of relapses and the nutritional state, as defined by percent of the 50th percentile weight-for-height; this was most marked in patients who had solid tumors.

## THE ETIOLOGY OF MALNUTRITION IN CHILDREN

All insults related to food intake, food absorption, and assimilation that occur in cancer patients occur in adults as well as in children. In general, the total demand per body surface area is higher in children than it is in adults. Therefore, specific insults manifest themselves more quickly. In addition, a number of phenomena are especially pronounced in pediatric cancer patients.

### Learned Food Aversion

It is easy to demonstrate in animals the phenomenon of learned food aversions. Thus, animals that eat a particular food before receiving radiotherapy will later avoid that food because they associate it with radiation sickness (21). It is possible to demonstrate the same phenomenon in children. Bernstein et al. (3), on evaluating food preferences for each patient receiving chemotherapy, found that aversions to foods in the diet occurred in 44% of the children who received gastrointestinally toxic chemotherapy and in only 7% of the children who received vincristine or no drugs. A controlled experiment, using an unusual ice cream, demonstrated that only 21% of the children would choose the ice cream again if it was given paired with gastrointestinal toxicity, whereas children who had no such toxicity after the first session selected the ice cream in 73% of the cases (2). The very young child, who has not yet experienced all potential food elements that will become common in the diet later, is especially prone to the dangers of learned food aversions during cancer chemotherapy. As yet, this is still a neglected area of management of children.

## Malabsorption

Malabsorption is a serious problem associated with cancer in children. It is most important to remember that malnutrition per se is a cause of malabsorption. Chronic diarrhea is a common accompaniment to malnutrition (1). Supplying adequate amounts of nutrients will return the bowel rapidly to a more normal pattern; however, this may require total parenteral nutrition. Therefore, malnutrition can generate a vicious cycle if this is not recognized.

Certain tumors have a specific association with protein-losing enteropathy. In the pediatric age group, such enteropathy is most often secondary to intestinal lymphoma (54). Neuroblastoma, also, can occasionally cause therapy-resistant diarrhea. In this case, it is not the result of direct involvement of the intestinal tract with tumor, but rather of the distant effect of excessive catecholamine excretion (18).

A major malabsorption problem arises from the effects of therapy. It is simple to show in an animal model that modest amounts of drugs such as methotrexate or 5-fluorouracil have a significant effect on the intestinal mucosa. This is not only morphologically demonstrable but is corroborated by the demonstration that intestinal disaccharidases are rapidly diminished in rats after even a short period of methotrexate treatment (25). This same sensitivity to chemotherapy is quite evident in the human patient. There are, in fact, a number of commonly used chemotherapeutic agents for which gastrointestinal toxicity may be dose-limiting, such toxicity being manifest as anorexia, nausea, vomiting, and mucositis. Children, again, are especially prone to this kind of toxicity (15).

Radiotherapy to the abdomen is also a serious challenge to the ability to absorb. The problem is most accentuated in children. Children as a group tolerate radiotherapy poorly, and their gastrointestinal tracts are no exception (13,15). The main point that must be remembered in malabsorption is that oral intake is not necessarily a measure of absorption and assimilation, nor are the manifestations of malabsorption always the overt signs of gross diarrhea. This is especially true because malabsorption is often coupled with anorexia.

## Anorexia

Anorexia is very frequent indeed in children with cancer. It results from a combination of gastrointestinal toxicity of a variety of drugs, the association of nausea with eating, and the general listlessness and malaise that can occur in malnutrition. Furthermore, many children are, in fact, depressed. Because it is very difficult to diagnose depression objectively in children, it is often overlooked as an etiologic factor in anorexia. Finally, issues about eating are very common in children. The presence of cancer heightens the anxiety of the parents about inadequate food intake. As a result, issues can readily be fought out between the child and the mother who is overfeeding. In the last two years at M. D. Anderson Hospital and Tumor Institute, we have seen one case of anorexia nervosa in a teen-age girl who had a brain tumor, and a case of failure to thrive secondary to maternal deprivation, again superimposed on a brain tumor. All objective evidence demonstrated that the brain tumor was in remission in both children, but the progressive weight loss and starvation were initially attributed to tumor, without consideration of the psychiatric problems that were present.

### Increased Demands

There is a question as to whether weight loss in patients with cancer can occur despite otherwise adequate calorie inake—in other words, whether tumors, in fact, require a higher calorie intake than an equivalent mass of normal tissue. There are also paraneoplastic consequences of tumor. The distal effects of ectopic hormone production are now well known. It is tempting to speculate, although by no means is it proved, that the high incidence of malnutrition seen in neuroblastoma results at least in part from the catabolic effects of catecholamines. There is little information to support such a speculation. Nevertheless, it must always be remembered that the tumor burden of hematologic malignancies can be extraordinarily large. Lactic acidosis, as evidence of inadequate oxidative utilization of carbohydrate, is very common in such instances. Therefore, the inefficient utilization and generation of usable energy by tumor cells when large tumor masses are present makes it very likely that an extracaloric demand exists on the basis of tumor burden (49). The only proof that this is a significant factor would be the demonstration of overall poor energy utilization by the tumor-bearing host. Waterhouse (56) has attempted to evaluate this. Components of both starvation- and stress-induced changes in metabolism are seen, contributing to a relative rigidity of the glucose metabolism in tumor-bearing hosts. There appears to be relative stability of protein utilization and therefore no excessive protein wastage. Again, this fits the picture of calorie but not protein–calorie malnutrition that is most frequently seen.

The data are not adequate to demonstrate that there is a major increased calorie demand. Some early data from a prospective evaluation of all children with cancer do seem to suggest that dietary intake is mostly related to the presence of malnutrition in nontumor or benign tumor-bearing children, whereas often there is a higher degree of nutrient intake than would be expected from the clinical status of the children (Table 7). These data are very preliminary, but they are the first suggestion that it might be possible to demonstrate in practice an increased calorie need.

## THERAPY OF MALNUTRITION IN CHILDREN

### Age-related Dietary Advice

Nutritional support even of the well child is more complex than that of adults. Dietary requirements change rapidly with changing age, ranging from infant formulas to full adult diets within the age range of the usual pediatric

TABLE 7. *Relationship between nutritional state and caloric intake*

|  | Wt/Ht Percentile | No. | No. missing Dietary data | RDAs Percentiles | | Total |
|---|---|---|---|---|---|---|
|  |  |  |  | Calories | Proteins |  |
|  | Unknown | 1 |  |  |  |  |
| Benign | <25% | 3 | 0 | 30–59% | Above 90% | 13 |
|  | >25% | 9 | 4 | 60–90% | Above 90% |  |
|  | Unknown | 0 | 0 | 60–90% | Above 90% |  |
| Leukemia | <25% | 4 | 0 | 60–90% | Above 90% | 20 |
|  | >25% | 16 | 3 | 60–90% | Above 90% |  |
|  | Unknown | 1 | 1 |  |  |  |
| Other Tumors | <25% | 20 | 6 | 60–90% | Above 90% | 61 |
|  | >25% | 40 | 11 | 60–90% | Above 90% |  |
| Total |  | 94 | 26 |  |  | 94 |

population. It has already been mentioned that parental anxiety is a big factor in the treatment of children. It is exceedingly important that there be a relaxed atmosphere associated with eating for the child with cancer in the hospital setting. If the child has inadequate intake, supplements are used extensively in our institution. Major emphasis is placed on snacking and extra calories at parties (7).

A major asset is the presence of a "mother's kitchen" at M. D. Anderson Hospital (7,44,45). There, mothers can actively participate in the nutritional care of their children, providing the diet they are most familiar with. In addition, meals can be adjusted to alterations in the child's schedule which have been imposed by diagnostic and therapeutic routines. The new pediatric floor at M. D. Anderson Hospital will have a communal dining room in which children can eat their meals in a less institutionalized setting. All of these approaches have the major goal of preventing malnutrition, which is far more effective than any nutritional rehabilitation.

## NUTRITIONAL INTERVENTION

### Enteral Nutrition

Whenever nutritional intervention is indicated, it is highly preferable to use the gastrointestinal route, if at all possible. Although children often do not tolerate nasogastric feeding well, an attempt at nasogastric feeding should be made before more serious interventions are considered. Ordinary blenderized diets or commercially prepared formulas can be used if the reason for nasogastric feeding is the inability to swallow or tolerate food in the mouth. More frequently, there is an element not only of difficulty with swallowing but also of malabsorption. Therefore, chemically defined formulations have begun to be used (36, 37,40). Such diets have, of course, been used in pediatrics for a long time, especially in the treatment of inborn errors of metabolism. The so-called Lofenalac diet used in the treatment of phenylketonuria has had significant beneficial effect on the growth and development of such children. It is now even possible to utilize chemically defined diets without having to resort to total parenteral nutrition in patients who have surgically induced ileus. The main advantage of chemically defined diets in children is the avoidance of the complications of total parenteral nutrition. These diets are also hypoallergenic. However, the diets are often hypertonic and may require dilution before they can be safely used in children. They have a very poor taste, and therefore usually require nasogastric feeding in children. Nevertheless, they are undoubtably effective (40).

## Parenteral Nutritional Support

Practical hyperalimentation had its genesis in pediatric patients (17). The use of hyperalimentation in the patient with cancer has been reviewed extensively on many occasions (8,9,10). Parenteral hyperalimentation is the most invasive mode of intervention, and therefore requires justification as to efficacy and safety. There is no doubt that intravenous hyperalimentation (IVH) is effective in restoring the nutritional state. Complications of hyperalimentation can occur, such as infection, metabolic derangements, and surgical complications, such as pneumothorax. However, the risk is acceptable as long as careful surgical insertion techniques and rigid attention to septic management of the catheter are maintained. Under such conditions, the incidence of sepsis can be kept within acceptable limits (48). In a multi-institutional prospective randomized trial of IVH, infections and other complications were seen in both control and IVH groups (51). This acceptable infection rate was also found in children by Filler et al. (19,20).

There are peculiar pediatric complications of IVH. For instance, a 23-month-old boy admitted to M. D. Anderson Hospital with recurrent neuroblastoma was placed on central IVH, which he received initially without complication. Fourteen days after his central venous catheter was placed, he bit through the line. An abrupt oral temperature rise to 102°F occurred. Cultures of the blood were positive for *Streptococcus mitis*. This occurred at the time of moderately severe granulocytopenia, with a white count of 1,000/mm³ and a differential count of 20% granulocytes. The central line was discontinued, but was reinserted after almost three weeks of peripheral hyperalimentation and therapy with appropriate antibiotics. The child tolerated central hyperalimentation without further incident through further hospitalizations for chemotherapy.

Long-term hyperalimentation presents special problems in its own right. Although most reports of essential fatty acid and zinc deficiency precipitated by hyperalimentation with solutions deficient in such nutrients have appeared in the neonatal literature and literature on children with gastrointestinal defects, the same complications can occur in children with cancer. It is quite feasible to keep children on prolonged hyperalimentation in the face of severe marrow depression; however, under such circumstances, in our experience, at least one incidence of zinc deficiency was seen in a child who had a gastrointestinal fistula. This occurred despite maintenance zinc supplementation in the IVH fluid.

## NUTRITION AND OUTCOME OF CANCER THERAPY IN CHILDREN

### Malnutrition and Cancer Prognosis

As already mentioned, malnutrition is a poor prognostic factor in its own right. It is far more frequently associated with metastatic and advanced disease than it is with early disease. At this time, it is impossible to ascertain the cause and effect of this correlation. The incidence of infection is highest in children who are malnourished and still remains the major cause of death among children with malignant disease. Early observations of vigorous nutritional intervention by hyperalimentation seem to suggest a beneficial outcome (19,20); however, to prove this assertion, cooperative prospective randomized trials had to be executed.

## THERAPY DELIVERY AND NUTRITIONAL INTERVENTION

### General Observations

Objective data on the advantage of IVH as an early mode of intervention in children with malignancies are sparse. In a controlled randomized prospective clinical trial, the utility of IVH and the intolerance to administration of chemotherapy was tested in a number of children who had metastatic disease to and from bone. In that study, IVH was safe at the tolerable infection rate already mentioned, and the infectious complications correlated significantly with the nutritional status of the patient, with the presence of IVH being only a secondary factor. The IVH was effective in nutritional rehabilitation even of patients on intensive chemotherapy. There was an indication that the ability to deliver chemotherapy to patients seemed to be improved by IVH, especially in malnourished patients and in patients with late stages of disease. Among 20 patients, the 10 randomized controls had 7.6 adjustments in their chemotherapy course per 100 episode days, whereas patients randomized on IVH had 2.8 course adjustments per 100 episode days. This difference was significant. Patients who were treated with IVH without being randomized because they were overtly malnourished still had fewer course adjustments than did control patients not so treated (52). A prospective randomized clinical trial of the value of total parenteral nutrition in children with cancer who were undergoing radiotherapy to the abdomen showed good tolerance to IVH and maintenance of weight on IVH without oral intake. However, there were no significant differences in dose adjustments in these children when IVH and controls were compared (14). The difference in results between these two series of patients could be explained by the fact that the patients receiving irradiation were at initial diagnosis, whereas the patients on chemotherapy were advanced in their disease and had overt metastases.

It is unreasonable to expect a specific cancer-directed therapeutic effect from IVH. All that one can hope is that the development of malnutrition is inhibited, or that overt malnutrition is counteracted. Therefore, the application of IVH to patients who are well nourished is unlikely to give additional benefit. In patients who were to receive abdominal irradiation, part of the question of IVH was whether putting the bowel to rest might prevent some of the consequences of abdominal irradiation. It did not improve the rate of dose delivery that could be given. However, it is more likely that marginal malnutrition could be found among the patients with metastatic disease. Furthermore, in certain diagnoses, marginal malnutrition can be inferred on clinical grounds. It is therefore especially instructive to look at such particular patients.

### Specific Diagnoses and Therapies

Illustrative of what can be accomplished with hyperalimentation in pediatric oncology are the experiences with children who are receiving therapy for neuroblastoma or who are undergoing bone marrow transplantation.

The experience with neuroblastoma at M. D. Anderson Hospital can be summarized by evaluating the outcome of treatment of 10 children. The median age of these children was 4.6 years, and all had disseminated neuroblastoma. Their nutritional status was evaluated and carefully monitored during treatment with intensive courses of cyclophosphamide, vincristine, trifluoromethyl-deoxyuridine, and papavarine. Six patients also received IVH. Four were malnourished at the time of initiation of chemotherapy, one became malnourished within two months, and one was given IVH as part of the above-mentioned randomized study, although he was well nourished. The nutritional status of the remaining four was maintained by oral feeding. Although severe neutropenia occurred in all patients, there was adequate recovery to permit administration of chemotherapy on schedule. Responses were observed in nine of those ten patients, including healing of bone lesions. Six of the responding patients were re-explored for removal of the primary tumors. One demonstrated complete maturation to ganglioneuroma and in the remaining five 90% maturation was observed. The six patients were symptom-free and surviving six to 60 months from diagnosis at the time of tabulation of this information. Delivery of antitumor treatment was facilitated by maintaining an adequate nutritional state, and supported the continued use of nutrition as a valuable adjunct in cancer management. When the outcome of such patients was compared to patients treated by the Southwest Oncology Group with equivalent therapy, the outcome was improved over the non-nutritionally supported cohort (6) though ultimate survival was unaffected by IVH.

Marrow transplantation in childhood cancer is indicated for acute granulocytic leukemia early during the course, and for relapsing acute lymphocytic leukemia when a suitable donor is available. It has been the experience that transplantations have a far better outcome if performed when the child is in remission. An additional indication for bone marrow transplantation in childhood is severe aplastic anemia. Recently, the concept of autologous bone marrow rescue after near-lethal chemotherapy has become prominent. In our experience, continued support of the patient with IVH is a significant modality in the successful completion of a bone marrow transplant. In one child with aplastic anemia, a central venous catheter was maintained despite periods of profound granulocytopenia and sepsis in excess of 120 days. In addition, the administration of melphalan as a chemotherapeutic agent, to be administered in near-lethal doses with bone-marrow rescue, frequently results in profound protein-losing enteropathy. Intravenous hyperalimentation has made this modality of therapy feasible (Culbert, unpublished observations). Thus, the degree of myelosuppression is no contraindication to IVH and it, in turn, makes survival possible despite the profound iatrogenic complications induced by the preparatory regimens of allogeneic transplantation and the very high doses of chemotherapy used with autologous transplantation.

### Nutritionally Based Therapy in Childhood

Children are totally dependent on their parents; therefore, they are the passive subjects of attempts at administration of unusual remedies. Among all the claims that specific nutrients might be therapeutic, only two should be mentioned. The first is the use of high-dose vitamin C. Claims that vitamin C may be effective in cancer therapy have been widely publicized. In our hands, the administration of high-dose vitamin C, in the order of 6 g/M², was not toxic but did not result in any therapeutic effect among five children in whom it was tried.

There is, however, a potential use of vitamin E in the prevention of Adriamycin-induced cardiotoxicity. This protective effect can be demonstrated in rabbits as an animal model and is currently being investigated in the clinical setting (55).

### ETHICAL CONSIDERATIONS

The child, in effect, is totally dependent on parents for care, from the support of the body to the development of the mind, but of these two, the physical care of the child is primary. Among all the concepts of care, feeding is the most basic, beyond shelter and protection. It is so basic that the psychological concept of nurture is derived from that root. Therefore, the very sick child is surrounded by nutritional support from the parents. It is so much a concept of basic care that its importance is underplayed in medical circles. Just as the hospital should give shelter, so should it feed as a necessity and not as part of the medical care concept. Most orders from physicians are, in fact, negative orders. They are likely to start with diet for age, but diet orders will be made more specific only if the physician wants to place the child on a restricted diet from "NPO" to fat-free, salt-free, or other specialized diet.

The question of using IVH sometimes arises at times when the child is severely malnourished and has no other available modes of nutritional rehabilitation; however, at the same time, no further medical intervention can be expected to be successful. The question of using IVH as intervention can be posed in one of two ways: "Do you want your child to starve to death?" or "Do you want your child to be kept alive by artificial means?" The answer very likely will be "of course not" to either question. To feed or not to feed the young dying child is a decision that lies with the parents, but it is not a decision for which physicians present facts to help parents make up their mind. Physicians have concepts on which their decisions are based. Such dialogue is not simple. There is no ethical structure that allows the decision to be easy and obvious. This must be understood, since the question of extraordinary care will frequently revolve around hyperalimentation (50).

## CONCLUSION

The treatment of children with cancer who are malnourished is clearly a team effort. Malnutrition is becoming the major terminal complication contributing to death in children with cancer. To prevent this complication, early and continuous support of the nutritional state of the patient is necessary. The team for pediatric oncology is, in principle, no different from the team for any patient with cancer. It should contain at least a physician, a nurse clinician, a dietitian, and a laboratory that can do the necessary nutritionally oriented analyses. There is, however, a specific need for pediatric orientation from the primary physician, nurse, and dietitian alike. The dietitian should be schooled in the nutritional needs of the developing child. Only by this continual vigilance will malnutrition ultimately disappear as a complicating factor in childhood oncology.

## ACKNOWLEDGMENT

Original data in this paper were obtained under the support of contracts NO 1-CP-65794 and NO 1-CP-85655 from the Diet, Nutrition, and Cancer Program of the National Cancer Institute, and by grant CA-3713 from the National Cancer Institute.

The observations and experiences recorded here would not have been possible without the help of our dietitians Brenda Becker, Patricia Carter, and Karen Gallagher, research dietitian assistant Diane Carr, our surgical support through Drs. E. M. Copeland and J. Daly, our hyperalimentation nurses Betsy Cohen Teitell and Chris Ortiz, our nutritional assessment nurse Deborah Coody, our data manager Pat Bingham, and the many people who make our nutritional team functional.

## REFERENCES

1. Alleyne, G. A. O., Hay, R. W., Picou, D. I., Stanfield, J. P., and Whitehead, R. G. (1977): *Protein Energy Malnutrition.* Edward Arnold Publishers Ltd., London.
2. Bernstein, I. L. (1978): Learned taste aversions in children receiving chemotherapy. *Science,* 200:1302–1303.
3. Bernstein, I. L., Wallace, M. J., Bernstein, I. D., Bleyer, W. A., Chard, R. L., and Hartmann, J. R. (1979): Learned food aversions as a consequence of cancer treatment. In: *Nutrition and Cancer,* edited by J. van Eys, M. S. Seelig, and B. L. Nichols, pp. 159–164. S. P. Medical and Scientific Books, New York.
4. Brown, R. E. (1977): Interaction of nutrition and infection in clinical practice. *Pediatr. Clin. North Am.,* 24:241–252.
5. Brunell, B. A. (1977): Immunologic response of immunosuppressed children to influenza vaccine. *Morbidity–Mortality Weekly Report,* 26:54.
6. Cangir, A., van Eys, J., and Teitell-Cohen, B. (1979): Role of nutrition in the management of patients with neuroblastoma. *Proceedings of the American Society for Clinical Oncology and American Association for Cancer Research,* 20:392.
7. Carter, P. (1979): Nutrition in the pediatric cancer patient. In: *Nutritional Management of the Cancer Patient,* edited by J. Wollard, pp. 131–139. Raven Press, New York.
8. Copeland, E. M., Daly, J. M., and Dudrick, S. J. (1977): Nutrition as an adjunct cancer treatment in the adult. *Cancer Res.,* 37:2451–2456.
9. Copeland, E. M., Daly, J. M., Ota, D. M., and Dudrick, S. J. (1979): Nutrition, cancer and intravenous hyperalimentation. *Cancer,* 43:2108–2116.
10. Copeland, E. M., Rodman, C. A., and Dudrick, S. J. (1979): Nutritional concepts of neoplastic disease. In: *Nutrition and Cancer,* edited by J. van Eys, M. S. Seelig and B. L. Nichols, pp. 133–156. S. P. Medical and Scientific Books, New York.
11. Cravioto, J., Hambraeus, L., and Vahlquist, (editors) (1974): *Early malnutrition in mental development: Symposium of the Swedish Nutrition Foundation XII.* Almqvist and Wiskell, Uppsala, Sweden.
12. Darby, W. J., Salsbury, C. G., McGanity, W. J., Johnson, H. F., Bridgforth, E. B., and Sandstead, H., R. (1956): A study of the dietary background and nutriture of the Navajo Indian. *J. Nutr.,* 60 (suppl. 2):3–85.
13. Donaldson, S. S. (1977): Nutritional consequences of radiotherapy. *Cancer Res.,* 37:2407–2413.
14. Donaldson, S. S., DeWys, W. D., Ghavimi, F., Knox, K. D., Suskind, R. M., Shills, M. E., and Wesley, M. N: A prospective randomized clinical trial of the value of total parenteral in children with cancer (in preparation).
15. Donaldson, S. S., and Lenin, R. A. (1979): Alterations of nutritional status: Impact of chemotherapy and radiation therapy. *Cancer,* 43:2036–2052.
16. Donaldson, S. S., Wesley, M. N., DeWys, W. D., Suskind, R. M., and van Eys, J: A nonconcurrent prospective study of the nutritional status of pediatric cancer patients. *Am. J. Dis. Child. (in press).*
17. Dudrick, S. J. (1977): The genesis of intravenous hyperalimentation. *J. Parent. Ent. Nutr.,* 1:23–29.
18. Fernbach, D. J., Williams, T. E., Donaldson, M. H. (1977): Neuroblastoma. In: *Clinical Pediatric Oncology,* second edition, edited by W. W. Sutow, T. J. Vietti, and D. J. Fernbach, pp. 506–537. C. V. Mosby Co., St. Louis.
19. Filler, R. M., Dietz, W., Suskind, R. M., Jaffe, N., and Cassady, J. R. (1979): Parenteral feeding in the management of children with cancer. *Cancer,* 43:2117–2120.
20. Filler, R. M., Jaffe, N., Cassady, J. R., Traggis, D. G., and Das, J. B. (1977): Parenteral nutritional support in children with cancer. *Cancer,* 39:2655–2669.
21. Garcia, J., Hankins, W. G., and Rusiniak, W. (1976): Flavor aversion studies. *Science,* 197:192–265.
22. Garner, S. M., and Clark, D. C. (1975): Nutrition, growth, development and malnutrition: Findings from the ten state nutrition survey 1968–1970. *Pediatrics,* 56:306–319.

23. George, S. L., Aur, R. J. A., Mauer, A. M., and Simone, J. V. (1979): A reappraisal of the results of stopping therapy in childhood leukemia. *N. Engl. J. Med.,* 300:269–273.
24. Good, R. A., Fernandes, G., and West, A. (1979): Nutrition, immunity and cancer—a review: Part I. Influence of protein or protein calorie malnutrition and zinc deficiency on immunity. *Clin. Bull.,* 9:3–12.
25. Green, H. L., Hulsey, T., Hoffman, L. H., and Bennett, S. (1979): The effects of malnutrition and cancer therapy agent on small bowel. In: *Nutrition and Cancer,* edited by J. van Eys, M. S. Seelig, and B. L. Nichols, pp. 71–90. S. P. Medical and Scientific Books, New York.
26. Guthrie, H. A., and Guthrie, G. M. (1976): Factor analysis of nutritional status data from ten state nutrition surveys. *Am. J. Clin. Nutr.,* 29:1238–1241.
27. Hamill, P. V. V., Drizd, T. A., Johnson, C. L., Reed, R. B., Roche, A. F., and Moore, W. M. (1979): Physical growth: Nutritional center for health statistics percentiles. *Am. J. Clin. Nutr.,* 32:607–629.
28. Health Examination Survey Data from the Nutritional Center for Health Statistics (N.CH.S.) (1976), *Supplement to Monthly Vital Statistics Report,* Volume 25, Number 3.
29. Johnson, C. L. (1979): Hemoglobin and selected iron-related findings of persons 1–74 years of age: United States, 1971–74. *Advanced Data from Vital and Health Statistics of the National Center for Health Statistics, Public Health Service booklet No. 46.*
30. Joint FAO/WHO Expert Committee on Nutrition (1971): *World Health Organization Technical Report Series,* No. 477. WHO, Geneva.
31. Meadows, A. T., Krejmas, N., and Belasco, J. (1980): The medical cost of cure: Sequelae in survivors of childhood cancer. In: *Status of Curability of Childhood Tumors,* edited by J. van Eys and M. P. Sullivan, pp. 263–275. Raven Press, New York.
32. National Academy of Sciences (1974): *Recommended dietary allowances.*
33. Pearson, H. A., and Robinson, J. E. (1976): The role of iron in host resistance. *Adv. Pediatr.,* 23:1–33.
34. Richie, E., and Copeland, E. M. (1979): Nutrition and immunity. In: *Nutrition and Cancer,* edited by J. van Eys, M. S. Seelig, and V. L. Nichols, pp. 55–69. S. P. Medical and Scientific Books, New York.
35. Schloen, L. H., Fernandes, G., Garafalo, J. A., and Good, R. A. (1979): Nutrition, immunity and cancer—a review: Part II: Zinc, immune function and cancer. *Clin. Bull.,* 9:63–75.
36. Shils, M. E. (1977): Enteral nutrition by tube. *Cancer Res.,* 37:2432–2439.
37. Shils, M. E. (1978): Enteral nutritional management of the cancer patient. *Cancer Bull.,* 30:98–101.
38. Smithson, W. A., Siem, R. A., Ritts, R. E., Gilchrist, G. S., Burgert, O., Jr., Ilstrup, D. M., and Smith, T. F. (1978): Response to influenza virus vaccine in children receiving chemotherapy for malignancy. *J. Pediatr.,* 93:632–634.
39. Suskind, R. M., (editor) (1977): *Malnutrition and Immune Response.* Raven Press, New York.
40. Suskind, R. M., and Gordon, D. (1979): The use of elemental diets in the cancer patient. In: *Nutrition and Cancer,* edited by J. van Eys, M. S. Seelig, and B. L. Nichols, pp. 111–132. S. P. Medical and Scientific Books, New York.
41. Sutow, W. W. (1977): General aspects of childhood cancer. In: *Clinical Pediatric Oncology,* second edition, edited by W. W. Sutow, T. J. Vietti, and D. E. Fernbach, pp. 1–15. C. V. Mosby Co., St. Louis.
42. Teitell, B. C., Herson, J., and van Eys, J. (1979): Comparison of techniques assessing malnutrition in children with cancer (abstract). *J. Parent. Ent. Nutr.* 3:514.
43. Teitell, B. C., Herson, J., and van Eys, J. (1980): Recall antigen response in pediatric cancer patients receiving parenteral hyperalimentation. *J. Parent. Ent. Nutr.,* 4:9.
44. van Eys, J. (1977): Nutritional therapy in children with cancer. *Cancer Res.,* 37:2457–2461.
45. van Eys, J. (1978): Nutrition and cancer in children. *Cancer Bull.,* 30:93–97.
46. van Eys, J. (1979): Nutritional therapy in childhood malignancies: A historical perspective. In: *Nutrition and Cancer,* edited by J. van Eys, M. S. Seelig, and B. L. Nichols, pp. 91–110. S. P. Medical and Scientific Books, New York.
47. van Eys, J. (1979): Malnutrition in children with cancer, incidence and consequence. *Cancer,* 43:2030–2035.
48. van Eys, J. (1979): Nutritional management as adjuvant in pediatric cancer therapy. In: *Care of the Child with Cancer,* pp. 86–92. American Cancer Society, New York.
49. van Eys, J. (1979): The metabolic consequences of cancer. In: *Nutritional Management of the Cancer Patient,* edited by J. Wollard, pp. 1–11. Raven Press, New York.

50. van Eys, J. (1979): Feeding the dying child: Ethical considerations in a new guise. Presented at the Foundation for Thanatology, New York.
51. van Eys, J., Cangir, A., Copeland, E. M., Suskind, R., Jaffe, N., Filler, R., Chavinio, G., Shils, M., Donaldson, S. S., and Wesley, M. M.: The safety of intravenous hyperalimentation in children with malignancies: A cooperative hospital trial. *J. Parent. Ent. Nutr. (in press)*.
52. van Eys, J., Copeland, E. M., Cangir, A., Taylor, G., Teitell, B. C., Carter, P., and Ortiz, C. (1980): A randomized controlled clinical trial of hyperalimentation in children with metastatic malignancies. *Med. Pediatr. Oncol.,* 8:63–73.
53. van Eys, J., and Hilliard, J.: Nutritional status and immune function in childhood cancer. In: *Nutrition and Cancer,* Vol. II.
54. Waldmann, T. A., Broder, S. and Strober, W. (1974): Protein-losing enteropathies in malignancy. *Ann. N.Y. Acad. Sci.,* 230:306–317.
55. Wang, Y. M., Madanat, F. F., Kimball, J. C., Gleiser, C. A., Ali, M. K., Kaufman, M. W., and van Eys. J. (1980): Effect of vitamin E against Adriamycin-induced toxicity in rabbits. *Cancer Res.,* 40.
56. Waterhouse, C. (1979): Metabolism in the cancer patient. In: *Nutrition and Cancer,* edited by J. van Eys, M. S. Seelig, and B. L. Nichols, pp. 49–53. S. P. Medical and Scientific Books, New York.
57. Waterlow, J. C. (1972): Classification and definition of protein calorie malnutrition. *Br. Med. J.,* 3:566–569.
58. Winick, M. (1976): Malnutrition and brain development. Oxford University Press, London.
59. Woodruff, C. W. (1977): Iron deficiency in infancy and childhood. *Pediatr. Clin. North Am.,* 24:85–94.
60. Zerfos, A. J., Shorr, J. J., and Neumann, C. G. (1977): Office assessment of nutritional status. *Pediatr. Clin. North Am.,* 24:253–272.

# Subject Index